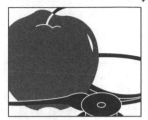

# Teaching Nursing:
## The Art and Science
## Volume 1

Linda Caputi, MSN, EdD, RN, CNE
Professor of Nursing
College of DuPage
Glen Ellyn, Illinois

College of DuPage Press

2nd EDITION

College of DuPage Press
425 Fawell Blvd.
Glen Ellyn, Illinois 60137

Project Manager: Joseph Barillari
Designer: Janice Walker
Typesetter: Janice Walker
CD Design: Kevin Dudey

**About College of DuPage:** For more than 20 years College of DuPage has been a leader in publishing learning materials for nursing education including multimedia computer programs, videos, books, other print materials, and educational computer and board games. We are committed to providing the highest quality products in the most appropriate format for our colleagues. Visit the College of DuPage website at www.dupagepress.com for information on all our products.

# Teaching Nursing:
## The Art and Science
## Volume 1

2nd EDITION

## Acknowledgements

My sincere thanks and appreciation to the over 100 esteemed colleagues who contributed to the 2nd edition of Volumes 1 through 3 of this book. I am amazed and in awe of all the talented authors and nurse educators who contributed to this book. I sincerely appreciate the time and knowledge they each shared with me and all who read these books.

It would be impossible to list all the people at College of DuPage who made this 2nd edition of these 3 volumes possible. I would like to thank the college leadership and my college colleagues for their support. I would especially like to acknowledge Joseph Barillari, Director of the College of DuPage Press, for his support; it is a privilege to work with such an administrator. As always, I appreciate the work of the support staff who helped maintain a smooth, efficient production process: Gail McPike, Cathy Russo, and Susan Puccinelli. I am also grateful for the hard work of my book designer Janice Walker. Finally, I would like to thank my husband Victor for his endless support, patience, and trips to the office supply store.

# Preface

Nursing practice is a demanding profession – the serious nature of the work, a tiresome work schedule, need to juggle many tasks simultaneously, breadth of knowledge, and cognitive abilities necessary for safe practice.

Teaching nursing mirrors the practice field, requiring skills that all teachers have, plus a lot more! Nursing faculty must deal with college and hospital administration, legal challenges, funding deficits, and much, much more. Entering the world of nursing education is a complex, multifaceted journey. These volumes were written to help with this journey, whether you're at the beginning of the journey or nearing its end.

Because of the complex nature of nursing education, I have drawn upon the knowledge of over 100 experts to assist in writing these 3 volumes, bringing their personality and expertise to the subject at hand. I am proud of the many experts who graciously contributed chapters. These authors bring a wealth of information and a wide diversity in background and style. To maintain the integrity of each author's personality, I have made every effort to preserve individuality in writing style, allowing each author to set the tone for his or her chapter. With this approach, the reader can experience the true spirit of the author's personal expertise. In addition, my three reviewers also represent diverse backgrounds, providing unique perspectives in their review of each chapter.

The overall character I strive to set is friendly, yet professional, so sit back and enjoy!

# Forward

As you read this book, you will no doubt be thinking about how the content might apply to you, your students, and your teaching philosophy. To take full advantage of the varied backgrounds and expertise of the chapter authors, I have asked them to share their teaching philosophy with you. The authors' philosophies appear at the end of each of their chapters – providing an array of teaching perspectives for you to ponder.

*Teaching Nursing: The Art and Science, (2nd ed.) Volumes 1 through 3* are books whose value lies in both its practical and theoretical application. To that end, each volume includes a CD that holds valuable supplemental material the authors have designed. Please feel free to use these tools in your role as a nurse educator. You may wish to use these materials as a springboard for your own development of educational materials. These items are copyrighted, as noted.

# EDITOR

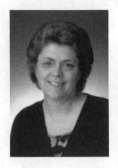

**Linda Caputi, MSN, EdD, RN, CNE**

Dr. Caputi is certified as a Certified Nurse Educator (CNE) from the National League for Nursing. She has authored over 25 educational multimedia programs, nursing education books, produced and developed videotapes, and published book chapters, journal articles, and board games for nursing education. She is editor of *Teaching Nursing: The Art and Science (Volumes 1, 2, and 3 – 2nd ed.)* and coauthor of *Teaching Nursing: The Art and Science (Volume 4: It's All About Student Success)* and *Teaching Nursing Using Concept Maps.* Dr. Caputi also authored *Little Lessons for Nurse Educators.* She has presented her work nationally for over 15 years on many nursing education topics. Her work has won six awards from Sigma Theta Tau, two from American Journal of Nursing Company, and one from The Association for Educational Communication and Technology. Dr. Caputi was acknowledged for teaching excellence in the 1998, 2002, and 2005 editions of *Who's Who Among America's Teachers* and the 2008 *Who's Who Among Executives and Professionals.* Dr. Caputi was named Educator of the Year for 2004 by the National Organization of Associate Degree Nursing. She serves on the Board of Governors for the National League for Nursing. She is a member of Sigma Theta Tau International Honor Society of Nursing. She was an invited member to the National League for Nursing's Think Tank on Transformation of Clinical Instruction. She is a Professor of Nursing at College of DuPage in Glen Ellyn, Illinois with 25 years of teaching experience.

Dr. Caputi is a consultant to all levels of nursing programs in the areas of curriculum, student success, getting ready for accreditation, and effective teaching strategies in the classroom, the nursing laboratory, and clinical; and, has developed curriculum for Practical Nursing, Associate Degree Nursing, Baccalaureate Nursing, and RN-to-BSN Programs.

# AUTHORS

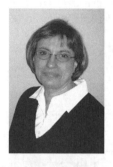

**Rosemarie O. Berman, PhD, RN**

Dr. Berman is an Assistant Professor of Nursing in the School of Professional Studies at Trinity (Washington) University. As one of the inaugural nursing faculty, she has been actively involved in program and curriculum development of the nursing programs, teaching the transition course and nursing research for RN-to-BSN students. She is a member of Sigma Theta Tau International (Kappa Chapter), Lamaze International and AWHONN.

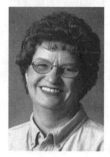

**Carol Boswell, EdD, RN, CNE, ANEF**

Dr. Boswell received a diploma from Methodist Hospital School of Nursing in Lubbock, Texas, a BSN from Texas Tech University Health Sciences Center in Odessa, an MSN from Texas Tech University Health Sciences Center in Lubbock, and an EdD in curriculum development from Texas Tech University in Lubbock. Dr. Boswell frequently speaks at local, state, national, and international conferences on topics ranging from health literacy, research, ethics, evidence-based practice, and leadership. She has authored multiple publications related to healthcare literacy, online teaching, research, and diabetes. Dr. Boswell has co-authored the textbook entitled "Introduction to Nursing Research: Incorporating Evidence-Based Practice". She is the co-director for the Texas Tech University Health Sciences Center School of Nursing and Medical Center Hospital Center of Excellence in Evidence-Based Practice. She has been an educator for more than 15 years, working at multiple levels, including ADN, RN-to-BSN, graduate, and continuing education. She teaches online RN-BSN and graduate courses.

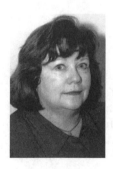

**Lynne Bryant, MSN, EdD, RN**

Dr. Bryant is a diploma graduate of The Johns Hopkins Hospital School of Nursing. She received a BSN from the University of Maryland, an MSN from University of Pennsylvania, and a Doctorate in higher education from Florida International University.

Dr. Lynne Bryant is currently an Assistant Professor and Director of the Nurse Educator and Nurse Administration Programs at Barry University in Miami Shores, Florida. She has been a nurse educator for 20 years in both undergraduate and graduate programs. Dr. Bryant has a diverse background in education, administration, and critical care. She has presented at national conferences on a variety of topics related to nursing education.

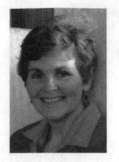

### Kathleen M. Buckley, PhD, RN, IBCLC

Dr. Kathleen M. Buckley received a Masters of Science degree in maternal/child health from the University of Maryland and a Masters of Arts and PhD in medical anthropology from the Catholic University of America. She is currently an Associate Professor in the School of Nursing at the Catholic University of America, where she has taught in traditional and accelerated nursing programs.

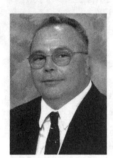

### Ken Burns, MS, PhD, RN

In 2005, Dr. Burns accepted a position at Martin Methodist College to establish a Baccalaureate Nursing program in rural south central Tennessee, a region that previously did not have on-site baccalaureate education available. From 1998 to 2005, Ken was associate chair of the School of Nursing at Northern Illinois University as well as director of graduate studies. Prior to this time, he was a faculty member and director of the family nurse practitioner program (1996-1998) at Drake University. Ken was at the University of Minnesota from 1974 - 1996. Dr. Burns has published in the areas of depression, stress appraisal, therapeutic hand message to promote relaxation and decrease agitation behaviors in individuals with Alzheimer's disease. He has received approximately 4 million dollars in funding and is an active member of the Midwest Nursing Research Society.

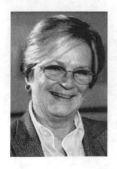

### Sharon Cannon, MSN, EdD, RN

Dr. Cannon received a BSN from St. Louis University, and an MSN and EdD from Southern Illinois University, Edwardsville. Dr. Cannon is a professor and regional dean for Texas Tech University Health Sciences Center in Odessa. She has been a nurse educator for more than 20 years in various settings, including ADN, BSN, graduate, and continuing education. She has presented at local, state, national, and international conferences with an emphasis on healthcare literacy, leadership, curriculum, instruction, and online education. She has authored multiple publications on topics ranging from healthcare literacy to politics in nursing. Dr. Cannon has co-authored the textbook *Introduction to Nursing Research: Incorporating Evidence-Based Practice*.

### Linda Caputi, MSN, EdD, RN, CNE

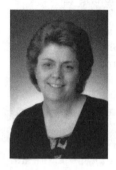

Dr. Caputi is certified as a Certified Nurse Educator (CNE) from the National League for Nursing. She has authored over 25 educational multimedia programs, nursing education books, produced and developed videotapes, and published book chapters, journal articles, and board games for nursing education. She is editor of *Teaching Nursing: The Art and Science (Volumes 1, 2, and 3 – 2nd ed.)* and coauthor of *Teaching Nursing: The Art and Science (Volume 4: It's All About Student Success)* and *Teaching Nursing Using Concept Maps*. Dr. Caputi also authored *Little Lessons for Nurse Educators*. She has presented her work nationally for over 15 years on many nursing education topics. Her work has won six awards from Sigma Theta Tau, two from American Journal of Nursing Company, and one from The Association for Educational Communication and Technology. Dr. Caputi was acknowledged for teaching excellence in the 1998, 2002, and 2005 editions of *Who's Who Among America's Teachers* and the 2008 *Who's Who Among Executives and Professionals*. Dr. Caputi was named Educator of the Year for 2004 by the National Organization of Associate Degree Nursing. She serves on the Board of Governors for the National League for Nursing. She is a member of Sigma Theta Tau International Honor Society of Nursing. She was an invited member to the National League for Nursing's Think Tank on Transformation of Clinical Instruction. She is a Professor of Nursing at College of DuPage in Glen Ellyn, Illinois with 25 years of teaching experience.

Dr. Caputi is a consultant to all levels of nursing programs in the areas of curriculum, student success, getting ready for accreditation, and effective teaching strategies in the classroom, the nursing laboratory, and clinical; and, has developed curriculum for Practical Nursing, Associate Degree Nursing, Baccalaureate Nursing, and RN-to-BSN Programs.

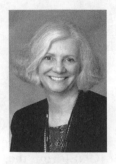

### Sharon M. Coyer, PhD, RN, CPNP, APRN

Dr. Coyer has taught at the Northern Illinois University, School of Nursing and Health Studies for 12 years. She has also taught for Marcella Niehoff College of Nursing of Loyola University Chicago. Dr. Coyer began her career as a staff nurse and has worked at multiple hospitals in the Chicago area. She has practiced nursing in the area of adult medical/surgical nursing, pediatrics, neonatal intensive care, well baby nursery, and mother-baby nursing care. Currently, Dr. Coyer teaches both graduate and undergraduate students. She also works as a pediatric nurse practitioner at DeKalb County Health Department.

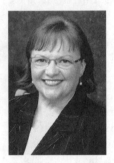

### Diann DeWitt, BS, MS, DNS, RN, CNE

Dr. DeWitt has 28 years of teaching experience in adult health and critical care nursing. She is a Professor of Nursing at Colorado Christian University in Lakewood, Colorado developing a pre-licensure BSN program that integrates faith and nursing. Previously she was an Associate Professor of Nursing at St. John's College in Springfield, Illinois. Dr. DeWitt is very active in Nurses Christian Fellowship and serves on committees related to Spiritual Care Research.

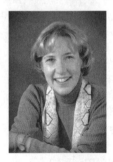

### Susan Diehl, EdD, RN, FNP, APRN

Dr. Diehl received a BSN from Cedar Crest College in Pennsylvania, an MSN from St. Joseph College in Connecticut, and an EdD in the Doctoral Program of Educational Leadership at the University of Hartford in Connecticut.

Susan is a Family Nurse Practitioner and Associate Professor at the University of Hartford. She is a research consultant and grant reviewer for the State of Connecticut Children's Trust Fund, and is engaged in research involving testing of relationship building models for mothers and infants.

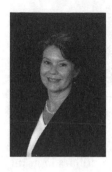

### Joanne R. Duffy, MSN, PhD, RN

Dr. Duffy is a graduate of St. Joseph's Hospital School of Nursing in Providence, Rhode Island. She received a Bachelor's degree at Salve Regina College in Newport, Rhode Island, and holds Master's and Doctoral degrees from The Catholic University of America where she is a tenured Associate Professor. Dr. Duffy received the First Annual Health Care Research Award from the National Institute of Health Care Management. She developed the Cardiovascular Center for Outcomes Analysis at INOVA Fairfax Hospital, and developed the Quality-Caring Model© which integrates the relationship-centered nature of nursing with the evidence-based culture of modern-day health care.

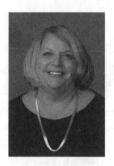

### Stacie Elder, PhD, RN

Dr. Elder earned a Bachelor of Science in Nursing from Aurora University, Aurora, Illinois; a Master of Science in Nursing (Adult Health) from Northern Illinois University; and a PhD in Nursing (Research and Education) from Barry University in Miami Shores, Florida. She is an Associate Professor of Nursing at Lewis University in Romeoville, Illinois. She has been a critical care nurse for over 20 years.

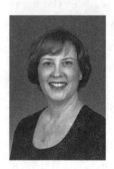

### Lynn Engelmann, MSN, EdD, RN, ANEF

Dr. Engelmann is Coordinator of the Associate Degree Nursing Program and Professor of Nursing at College of DuPage, Glen Ellyn, Illinois and has been a faculty member in nursing education for over 20 years. Lynn is co-editor of *Teaching Nursing: The Art and Science* (First Editions, Volumes 1, 2, and 4). She has presented at national conferences on a number of topics. Lynn has served on the National League for Nursing (NLN) task force on excellence in nursing education, and serves as an NLN Ambassador. She is Associate Editor for *Teaching and Learning in Nursing* and is a member of Sigma Theta Tau International Honor Society of Nursing and Kappa Delta Pi, International Honor Society in Education. Lynn was acknowledged for teaching excellence in Who's Who Among America's Teachers, 2005 and was acknowledged in Who's Who of American Women, 2007.

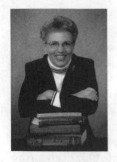

### Marilyn Frank-Stromborg, MS, EdD, JD, RN, ANP, FAAN

Dr. Frank-Stromborg was awarded a BS from Northern Illinois University, an MS from New York Medical College, School of Nursing, and a Doctorate in Educational Psychology, and a JD, from Northern Illinois University. Prior to retirement in 2003, Marilyn was Presidential Research Professor and Chair, School of Nursing, at Northern Illinois University. Dr. Frank-Stromborg has presented 176 papers at national and international conferences, published 76 journal articles, 33 book chapters, and 6 books, and has received over 3 million dollars in grant funding. Dr. Frank-Stromborg is the coordinator of the DeKalb County Drug Court (DeKalb County Illinois) and part-time attorney with the State's Attorney Office in DeKalb County.

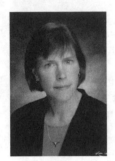

### Jean Giddens, PhD, RN

Dr. Giddens, is an Associate Professor and Coordinator for the Nursing Education Concentration in the Master's Degree Program at the College of Nursing, Health Sciences Center, The University of New Mexico in Albuquerque. She has 24 years of teaching experience in higher education. Dr. Giddens has conducted numerous national and international presentations, has multiple publications (including nursing textbooks, electronic media, and journal articles), and has been an education consultant over the past several years in the areas of instructional design, curriculum development, and conceptual learning.

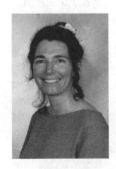

### Kathleen T. Heinrich, PhD, RN

Dr. Heinrich has taught in Masters, Doctoral, and RN-to-BSN programs in her 25-year teaching career. She created **K T H Consulting** in 2004 to help educators turn their everyday experiences into scholarship. The author of *A Nurse's Guide to Presenting and Publishing: Dare to Share*, Dr. Heinrich now shares best practices for presenting, publishing, and partnerships with faculty groups to enhance their careers, renew their passion for the profession, and foster zestful workplaces.

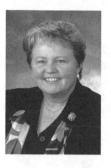

### Christine Henshaw, EdD, RN, CNE

Dr. Henshaw is Associate Dean and Assistant Professor in the School of Health Sciences at Seattle Pacific University. Dr. Henshaw earned a Bachelor of Science degree in nursing in 1978 from Washington State University, a Master's of Nursing in physiological nursing in 1987 from University of Washington, and a Doctorate in educational leadership in 2004 from Seattle University. Christine has taught at the LPN-to-BSN, Associate degree, Baccalaureate, and Master's levels.

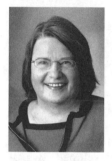

### Judith E. Hertz, PhD, RN

Dr. Hertz holds a diploma in nursing from the Geisinger Medical Center School of Nursing, Danville, Pennsylvania, a BSN from the University of San Diego, an MSN in Family Health Nursing with a functional role focus on Education, a Doctorate in Adult Health Nursing from The University of Texas at Austin, a graduate certificate in Gerontology from Northern Illinois University. She has taught in all types of nursing programs for over 25 years and is currently Associate Professor of Nursing and Director of Nursing Graduate Studies at Northern Illinois University, DeKalb, Illinois. From 2002 to 2004, Dr. Hertz served as a John A. Hartford Foundation Building Academic Geriatric Nursing Capacity Postdoctoral Scholar. She is also the 2007-9 President of the National Gerontological Nursing Association.

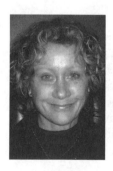

### Stephanie Holaday, DrPH, RN

Dr. Holaday received a Bachelors Degree in Nursing Science from The Catholic University of America, a Masters Degree in Nursing administration from Georgetown University, and a Doctorate in Public Health with a concentration in international program development from the University of Hawaii. Dr. Holaday is the Director of Nursing Programs at Trinity University in Washington, D.C. She has over 16 years of teaching experience in graduate and undergraduate nursing programs. Prior to her Director of Nursing role at Trinity University, she was Assistant Professor of Nursing at the University of Hawaii at Manoa, The Catholic University of America in Washington, D.C., and George Mason University in Fairfax, Virginia. In addition to her role as a nurse educator, she has worked with faculty from schools of nursing and public health throughout the nation and internationally for over 15 years as a consultant in healthcare education.

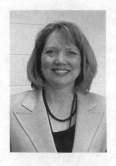

**Barbara Hunt, MS, RN, APRN-CNS, AOCN**

Ms. Hunt is a professor of nursing at the College of Lake County in Grayslake, Illinois. She received a BSN from the University of Minnesota, an MS from North Park University, Chicago, and is currently enrolled in a PhD program in nursing at Loyola University, Chicago. She has presented at local and national seminars and workshops. Barbara is a clinical nurse specialist in oncology and was awarded the ONS Excellence in Patient/Public Education Award by the Oncology Nursing Society in 2006.

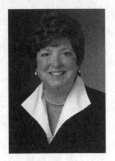

**Jane M. Kirkpatrick, MSN, PhD, RNC-OB**

Dr. Kirkpatrick is an Associate Professor, Interim Head of the School of Nursing, and an Associate Dean in the College of Pharmacy, Nursing, and Health Sciences at Purdue University in West Lafayette, Indiana. She has authored numerous articles and book chapters on various aspects of nursing education. She recently served as the chair of the university's Teaching Academy, which promotes excellence in scholarly teaching across the university. She designed and developed award-winning multimedia programs on the topics of teaching nursing care in Labor and Delivery, newborn assessment, gestational age assessment, and APGAR scoring.

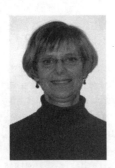

**Mary Elaine Koren, PhD, RN**

Dr. Koren received a Bachelor in Nursing degree from Saint Xavier University, Chicago and a Master's in Medical Nursing degree from Loyola University, Chicago. She earned a Doctorate in nursing from Rush University, Chicago with a specialty in the older adult. She has held positions in both the clinical and academic areas. Her teaching career spans almost two decades where she has taught in both the classroom and clinical setting. She is an active member of Sigma Theta Tau International, National Gerontological Nurses Association, and Midwest Nursing Research Society.

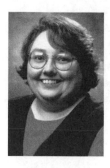

### Fran London, BS, MS, RN

Ms. London is currently the health education specialist at Phoenix Children's Hospital. She has worked as a staff nurse, school nurse, and psychiatric consultation liaison nurse. Fran has taught nursing and published articles and books, including *No Time to Teach? A Nurse's Guide to Patient and Family Education*. For five years she served as editor of the *Journal of Nursing Jocularity*.

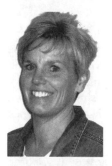

### Susan Luprell, PhD, RN, CNS-BC, CNE

Dr. Luprell teaches at Montana State University in both the undergraduate and graduate nursing programs. She earned a PhD from the University of Nebraska-Lincoln, majoring in Administration, Curriculum, and Instruction. Dr. Luprell provides faculty development workshops on the topic of incivility in nursing and nursing education. Prior to teaching, Susan was a Clinical Nurse Specialist specializing in adult health and critical care.

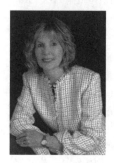

### Donna Carol Maheady, MS, EdD, RN, CPNP

Dr. Maheady graduated from the University of Bridgeport School of Nursing in Bridgeport, Connecticut. She received a certificate as a Pediatric Nurse Practitioner from the University of Texas Medical Branch at Galveston, an MS in Nursing from the State University of New York at Buffalo, and an EdD in Educational Leadership from Florida Atlantic University. Donna is an Adjunct Assistant Professor in the Christine E. Lynn College of Nursing at Florida Atlantic University. She has been a faculty member in nursing education for more than 25 years. Dr. Maheady authored *Nursing Students with Disabilities Change the Course*, the winner of the 2004 AJN Book of the Year Award, and *Leave No Nurse Behind: Nurses working with disabilities*.

Donna is the founder of a nonprofit resource network for nurses and nursing students with disabilities (www.ExceptionalNurse.com). In collaboration with Washington State University, she developed and co-sponsored a DVD called "Nursing with the Hand you are Given: A Message of Hope for Nursing Students with Disabilities". Donna has also been a featured guest on the radio show "Disability Matters" on the Voice of America Channel.

### Marilyn McDonald, BSN, MSN, DHSc, RN

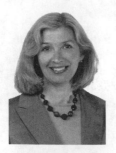

Dr. McDonald holds a BSN from The Massachusetts College of Pharmacy and Allied Health Sciences, an MSN from Yale University, and a Doctor of Health Science from Nova Southeastern University. She has practiced nursing for 30 years and has been a nurse educator and nurse practitioner for the past 15 years.

### Margaret A. Miklancie, PhD, RN

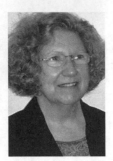

Dr. Miklancie earned a Practical Nursing degree from the Catherine McCauley Practical Nursing School in Pittsburgh, Mercy Hospital, an Associate Degree in Nursing for Northern Virginia Community College, and a BSN, an MSN with a Certificate in Nursing Education, and a PhD from George Mason University. Dr. Miklancie has experience teaching in a Practical Nursing program. She has also taught at George Mason University and Columbia Union College in Maryland. She served as Coordinator for the Undergraduate Program at George Mason University from 1995-2000. Since 2002 has taught in the one-year Accelerated Track for second degree students.

### Arlene H. Morris, MSN, EdD, RN

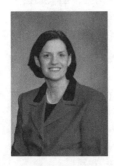

Dr. Morris is an Assistant Professor of Nursing at Auburn University Montgomery, Alabama. She has taught nursing for 15 years, and currently teaches in both the BSN and RN-to-BSN programs. Arlene received the Distinguished Teaching Professor Award from Auburn University Montgomery and the Outstanding Nurse Educator Award from the Alabama State Nurses Association. She has published and presented nationally and internationally regarding nursing education and gerontological issues.

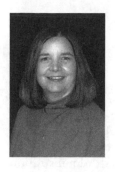

### Lynn Norman, BSN, MSN, EdD, RN

Dr. Norman was awarded a BSN and MSN from the University of Alabama at Birmingham, School of Nursing. She earned an EdD in educational foundations, leadership, and technology with a focus on adult education from Auburn University. She is a clinical faculty member with Auburn Montgomery School of Nursing and Troy University School of Nursing. Dr. Norman was an education consultant with the Alabama Board of Nursing and served on the National Council of State Boards of Nursing Examination Committee. She has taught in Associate and Baccalaureate Degree nursing education programs for 15 years.

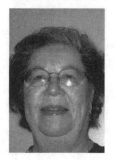

### Kathleen F. O'Connor, PhD, RN, CNE

Dr. O'Connor is Professor and Nurse Educator Role Option Coordinator in the School of Nursing at California State University, Dominguez Hills, in Carson, California. Dr. O'Connor holds a Baccalaureate Degree in Medical Technology from St. Mary's College, Notre Dame, Indiana, a generic Master's Degree in Nursing from New York Medical College, Graduate School of Nursing, a Master's Degree in Physiological Nursing from the University of California, San Francisco, and a Doctorate from Claremont Graduate University. She is a member of the National League for Nursing's Nursing Educator Research Advisory Council (NERAC), and an NLN Ambassador for her school. She has earned the designation of Certified Nurse Educator (CNE) from the National League for Nursing.

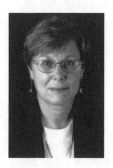

### Marilyn H. Oermann, PhD, RN, FAAN, ANEF

Dr. Oermann is a Professor and Division Chair in the School of Nursing at the University of North Carolina at Chapel Hill. She is author/co-author of 10 nursing education books and more than 160 articles and chapters. She edited 6 volumes of the *Annual Review of Nursing Education*. Her current books are *Evaluation and Testing in Nursing Education* (2nd ed.), *Clinical Teaching Strategies in Nursing Education* (2nd ed.), and *Writing for Publication in Nursing*. Dr. Oermann has written extensively on educational outcomes, teaching and evaluation in nursing education, and writing for publication as a nurse educator. She is the Editor of the *Journal of Nursing Care Quality* and past editor of the *Annual Review of Nursing Education*. She is a member of the American Academy of Nursing and NLN's Academy of Nursing Education.

### Kathleen Ohman, MS, EdD, RN, CCRN

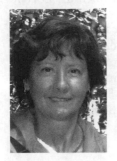

Dr. Ohman earned a BS in Nursing from the College of St. Benedict in St. Joseph, Minnesota, an MS from St. Cloud State University with a focus in Health Care Education, an MS in Nursing from the University of Minnesota, and an EdD in Educational Policy and Administration from the University of Minnesota. Dr. Ohman has taught at the College of St. Benedict for the past 20 years. She has also taught in a diploma program, and an ADN program, and worked as an education specialist at the University of Minnesota. Dr. Ohman has presented nationally and internationally on topics such as teaching-learning strategies, transformational leadership, family presence during resuscitation, and ventilator associated pneumonia. She has twelve manuscripts published (two for which she received writing awards), contributed to six software programs and two NCLEX-RN review books, and twice served as item writer for NCLEX-RN. Dr. Ohman is currently writing a NCLEX-RN Q&A book to be published by F.A. Davis.

### Thena E. (Wilson) Parrott, MS, PhD, RN

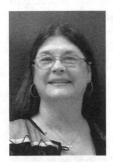

Dr. Parrott was educated at Baylor University (BSN), Texas Woman's University (MS), and Texas A&M University (PhD). She is currently Allied Health Division Chair at Blinn College in Bryan, Texas. She is a long-time nurse educator, who has taught in Baccalaureate, Vocational, and Associate Degree Nursing programs. She has presented and published on a variety of topics.

### Daniel J. Pesut, PhD, RN, FAAN

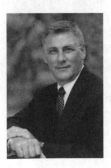

Dr. Pesut is Professor of Nursing and Associate Dean for Graduate Programs at Indiana University School of Nursing. Dr. Pesut earned a Bachelor of Science degree in nursing from Northern Illinois University, a Master of Science degree in psychiatric mental health nursing from the University of Texas Health Science Center, San Antonio, Texas, and a doctorate in Nursing from the University of Michigan. In addition, he holds a certificate in management development from the Harvard

Institute for Higher Education and is pursuing a certificate in Integral Studies from the Fielding Graduate University in Santa Barbara, California.

Dr. Pesut served as President (2003-2005) of the Honor Society of Nursing, Sigma Theta Tau International. He is a Fellow in the American Academy of Nursing. He is the recipient of many awards including an Army Commendation Award while on active duty (1975-1978) in the US Army Nurse Corps; the Honor Society of Nursing, Sigma Theta Tau International Edith Moore Copeland Founder's Award for Creativity; The American Assembly for Men In Nursing Luther Christman Award; Distinguished Alumni Awards from Northern Illinois University School of Nursing-College of Health and Human Services; as well as a number of other distinguished alumni, teaching, mentoring, and leadership awards. Dr. Pesut is a popular author, speaker, and consultant, and is internationally known for his work in nursing education related to creative-teaching learning methods; self-regulation of health status, clinical reasoning, futures thinking, and leadership development.

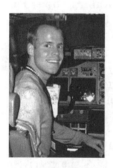

**Elliott Z. Pesut, BSAS**

Elliott Z. Pesut graduated from Embry-Riddle Aeronautical University's Prescott, Arizona campus with a Bachelors Degree in Aeronautical Science. He is experienced in the design and development of contextually-based aviation curriculum learning experiences. Mr. Pesut is currently a Courseware Developer for Alaska Airlines and is responsible for developing Computer Based Learning Experiences for the pilots that fly the Boeing 737. Elliott is a consultant and knowledge broker. He consults with companies and educational institutions about future applications of emerging technology platforms that support the design and development of teaching/learning products and services.

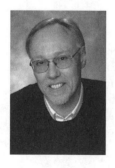

**Bradley Peters, MS, EdD, PhD**

Dr. Peters is an Assistant Professor of English and Coordinator of Writing Across the Curriculum at Northern Illinois University. His scholarly interests include assessment, ongoing professional development, and disciplinary rhetorics.

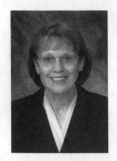

### Julie Fisher Robertson, BSN, MSN, EdD, RN

Dr. Robertson has a Baccalaureate in Nursing from Cornell University, a Master's degree in community health nursing from the University of Rochester, and a Doctorate in educational psychology from Northern Illinois University. Dr. Robertson has been teaching for 22 years and is a Professor of Community Health Nursing at Northern Illinois University where she was also the project director for the revision of nursing's undergraduate portfolio program and co-developer of the undergraduate assessment program. Dr. Robertson has published and presented nationally on portfolio and critical thinking assessment. In 2007, Dr. Robertson received the Excellence in Undergraduate Teaching Award from Northern Illinois University.

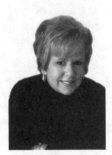

### Jeanette Rossetti, BSN, MS, EdD, RN

Jeanette was awarded a BSN from Lewis University in Romeoville, Illinois, an MS from St. Xavier in Chicago, and an EdD in adult education from Northern Illinois University in DeKalb, Illinois. Dr. Rossetti is an assistant professor at Northern Illinois University School of Nursing and Health Studies. Her specialty area is mental health psychiatric nursing. In addition to her teaching experience Dr. Rossetti worked at Riveredge Psychiatric Hospital for 12 years in a variety of nursing and administrative positions. Dr. Rossetti is a member of the Illinois Guardianship and Advocacy Commission, Human Rights Authority, Sigma Theta Tau International Honor Society, and the American Psychiatric Nurses Association. In 2007 she was awarded Northern Illinois University's College of Health and Human Sciences Lankford Award for Teaching Excellence, and in 2006 she received the Outstanding Teacher of the Year Award from Northern Illinois University School of Nursing.

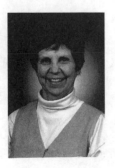

### Enid A. Rossi, MSN, EdD, RN

Dr. Rossi earned a BSN and MSN from California State University at Los Angeles and an EdD in Curriculum and Instruction from Northern Arizona University. Dr. Rossi is an assistant professor in the School of Nursing at Northern Arizona University. In the past five years Enid has presented four professional papers and one poster about how action research impacts teaching, developing teaching strategies that engage the learner through action research, and bridging the gap between education and practice. She has produced two cultural videotapes for Navajo Community College.

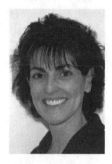

**Dianne M. Ryan, MA, RN, BC**

Ms. Ryan has worked in staff development at New York-Presbyterian Hospital (formerly New York Hospital) for 18 years. As director, Dianne's role was to plan, develop, implement, and evaluate orientation, in-services, staff development programs, and continuing education for all levels of nursing staff. Dianne is currently a Six Sigma Black Belt responsible for coordinating and conducting process improvement initiatives around enhancing patient throughput and quality of care at the hospital. For the past 15 years Dianne has lectured on various staff development-related topics at Drexel University's National Staff Development Conferences, and at hospitals and healthcare-related organizations. Dianne authored book chapters on the creation and use of visual aids for the Emergency Nurses' Association.

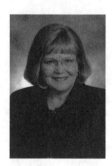

**Cathy Shultz, PhD, RN, CNE, FAAN**

Dr. Shultz completed a 3-year diploma program (now part of Kent State University) in East Liverpool, Ohio, a BSN at the University of South Carolina, an MSN as a clinical nurse specialist in Family-Community Health Nursing from Emory University in Atlanta, Georgia. She was awarded the Distinguished Alumna Award from the University of South Carolina. She earned a nurse practitioner certification from Case Western University in Cleveland, Ohio and a PhD in Higher Education Administration and Nursing from Vanderbilt University in Nashville, Tennessee. She is the Dean of the College of Nursing at Harding University in Searcy, Arkansas. Dr. Shultz is a Certified Nurse Educator through the National League for Nursing. She is the current President-Elect of the National League for Nursing.

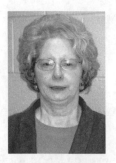

**Elizabeth N. Stokes, EdD, RN, CNE**

Dr. Stokes has an educational and experiential background in adult health and gerontological nursing. Her primary teaching areas are research, role development, and the care of the chronically ill. She is also a consultant on curriculum, instruction, and evaluation to both undergraduate and graduate nursing programs. A Professor Emeritus, Dr. Stokes is currently teaching as adjunct faculty at Arkansas State University, and continuing professional service and scholarship activities.

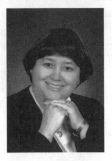

**Leonie Sutherland, PhD, RN**

Dr. Sutherland holds a Master's and Doctoral degree in Nursing with current research focusing on health promotion for ethnically diverse populations. She is an Associate Professor at Boise State University, Boise, Idaho and teaches in both the undergraduate and graduate nursing programs.

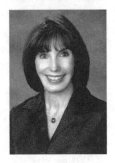

**Diane Whitehead, BSN, MSN, EdD, RN, ANEF**

Dr. Whitehead has a BSN from Florida State University, an MSN from University of Miami, and a doctorate from Florida International University. Dr. Whitehead has been actively teaching and administering ADN, BSN, and MSN programs for many years. She was instrumental in developing the first fully online Associate Degree Nursing program in Florida. Currently Dr. Whitehead is the associate dean for nursing at Nova Southeastern University in Fort Lauderdale, Florida. She has published in the areas of nursing leadership and management, and online nursing education. Her textbook, *Essentials of Nursing Leadership and Management*, is widely used in Associate Degree Nursing programs. Dr. Whitehead is an active participant with the National League for Nursing. She serves as president for the Florida League for Nursing, chair for the NLN task group on leadership in nursing education, and is an Ambassador for the NLN. She was inducted as a fellow into the Academy of Nursing Education. Dr. Whitehead was selected as the South Florida Organization of Nurse Executives Leader of the Year in 2006, and a "Heavy Hitter in Healthcare 2007" by the South Florida Business Journal.

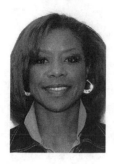

**Linda Wilson, MSN, PhD, RN**

Dr. Wilson has been involved in nursing education for over 25 years, and is currently a professor at Middle Tennessee State University. Honors and activities include NLNAC program reviewer, Outstanding Researcher, and distinguished lecturer for Sigma Theta Tau International, Honor Society of Nursing. Linda has conducted research, presented numerous times, as well as published several articles on cultural diversity.

# REVIEWERS

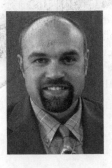

**Tim Bristol, PhD, RN, CNE**

Dr. Bristol is Director of Nursing at Crown College and an E-Learning specialist who has taught face-to-face and online courses in undergraduate and graduate nursing programs. He has provided faculty development for public and private colleges as well as healthcare institutions. Tim facilitates strategic planning for E-Learning, and serves as a coach for faculty and administrators. Dr. Bristol also assists organizations in developing effective instructional design for face-to-face, clinical, and lab resource centers.

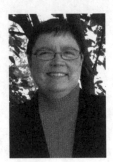

**Carmella Mikol, PhD, MN, RN-BC, CNE, CPNP**

Dr. Mikol earned a BSN from Loyola University of Chicago, a Masters in Nursing from the University of Pittsburgh, and a PhD in Nursing from the University of Wisconsin, Milwaukee. She is a board certified Pediatric Nurse Practitioner (NAPNAP), General Pediatric Nurse (ANCC) and Certified Nurse Educator (NLN). Dr. Mikol has been associated with nursing education for over twenty-five years. Currently, she is a professor in the Associate Degree Nursing Program at College of Lake County and practices as a Pediatric Nurse Practitioner.

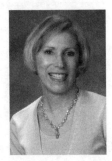

**Sally A. Weiss, MSN, EdD, RN**

Dr. Weiss earned a BSN from the American University in Washington, D.C., an MSN in community health and administration from the University of Miami in Coral Gables, Florida, and an EdD from Florida International University. Dr. Weiss has been a nurse educator for 30 years and presently holds the position of Associate Chair and Professor in the nursing department at Nova Southeastern University. Dr. Weiss remains active in clinical nursing and presents at the American Association of Critical Care Nurses regional meetings and at local hospitals.

| Key to Credentials | |
|---|---|
| Abbreviation | Definition |
| | |
| **Degrees** | |
| BA | Bachelor of Arts |
| BAN | Bachelor of Arts in Nursing |
| BS | Bachelor of Science |
| BSAS | Bachelor of Science Aeronautical Science |
| BSEd | Bachelor of Science in Education |
| BSN | Bachelor of Science in Nursing |
| DHSc | Doctor of Health Science |
| DM | Doctor of Management |
| DNP | Doctor of Nursing Practice |
| DNS | Doctor of Nursing Science |
| DNSc | Doctor of Nursing Science |
| DPA | Doctorate in Public Administration |
| DrPH | Doctoral Degree in Public Health |
| EdD | Doctor of Education |
| JD | Juris Doctor |
| MA | Master of Arts |
| MBA | Masters of Business Administration |
| MEd | Masters in Adult Education |
| MN | Master of Nursing |
| MPH | Master of Public Health |
| MS | Master of Science |
| MSN | Master of Science in Nursing |
| PhD | Doctor of Philosophy |
| | |
| **Certifications** | |
| ACNP-BC | Acute Care Nurse Practitioner Board Certified |
| ANP | Adult Nurse Practitioner |
| AOCN® | Advanced Oncology Certified Nurse |

| | |
|---|---|
| APRN | Advanced Practice Registered Nurse |
| APRN-CNS | Advanced Practice Registered Nurse, Clinical Nurse Specialist |
| APRN-P/MH | Advanced Practice Registered Nurse Psychiatric/Mental Health |
| BC | Board Certified |
| CAE | Certified Association Executive |
| CCAP | Certified Clinical Aromatherapy Practitioner/Instructor |
| CCRN | Critical Care Registered Nurse |
| CEN | Certified Emergency Nurse |
| CHC | Certified Healthcare Consultant |
| CHTP | Certified Healing Touch Practitioner |
| CNE | Certified Nurse Educator |
| CNS-BC | Clinical Nurse Specialist Board Certified |
| CPNP | Certified Pediatric Nurse Practitioner |
| CRRN | Certified Rehabilitation Registered Nurse |
| FNP | Family Nurse Practitioner |
| IBCLC | International Board Certified Lactation Consultant |
| RNC-OB | Register Nurse Certified in Inpatient Obstetric Nursing |
| | |
| **Fellows** | |
| ANEF | Academy of Nursing Education Fellows |
| FAAN | Fellow of the American Academy of Nursing |
| | |
| **Licensure** | |
| LPN | Licensed Practical Nurse |
| RN | Registered Nurse |

# TABLE OF CONTENTS

## UNIT 1: AN OVERVIEW OF TEACHING ROLES AND RESPONSIBILITIES

## UNIT 2: FOCUS ON STUDENTS

# UNIT 3: THE NURSING CURRICULUM

# TABLE OF CONTENTS OF OTHER VOLUMES

## VOLUME 2

# VOLUME 3

## UNIT 1: TESTING AND ASSESSMENT

# UNIT 1: AN OVERVIEW OF TEACHING ROLES AND RESPONSIBILITIES

Chapter 1: Addressing the Competencies for Academic Nurse Educators
*Linda Caputi, MSN, EdD, RN, CNE*

Chapter 2: The Nursing Faculty Shortage
*Linda Caputi, MSN, EdD, RN, CNE*

Chapter 3: An Overview of the Educational Process
*Linda Caputi, MSN, EdD, RN, CNE*

Chapter 4: So You're a Teacher, Now What Do You Do?
*Lynn Engelmann, MSN, EdD, RN, ANEF*

Chapter 5: Motivating Students to Learn
*Jane M. Kirkpatrick, MSN, PhD, RNC-OB*

Chapter 6: Inspiring Students
*Jeanette Rossetti, BSN, MS, EdD, RN*

Chapter 7: Defining the Boundaries of the Faculty-Student Relationship
*Christine Henshaw, EdD, RN, CNE*

Chapter 8: Evidence-Based Nursing Education
*Cathy Shultz, PhD, RN, CNE, FAAN*

Chapter 9: Action Research to Develop Evidence-Based Teaching
*Enid A. Rossi, MSN, EdD, RN*

Chapter 10: Writing for Publication in Nursing: What Every Nurse Educator
Needs to Know
*Marilyn H. Oermann, PhD, RN, FAAN, ANEF*

Chapter 11: Can-do Strategies for Publishing Success: Dare to Share, Work Smart,
Ask for Help
*Kathleen T. Heinrich, PhD, RN*

# CHAPTER 1
# ADDRESSING THE COMPETENCIES FOR ACADEMIC NURSE EDUCATORS

Linda Caputi, MSN, EdD, RN, CNE

## Introduction

Many nurses struggle when entering academia as nurse educators. Most arrive from clinical backgrounds as strong practitioners, but have very little knowledge in the field of education. These new faculty aspire to be excellent teachers, but have no direction in the role of the academic nurse educator.

There remained a void – a void that was noticed by colleges and universities. According to Adams (2002), higher education is acknowledging that being knowledgeable in one's field of study is not sufficient for preparing the next generation of practitioners. Teacher preparation, required to teach in primary and secondary education, has moved to higher education. The primary role for faculty, to facilitate student learning by creating learning experiences that develop students into practicing nurses (Valiga, 2007), is not intuitive; it takes study and experience to learn this role.

Many of these teachers pursued advanced degrees in education. These degrees provided educational theory and enhanced one's teaching ability, but did not necessarily relate specifically to nursing education. Yet there was no universally accepted role of the academic nurse educator. The roles of a teacher in general certainly apply, but there are subsets that are quite different for an academic nurse educator. However, all this was prior to 2005. Since then changes have occurred.

## Identifying the Changes

Since the first edition of this publication (*Teaching Nursing: The Art and Science*), several significant events have occurred. These include:
- National League for Nursing's publication of *The Scope of Practice for Academic Nurse Educators*
- National League for Nursing's Certified Nurse Educator (CNE) credential
- Colleges and universities offering graduate programs in nursing education

The first two changes represent a significant contribution to the field of nursing education and an evidence base for the curricula of graduate level programs in nursing education. What an exciting time to be an academic nurse educator! Finally, our role has have been uniquely described and our contributions validated. These efforts provided just what nursing faculty and institutions offering nursing education needed.

## The Scope of Practice for Academic Nurse Educators

"Outlining nurse educator competencies is a foundational step in achieving excellence in nursing education" (Valiga, 2007, p. 173). This is the specificity that is needed for nurse educators to understand their unique role in educating nurses. The core competencies identified in **The Scope of Practice for Academic Nurse Educators** serve as the seminal work for development of the Certified Nurse Educator (CNE) credential. They also provide the basis for studying the evidence base for nursing education.

The National League for Nursing (NLN) tackled the noble challenge of identifying these core competencies for academic nurse educators. The NLN assembled a group of distinguished nursing educators with decades of nursing education experience. The results were stellar.

The first task the group identified was to define nursing education. The definition that emerged is as follows: "Nursing education is the process of facilitating learning through curriculum design, teaching, evaluation, advisement, and other activities undertaken by faculty in schools of nursing. Academic nursing education is a specialty area and an advanced practice role within professional nursing" (NLN, 2005, p. 2).

From this definition the group worked to identify eight core competencies that provide a listing of the responsibilities of the academic nurse educator. The competency statements developed by the NLN were based on the results of an extensive search of research-based literature. These competencies characterize the knowledge, skills, and attitudes required of nurse educators (Ortelli, 2010). These competencies are:

- Competency I: Facilitate Learning
- Competency II: Facilitate Learner Development and Socialization
- Competency III: Use Assessment and Evaluation Strategies
- Competency IV: Participate in Curriculum Design and Evaluation of Program Outcomes
- Competency V: Function as a Change Agent and Leader

- Competency VI: Pursue Continuous Quality Improvement in the Nurse Educator Role
- Competency VII: Engage in Scholarship
- Competency VIII: Function within the Educational Environment (NLN, 2005)

These eight competencies provide the foundation for educational expertise. Faculty can look to these to provide guidance on their scope of practice and continuing education needs. Table 1 provides a tool that faculty can use to identify how these eight competencies are used in their daily teaching and to identify areas of faculty development. Using such a tool keeps these core competencies front and center in the minds of academic nurse educators, providing a constant reminder of their professional role.

| **Philosophy Statement:** The nursing faculty acknowledge the core competencies of The Scope of Practice for Academic Nurse Educators (NLN, 2005) and aspire to incorporate the eight competencies in their daily practice. | | |
| --- | --- | --- |
| **Competency** | **Examples of How I Use the Competency in My Practice** | **Identified Areas for Faculty Development** |
| 1. Facilitate Learning | | |
| 2. Facilitate Learner Development and Socialization | | |
| 3. Use Assessment and Evaluation Strategies | | |
| 4. Participate in Curriculum Design and Evaluation of Program Outcomes | | |
| 5. Function as a Change Agent and Leader | | |
| 6. Pursue Continuous Quality Improvement in the Nurse Educator Role | | |

**Table 1.** Sample Faculty Development Tool

| 7. Engage in Scholarship | | |
| 8. Function within the Educational Environment | | |

## The Certified Nurse Educator (CNE) Credential

*The Core Competencies of Nurse Educators*© provided a foundation for the *Academic Nurse Educator Practice Analysis*, the *Certified Nurse Educator (CNE) Detailed Test Blueprint*, and *The Scope of Practice of Academic Nurse Educators* (NLN, 2005). The NLN conducted the practice analysis through the administration of a survey to nursing faculty. The activities identified in the Practice Analysis linked together the core competencies, the practice of academic nurse educators, and the detailed test blueprint of the CNE examination (Ortelli, 2010). The Practice Analysis provided evidence of the validity of the content of the examination. It also provided evidence of the activities of academic nurse educators as written in the Core Competencies of Nurse Educators (NLN, 2006).

## Colleges and Universities Offering Graduate Programs in Nursing Education

The nursing faculty shortage is upon us. To meet the demand to fill vacant faculty positions and increase the number of students admitted to nursing programs, there has been an increase in the number of graduate programs with an emphasis on preparing nurse educators. These programs are sorely needed. Many of these programs use publications focusing on nursing education, such as the first edition of *Teaching Nursing: The Art and Science*, as their course textbooks. Doing so provides direct application of educational theory to nursing education.

With the development of *The Scope of Practice for Academic Nurse Educators* and the CNE credential, these programs have a framework for their curricula. This framework provides standards for the academic nurse educator and focuses on the nurse educator as a specialty area in nursing. General educational principles can be taught and applied to the work of academic nurse educators; however, there is an additional body of knowledge necessary for an evidence-based practice for nurse educators. Using the core competencies of academic nurse educators as expressed in the CNE detailed test blueprint, provides an evidence base for the education of nursing faculty.

## Relating these Initiatives to the Content of this Book

These initiatives laid the groundwork for the education and professional role of an academic nurse educator. As members of that group, this work must permeate our professional being. To that end, I have related the content of each chapter in Volumes 1 through 3 of this book to the detailed test blueprint of the CNE examination. At the beginning of each chapter I relate the specific activities as provided in the detailed test blueprint to the content of the chapter. The purposes of this linking of content to activities of the academic nurse educator are to:

1. Demonstrate application of the literature that supports the core competencies of academic nurse educators
2. Assist nurse educators to understand their role and how their role relates to the core competencies
3. Assist readers who are preparing to write the CNE examination
4. Continue to build the evidence base for nursing education
5. Assist faculty in graduate programs in nursing education to incorporate this book into a framework built on the core competencies published in *The Scope of Practice for Academic Nurse Educators*

The work published in these seminal documents must be put to use to validate their important contribution to nursing education, and to provide current and future academic nurse educators a role identity as an advanced practice nurse with an evidence-based practice. The time has finally arrived.

## Educational Philosophy

My educational philosophy is succinct: Give the best educational experience possible. I believe faculty should continuously challenge themselves to provide creative, interesting, and sound education—students soon learn that education doesn't have to be boring; they become self-motivated, enthusiastic, and interested…learning then follows. — Linda Caputi

# References

Adams, K. A. (2002). *What colleges and universities want in new faculty*. Washington, DC: Association of American Colleges & Universities.

National League for Nursing. (2005). *The scope of practice for academic nurse educators*. New York: Author.

National League for Nursing. (2006). *Core competencies of nurse educators® with task statements*. Retrieved March 13, 2009 from www.nln.org/profdev/corec-ompetencies.pdf

Ortelli, T. (2010, in press). The certified nurse educator credential. In L. Caputi (Ed.). *Teaching Nursing: The Art and Science, Volume 3*, (2nd ed.). Glen Ellyn, IL: College of DuPage Press.

Valiga, T. (2007). Creating an evidence-based practice for nurse educators. In J. Halstead, (Ed.). *Nurse educator competencies: Creating an evidence-based practice for nurse educators* (p. 169-174). New York: National League for Nursing.

# CHAPTER 2

# THE NURSING FACULTY SHORTAGE

Linda Caputi, MSN, EdD, RN, CNE

---

The content of this chapter relates to the following major content areas and subconcepts on the Certified Nurse Educator Examination Detailed Test Blueprint:

**Pursue Continuous Quality Improvement in the Academic Nurse Educator Role**
- Engage in activities that promote one's socialization to the role
- Participate in professional development opportunities that increase one's effectiveness in the role
- Mentor and support faculty colleagues in the role of an academic nurse educator

**Engage in Scholarship of Teaching**
- Share teaching expertise with colleagues and other

**Function Effectively within the Institutional Environment and the Academic Community**
- Integrate the values of respect, collegiality, professionalism, and caring to build an organizational climate that fosters the development of learners and colleagues

---

## Introduction

*"As nursing looks forward to providing care for an increasingly chronically ill, dependent population with demands for nursing care, will the educators be available to prepare future generations of nurses?"*

*"Rising nurse salaries in practice settings have attracted potential new nurse educators into nursing service. A PhD heading a hospital's nurse education and research department is no longer an oddity."*

*"The term faculty shortage however does not adequately capture the entire problem. The problem is not only that there are faculty shortages but rather shortages of faculty who are educated as teachers, let alone experienced educators of nursing. The shortages nonetheless are as severe as they have ever been, due to the complicated interplay between the need to increase student enrollments (to increase the numbers of practicing nurses),*

*and the need to turn qualified applicants away from many schools due to limited faculty and financial resources."*

Reading these quotes, it may appear you are reading from the latest nursing education journal. Actually, the first two were published in the *Journal of Professional Nursing*, 1990, written by Mullinix (p. 133), and the last appeared in *Nurse Educator*, 1992, written by Princeton (p. 34).

The *American Journal of Nursing* reported in 1991 that the National League for Nursing (NLN) estimated that about 5 percent of the full-time teaching positions were vacant in all kinds of nursing programs (*News*, 1991). In 2002 the *American Nurse* reported that an October, 2000 survey by the American Association of Colleges of Nursing (AACN) found that 7.4 percent of faculty positions were vacant (Trossman, 2002). These vacancies are for "heavy lifting" faculty positions; that is, positions that require both classroom and clinical teaching. In 2006 the NLN estimated the unfilled, budgeted positions for full-time faculty was 1,390 positions, a 7.9 percent vacancy rate in baccalaureate and higher degree programs and a 5.6 percent vacancy rate in associate degree programs.

"The 'writing's been on the wall' for many years, so to speak, in terms of documenting the need for more well-prepared teachers of nursing and anticipation of future needs.... It is clear what measures need to be taken immediately to turn the teacher crisis in nursing around to prevent it from becoming more severe. What we must do is obvious; the challenge is to begin, now" (Princeton, 1992, p. 37). This quote, too, is from 1992 – more than 15 years ago! Clearly, it is time for all stakeholders to get off the mark and do something!

The American Academy of Colleges of Nursing (AACN) statistics indicate that in baccalaureate and graduate nursing programs in 2001, the mean age of full-time, doctorally prepared faculty was 53.2; it was 48.7 years for master's prepared faculty (Berlin & Sechrist, 2002). With the average age at retirement for nursing faculty at 62.5 years, this indicates a tremendous need for nurse educators over the next 10 years as further retirements occur. The shortage that existed a decade ago is still with us.

This chapter discusses the current nursing faculty shortage and ways to minimize its impact.

## Causes of the Current Faculty Shortage

Interestingly, many of the basic causes of the current faulty shortage are the same as those indicated in the literature 10 years ago (Berlin & Sechrist, 2002; DeYoung & Bliss, 1995). The primary causes are:

- **Aging of the present faculty.** According to AACN (2003) the mean age of full-time doctorally prepared nursing faculty rose to 53.5 in 2002 from 49.7 in 1993; for master's prepared, the mean age rose to 48.8 in 2002 from 46 in 1993. At the same time, the percent of faculty aged 36 to 45 dropped to only 10 percent in 2002 from 30 percent in 1993. The faculty are aging with no younger faculty taking their place. The National League for Nursing (NLN) reported in 2005 that 75 percent of the current nursing faculty will retire by 2019.
- **Fewer graduate students choosing teaching careers.**
  - In 1977, 24.7 percent of graduates from nursing master's programs were education majors.
  - In 1994, 11.3 percent of graduates from nursing master's programs were education majors.
  - In 2002, 3.5 percent were education majors (AACN, 2003).

However, since 2002 there has been a major increase in the number of master's nursing programs preparing nurse educators. A quick search of the Internet yielded over a dozen programs offering an education track in a master's degree program (www.mastersinnursing.com). Many of these programs are offered totally online.

- **An exit of master's and doctorally prepared nurses from academia to clinical and private sectors offering greater financial rewards.** Over the last decade, considerable budget cuts at academic institutions have placed constraints on faculty salaries. Academia cannot compete with private-sector healthcare organizations competing for nurses educated at the graduate level (AACN, 2003). Nurse practitioners educated at the master's level earn approximately 12 percent more than master's-prepared faculty (Kaufman, 2007) and an independently employed nurse practitioner's salary is 150 percent greater than a full professor's salary (NLN, 2005). However, Garbee and Killacky (2008) report that low pay was not the most frequent dissatisfaction of faculty who leave teaching positions. These researchers found time demands and extremes in leadership were more frequently cited as causes of faculty dissatisfaction.
- **Workload and workplace issues.** It is not unusual for nursing faculty to have the heaviest teaching load in terms of contact hours among college or

university faculty. This is often because clinical hours are not assigned a one-to-one ratio; that is, one clock hour of clinical instruction is not considered one contact hour of teaching load. Some faculty must teach two or more hours to equal one hour of teaching load. Clinical teaching is extremely labor-intensive and should merit one hour of contact for one clock hour of teaching. New faculty will find this more attractive. Additionally, to retain older faculty, clinical teaching assignments may need to be adjusted relative to faculty's physical and energy limits (Brendtro & Hegge, 2000).

- **Unrealistic role expectations.** New faculty struggle to fill all the roles expected of them by administrators, colleagues, and students. Because most new faculty do not have a background in nursing education, it is impossible for them to meet expectations, which contributes to the stress of new faculty.

- **Advanced practice registered nurses (APRNs) are unable to maintain their clinical practice and certification while in full-time faculty positions.** Perhaps more APRNs would consider a teaching position if they had time to maintain their certification.

In addition, other contemporary factors are impacting the workload and role expectations of faculty teaching undergraduate nursing students. Health care has changed dramatically, requiring more education in the same amount of time. Faculty struggle to find ways to teach all that needs to be taught. Additionally, the passing standard for the NCLEX® continues to rise. Although this is justified in terms of preparing safe practitioners, it nevertheless puts pressures on nursing faculty. When a student fails the NCLEX, faculty often feel responsible. This contributes to faculty not enjoying their positions.

## Consequences of the Faculty Shortage

### Inability to Accommodate Burgeoning Student Applications

The consequences of the faculty shortage are both obvious and subtle. The most obvious consequence of the faculty shortage is the inability to accommodate all students applying for admission to undergraduate nursing programs. This, in turn, exacerbates the nursing shortage, threatening the health care of all citizens.

In recent years the number of applicants to schools of nursing has increased dramatically. Schools can not accommodate all the qualified applicants. The NLN (2009) reports that in the 2006-2007 academic year, 33 percent of applicants were not qualified, 41 percent of applicants were accepted into nursing programs, and 26 percent were qualified but not accepted. At the same time there is an acute nursing shortage that is predicted to worsen as the baby-boomers become senior citizens.

## Nursing Research

A less noticeable result of a faculty shortage is its effect on nursing research. Research in all areas of nursing will be affected. Traditionally, doctorally-prepared faculty produce the lion's share of nursing research. Only about half of the full-time faculty teaching in baccalaureate and higher degree programs are educated at the doctoral level (NLN, 2005). Institutions employing low numbers of doctorally-prepared educators may be less likely to secure funds to conduct research. With senior faculty retiring and an insufficient number of junior faculty taking their places, who will conduct this research?

Another important consideration relative to nursing research is the degree required for tenure. Many institutions require a doctorate in nursing. These credentials are extremely helpful to generate research that will enhance the knowledge base of nursing. However, these programs generally do not develop effective teachers because they do not typically include education courses in their curricula (Brendtro & Hegge, 2000). There is a real need for **educational** research. The NLN (2003) has published a position statement noting the need for the design of "evidence-based curricula." Among its recommendations for faculty were:

- Explore new pedagogies and new ways of thinking about nursing education.
- Conduct pedagogical research to document the effectiveness and meaningfulness of innovations being undertaken.
- Create an evidence base for nursing education that embraces innovation, identifies best practices, and serves to prepare a diverse nursing population that can transform nursing practice (p. 5).

Educational research is indeed important to the development of evidence-based nursing education. The NLN advocates the development of evidence-based nursing education as a science base for academic nurse educators (Shultz, 2010). To this end, it is imperative that faculty hold doctorates in education. Institutions should not limit tenured faculty positions to those holding nursing doctorates. A mix of doctorates would be ideal. "There also continues to be a need in our academic communities for scholars and researchers in education.... As a discipline, nurse educators need research in nursing education." (Tanner, 1999, p. 51).

Opening tenure-track positions to nurses doctorally prepared in education would add to the pool of potential faculty and bring into the profession scholars in the art and science of education who can develop an evidence-based science of nursing education. Additionally, it may be a worthwhile experiment for universities to grant doctorates in nursing education.

## Solutions for the Nursing Faculty Shortage

The solution to this shortage will be as multifaceted as the causes. One approach to conceptualizing solutions is to consider the causes of the shortage and the environment in which nursing faculty work.

The causes of the shortage are an obvious area of concern and will be addressed throughout this chapter. The problems with the environment in which nursing faculty work is equally important, but solutions are perhaps more elusive. However, it will be difficult to attract new faculty if the current faculty "....don't enjoy their day" (Berlin & Sechrist, 2002, p. 55). AACN (2003) reports that 54.7 percent of faculty at the assistant professor, instructor, or lecturer levels reported dissatisfaction with their workloads. Many of these faculty leave teaching due to this dissatisfaction, and, more disconcerting, would not recommend teaching to nurses considering entering the teaching profession. Schools of nursing with a "good work climate" will have greater success recruiting and retaining faculty (Hinshaw, 2001).

Several changes that have occurred over the last decade may contribute to this dissatisfaction (AACN, 2003). They include:

- **Changes in the way higher education is conducted.** The triad of teaching, service, and research remains. However, the service and research requirements are becoming more intense as faculty are required to obtain extramural funding and publish extensively. These requirements put additional pressure on the shrinking faculty workforce.
- **Changes in the characteristics of today's students.** Today's college students are increasingly diverse and represent many different cultures. For many students, English is a second, third, or foreign language (Sutherland, 2004). This diversity enriches the classroom, but requires additional skills for the teacher. In addition, students now are more likely to be at different stages of life as they enter undergraduate nursing programs; 73 percent of undergraduate nursing students are considered nontraditional. With an average age of 30.9 years, more students are delaying their entry into higher education or changing their careers, and have jobs and families competing for their time and attention. Although adult learners bring a multitude of talents and

skills, they challenge the faculty to develop creative, relevant, critical thinking, and problem solving experiences. Faculty must relate to students with varying learning styles and needs (Forrest, 2010).

These changes create challenges for faculty. Junior faculty who were prepared as nurse practitioners, rather than as nurse educators, may find they are not prepared to fill all these roles and ultimately leave teaching.

## Faculty Mentors

How does a nurse with little or no teaching experience learn to teach? How would a new teacher know **how** to teach without any formal coursework? For many, teaching is like parenting: One parents as one was parented and one teaches as one was taught. In this case, the new teacher may emulate a teacher from the distant past; the teaching approach may be decades old and not reflective of current educational theory. Then how should a new teacher learn? One of the best resources for practitioners entering teaching is a faculty mentor.

The faculty mentor facilitates the orientation and enculturation of the new teacher into the specific academic setting. This person provides guidance, assistance, and positive feedback, and is a friend who is willing to listen and offer support. However, the mentor does not provide a graduate degree in nursing education. Unfortunately, many faculty who are asked to be mentors are expected to teach the new faculty everything the mentor knows about teaching. This approach tends to cause resentment and disdain among the experienced faculty, and could eventually diminish the pool of willing mentors (Smith & Zsohar, 2007).

One way to avoid overloading senior faculty with additional mentoring duties is to hire new faculty a year before the date another faculty member retires. The junior faculty can work side by side with the retiring teacher. This allows time for both people to achieve a successful mentoring experience.

## The New Faculty Team

The idea of a faculty team is one that has been employed in clinical nursing for many years. Some institutions provide newly employed nurses with educational time, a preceptor, and extended orientation. Schools of nursing might benefit from such a plan tailored to the needs of new faculty. A new-faculty team would be comprised of the following members:

- The new faculty

- The mentor, a senior faculty
- The department administrator

Together, this three-person team develops an action plan that outlines the specific needs of the new teacher and the means to meet those needs. This plan may cover a period of several years, and should be **individualized** to each new teacher. The plan should focus first on the teaching aspect of the triad of faculty responsibilities – teaching, research, and service – and should be designed so the new faculty first becomes a competent, able teacher. Research and service can then be addressed after a few years of teaching experience. To expect the new teacher to perform all aspects of the position while learning to be a teacher may very well drive the new person out of education completely. New teachers' committee responsibilities should also be minimized for their first three years.

The tenure clock should be paused for those finishing doctoral degrees to allow time to complete their coursework and dissertation. It is nearly impossible for a master's-prepared teacher to fill the triad of service, teaching, and research while also completing a doctoral degree. The tenure clock can be reset when the teacher has completed the doctoral work.

## Developing the Individualized Plan of Action

When deciding what areas of content to include in the action plan for the new faculty, the team should start by considering core competencies. The NLN (2006) has developed a list of core competencies for nurse educators that serve as the basis for the Academic Nurse Educator. The complete list can be found at www.nln.org/profdev/competency.htm. The major categories of competencies include:
- Facilitate learning
- Facilitate learner development and socialization
- Use assessment and evaluation strategies
- Participate in curriculum design and evaluation of program outcomes
- Function as change agents and leaders
- Develop educator role
- Engage in scholarship
- Function within the educational environment

Although it is important for all educators to acquire each of the competencies listed within each of the above categories, the list may appear somewhat daunting to the novice educator. Among the many new faculty with whom I have worked and consulted over the last decade, several common areas emerge as priorities:

- Curriculum development
- Conducting classroom sessions
- Grading term papers
- Test item writing

Following are some suggestions to help the novice educator in each of these areas.

**Curriculum Development.** An important first endeavor for the new faculty is to gain an understanding of the nursing program curriculum. This helps the teacher appreciate the bigger picture, and understand how all the pieces fit together to make the whole. It is important for the new faculty to understand basic concepts such as:
- Program philosophy
- Major concepts
- Program outcomes
- Course structure and sequencing
- Content flow

A sound understanding of these points will provide a framework within which the new teacher can develop educational experiences (Caputi, 2010).

**Conducting Classroom Sessions.** A common learning need of new faculty is how to conduct classroom sessions, whether in lecture, case study discussion, or small group settings. Students may complain the new teacher only talks about the topic without providing visuals, examples, or application to patient care. These deficiencies may stem from a lack of knowledge about instructional design. Therefore, it can be extremely helpful to focus the action plan on instructional design, steps of the design process, and application to the classroom.

**Grading Term Papers.** A common complaint of students is the inconsistency among teachers when grading term papers and other subjective assignments; inexperienced teachers often struggle with this task. The teacher can use a grading grid to determine topics the students must cover in an assigned paper. See Figure 1 for an example of such a grid for grading a term paper. To provide enhanced specificity, the faculty can develop a rubric that provides specific information about what constitutes a passing grade and what constitutes a failing grade. When a grid and rubric are used, the teacher can be confident with the grade awarded and is empowered when discussing the grade with the student.

**Test Item Writing.** One of the most difficult tasks for a new teacher is constructing valid and reliable multiple-choice tests. Currently in undergraduate nursing education, there is a need not only for valid and reliable multiple-choice test items, but also for tests to be written at the application and analysis levels.

Writing valid and reliable questions is also important because poorly written questions can lead students to fail, even if they understand the subject matter. Teachers must take the responsibility for ensuring that items are well-written, fair, valid, and reliable so they can be confident that students who fail do so because of deficient knowledge and not because of poorly constructed tests.

The National Council of State Boards of Nursing offers two Internet courses for nursing faculty on test item writing at www.ncsbn.org. These courses are:

- **Basic assessment strategies: test development and item writing.** This course offers information about measurement statistics, principles of multiple-choice item writing, basic techniques for writing items that assess higher-order cognitive processes, guidelines regarding potential item bias, and a critique of sample NCLEX® examination questions.
- **Advanced assessment strategies: assessing higher-level thinking.** This course teaches nursing educators how to write items that assess critical thinking. It also offers suggestions for converting items to a higher cognitive level.

It may be best to take a basic course on general test construction and measurement before beginning these courses.

## Helping New Faculty Navigate Conferences

Although new faculty can learn much from their colleagues at their home institutions, it is important for them to tap the wealth of information and learn the value of networking that comes from attending conferences. The mentor should encourage the new teacher to take advantage of such opportunities. At a recent nurse educators conference, I spoke with a senior faculty from another college whom I had met at a previous conference. As I approached her, I noticed a young woman with her. I remarked, "How nice to bring your daughter with you!" She replied, "Oh, this isn't my daughter! This is one of our new faculty."

After the blushing subsided, I commented that it was wonderful to see a seasoned faculty attending a conference with a novice faculty. What a great way for the new person to learn how to get the most out of a conference. Fitzpatrick (2003) offers these suggestions for deriving the greatest benefit when attending a conference:

- Attend the keynote. This sets the stage for the conference.

| Total Points: 25 | Points Allowed | Points Deducted | Points Given |
|---|---|---|---|
| I. Introduction | 1 | | |
| II. Assessment: Effects of Illness on Growth & Development | 6 | | |
| III. Nursing Diagnoses | 1 | | |
| IV. Planning and Intervention | | | |
|    A. Goals and outcome criteria | 1 | | |
|    B. Nursing management | | | |
|       1. Care during admission | 5 | | |
|       2. Child/family teaching and discharge planning; evaluation for long-term management | 3 | | |
|       3. Activity therapy appropriate to child's age | 3 | | |
| V. Conclusion | 1 | | |
| VI. Format | | | |
|    A. Composition | 2 | | |
|    B. APA Format | 2 | | |
|    C. One point off for each page over 12 pages | | | X |
|    D. One point off for each of four professional nursing journals not used. | | | X |
|    E. Two points off if submitted after due date and time. | | | X |
|    F. Any paper received more than one week late will receive zero points. Failure to submit a paper will result in a failing grade for the course. | | | X |
|    G. Plagiarism – See syllabus. | | | X |
| Additional Comments: | | | |
| TOTAL POINTS: | 25 | | |

**Figure 1.** Grid for Grading a Term Paper

- Attend informal activities and network with other attendees.
- Attend the poster sessions and discuss the work of these presenters; collect the abstracts.
- Make connections and network during educational offerings.

When I attend a conference, I make a point to meet at least one new person. Over the years, the people I have met at conferences have become colleagues and have provided an invaluable network. Staying in touch with them has provided a continual source of new thoughts and innovative ideas, none of which I would have gained without first having met them at conferences.

## Retirees: A Resource to Deal with the Faculty Shortage

Once the experienced faculty has successfully mentored the new teacher, it may be time for the senior faculty to retire. As is the case in private industry, many faculty are being offered attractive retirement packages – this is good for them, but not good for the system. In some cases, administrators, fueled by the bottom line, actually encourage their faculty to retire. After all, a doctorally prepared professor with 25 years of tenure earns twice as much as an assistant faculty with a master's degree (Acord, 2000). But this practice is very short-sighted.

The traditional all-or-nothing retirement approach needs an overhaul. Senior faculty have much to offer. Administrators and faculty must develop strategies for retaining the senior faculty's expertise. The aging professorate may not have the physical energy of their more youthful junior faculty, but their intellect and wisdom are qualities that should not be retired.

As an eager student of nursing education in the early 1980s, I studied at Loyola University, Chicago. I witnessed the value of our aging experts in nursing. Ann Zimmerman, a retired professor and former president of the ANA, was invited to teach a class in the graduate school. At that time Dr. Zimmerman was in her 70s. It was most exciting to learn about her early years in nursing and listen to her wisdom on nursing education. She was inspiring and an outstanding role model. Retired faculty serving in this capacity should be the norm throughout nursing education.

By phasing a person's retirement, the exiting faculty enjoys all the benefits of their retirement with an opportunity for part-time employment as an expert member in nursing academia (AACN, 2003).

It would be wonderful for schools of nursing to bring back retired faculty in an expert advisory role. The professor emeritus might do the following:
- Attend lectures and critique the teacher's delivery

- Facilitate case study discussions and concept mapping
- Guide new faculty in grading subjective assignments such as research papers
- Help new faculty complete clinical evaluations
- Tutor at-risk students

This list is only a beginning. What a valuable resource – those entering the ranks of professor emeritus. These faculty would not only assist novice faculty in developing quality instruction and learning experiences, but they also can play a valuable role in helping students succeed. The end results – novice faculty who are truly mentored and at-risk students assisted to complete the nursing degree – are outcomes no one could fault.

Additional roles for retired faculty that would help lessen the workload of full-time faculty include:
- Supervise in the nursing skills laboratory
- Assist with research projects
- Teach selected classes
- Attend conferences and share information and proceedings with faculty

An interesting way to utilize the knowledge of senior faculty is a faculty development center for nursing. This center can be staffed by a cadre of retired faculty who may have retired from other institutions within a community or region. Such a consortium can provide the benefit of varied faculty interests and expertise and a pooling of resources for new faculty. Workshops, seminars, and Web-based courses can be developed by these faculty and offered as a means of financial support for the center.

## Teaching Web-Based or Hybrid Courses

Another exciting area for retired faculty is teaching web-based courses. Many schools have completely shifted the theory portion of their courses to web course or are developing hybrid courses that employ a mix of face-to-face and online instruction. Retired faculty may be interested in teaching the online portion of the course. This also can decrease the full-time faculty's workload.

## Part-Time Faculty

The shortage of faculty often is met with an increase in part-time faculty. Budget cuts in higher education are also fueling the trend toward hiring part-time teachers. Currently, there is one part-time nursing faculty for every 1.7 full-time faculty (Zungolo, 2003). Employing part-time faculty is a short-sighted solution because part-time faculty typically have a very limited role. It is helpful to employ part-time faculty to avoid cancellation of a class; however, the increased use of part-time faculty puts an increased burden on the smaller core of full-time faculty (DeYoung, Bliss, & Tracy, 2002). As more part-time faculty are used as replacements, the work of the decreasing number of full-time faculty increases proportionately. The work of academia continues with fewer people to carry the increased workload. The work this entails includes:

- Reviewing prospective student files. In one nursing program, the number of applicants has increased from 200 per year in the late 1990s to nearly 1,200 in Fall, 2004. However, the school employs no additional assistance to sort through all these student files. Implementing an office of selective admissions is a strategy used by some nursing programs to provide needed assistance.
- Reviewing program policies and procedures
- Updating curriculum to meet the changing practice arena
- Developing weekend and fast-track programs to accommodate more students
- Integrating technology, such as developing Web-based courses, to meet the needs of changing student populations

And the list goes on. This can lead to an overworked full-time faculty, and might prompt early retirement for some who might otherwise work beyond the usual retirement age. Unfortunately, disgruntled full-time faculty often paint an unpleasant picture of the workload, which can further discourage nurses from entering the teaching profession.

## Attracting Younger Faculty

A problem commonly cited in the literature is that nurses enter faculty positions at a much older age than faculty in other disciplines. On average, a person entering nursing academia is 10 years older than teachers of other disciplines (DeYoung, Bliss, & Tracy, 2002). This typically leaves 15 to 20 years before reaching retirement age (Hinshaw, 2001). "Thus, a new professional tradition needs to be considered in order to lengthen the number of years nursing faculty have to be productive in academia" (Hinshaw, 2001, p. 11). We must entice nurses to enter teaching at a much younger age so they can provide more years of teaching throughout their careers.

One suggestion is to entice younger nurses into graduate education with a focus on nursing education. We must guide and mentor these students into academia or risk losing them to the practice arena. Additionally, the idea that a nurse must practice for several years before entering a master's program further discourages students from earning graduate degrees during the early years of their careers. Institutions should create fast-track programs that allow students to move from bachelor's to doctorate degrees in a reduced time. These programs are necessary to ensure master's graduates advance into doctorate programs. Accessibility is also important. Web-based master's and doctoral programs may create more opportunities for nurses to join the teaching profession, regardless of their proximity to colleges and universities.

Young, promising nurses should be encouraged to consider careers in education, but this may be difficult given today's nursing shortage. Many nurses are enjoying attractive salaries and benefits. They may be deterred from entering graduate programs to eventually teach, when they might earn less than they are earning in a staff nurse position. In fact, Trossman (2002) reports that some new graduates accept clinical positions at which they earn more than the faculty who taught them. Interestingly, this creates a self-destructive cycle for the teaching profession. If nurses do not continue their education to become nurse educators, the number of students denied admission to nursing schools will continue to increase.

Faculty would do well to share with potential nurse educators the satisfying aspects of a career in academia which include opportunities to (Hinshaw, 2001, p. 7):

- Develop and shape new professionals
- Engage in creative, intellectual discussions with faculty colleagues and students
- Pursue a research and/or scholarly program of professional and personal interest
- Contribute to improving health care through student education and the generation of new knowledge
- Provide professional, disciplinary, and interdisciplinary leadership
- Shape health policy based on professional and scholarly expertise

## Summary

The causes of the nursing faculty shortage are multifaceted and complex. Both short-term and long-term strategies must be considered if the shortage is to be reversed. Reversing the faculty shortage is imperative to increasing the number of practicing nurses providing direct patient care. Unfortunately, the faculty shortage has been present for more than a decade and continues to grow. To date, attempts to change the situation either have not worked or have not been seriously considered.

## Learning Activities

1. AACN provides more suggestions for relieving the faculty shortage in its 2003 white paper, *Faculty Shortages in Baccalaureate and Graduate Nursing Programs: Scope of the Problem and Strategies for Expanding the Supply* – www.aacn.nche.edu/Publications/WhitePapers/FacultyShortages.htm. Analyze the suggestion to use non-nursing faculty and courses to satisfy nursing course requirements. Discuss this option with a colleague.
2. Survey the nursing schools in your state. How many full-time faculty do they employ? How have the schools handled faculty retirements? How many faculty will be retiring in the next five years? Are these schools experiencing difficulty hiring new faculty? If so, are they implementing any policy changes to address this problem?

## Educational Philosophy

My educational philosophy is succinct: Give the best educational experience possible. I believe faculty should continuously challenge themselves to provide creative, interesting, and sound education—students soon learn that education doesn't have to be boring; they become self-motivated, enthusiastic, and interested...learning then follows. — Linda Caputi

## References

Acord, L. G. (2000). Education. Help wanted—faculty. *Journal of Professional Nursing, 16*(1), 3.

American Association of Colleges of Nursing. (2003). *Faculty shortages in bacca-laureate and graduate nursing programs*. Washington, DC: Author.

Anderson, C. A. (2002). From the editor. Nursing faculty—going, going, gone. *Nursing Outlook, 50*(2), 43-44.

Berlin, L. E., & Sechrist, K. R. (2002). The shortage of doctorally prepared nursing faculty: A dire situation. *Nursing Outlook, 50*(2), 50-56.

Brendtro, M. J., & Hegge, M. (2000). Nursing faculty: One generation away from extinction? *Journal of Professional Nursing, 16*(2), 97-103.

Caputi, L. (2010, in press). Curriculum design and development. In L. Caputi (Ed.). *Teaching Nursing: The Art and Science, Vol. 1*. Glen Ellyn, IL: College of Du-Page Press.

DeYoung, S. (1995). Nursing faculty—an engendered species? *Journal of Professional Nursing, 11*(2), 84-88.

DeYoung, S., Bliss, J., & Tracy, J. P. (2002). The nursing faculty shortage: Is there hope? *Journal of Professional Nursing, 18*(6), 313-319.

Fitzpatrick, J. (2003). Professional development: Getting the most from the summit. *Nursing Education Perspectives, 24*(3), 221.

Forrest, S. (2010, in press). Learning styles. In L. Caputi (Ed.). *Teaching Nursing: The Art and Science, Vol. 2*. Glen Ellyn, IL: College of DuPage Press.

Garbee, D. D., & Killacky, J. (2008). Factors influencing intent to stay in academia for nursing faculty in the southern United States of America, *International Journal of Nursing Education Scholarship, 5*(1), www.bepress.com/ijnes/vol5/iss1/art9

Hinshaw, A. (2001). A continuing challenge: The shortage of educationally prepared nursing faculty. *Online Journal of Issues in Nursing, 6*(1). Retrieved March, 2004, from http://www.nursingworld.org/ojin/topic14/tpc14_3.htm

Mullinix, C. F. (1990). The next shortage—the nurse educator. *Journal of Professional Nursing, 6*(3), 133.

National League for Nursing. (2003). *Position statement: Innovation in nursing education: A call to reform*. New York: Author.

National League for Nursing. (2005). *Nurse faculty shortage fact sheet*. Retrieved March 13, 2009 from www.nln.org/governmentaffairs/pdf/NurseFacultyShort-age.pdf

National League for Nursing. (2006). *Core competencies of nurse educators® with task statements*. Retrieved March 13, 2009 from www.nln.org/profdev/corecompetencies.pdf

National League for Nursing. (2006, July 24). *Nurse faculty support continues to fall short; NLN's 2006 faculty census survey shows increased vacancy rates*. Available at http://www.nln.org/newsreleases/nurseeducators2006.htm

National League for Nursing. (2009). *Disposition of applications to basic RN programs, 2006-07* Retrieved March 13, 2009 from www.nln.org/research/slides/index.htm

News, As enrollments rebound, schools face a growing faculty shortage. (1991). *American Journal of Nursing, 91*(4), pp. 108,112-113.

Princeton, J. C. (1992). The teacher crisis in nursing education—revisited. *Nurse Educator, 17*(5), 34-37.

Shultz, C. (2010, in press). Evidence-based nursing education in L. Caputi, (Ed.). *Teaching nursing: The art and science, Vol. 1*. Glen Ellyn, IL: College of DuPage Press.

Smith, J. A., & Zsohar, H. (2007). Essentials of neophyte mentorship in relation to the faculty shortage. *Journal of Nursing Education, 46*(4), 184-186.

Sutherland, L. (2010, in press). Teaching Students from Culturally-Diverse Backgrounds. In L. Caputi & L. Engelmann (Eds.), *Teaching nursing: The art and science Vol. 1*. Glen Ellyn, IL: College of DuPage Press.

Tanner, C. A. (1999). Developing the new professorate. *Journal of Nursing Education, 38*(2), 51-52.

Trossman, S. (2002). Who will be there to teach? Shortage of nursing faculty a growing problem. *American Nurse, 34*(1), 22-23.

Zungolo, E. (2003). President's message. The predicament of nursing education: The faculty censes. *Nurse Education Perspectives, 24*(2), 62.

# CHAPTER 3

# AN OVERVIEW OF THE EDUCATIONAL PROCESS

Linda Caputi, MSN, EdD, RN, CNE

---

The content of this chapter relates to the following major content areas and subconcepts on the Certified Nurse Educator Examination Detailed Test Blueprint:

**Facilitate Learning**

- Implement a variety of teaching strategies appropriate to content, setting, learner needs, learning style, desired learner outcomes
- Use teaching strategies based on educational theory and evidence-based practices related to education

**Facilitate Learner Development and Socialization**

- Identify individual learning styles and unique learning needs of learners with a variety of diverse characteristics
- Provide resources for diverse learners to meet their individual learning needs
- Adapt teaching styles and interpersonal interactions to facilitate learner behaviors

---

## Introduction

This chapter explores the teaching-learning process (also called the educational process) – what it is and how to use it to achieve optimal results from both the teacher and the learner. This chapter reflects the essence of the title of this book, *Teaching Nursing: The Art and Science*. The science refers to teaching-learning as a process comprised of steps, each with their related activities. The art is in the doing, the creativity each teacher brings to each of those steps and takes into the class with the end goal of producing unique, unforgettable educational experiences.

## A Look at the Educational Process

The educational process involves two complementary elements: teaching and learning. Therefore, the educational process is often known as the teaching-learning process. A basic premise underlying the teaching-learning process is that teaching exists to support learning. Teaching is not a solitary activity, an activity that exists by itself. If it were not for learning, there would be no need for teaching. This reflects the major paradigm shift of the last decade – a shift from focusing on the teacher to focusing on the student.

The teaching-learning process is multifaceted. It involves ideas and concepts from many disciplines, including nursing, educational psychology, instructional technology, instructional design, tests and measurements, and evaluation theory. It is a wise educator who puts all this theory together and emerges with a plan in hand to develop and deliver outstanding teaching that results in high levels of relevant, meaningful learning.

At the same time, the wise educator realizes that a lock-stop, prescriptive approach is counterproductive in the ever-changing world of nursing education. The teacher must be ready to adjust and adapt as the student body changes and new educational delivery methods evolve. The teacher must be imaginative, flexible, and proficient at using a variety of teaching methods. The teacher must also be a skilled communicator with an ability to motivate others (Bastable, 2008). Many of the chapters in this book provide valuable information to help teachers develop these skills.

If this sounds like a plan, it may also sound like a formidable task requiring continuous updating and faculty development. The key to handling all that is required to become an expert at implementing the teaching-learning process is to have a cognitive schemata – a way of looking at the elements that provide a framework for the implementation of the process – something similar to the nursing process. For example, by the time nurses are at the point of becoming faculty, they are very familiar with the nursing process – they are experts. Application of the nursing process to patient care is fluid and intuitive. The nurse easily applies any of the five steps when faced with a patient situation. Revising and refining the patient care plan using the nursing process becomes innate for expert nurses – they often do not consciously consider the process itself. Rather, they operate from a deep understanding of the total situation. Rules and procedures are no longer used to guide decisions. Patient care is fluid, flexible, and highly proficient (Benner, 2001). This is not to say that experts never use analytic tools. They use those tools when faced with new, unfamiliar situations.

Nurses as faculty apply the same type of thinking to the teaching-learning process when educating students. Traditionally, this process has been called the instructional design process. The name of the process – instructional design – is somewhat outdated for a couple of reasons: (1) the educational paradigm shift from a focus on instruction to a focus on learning, and (2) the implication of the word design, that the process only addresses how to design instruction, when in fact, the instructional design process actually encompasses all steps of the educational process.

Therefore, this author prefers the term **educational process**. Throughout this chapter, the terms educational process and teaching-learning process are used interchangeably to describe the steps in this process. Readers familiar with the instructional design process will note how the educational process is very similar to the process widely described in educational literature of the past. Yet they may soon realize that the term educational process has a much broader focus, encompassing all aspects of teaching and learning rather than just the design of instructional materials. However, the shift in education from a focus on the teacher (instruction) to a focus on the student (learning) makes the naming of the process – the teaching-learning process – much more congruent with the present-day paradigm.

## Steps in the Educational Process

Some basic elements must be in place before invoking the educational process. Nursing programs must have an established curriculum. The curriculum tells the faculty **what** to teach. The teaching-learning process then guides faculty in **how** to teach the curriculum. The teaching-learning process provides a systematic design for teaching and learning – with an emphasis on the word **specific**– a plan for developing **specific** teaching-learning materials **specifically** for your **specific** learners.

The five steps in the traditional instructional design process are used to explain the teaching-learning process. These steps are:
- Step 1: Assess and analyze
- Step 2: Design
- Step 3: Develop
- Step 4: Implement
- Step 5: Evaluate

## Step 1: Assess and Analyze

The first step – assess and analyze – is extremely important. This step provides information relative to the learners, the content, and the available resources. First, consider the learner.

**Learner analysis.** Learner analysis, sometimes referred to as audience analysis, is focused on becoming familiar with the characteristics of the learners. It is important to have a good sense of the characteristics of the students in a class. One method for ascertaining the characteristics of students is to conduct a self-assessment. The self-assessment can include many dimensions such as: number of hours worked each week, previous college education, number of people depending on the student for support, learning style, familiarity with NCLEX® style questions, and many others. The easiest way to collect this information is to use a software program such as that offered by College of DuPage titled *StartRight in Nursing School* (www.dupagepress.com/nursing/start-right). Collecting this data when the student begins the nursing program assists both the student and the faculty with analyzing information about the student and developing a plan of action to use the strengths noted in the assessment to improve retention and to correct areas that may interfere with success. Sample reports generated by *StartRight* are included on the CD accompanying this book.

A superficial assessment of nursing students may, at first glance, reveal a fairly homogenous group. Most nursing programs have entrance requirements that all students must meet, therefore nursing students tend to be similar in many ways. Students must pass prerequisite courses, often with the requirement that a specific grade be earned, prior to enrolling in nursing courses as well as meet other entrance requirements. This, however, is probably where the homogeneity ends.

Nursing students no longer resemble the traditional college student. They vary in many ways. Some of these diverse characteristics include the following:

- **Age:** Nursing students range in age from 18 to 55 plus years. Students in any one nursing course may represent as many as three developmental stages and three generations – from the baby-boomers (born 1946-1960) to the generation Xers (born 1960s-1982) to the millennials (born 1982+). The developmental stage and generational influences impact the meanings students derive from instruction. For example, baby-boomers live to work, maintain a general sense of optimism, and are team- and process-oriented. Generation Xers work to live, not live to work; believe in clear, consistent expectations; and look for jobs with opportunities for growth. And finally, millennials live in the moment, rely on the immediacy of technology, question everything, demand clear and consistent expectations, and believe that earning money translates into immediate consumption (Johnson & Romanello, 2005; McDonald, 2010; Oblinger, 2003; Stokes, 2010). A multigenerational classroom presents unique challenges for appealing to the needs of all learners.
- **Ethnic diversity:** Several chapters in this book discuss the culturally diverse student body in nursing education (see *Teaching Faculty to Provide Culturally-Competent Nursing Education* by Leonie Sutherland and *Cultural Diversity: Teaching Students to Provide Culturally-Competent Nursing Care* by Linda Wilson). Teaching to a group of culturally diverse students is not only challenging but growth-enhancing for faculty. Students share their beliefs and concerns, enriching the learning experience for all students. Par-

ticularly challenging is the language barrier that many students face. Just as faculty were becoming more skilled in assisting students with English as a second language, students with English as a foreign language are becoming more common in nursing programs. These students may have English as their third or fourth language, making their understanding of nursing content even more difficult to comprehend (Sutherland, 2010).

- **Progression through the nursing program:** Teaching students in the beginning nursing courses is much different than teaching students in advanced courses. Beginning students are still learning the language of the profession, developing a nursing attitude, and in general, just "getting their feet wet." Lessons developed for these students take on a more basic nature than lessons for advanced students. Using instructional strategies such as storytelling and humor must be accomplished at a level beginning students can understand and advanced students can appreciate.

- **Learning styles:** Assessing learning styles is helpful so the teacher can design and develop instruction that best meets the learners' needs. There are many definitions in the literature of learning styles. One definition is: Personal qualities that influence a student's ability to acquire information to interact with peers and the teacher and otherwise to participate in learning experiences (Grasha, 1996; Haar, Hall, Schoepp, & Smith, 2002). There are also many inventories that can be used to assess the student's learning style. Forrest (2010) provides a listing of such sites. Most inventories are free for students to use and provides both students and faculty with valuable information. *StartRight in Nursing School* discussed earlier in this chapter includes a learning styles inventory.

- **Motivation or attitude about nursing content:** It may seem difficult to believe, but not all nursing students are interested in every topic, no matter how excited the teacher is about teaching it! This presents one of teaching's greatest challenges – making a class interesting for students not particularly excited about a topic. Assessing students' motivations and attitudes about course content can be accomplished through questionnaires and small-group discussions. Humor can be used to introduce a topic to a new group of students when the topic has historically not been a favorite. For example, the first topic area I often cover in an advanced medical/surgical nursing course is care of patients with alteration in the urinary system. At the beginning of the first of three lectures, I start with the following comment, "I'll bet it was difficult driving to class today." At this point, the students look at each other and wonder what I'm talking about. I continue on, "I know you have been working hard for years to get to this point in your nursing studies. Well, the time has finally arrived. We will be discussing the renal system today. How many of you are feeling excited?" I then wait for a hand to raise, then slowly another one, and, with a little encouragement, all the students raise their hands. Then I end the introduction with, "Well, I'll try to be worthy and not let you down after you have waited so long for this day to arrive!" Of course, the ultimate challenge facing me at this point is to make the next three class sessions unforgettable learning experiences, but that is the challenge teachers face every day when entering the classroom.

- **Anxiety:** Anything that affects psychological comfort can affect the students' ability to learn. As the level of anxiety rises, the ability to learn decreases (Bastable, 2008). Nurses have long applied this fact to patient teaching. The teacher considers this when designing the instruction and remembers that a learner who is unreceptive to instruction when anxiety is high is more receptive to the same instruction when anxiety is decreased. Many instructional strategies discussed later in this chapter are aimed at increasing the students' psychological comfort which in turn increases their readiness to learn.

**Content analysis.** A content analysis determines exactly what the faculty will teach. The overall content taught in the course stems from the nursing program curriculum. It is important that all faculty have a good understanding of the curriculum, that is, how the curriculum was established, its overall framework, and how it is implemented in the classroom, skills laboratory, and clinical. Remember, curriculum is developed by the total faculty; all faculty use the curriculum as the basis for individual courses. The syllabus for each course reflects the program curriculum, specifically reflecting course outcomes and competencies then specific unit objectives that support those outcomes. The content is revised even further when specific content objectives are written for each unit. These content objectives guide the design and development of the teaching that takes place in the classroom, clinical, and skills lab. Finally, test blueprints are developed based on these objectives.

Content analysis in nursing education is typically a function of curriculum development. Once the curriculum is in place, all faculty take responsibility for updating content. This is an important aspect of the teaching-learning process – keeping content up-to-date. Content must be analyzed and modifications made to incorporate the latest nursing care and healthcare initiatives. This requires all teachers to be current in the areas they teach. This is often a challenging task in undergraduate education, where nursing faculty are frequently required to teach content outside their areas of expertise.

Another challenge for faculty developing nursing curricula is the likelihood the curriculum will become bloated with content. This is termed the additive curriculum and is a common occurrence in undergraduate nursing education (Ironside, 2004). In their efforts to be conscientious and include all important information in their teaching, faculty keep adding more content but often fail to eliminate content. This provides a major problem for both faculty and students. The challenge for faculty is to determine what to leave in and what to take out.

**Resource analysis.** Resource analysis refers to both time and materials. One hour of classroom instruction can take from 20 to 40 hours of preparation, not including time to develop test items. Creating an exciting, effective learning experience requires many hours of planning and preparation. Educational materials such as videos, computer programs, case studies, electronic presentations, web-based support materials, and practice critical thinking test items, all take time and money to create or purchase.

Teachers also need to look at their own skill set asking questions such as:
1. Do I have the skill to create electronic presentations, graphics, or computer modules?
2. Is there a faculty development center that can assist with production of these materials?
3. If others will be creating instructional materials for me, what is the lead time needed for getting this work completed?

The amount of resources available needs to be analyzed prior to designing the educational experience.

The assessment and analysis phase yields much information about the student, the teacher, the content, and the resources available. Once this phase is complete, the teacher is ready to proceed to the next step, designing the instruction.

## Step 2: Design the Instruction

**Learning theories.** Learning theories provide a theoretical framework when designing instructional materials. These theories explain how individuals acquire, process, and use information to change their way of thinking and behaving (Bastable, 2008). A review of these theories indicates that learning is a complex process. Taking an eclectic approach by using each of these theories as they apply to a specific student body to guide the design of instruction facilitates learning. Following is a brief overview of learning theories relevant to nursing students.
- **Behavioral learning theory:** Early behavioral psychologists contributed to learning theory still in use today. Behavioral learning theory focuses on the learner's response to stimuli. B. F. Skinner (1974), a leader in this move-

ment, differentiated behaviorism as applied to learning as voluntary behavior rather than the reflexive behavior demonstrated by Pavlov's salivating dog. Behaviorists rely on observable behaviors that explain simple learning tasks. Behaviorism does not explain what happens internally as learners process information.

Reinforcement in Skinner's learning theory describes techniques to lead a learner through a series of instructional steps to a desired level of performance (Smaldino, Russell, Heinich, & Molenda, 2006). Skinner's reinforcement theory includes:

o   Programmed learning, consisting of small steps carefully sequenced with reinforcement for the learner
o   Behavior modification, the shaping of behavior using principles of reinforcement
o   The technique of writing measurable learning objectives in conjunction with programmed instruction

Skinner's programmed instruction, as it was known in the early years, fell from favor mostly due to its boring nature. However, some of the instructional strategies derived from behavioral psychology are still useful when designing instruction. These strategies include:

o   Chunking or breaking the content into small segments
o   Using frequent practice activities
o   Providing immediate feedback
o   Using positive reinforcement
o   Keeping learners informed about their progress and success in the lesson

• **Cognitive learning theory:** Cognitive psychologists believe that learning is an active, constructive process. During the learning process, changes in the individual's internal representation of knowledge occur. Learning is greater when the learner is actively responding to the instruction. Learners need to focus on the learning situation, fit the new information into their existing knowledge schemata (which are mental structures individuals use to organize their perceptions), change the structure of their knowledge base, and then encode all this learning into memory. Later, the student should be able to explain and interpret this learned information. The meaning of the newly learned information is generated and constructed by the individual student as it relates to past experiences.

Instruction designed using a cognitivist perspective is less structured than instruction based on behavioral learning theory. Learners are encouraged to use their own cognitive strategies and interact with other students. Instructional materials that require problem solving, critical thinking, and creative behaviors are best created using a cognitive instructional approach (Smaldino, Russell, Heinich, & Molenda, 2006). Instructional strategies based on cognitive learning theory include:

o  Making the instruction as interactive as possible
o  Requiring the learner to actively process the new information
o  Giving control over the lesson to the learner
o  Designing the instructional environment to be as similar as possible to the environment in which the learner is to apply the knowledge
o  Making the learner aware of relationships among the concepts and principles presented
o  Adjusting the learning environment to the individual students' knowledge and skill level
o  Building new experiences based on old ones
o  Using simulations to help the learner experience the new role

Simulations, case studies, critical thinking activities, and concept mapping are examples of learning experiences based on cognitive learning theory.

- **Social learning theory:** Social learning theory explains learning in a social context. People learn by watching others and observing what happens to them. Role models and significant others provide compelling examples of how to think, feel, and behave. Role modeling is the central theme in this theory (Bastable, 2008). Nursing faculty and experienced nurses serve as role models for students. Powerful instructional materials can be developed based on social learning theory because it often appeals to the affective domain. Affective domain refers to the learner's attitude about the topic under study. An example of using social learning theory is a video titled *Tucked in Tight* (Caputi, 2000). This video presents a series of photographs of a nurse caring for an elderly patient. A soft, gentle voice sings about the elderly female in the video and the special relationship she has with her nurse. Students watching this video observe a very positive image role modeled by the nurse providing care to an elderly patient. After viewing the video, students are asked to write a one-page reflection paper describing what they saw and the lessons they learned. A version of this video with the instructional strategies used to develop it is included on the CD accompanying this book.

- **Adult learning theory:** Most nursing students are considered to be adult learners, albeit in various developmental stages – young adulthood (18 to 25 years) and middle adulthood (25 to 65 years). Characteristics that influence learning in adults are different from those that influence learning in children (Lee & Owens, 2000). These differences have been explained by Knowles (2005) in his theory of androgogy – the study of how adults learn. When developing instruction for adult learners, these adult characteristics should be considered throughout the design process. Following are some of these characteristics:
    o Adults must see a direct relationship between what is being learned and application to the real world. Adults focus on dealing with problems they encounter in real-life situations.
    o Adults want to participate in the learning process; they want to be actively involved.
    o Adults bring a wide variety of life experiences to a new learning situation.
    o Adults are independent, self-reliant learners; they want independence to learn in the way that best suits their learning styles.
    o Adults prefer self-paced, individualized instruction so they can learn at their own rate.

**Planning instructional strategies.** After the above assessments have been completed, the teacher now has a good idea of the characteristics of the learners, the content to be taught, and the available resources. Learning theories provide a theoretical basis and guide for developing instruction, and learning objectives delineate what is to be taught. The next step is to plan the learning experience. Learning is an internal event influenced by the external events of teaching. Gagne, Briggs, and Wager (2004) provided the events of instruction that influence learning. These can be used to develop most types of educational experiences:

- **Gaining attention:** This involves appealing to the learners' interest; capturing their attention and curiosity; asking a question; posing a problem; and using humor.
- **Informing the learner of the objective:** The objectives for the lesson are often listed in the course syllabus.
- **Stimulating recall of prerequisite learning:** New learning is connected to prior learning; helping students fit new learning into existing schemata.

- **Presenting the stimulus material:** The nature of the material depends on the type of objective – psychomotor, cognitive, or affective. Examples of ways to present stimulus material include lecture, small-group discussion, case studies, demonstrations, interactive games, computer modules, and web-based exercises.
- **Providing learning guidance:** The type of guidance depends on the type of objective. A knowledge/comprehension objective might require only telling whereas an application/analysis objective may require prompting the learner to use critical thinking and problem solving. Highly didactic instruction and direct, low-level questions are looked upon favorably among learners experiencing high anxiety. Less anxious learners are much more positive about challenging, guided learning experiences (Gagne, Briggs, & Wager, 2004). A common characteristic of nursing students is a high degree of anxiety, which may explain why many nursing students prefer lectures in which they are told what to know, rather than experiential learning environments, where they must discover the answers. However, discovery learning leads to more permanent learning than purely didactic instruction (Gagne, Briggs, & Wagner, 2004).
- **Eliciting performance:** This implies a "show me" or "do it" strategy. Teachers who periodically challenge students with application, analysis, or higher-level questions throughout a lecture is one example of eliciting performance.
- **Providing feedback about performance correctness:** Students need immediate feedback on their performance to correct any misunderstandings.
- **Assessing the performance:** Students are provided the opportunity to use the information learned when teachers use strategies such as practice test questions, patient scenarios, or concept maps. The teacher can then assess the students' application of their learning while the learning is taking place. Classroom examinations and clinical evaluations provide summative evaluations of learning.
- **Enhancing retention and transfer:** The ultimate goal is for students to retain the lessons taught and apply that information to nursing care.

An important aspect in the planning process is to design instruction so students retain what is taught. Bastable (2008) offered the following suggestions to ensure that learning becomes permanent:
- Organize the learning experience
- Make the learning experience meaningful and pleasurable

- Pace the presentation according to the learners' abilities to process information
- Help learners practice using new information and skills under varied conditions soon after the learning has occurred
- Provide opportunities for learners to continue to use the learned information periodically to ensure retention and recall

Only the imagination and creativity of the teacher can limit the type of instruction designed to meet the learning objectives. When creative teachers apply learning theories, the events of instruction, and the above suggestions to the design of educational experiences, the needs of the students are more readily met.

## Step 3: Develop the Instruction

After the instruction has been conceptualized and designed, the teacher then develops and assembles the materials for the learning experience. Incorporating a variety of instructional strategies into the learning experience appeals to the learners' interests and keeps their attention focused on what is being taught. Following is an example of a renal lecture prepared by the author for second-level nursing students using a variety of instructional strategies and incorporating principles from learning theory and the events of instruction.

As students enter the classroom, they are given a lecture packet containing pertinent handouts. The first page contains a one-page outline of the lecture. On this page is a cartoon of a nurse in a physician's office with a sign: Urinary Clinic. The nurse is on the phone and is saying, "Can you hold?" A review of this outline gives the students an overview of the two-and-a-half-hour session, informing the learner of the content to be covered. This content follows the objectives in the syllabus.

To gain attention at the beginning of the first lecture, I play a song titled *Doin' the Incontinence Rag* by Too Live Nurse (www.toolivenurse.com). (See Figure 1.) While students listen to this song, I hold up equipment and cards with words that relate to previous units on elimination covered in the first year, thus stimulating recall of prerequisite learning. Here are a few verses from this song.

There's a new dance sensation
That's flooding the nation,
Done by nurses from Maine to L.A.
And we sign all the louder
As we wash, wipe, and powder,
And our patients stay dry all the day,
All the day.

Always cause for celebration,
When you catch that micturation,
It really blows your I and Os,
When you're doing the inconcentence rag.

Gosh, oh gee, and holy, moly,
Can I please insert a foley?
It's depends or Attends,
When you're doing the incontinence rag.

**Figure 1.** Sample "The Incontinence Rag" Lyrics

This song encourages laughter, relaxes the students, and puts them in a "urinary" mindset. It is very effective in meeting all three of these instructional objectives.

Presentation of the stimulus material includes a variety of strategies. A lecture packet is distributed containing extensive notes from the lecture. The lecture begins with a PowerPoint® presentation containing cartoons. Students follow along with the lecture packet, adding notes to their handouts as needed. Students report this lecture packet helps them focus on what is being said rather than on frantically writing down every word.

As the normal physiology of the kidneys is discussed, selected parts of the software program *The PhysWhiz: The Renal System* are projected (Caputi, 1997). This program contains graphics and animations that demonstrate visually what is being explained verbally. Many of the screens have additional thinking questions or practice items used to engage student participation. These items elicit student performance. Items are written at both knowledge/comprehension and application/analysis levels. All students must answer the multiple-choice questions using electronic response devices (iClicker®). The teachers can then offer feedback and correct any misunderstandings, providing learner guidance.

To provide further learning guidance in application of the content, a patient in the software program *TLC Medical Center* (Caputi, 1999) is presented. This program contains the records of a patient with urolithiasis. Students are presented with questions about the patient. The record is then examined and relationships made to the clinical picture of this patient. This strategy enhances transfer of learning to patient care.

For fun and to keep the students' attention, throughout the lecture the students are periodically challenged with a hinky-pinky. A hinky-pinky is a definition for 2 or 3 words that rhyme. Some of the hinky-pinkies used in this lecture are the following:

Definition: What urologists spend their day doing.
Answer: Curin' urine.

Definition: An overdistended urinary drainage bag.
Answer: A roly-poley foley.

For additional examples of hinky-pinkies refer to the CD that accompanies this book.

A 15-minute break is provided after the first hour. Soft, relaxing music is played during the break for students who remain in the room and while students are returning from break. The intent of this music is to decrease anxiety.

A top-10 list is used to start the session after break. Following is an example of a renal-related top-10 list:

**Top 10 Reasons to Be Thankful We Have Kidneys**
10. Without them, a couple of cans of pop and we'd explode.
9. Kidneys promote family harmony. Better be nice to your siblings; some day you may need one of their kidneys.
8. Dialysis Rotation Observation Day: Stress-free clinical day.
7. To provide the opportunity to relate nursing skills to culture, such as inserting a 16 French foley catheter.
6. Without kidneys, what would you call kidney bean salad?
5. Studying the renal system gives you another chance to figure out all that electrolyte stuff!
4. Without kidneys and the formation of urine, your lecture would go on and on for the full two-and-a-half hours. Kidneys mean a potty break!
3. Provides the opportunity to use the word micturate.

2. Using the restroom to micturate provides some challenges in your life, such as how to use those dryers. Instructions: wash hands; rub vigorously under dryer; wipe hands on pants.
1. Without kidneys we would look like this:

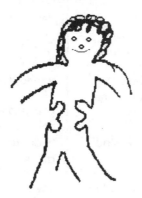

The top-10 list helps increase student endorphin levels through laughter, thereby further reducing stress. For additional top-10 lists refer to the CD that accompanies this book.

The lecture then continues with a variety of materials, including videos from the National Kidney Foundation on peritoneal dialysis and colored graphics of various pathologies such as polycystic kidney disease.

Finally, when the lecture is over, the students receive a rap that incorporates many of the topics discussed in the class. Figure 2 contains The Renal Rap. For additional raps refer to the CD that accompanies this book.

## Step 4: Implement

During the implementation step of the educational process, the teaching comes to life. The classroom is transformed into an educational environment. The teacher's personality interacts with the content being taught, making a unique, personalized experience. Whatever the setting, the purpose of this step is to ensure the effective and efficient delivery of instruction with the intent that learning takes place. This phase must promote the students' understanding of the material, support the students' mastery of objectives, and ensure the students' transfer of knowledge from the instructional setting to practice.

Now that it's test time, Let's review. Bladder, ureters, And kidneys, too.

Let's start with the nephron, That's where the action's at. 125 mLs a minute – Can't beat that! The blood pH is dropping, The kidneys play a part. Secrete that extra hydrogen, Before acidosis even starts.

How are the kidneys working? Let's check out the labs today. We could look at the BUN, But creatinine's a better way.

Now that it's test time, Let's review. Bladder, ureters, and kidneys, too.

Pathologies can happen, In every part of the urinary tract. Like urinary tract infection, E. coli knows about that!

Let's eradicate those bugs, Get a C & S for UT's sake. Culture to see what's growing, Sensitivity shows the right drug to take.

Diuretics are helpful drugs When too much fluid you retain. Works on what part of the kidney nephron? Tubule is the name.

Now that it's test time, Let's review. Bladder, ureters, And kidneys, too.

Acute pyelonephritis Isn't so cute you say. Bring on those IV antibiotics, That'll make it go away.

Oh, my, what a pain! Stones caught in the tract. Better strain all that urine, Diet changes so they don't come back!

Remember specific gravity? What's ARF's affect? Can't concentrate or dilute, At 1010, spec grav gets fixed.

Now that it's test time, Let's review. Bladder, ureters, And kidneys, too.

CRF, that's the path, That's really most severe. Some of the things that can go wrong, Is what you're about to hear.

Phosphate really takes to task All the calcium in the bones. Mealtime aluminum hydroxide, then it'll leave the calcium alone.

The skin is so very itchy, Makes him angry and cross. Look closer and you'll see Crystals of uremic frost!

Now that it's test time, Let's review. Bladder, ureters, And kidneys, too.

Tuberculosis, you might think, Is in the lungs for sure. Did you think it's in the kidney? Rifampin could be a cure.

Kidney transplants now are common. Happens every day. So to not reject that kidney, Cyclosporine on the way!

Now it's almost test time, That's the end of the review. My advice is to really study, And good luck to you!

**Figure 2.** The Renal Rap

## Step 5: Evaluate

The purpose of the last step of the educational process is to measure the effectiveness of the instruction. Two types of evaluation are used.

**Formative evaluation.** Formative evaluation is conducted as the instruction is being formed. The purpose of this type of evaluation is to improve the instruction as the course is progressing to ensure students are learning before the end of the term when it is too late to make adjustments. Examples of formative evaluation include midterm clinical evaluation and practice exams for the classroom.

The faculty may also evaluate their teaching prior to the end of the course. One type of evaluation is the Critical Incident Questionnaire (CIQ) (Brookfield, 1995). See Figure 3 for the types of questions you may ask of students.

---

Critical incidents are vivid happenings that people remember as being significant. The CIQ focuses the students on specific, concrete happenings that were significant to them. Students answer these questions at the end of the week:
1. At what moment in the class this week did you feel most engaged with what was happening?
2. At what moment in the class this week did you feel most distanced with what was happening?
3. What action that anyone (teacher or student) took in class this week did you find most affirming and helpful?
4. What action that anyone (teacher or student) took in class this week did you find most puzzling or confusing?
5. What about the class this week surprised you the most? (This could be something about your own reactions to what went on, or something that someone did, or anything else that occurs to you.)

---

**Figure 3.** Critical Incident Questionnaire

**Summative evaluation.** Summative evaluation is conducted after the teaching is complete. This could be at the end of a unit or at the end of the course. The information from the summative evaluation is used not only to assign a grade to the student's performance, but also to revise and refine the course – making it better for future students. This can occur both formally, during pre-scheduled curriculum evaluation meetings, or informally as needed by individual faculty.

Typically, summative evaluation is conducted using some form of testing which may include written work such as care plans and term papers; return demonstration of psychomotor skills; and objective, multiple-choice tests. The multiple-choice format is extremely popular because the NCLEX® uses the format as well as the newer alternative item types.

One issue facing nursing faculty relates to the passing level assigned to each course. Although most colleges and universities use an established grading scale, nursing programs often have their own versions, which are typically more stringent. For example, a C grade is often 70% to 79%, and a D is from 60% to 69%. D is a passing grade in most courses. However, in nursing, it is commonplace that a C must be earned to advance to the next nursing course or to graduate, with the minimum C ranging from 75% to 80%. Because of this higher-level grading scale, it is imperative that all evaluation methods including multiple-choice exams are valid and reliable. Whether a student passes or fails, the teacher must be very certain the score the student earns is based on quality evaluation methods.

Additionally, many faculty require the minimum percent be earned prior to adding "soft" grades, such as those earned on term papers, care plans, projects, and extra credit. In other words, these additional assignments may increase the grade but cannot be a factor in determining if the student passes the course. However, grades on these assignments may in fact drop a passing grade to a failing grade, preventing the student from enrolling in the next nursing course.

Clinical grading is an often debated issue. Should clinical performance be assigned a pass/fail grade or a letter grade? Should the clinical performance grade be factored into the overall percentage? Is the clinical performance grade a soft grade added after the passing percentage has been calculated? Faculty discussions addressing these questions are important so all faculty use the same guidelines for grading within the nursing program.

Another grading issue is whether or not to "round up." Some faculty decide to round up at .45 or .5, but others do not round up at all. This is an interesting concept because if the minimum passing grade for a course is 78%, the actual passing grade might be 77.45%. Whatever grade is determined as passing, students must be made aware of the grade, including the rounding-up policy.

Faculty must determine this grading policy based on the needs and philosophy of their specific nursing program. Whatever is decided, the decision should be made after careful consideration by the total faculty.

## Seven Principles of Good Practice

In 1987 Chickering and Gamson published a classic work titled "Seven Principles for Good Practice in Undergraduate Education". These seven principles may appear to be common sense, but surprisingly many faculty do not routinely consider them when planning instruction. The seven principles are:

1. Encourages contacts between students and faculty
2. Develops reciprocity and cooperation among students
3. Uses active learning techniques
4. Gives prompt feedback
5. Emphasizes time on task
6. Communicates high expectations
7. Respects diverse talents and ways of learning

Applying these seven principles can improve both teaching and learning and are based on over 50 years of research (Chickering & Gamson, 1987). These principles can also be applied to online teaching. They are simple guidelines that can have a tremendous impact on the educational process.

## Summary

The educational process is a useful framework for developing learning experiences. Application of this process ensures that all aspects of teaching and learning are considered, leading to quality education. As you read this book, consider how the content of each chapter fits within this framework. In so doing, you will capture the essence of the art and science of teaching nursing.

## Learning Activities

1. Choose a unit of content that you typically teach. Apply the educational process to the content and develop a plan for teaching that content.
2. Analyze your student body. Identify commonalities and differences.
3. Consider the seven principles of good practice in undergraduate education. How would you apply them to your teaching?

## Educational Philosophy

My educational philosophy is succinct: Give the best educational experience possible. I believe faculty should continuously challenge themselves to provide creative, interesting, and sound education—students soon learn that education doesn't have to be boring; they become self-motivated, enthusiastic, and interested...learning then follows. — Linda Caputi

## References

Bastable, S. B. (2008). *Nurse as educator: Principles of teaching and learning for nursing practice*. (3rd ed.). Boston: Jones and Bartlett.

Benner, P. (2001). *From novice to expert:* Excellence and power in clinical nursing practice, Commemorative Edition, Menlo Park, CA: Addison-Wesley.

Brookfield, S. (1995). *Becoming a critically reflective teacher*. San Francisco: Jossey-Bass.

Caputi, L. (1997). *The physwhiz: The renal system* [computer program]. Glen Ellyn, IL: College of DuPage Press.

Caputi, L. (1999). *TLC medical center* [computer program]. Glen Ellyn, IL: College of DuPage Press.

Caputi, L. (2000). *Tucked in tight* [videotape]. Glen Ellyn, IL: College of DuPage Press.

Chickering, A. W., & Gamson, Z. F. (1987). Seven principles for good practice in undergraduate education. *American Association for Higher Education Bulletin*, March, 3-7.

Forrest, S. (2010, in press). Learning styles. In L. Caputi (Ed.). *Teaching nursing: The art and science*, Vol. 2. Glen Ellyn, IL: College of DuPage Press.

Gagne, R. M., Briggs, L. J., & Wager, W. W. (2004). *Principles of instructional design*. New York: Holt, Rinehart and Winston.

Grasha, A. F. (1996). *Teaching with style*. Pittsburgh, PA: Alliance.

Haar, J., Hall, G., Schoepp, P., & Smith, D. H. (2002). How teachers teach to students with different learning styles. *The Clearing House, 3*, 142-145.

Ironside, P. M. (2004). "Covering content" and teaching thinking: Deconstructing the additive curriculum. *Journal of Nursing Education, 43*, 5-12.

Johnson, S.A., & Romanello, M.L. (2005). Generational diversity: Teaching and learning approaches. *Nurse Educator, 30*(5), 212-216.

Knowles, M. (2005). *The adult learner: The definitive classic in adult education and human resource development*. (6th ed.). San Diego, CA: Elsevier.

Lee, W., & Owens, D. (2000). *Multimedia-based instructional design: Computer-based training, web-based training, distance broadcast training.* San Francisco: Jossey-Bass.

McDonald, M. (2010, in press). Understanding and teaching the millennial generation of nursing students, In L. Caputi (Ed.). *Teaching nursing: The art and science, Vol. 1.* Glen Ellyn, IL: College of DuPage Press.

Oblinger, D. (2003). Boomers, gen–xers & millennials: Understanding the new students. *Educause Review.* July/August, p. 37-47.

Skinner, B. F. (1974). *About behaviorism.* New York: Random House.

Smaldino, S., Russell, J., Heinich, R., & Molenda, M. (2006). *Instructional technology and media for learning.* Columbus, OH: Allyn & Bacon.

Stokes, E. (2010, in press). Teaching the generations: Coping with the differences. In L. Caputi (Ed.). *Teaching nursing: The art and science, Vol. 1.* Glen Ellyn, IL: College of DuPage Press.

Sutherland, L. (2010, in press). Teaching faculty to provide culturally-competent nursing education. In L. Caputi (Ed.). *Teaching nursing: The art and science, Vol. 1.* Glen Ellyn, IL: College of DuPage Press.

Wilson, L. (2010, in press). Cultural diversity: Teaching students to provide culturally-competent nursing care. In L. Caputi (Ed.). *Teaching nursing: The art and science, Vol. 1.* Glen Ellyn, IL: College of DuPage Press.

# CHAPTER 4

## SO YOU'RE A TEACHER: NOW WHAT DO YOU DO?

Lynn Engelmann, MSN, EdD, RN, ANEF

---

The content of this chapter relates to the following major content area and subconcepts on the Certified Nurse Educator Examination Detailed Test Blueprint:

**Pursue Continuous Quality Improvement in the Academic Nurse Educator Role**

- Engage in activities that promote one's socialization to the role
- Participate in professional development opportunities that increase one's effectiveness in the role
- Select professional development activities to continue to grow and evolve in the role
- Balance the teaching, scholarship, and service demands inherent in the role of the educator and as influenced by the requirements of the institutional setting
- Use feedback gained from self, peer, learner, and administrative evaluation to improve role effectiveness
- Mentor and support faculty colleagues in the role of an academic nurse educator
- Engage in self-reflection and continued learning to improve teaching practices

---

## Introduction

This chapter presents an overview of general information that faculty need to consider as they evaluate terms of employment and accept or continue positions in nursing education. The responsibilities that educators face are reviewed to provide a clear picture of what it is that nurse educators **do** in these roles. This chapter provides an overview. Other chapters in this three volume set provide in-depth discussions on most of the topics presented in this chapter.

## Educational Delivery System

Roles and responsibilities for faculty are similar among different educational settings. However, just as nursing care delivery systems differ, so do nursing education delivery systems. For example, faculty members may be expected to teach an entire nursing course by themselves or a section of a course in conjunction with several faculty who divide content, such as the case with team teaching. Faculty may also be expected to teach on multiple program levels. For example, a medical-surgical faculty member might teach a fundamentals course with beginning students the first term and an advanced medical-surgical course with graduating students the last term. Additionally, faculty may be called upon to teach across levels, such as bachelors, masters, and doctoral programs within a school of nursing.

Faculty in staff development positions are called to teach content to new graduates as well as to experienced nurses, requiring a broad repertoire of skill and knowledge. While it is generally understood that all staff development educators plan and teach educational programs, it may not be well known that staff development educators also participate in management, consultation, and research activities. Grasmick (2002) describes six aspects of the staff development educator's role: educator, facilitator, change agent, consultant, researcher, and leader. Any one of these roles may predominate, depending upon particular circumstances, and the immediate needs of the organization and its personnel.

Brunt (2007) discusses the need to ensure use of evidence of best practices in all aspects of nursing, including education. Activities germane to professional nursing development include continuing education, staff development, and academic education. Some aspects of the educational role are similar across all settings. At any given point in time, both the staff development educator and the faculty member teaching in a program of nursing must be sensitive to the educational needs of those who are involved in learning.

Instructional modes may vary widely and include several approaches:
- Online, course is conducted via the Internet
- Hybrid, a combination of online and face-to-face instruction
- Simulation, with a patient care focus outside the traditional clinical setting, in a specially designed and equipped nursing skills laboratory
- Real time, face-to face contact in the classroom setting

## General Information

This section addresses terms of employment and aspects of the work environment that faculty may want to consider before committing to or continuing in a position.

## Work Climate

Prior to beginning a position, it is wise to find out as much as possible about the environment in the potential work setting. For instance, try to meet the faculty you will be working with and gain a sense of their experience and reputation, and the type of support you might expect to receive from them. If possible, make note of collegial relationships apparent in the climate of the institution, and if this collegiality is discernable at all levels within the institution. Explore the nature and breadth of faculty expertise. Talk with the administrators about the ways in which support is provided to faculty within the institution. For example, you might explore how personal development is fostered, such as support for attendance at conferences, graduate coursework, assistance with grant writing, or time away for professional pursuits. If there has been a recent turn-over in faculty, find out if it is due to natural causes, such as retirement, or some other factor. Ask if there is a strategic plan that has been developed for the nursing program or the institution, to better understand departmental and institutional priorities. It is also important for you to know that your personal philosophy of education and teaching meshes with that of the institution in which you would accept employment. And, of course, inquiry about a formal mentoring program for new faculty.

## Teaching Assignments

Faculty need to know what their teaching assignments entail and what is likely to affect their assignments. Typically, schools maintain an established reaching assignment relative to the number of courses that constitute the full-time faculty member's teaching assignment. This equates to a certain number of clock hours in the classroom, skills laboratory, or clinical teaching setting. Actual clock hours are then calculated. For example, an 18 hour load requires that faculty devote 18 actual clock hours of teaching per week. These 18 hours might entail 12 hours of clinical, 3 hours of skills laboratory, and 3 hours of lecture per week. In some schools, these hours may be calculated based on where the teaching occurs. Thus, one hour of teaching in the clinical setting may be different, in terms of actual clock hours, than one hour of classroom instruction. To illustrate, for one contact hour in the clinical, the faculty may have to teach 2 clock hours. In this case the assignment is 2 hours of teaching equals 1 contact hour. Workloads may vary, depending upon the type of educational institution, but considerations often include number of courses and necessary preparations for those courses in any given academic year. In addition, faculty may be compensated for teaching a larger class size (overload) than usually stipulated.

The teaching roles that faculty perform and the expectations for meeting these roles should be clearly delineated. Roles include:

- Preparation of course materials adapted for online instruction and monitoring of online course delivery
- Didactic teaching and presentation of course content in the classroom
- Supervision of students in the clinical setting
- Teaching nursing skills or designing and implementing simulation scenarios in the college laboratory

Roles also involve course organization, management, and leadership. Faculty are expected to structure and steer courses in a manner consistent with program goals and objectives. This sometimes involves close guidance and mentoring of other faculty. If a team-teaching approach is used, faculty members may share responsibility for executing the course. If a course leader, or team-coordinator approach is used, one faculty member may provide direction for the other faculty involved in the course. This may also include part-time or adjunct faculty teaching in classroom and/or clinical settings. See the CD-ROM that accompanies this book for a sample part-time faculty handbook that provides an overview of the expectations for part-time faculty.

The number of hours and times of day faculty teach each week in the classroom, skills laboratory, clinical setting, or online should be clearly established. It is important that faculty are clear about the process used to determine assignments and any factors that may influence this process. Faculty may or may not have a voice in this process. The rules and regulations that apply to teaching assignments may be impacted by seniority or tenure. Faculty assignments may be addressed with school coordinators, deans, or hospital administration. Circumstances that might alter faculty assignments should be discussed.

## Faculty Roles and Responsibilities

Faculty have varied roles and responsibilities, some of which include holding office hours; advising and supervising students and other personnel; working on committees, research, and publications; and performing service for the institutions in which they teach. Each of these is briefly explained.

## Office Hours

Faculty schedule office hours to meet with students, prepare or update lectures, or ready any materials related to the work faculty perform in their roles. Such work includes writing or grading tests, meeting committee responsibilities, or general organizational duties. New faculty, in particular, who are preparing course and lecture materials for the first time, will likely spend many hours outside of office hours, organizing and developing these materials.

Some institutions mandate a certain number of office hours per week, while other institutions do not. Office hours may be held in the faculty member's office, via e-mail or phone, online, or at an off-site location. It should be clearly communicated to students how they may access faculty. The location and times of faculty office hours are generally communicated in writing or online, and may be placed in the course syllabus or announced during orientation. Faculty must also explore expectations relative to how often they are to be on campus. Some institutions are unionized, and have explicit mandates concerning office hours and presence on campus.

## Advising Students

Faculty spend many hours each term working with students. Faculty need to know the resources available and expectations for their advising role. Typically, this is addressed during faculty orientation. For faculty in schools of nursing, advising students includes course selection, guidance to meet program and graduation requirements, and assistance to help students with academic problems. An advising worksheet may be used to guide faculty in their advisement and maintain a record of faculty student advising sessions. In addition, a student worksheet may be used by the institution to enable the student to track progress toward program and degree completion requirements.

## Supervising Other Personnel

Faculty work with many others in a supervisory capacity to effect teaching. These supervisory roles include work with:

**Ancillary personnel.** These personnel provide support to the faculty and should be accessed and utilized as appropriate. At the very least, faculty will want to gain a sense of the roles these individuals perform and where they fit into the scheme of overall program functioning. Faculty may have input as to job descriptions and responsibilities that ancillary personnel perform. There may also be student workers who meet a variety of program needs; however, these students require direction and guidance to perform their roles.

**Graduate assistants and preceptors.** Such assistance may be provided on a term-to-term basis and provide support for faculty via research and instruction. For example, research assistants gather data and help by researching information that faculty will use to write grants or publications. Teaching assistants provide contact hours teaching in the classroom or skills laboratory. Preceptors serve as a liaison, lending their expertise in the supervision and instruction of students in a variety of clinical settings. Faculty working with these assistants and preceptors need to establish expectations and guidelines for work and practice. Faculty should keep in mind the particular dictates of their state's nurse practice act which helps govern the role of preceptors.

**Other full-time, part-time, or adjunct faculty.** This work may involve orienting faculty to the course or to the program. In some cases, it may involve evaluation of part-time or adjunct faculty performance. Individual faculty, team leaders, or nursing deans/directors provide the orientation and support necessary for part-time or adjunct faculty to teach within a course. Specific roles of a course leader are discussed in a subsequent section of this chapter. Full-time faculty may also assume leadership or mentoring roles with part-time or adjunct faculty. It is of vital importance that faculty new to the institution, as well as new to teaching, be assigned a mentor (NLN, 2006).

## Committee Work

Whether faculty are teaching in programs of nursing or practice settings, committee work may be a major factor in terms of time commitment and workload. Committees may function solely within the nursing program, be institution wide, or a joint effort between the school of nursing and another institution, such as an advisory committee. In special circumstances, faculty may be given release time to accomplish committee work. There may be expectations for committee work with respect to advancement or tenure. In addition, it is expected that faculty periodically assume leadership roles within committees. It may be helpful for faculty to consult *Robert's Rules of Order Newly Revised* (2000) to guide smooth facilitation of a committee meeting.

## Research and Publications

Institutionally imposed requirements for research and publications as part of professional development and tenure also impact faculty roles and workload. Faculty teaching and working within an institution may not be granted tenure if consistent quality performance cannot be demonstrated. The number and sequencing of publications or grants relative to the timeline for tenure may impact the decision to grant tenure. For example, if a faculty member has written five articles, all in the last two years of a seven-year tenure track, productivity during the first five years might be questioned and tenure denied.

Faculty may seek grants or special funding to provide support for research activities. Professional organizations, among others, offer grants to foster research projects. Some institutions have individuals who function within the institution to help assist with grant writing and submission.

Faculty then disseminate findings of their research. This can be done through publishing articles or presenting at professional conferences.

## Service to the Institution

Faculty may be expected to participate in health fairs, career nights, and special events at which the profession of nursing is highlighted and promoted. Participating in these types of public services may be viewed as essential to the functioning and viability of the institution in which the faculty teaches.

## Procedure for Faculty Evaluation

Faculty are evaluated periodically and should determine from the onset, what the evaluation will address and how the evaluation will be used. Evaluation schedules vary from institution to institution, and will be impacted by the type of position the faculty member holds. For example, a tenure track position may necessitate periodic evaluations that are comprised of student, peer, and administrative feedback. However, the process is outlined, it is extremely important that faculty gain a sense of who takes part in the evaluation process, and how the evaluation will be used for personal growth, professional advancement, and remuneration. Faculty may wish to keep a portfolio that highlights personal accomplishments, any special letters, awards, or recognitions that are conferred, and documentation of service to community and professional organizations, such as involvement on a task force, advisory, or planning committee.

## Procedure for Grievance

Faculty must also explore their options relative to potential avenues for problem resolution, should conflict occur that can not be resolved using the usual pathways. In most cases, protocol for filing a grievance is listed in the faculty handbook, or union guidelines, so that faculty may follow the appropriate procedure. It may be helpful to keep a written account of events that are problematic and documentation of channels taken for resolution of the situation. When a conflict escalates, be aware of faculty rights and do not agree to discuss a situation without appropriate council or representation.

## Course Planning and Development

In addition to the roles that faculty perform that were highlighted in the previous section, faculty spend a large part of their time planning and developing courses. Such development entails preparation and delivery of content related to theory, clinical, and skills laboratory instruction. Teaching perspective, just as clinical expertise, develops over time, as experiences unfold and faculty come to understand the particular beliefs and principles that guide their teaching (Pratt, Boll, & Collins, 2007).

### Preparation for the Theory Component of a Course

As faculty prepare new or update course material, they should have a clear understanding of where the material fits within the entire curriculum. Faculty must keep in mind division, program, and course goals and objectives, so that components of every course are linked with what has come before, and what will come after that particular course. This preparation requires that faculty:

1. Attend and participate in course, level, and program meetings and share in the decision making process. Such decisions include curriculum development, implementation, and evaluation for each course on each level. Curriculum evaluation is an ongoing process. Faculty who lead a course or guide faculty in course planning should ensure that discussion regarding approaches to instruction is documented and communicated to all faculty teaching in that course.
2. Assist in the assignment of theory content, skills laboratory hours, and clinical placement before the beginning of the term.

3. Write objectives and other course materials, such as written assignments and assignment guidelines. These objectives and course materials lend to the overall program objectives and outcome criteria. In addition, evaluation of how well outcome criteria are met constitutes important data reviewed by accrediting agencies and professional organizations (Keating, 2006).

4. Prepare the course syllabus. The purpose of the syllabus is to provide students with a thorough understanding of material that is to be covered in each course. Typically this includes a course description, course outcomes, unit objectives, assignments, and evaluation methods. For example, expected clinical behaviors are communicated via a clinical evaluation tool that provides examples of student behaviors that must be evidenced for the student to meet the clinical objectives of the course. See the CD-ROM that accompanies this book for a sample syllabus that addresses these elements. Schools may include the nursing program philosophy, purpose, conceptual framework, and policies in individual course syllabi or in the student handbook that students receive upon entrance to the program. The student handbook and course syllabi establish legal contracts between faculty and students. In some cases, students are required to sign forms, indicating they have received and read the student handbook and course syllabus. See the CD accompanying this book for a sample student handbook.

5. Select class delivery methods and plan class activities. There are many options when designing course instruction. Faculty need to match teaching strategies with course outcomes. Faculty should also consider personal strengths and needs and seek assistance from appropriate resources as needed. For example, faculty may need assistance to learn how to implement a new technology. Such assistance may be available via information technology or faculty development via conference or workshop. Faculty who have mastered the technology may also be willing to share insights.

6. Establish criteria for and grade written assignments. Faculty need to follow the grading scale established by the institution or nursing program in which they teach. In addition, specific guidelines for the grading of assigned material should be established at the beginning of the course and communicated to the students. Assignments should flow from specific course objectives and serve a particular purpose. Consider inclusion of a rubric to guide students in completion of assignments (Caputi, 2006).

7. Write, analyze, revise, and refine tests. Faculty need to determine test content, item type, and how to score exams. This includes the weight each item and each test will have in determining the overall course grade. The amount of time allotted to test and whether or not to offer bonus points are also

important considerations, impacted by the nature of content and item difficulty. Typically, faculty choose to increase the number of higher level test items as students progress through the nursing program. Faculty should be familiar with the statistical analysis program available in their nursing program or within their institution. A test blueprint helps ensure test content reflects course objectives. Faculty may elect to create a test bank that is constructed and evaluated by all faculty teaching in a particular course. On the CD accompanying this book is a Part-Time Faculty Handbook with an example test blueprint.

## Preparation for the Clinical Component of the Course

Teaching in the clinical setting requires thoughtful and thorough preparation so that students and affiliating agencies understand roles and expectations. Guidelines are established at the onset, and clearly communicated to all involved: students, faculty, and agency personnel. This preparation requires that faculty:
- Establish clinical arrangements with the cooperating agency; ensure a clinical contract with the agency is in place
- Contact appropriate personnel of the clinical facility assigned before the beginning of the term
- Assume responsibility of self-orientation to the facility assigned
- Promote adherence to professional conduct and policies established by the cooperating agency
- Assume responsibility for planning learning experiences for students in the assigned facility in accordance with the objectives of the course and facility guidelines
- Promote open communication with the staff of the clinical facility, students, and the nursing program throughout the term and on an ongoing basis
- Evaluate the facility for its educational benefit to students and nursing program in cooperation with the program coordinator or dean
- Supervise students in the clinical area. Such supervision entails adherence to agency guidelines and policies
- Conduct pre- and post-conferences as specified by the nursing faculty
- Consult regularly with course leader, director, or dean about actual or potential problems with students and clinical agencies
- Evaluate student performance in the clinical setting

## Preparation for the Skills Laboratory Component of the Course

The skills laboratory is the "clinical away from clinical" that allows students to develop dexterity and mastery of skills in a safe environment that does not involve patients. In general, this preparation requires that faculty:

- Establish clear guidelines for safe use of the nursing skills laboratory
- Establish learning outcomes that relate to the course outcomes
- Design content that is to be taught
- Establish a procedure for and evaluation of skill demonstration. Clinical simulation is a viable educational design that may be used to teach concepts, assess skill competencies, implement nursing interventions, integrate technology, and foster development of problem-solving skills (Jeffries, 2006).
- Develop a procedure for skill remediation

## Organization for Course Planning and Development

Much preparation and organization is required both before the course begins and throughout the term. Course planning and organization tasks include the following:

- Arrange or verify classroom facilities
- Order textbooks for each nursing course and obtain desk copies for evaluation for possible adoption. Keep in mind that decision making about the selection of textbooks should be guided by curriculum philosophy and overall framework of the program. See sample tool for textbook evaluation, Figure 1. This tool may be accessed on the CD that accompanies this book.
- Verify course registration and develop attendance sheets
- Maintain a record of student grades
- Compile mid-term and final grades, submit a copy to the appropriate source (program coordinator, dean, or records office), and send warning or probation letters as indicated, per school policy.

**Category, Cost, and Physical Attributes**
Name of course(s) in which textbook will be used: _____
Name of textbook: _____
Publisher and date of publication: _____
Date of next publication for text: _____
Cost of textbook: _____
Size and durability of textbook: _____
*If new textbook is to be published soon, are galley copies available for students and faculty? yes __ no __
Cost of galley copy: _____
**Content**
Current yes _____ no _____
Accurate yes _____ no _____
Consistent with program philosophy and outcomes yes _____ no _____
Learning objectives clearly stated yes _____ no _____
Presence of chapter summaries yes _____ no _____
Suggested learning activities yes _____ no _____
Critical thinking activities yes _____ no _____
**Organization, Presentation, and Clarity**
Effective use of:
Tables, graphs, charts, and photographs yes _____ no _____
Indices yes _____ no _____
Glossary yes _____ no _____
Appendices yes _____ no _____
**Language and Readability**
Nonsexist language used yes _____ no _____
Reading level _____
Appropriate print size yes _____ no _____
Writing style:
Logical yes _____ no _____
Concise yes _____ no _____
Fluid yes _____ no _____
**Teaching Aids**
Test bank yes _____ no _____
Suggested learning activities yes _____ no _____

**Figure 1.** Textbook Review/Evaluation Form

Assessment tools yes _____ no _____
PowerPoint® slides yes _____ no _____
Case studies yes _____ no _____
Online resources with support yes _____ no _____
Additional comments: _____

**Figure 1 continued.** Textbook Review/Evaluation Form

The following websites may be consulted for an overview of textbook evaluation. These URLs are also located on the CD accompanying this book.
- www.project2061.org/newsinfo/research/articles/cbe.htm
- www.eiu.edu/~booth/about/fcbtc/old/EvaluatingTextbooks.html
- www.illinoisloop.org/scibook.html

• Develop a calendar of activities. See Figure 2 for a sample calendar.

## Working with Students

In addition to the roles listed above, faculty devote many hours to the students themselves. Such work includes student advising and interventions for academic support. Students may need advice regarding program and graduation requirements. Faculty maintain records and document advising sessions per institutional policy, such as through the use of specially designed worksheets for this purpose. Academic support includes sessions with faculty or tutors to discuss class content or test questions. Tutoring may involve use of peer tutors or part-time faculty who have been hired for tutoring purposes.

Referrals to academic support centers within the institution, which provide specific interventions for reading, writing, and math, may be indicated. In such centers, students may obtain one-on-one help from teachers or student tutors. Help with basic study skills and/or special topics may be of value for some students. Study skills include: listening, note taking, test taking, and reading techniques. Special topics may focus on math anxiety and aspects of writing such as punctuation, sentence structure, and paragraph construction.

Students may review tests with faculty in small group sessions or one-on-one. Students might also review tests during class times, which requires prior planning,

| Fall Semester 2007 | | | | | | | | |
|---|---|---|---|---|---|---|---|---|
| Week | SUN | MON | TUE | WED | THUR | FRI | SAT | Weeks Left |
| 1 | **August** 19 | 20 | 21 | 22 | <u>Class Begins</u> Orientation Endocrine 23 | 24 | 25 | 18 |
| 2 | 26 | 27 | 28 | 29 | Respiratory 30 | 31 | **September** 01 | 17 |
| 3 | 02 | **Labor Day No classes** 03 | 04 | 05 | Respiratory 06 | 07 | 08 | 16 |
| 4 | 09 | 10 | 11 | 12 | Test #1 13 | 14 | 15 | 15 |
| 5 | 16 | 17 | 18 | **In-service Day No classes** 19 | Cardiac 20 | 21 | 22 | 14 |
| 6 | 23 | 24 | 25 | 26 | Cardiac 27 | 28 | 29 | 13 |
| 7 | 30 | **October** 01 | 02 | 03 | PVD 04 | 05 | 06 | 12 |
| 8 | 07 | 08 | 09 | 10 | Test #2 11 | 12 | 13 | 11 |
| 9 | 14 | 15 | 16 | **End of first 8 week session** 17 | <u>Class Begins</u> Orientation Endocrine 18 | 19 | 20 | 10 |
| 10 | 21 | 22 | 23 | 24 | Test #1 Respiratory Content 25 | 26 | 27 | 9 |

**Figure 2.** Sample Course Calendar

| | | | | | | | | |
|---|---|---|---|---|---|---|---|---|
| 11 | 28 | 29 | 30 | 31 | **November** Respiratory 01 | 02 | 03 | 8 |
| 12 | 04 | 05 | 06 | 07 | Test #2 08 | 09 | 10 | 7 |
| 13 | 11 | 12 | 13 | 14 | Cardiac 15 | 16 | 17 | 6 |
| 14 | 18 | 19 | 20 | **Thanksgiving No classes** 21 | **Thanksgiving No classes** 22 | **Thanksgiving No classes** 23 | 24 | 5 |
| 15 | 25 | 26 | 27 | 28 | Cardiac 29 | 30 | **December** 01 | 4 |
| 16 | 02 | 03 | 04 | 05 | PVD 06 | 07 | 08 | 3 |
| 17 | 09 | 10 | 11 | 12 | Test #3 13 | 14 | 15 | 2 |
| 18 | 16 | 17 | 18 | <u>**End of semester**</u> 19 | 20 | 21 | 22 | 1 |

**Figure 2 continued.** Sample Course Calendar

Calendar reprinted with permission College of DuPage Associate Degree Nursing Program (2008).

to balance review needs with class time. Student review might entail students completing an analysis of their results and identifying why they answered questions incorrectly.

## Team Teaching

Some institutions choose to use a team approach, where more than one faculty member is involved in course delivery. Instruction of course content may be taught in tandem, by two or more team members. Alternatively, teams may opt to divide the course content into blocks, with faculty teaching the content in which they have expertise. Some institutions select team leaders, who help direct administrative tasks of the team. However duties are assigned, some members of the team will be responsible for:

- Orienting new or part-time faculty to the course, course outcomes, and expectations for their roles in the course
- Designing and submitting course materials for distribution to students and members of the team. These materials may include but are not limited to the course syllabus, communications between faculty and students, and a course schedule or calendar. (See Figure 2)
- Conducting regular course meetings, planning agenda for these meetings, and submitting minutes of these meetings
- Consulting regularly with team members regarding student progress, following the mechanisms established to alert appropriate faculty to actual or potential problems with students or clinical agencies
- Coordinating content of laboratory or simulation experiences
- Coordinating course evaluations

## Faculty Benefits

There are varying benefits of employment. These benefits are usually discussed prior to hiring. In general, faculty need to consider the following:

### Salary Schedule

Salary range and timetable are determined by individual institutions. Human resources should be consulted for discussion of pay scales for regular hours and overload or overtime. Faculty workload that exceeds the number of hours obligated to teach constitutes overload. Another type of overload is when the number of students exceeds the established class size. Generally, guidelines exist that govern circumstances that require overload and its associated remuneration. A differentiation between required and voluntary overload should be apparent.

## Savings and Credit Union

Many institutions provide special services, such as their own credit union. Such features might include low interest rate loans, savings and checking accounts, and home equity credit lines.

## Insurance Provisions

Health, dental, vision, and basic life insurance are generally available for full-time faculty. Eligibility, general provisions, exclusions, and exact nature of benefits are typically obtained from a human resources department. Faculty should consider insurance benefits for their impact during employment and upon retirement. If the college operates a health center, guidelines regarding use by faculty should be delineated.

## Leaves of Absence

Conditions that qualify for leave include sick leave, extended leave, and bereavement leave. Sabbatical leaves may also be granted after fulfilling the minimum number of years of service to qualify. Institutional policies that govern such leaves should be consulted.

## Educational Development

Funds for professional enhancement, attendance at conferences, and provisions for discounts on or loan of equipment, such as a personal computer, may be available.

## Retirement Schedule

Faculty should evaluate specific provisions for retirement, such as number of years of service and type of retirement package. In some instances, institutions may match employee retirement savings, offer early retirement incentives, and conduct retirement planning information sessions.

## Continuing Faculty Development

It is essential that faculty meet their own professional needs to have the energy, knowledge, and passion to sustain their teaching efforts. Faculty and students alike are lifelong learners. Nursing and teaching nursing are professional pursuits that have the distinct advantage of allowing an avenue to purse a wide variety of interests.

Faculty need to maintain currency in nursing specialties as well as in educational theory. One way to do this is faculty practice, in which faculty spend clinical hours in the field. Sometimes this work is donated to free clinics. Currency may also be gained when faculty share expertise at conferences or via publications.

The opportunity to discuss common concerns and interventions that are of benefit is rejuvenating and stimulating for faculty. Sharing expertise in content fosters personal growth and self-esteem. The opportunity to serve within nursing organizations is available at regional, state, and national levels and may be another avenue faculty wish to pursue.

Release time, reduced teaching load, or sabbatical leave are a few avenues faculty may wish to pursue which afford personal and professional growth. Typically, faculty must be full-time and have served the institution for a specified period of time before they are eligible for such benefits. Faculty may also consider grant writing, grant review, journal review, or consulting as an avenue to expand their horizons.

## Summary

Teaching nursing is indeed both an art and a science. It is challenging and rewarding, as those who teach have experienced. This chapter has detailed the roles and responsibilities educators face on a daily basis. The rich, human experience that faculty gain through work with students and clients evolves continuously and is all encompassing.

## Learning Activities

1. Outline a weekly plan. Include the hours you teach, advise, attend committees, and devote to personal development. Identify what changes you might like to make or what you might like to add. Include as possible options consulting, writing for publication, or presenting at conferences.

2. Consult with the human resources department at your institution. Determine the exact nature of your benefits in regard to sabbatical leave, retirement options, or other areas of interst.
3. Outline an ideal work environment, with delineation of hours for all aspects of teaching.
4. Design tools that streamline faculty workload, such as a standardized committee report form.
5. Design a tool that highlights the roles and responsibilities expected of a part-time faculty member working within your institution.

## Educational Philosophy

The teacher who artfully engages students in an atmosphere rich in trust, rapport, and resources is well on the way to developing a climate just right for learning. Students need to feel safe to explore and question in order to gain meaning from their experiences. Students also need focus, guidance, and perspective. In a collaborative atmosphere, both teacher and student are learners. This process is dynamic and ever unfolding. — Lynn Engelmann

## References

Brunt, B. A. (2007). *Competencies for staff educators: Tools to evaluate and enhance nursing professional development.* Marblehead, MA: HCPro, Incorporated.

Caputi, L. (2006). Grading papers: Pleasure or pain? *Teaching and Learning in Nursing, 1*(2), 35-42.

Grasmick, L. L. (2002). Roles of the staff development educator. In K. L. O'Shea (Ed.), *Staff development nursing secrets* (pp. 7-15). Philadelphia: Hanley & Belfus, Inc.

Jeffries, P. (2006). Designing simulations for nursing education. In M. H. Oermann & K.T. Heinrich (Eds.), *Annual review of nursing education, Vol 4, Innovations in curriculum, teaching, and student and faculty development.* New York: Springer.

Keating, S. B. (2006). *Curriculum development and evaluation in nursing.* Philadelphia: Lippincott Williams & Wilkins.

National League of Nursing. (2006). *NLN position statement. Mentoring of Nurse Faculty Pratt, D. D., Boll, S. L., & Collins, J. B. (2007).* Towards a plurality of perspectives for nurse educators. *Nursing Philosophy, 8*(1), 49-59.

*Robert's Rules of Order Newly Revised. (2000).*(10th ed.). Cambridge, MA: Perseus Publishing.

# CHAPTER 5

# MOTIVATING STUDENTS TO LEARN

Jane M. Kirkpatrick, MSN, PhD, RN, RNC-OB

The content of this chapter relates to the following major content areas and subconcepts on the Certified Nurse Educator Examination Detailed Test Blueprint:

**Facilitate Learning**
- Use teaching strategies based on: educational theory; evidence-based practices related to education
- Modify teaching strategies and learning experiences based on consideration of learners': cultural background; past clinical experiences; past educational and life experiences
- Create a positive learning environment that fosters a free exchange of ideas
- Show enthusiasm for teaching, learning, and the nursing profession that inspires and motivates students

**Facilitate Learning Development and Socialization**
- Adapt teaching styles and interpersonal interactions to facilitate learner behaviors

## Introduction

Have you ever asked yourself why students were surfing the Internet during your lecture or seemed less than engaged in the discussion you were leading? Have you thought to yourself that today's students just are not as interested in learning as you were as a nursing student? If these questions have crossed your mind or have dominated the lunch discussion with your faculty colleagues, then this chapter may give you a new way of reflecting on these issues. Maybe it is not just about the students…but it is also how we, as educators, design and develop the instructional experiences for our students.

## What do the Theorists Have to Say?

Motivation, by definition, is "the process whereby goal-directed behavior is instigated and sustained" (Pintrich & Schunk, 2002, p. 5). Educators agree that motivation plays an important role in learning and in learning environments (Driscoll, 2005; Miltiadou & Savenye, 2003; Paas, Tuovnien, van Merriënboer, & Darabi, 2005). Motivation to learn includes the processes that occur during learning as well as the ultimate performance. It is important to better understand the way that motivation to learn influences learning, and how the consequences of learning influences motivation for more learning.

There has been great interest over the years to better understand and explain what stimulates the "will" to learn and to identify the forces that contribute to motivation. This effort has resulted in a large body of research in educational psychology. Research findings with college students time and again have shown that motivational beliefs impact academic performance and the effort to achieve this performance (Paas, et al., 2005; Paulsen & Feldman, 1999).

There has been great interest over the years to better understand and explain the forces that contribute to both internal and external motivation. The challenge is that individuals have differences among each other as to what motivates them, and the same individual may not always be motivated in the same way (Gagné, Wager, et al., 2005). Because motivation is not a visible, tangible entity, we look at various measures of self-efficacy beliefs, goal orientation and task value beliefs to demonstrate motivation (Dembo &Eaton, 1997; McKeachie, Pintrich, Lin, Smith, & Sharma, 1990; Theall & Franklin, 1999; Stipek, 2002; Wlodkowski, 1999). Much of the literature on motivation has been informed by educational psychologists using a social cognitive perspective. Following is a review of the major constructs of social cognitive motivation theory.

### Social Cognitive Motivation Theory

The core of social cognitive motivation theory is that thoughts and beliefs affect the way people respond and react to the learning environment (Stipek, 2002). Miltiadou and Savenye (2003) grouped the major constructs of this theory into three broad categories.

- The first addresses the learner's question "Can I do this?" and includes the constructs of self-efficacy, locus of control, and attribution.
- The second category "Why should I do this?" addresses the purpose or reason for the learner to engage in the learning task. Constructs under this question include expectancies, intrinsic/extrinsic motivation, and goal orientation.

- The third category addresses the question "How do I go about doing this?" and includes the strategies used to accomplish the learning task that lead to self-regulation of learning. See Figure 1.

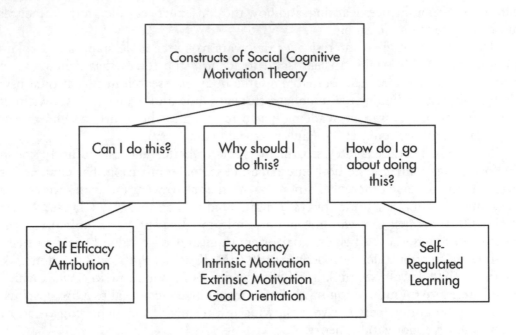

**Figure 1.** Concept model for social cognitive theory constructs (based on Miltiadou & Savenye, 2003).

## Self-Efficacy

Self-efficacy is defined as "peoples' judgments of their capabilities to organize and execute courses of action required to attain designated types of performances" (Bandura, 1986, p. 391). Self-efficacy expectations and outcome expectations (whether affirming or negative) contribute to the behaviors that lead to the anticipated outcome (Bandura, 1977; 1982). According to Bandura there are four ways to acquire an efficacy expectation. They include:

1. Performance accomplishments (i.e., success breeds success)

2. Vicarious experience (i.e., observing someone else achieving the goal and noting that it would be achievable "I can be that good")
3. Verbal persuasion from others (i.e., "You can do it!")
4. Physiological states (i.e., a "gut feeling" that tells whether you will succeed or fail)

Bandura's (1977) initial work with self-efficacy determined how much effort individuals would give in the face of a threatening activity. He found the higher the self-efficacy, the more the individual would persist and the less avoidance behavior was exhibited.

Research on self-efficacy in education has found that:
- Higher goals are set by persons who are high in self-efficacy (Zimmerman & Bandura, 1994 as cited in Stipek, 2002)
- More difficult tasks are chosen by people with high self-efficacy (Sexton & Tuckman, 1991)
- Individuals will persist longer at tasks if they are high in self-efficacy, even if the high self-efficacy is induced (Zimmerman, 1995)
- High self-efficacy students concentrate better on problem-solving while low self-efficacy students are more likely to spend energy on anxiety and fears of failing instead of concentrating on the learning task (Bandura, 1986; Bandalos, Yates, & Thorndike-Christ, 1995 as cited in Stipek, 2002; Zimmerman, 1995)
- Self-efficacy is a predictor of academic success (Pajares, 1996)

The implication of these research findings for nursing faculty is to consider methods which support and enhance self-efficacy, especially through performance accomplishment.

## Attribution Theory

Attribution Theory comes from the social psychology literature and focuses on how humans explain their behavior or the behavior of others. According to this theory, the interpretation of the outcome rather than motivational state or even actual outcome is the influence on future efforts (Eccles & Wigfield, 2002).

An external attribution assigns cause to something external to self while an internal attribution assigns cause to self (Driscoll, 2005; Keller, 2007; Stipek, 2002; Weiner, 2000). For example, if a learner's response to achieving a low test score focuses on the poor quality of the instruction, the inconvenience of the instructional method, and/or the lack of response from the teacher, it would be said that the learner was using external attribution. A learner who ascribes a low test score to an internal force, such as personal ability (e.g., I.Q.) or effort is using an internal attribution scheme (Driscoll, 2005; Stipek, 2002). Eccles and Wigfield (2002) reported when success is associated with an internal cause it can increase self-esteem and pride. However, when success is associated with an external cause, it creates a sense of gratitude. If failure is associated with an internal cause, it generates shame; whereas when failure is attributed to an external cause, it generates anger.

The most important attributions identified by Weiner (1992) include identified

- Ability
- Effort
- Task difficulty
- Luck

Attributions were also classified as being stable (not subject to change) or unstable (subject to change). For example, ability is classified in this scheme as a stable internal attribution. This means, ability cannot be controlled by the learner. In contrast, effort is classified as an unstable internal attribution and can be controlled by the learner. "Learners will have no motivation to participate in a learning experience without the belief that change is possible" (Hodges, 2004, p. 2). For this reason, faculty should strive to help students recognize the significance of their effort on the learning outcomes.

## Expectancy Value Theory

Expectancy Value Theory says that behavioral goals are a function of values and perceived ability to accomplish those goals. Expectation is mediated by the value of the task and the belief that success will come given a reasonable effort. Eccles and Wigfield (2002) identified four components of task values:

1. Attainment value (the value that accomplishing the task hold in terms of personal competency and definition of self)
2. Intrinsic value (the pleasure gained from the activity or level of interest about the activity)
3. Utility value (relationship to the individual's current and future goals)
4. Cost (effort, lost opportunities from the selection of this activity over other options, or risk of failure)

Motivation levels are found to increase as the value of the task increases and the learner's confidence increases (Atkinson, 1964; Brophy, 1987; Dembo & Eaton,

1997; Keller, 2004; Paulsen & Feldman 1999; Rodgers & Withrow-Thorton, 2005; Stipek, 2002).

## Intrinsic and Extrinsic Motivation

Does it matter if you are internally or externally motivated? It is certainly possible for learning to occur under both frameworks. The student who came to school to learn everything needed to be a competent nurse would be considered intrinsically motivated. Intrinsic theorists hold that learning and achieving is an inborn tendency; that individuals naturally seek opportunities to develop competence and desire to make choices about how they will engage, taking pleasure in accomplishment (Driscoll, 2005; Stipek, 2002). Intrinsic motivation has been identified by multiple researchers to be foundational to adaptive, self-regulated learning strategies in the context of achievement motivation (Deci & Ryan, 1985; Harackiewicz, 1989; Sansone, 1986 as cited by Rawsthorne & Elliot, 1999).

In contrast, the student who came to school to be the top achiever of the class and graduate magna cum laude would be considered to be externally motivated. Learners who are motivated by extrinsic motivation are those who work to achieve recognition by others based on external standards (Driscoll, 2005). Learners with extrinsic goal orientation are motivated by external rewards such as grades and competition. These learners are less interested in achieving the learning outcomes than in obtaining the rewards (Pintrich, Smith, Garcia, & McKeachie, 1991).

One of the challenges that have been identified is the impact of instruction on students who begin their learning experience intrinsically motivated. Deci and Ryan (1985) proposed that reward systems can undercut intrinsic motivation due to a change from internal to external locus of causality. Research has found that praise when provided in low effort and/or in the presence of low performance can actually contribute to future low effort and performance (Stipek, 2002). This means that the rewards actually interfere with self-determination because the learner perceives a loss of control.

Biggs (1987) looked at motivation to learn using a dichotomy of deep versus surface learning. The deep learner is described as intrinsically motivated, finding meaning in the learning task, seeking to incorporate the new knowledge into a meaningful way, and striving to develop competency. In contrast, the surface learner expects to meet the minimum requirement, views learning tasks as a requirement to be met, may be more focused on how much time the learning task is taking rather than the content of the learning and sees each learning task as distinct and separate. The deep learner reflects on the material and is able to relate the significance of the learning into a larger scheme and apply this information to other situations. In contrast, the surface learner may have memorized facts, but is at a loss to explain how these facts would be applied to a larger situation.

Biggs also considered achievement strategies (i.e., study habits, organization, methods of approaching the learning task). He reported that effective achievement strategies are used by both deep and surface learners. Students who take a deep learning approach without effective achievement strategies can easily become lost in the maze of content; while students who take a surface learning approach without effective achievement strategies can become dissatisfied and quickly bored.

## Goal Orientation

Goal orientation is the reasoning behind student engagement in a learning task (Pintrich, Smith, Garcia, & McKeachie, 1991). Because the terminology used by the key researchers varied, Murphy and Alexander (2000) used a review of literature and an eight member panel of experts, to develop conceptual definitions of mastery and performance goals. The term mastery goal "represents a desire to develop competence and increase knowledge and understanding through effortful learning" (p. 28). Reward for achieving a mastery goal is internal. A performance goal "represents a desire to gain favorable judgments and avoid negative judgments of one's competence, particularly if success is achieved through a minimum exertion of effort; Synonym: ego or ego-involved goal" (p. 28). The reward system for performance goals is external to the individual. Not only does the individual with a performance goal seek external recognition, it is also important to the performance goal oriented individual to avoid being viewed as incompetent.

Goal theorists have further delineated goal structure to distinguish between achievement and avoidance. Higher self-efficacy, higher level of personal goals, and higher level of effort are demonstrated by individuals with a mastery goal orientation as compared to those with a performance goal orientation (Phillips & Gully, 1997; Radosevich, Vaidyanathan, Yeo, & Radosevich, 2004; VandeWalle, Brown, Cron, & Slocum, 1999). When faced with ineffective results, learners with a mastery goal orientation will increase effort, persist, revise strategies, and generally refer to the experience as a challenge (Dweck & Leggett, 1988). When a performance goal was not readily achieved, low confidence learners demonstrated helplessness behaviors, avoidance, and were more likely to quit rather than persist. Low confidence learners attributed this performance goal failure to a lack of ability whereas high confidence learners attribute performance goal failures to poor choice of strategy. In general, performance-avoidance goal orientation is associated with disengagement and lack of persistence (Eccles & Wigfield, 2002).

## Self Regulated Learning

Self-regulated learners ask the question of themselves "How do I go about doing this learning activity?" These students actually construct their own strategies for learning and use them to regulate their behavior, cognition, and motivation as they seek to gain meaning from their learning experiences. Most models of self-regulated learning include the assumption that behavior is driven by goals and that learners modify their behaviors to meet these goals. In addition, these models also assume that individual performance, the context of the learning environment, and personal traits are mediated by the learner who self-regulates (Moos & Azebedo, 2006).

## How can I Conceptualize All of Theoretical Information into Something Usable?

Organizing the current knowledge about motivation to make informed decisions for instructional strategies can be challenging. Fortunately, the challenge to apply the best research about motivation to make informed decisions for instructional strategies was embraced by John Keller in the 1980's. The ARCS model of motivation synthesizes recent theories of motivation and presents a systematic model with recommended strategies for each of the four concepts (attention, relevance, confidence, and satisfaction – ARCS) that are needed to create a motivational learning environment (Huang, et al., 2004; Keller, 2004).

The model has been used effectively to develop educational projects for all ages of learners ranging from kindergarten through twelfth grade (e.g., Song & Keller, 2001) to college students (e.g., Means, Jonassen, & Dwyer, 1997) and even adult learners in an industry setting (e.g., Rogers & Withrow-Thorton, 2005). An interesting application of the ARCS model comes from Chyung, Winiecki, and Fenner (1999) who used the ARCS model along with an organizational model to redesign the framework for delivering online courses. This redesign dramatically improved the retention rate of online learners from 56% to 85% over a period of four years. The ARCS model has demonstrated multicultural effectiveness, as it has been used in at least five other countries around the world (Keller, 1999).

## Overview of the ARCS Components

As previously noted, ARCS stands for attention, relevance, confidence, and satisfaction. **Attention** refers to the process of gaining the interest or curiosity of the learner about the instruction and then maintaining that interest throughout the instruction. The attention component especially addresses the affective elements of motivation theories (Theall & Franklin, 1999). Expectancy, task value, and goal orientation are integrated in the **relevance** component. "Why do I need or want to know this?" or "What will I gain from this experience that will matter to me?" are two questions that are answered by the relevance component of the ARCS model. Self-efficacy, attribution, the learners' need for achievement, affiliation, and success are represented in both the relevance and confidence components (Clark, 2000; Driscoll, 2005; Keller, 1987a). **Confidence** occurs when the learner is able to navigate and successfully achieve the learning task. **Satisfaction** is the application of the new knowledge in a real or a simulated setting. Expectancy, task value, and goal orientation are again evident in the satisfaction component that follows successful completion of a challenging task. A summary of strategies for each of the four ARCS components can be found in Table 1.

| ARCS Component | Associated Motivational Strategies |
|---|---|
| Attention<br>• Perceptual arousal<br>• Inquiry arousal<br>• Variability | • Ask questions<br>• Create a sense of mystery<br>• Pose a problem<br>• Use boldface type or highlighting new words<br>• Use an unusual picture<br>• Provide background on the topic to be learned<br>• Compare an example to a non-example<br>• Tell a humorous story that relates to the topic<br>• Vary the instructional methods throughout the learning experience<br>• Use problem-based learning<br>• Use active learning strategies requiring student action or response<br>• Incorporate game-like features<br>• Include high level and divergent questions |

**Table 1.** ARCS Components with Associated Motivational Strategies

| | |
|---|---|
| Relevance<br>• Goal orientation<br>• Motive matching<br>• Familiarity | • Develop meaningful learning objectives<br>• Make abstract content more personal or concrete or familiar (use of analogy)<br>• Discuss how the new information relates to past learning<br>• Discuss how this learning activity will prepare learners for success in future experiences |
| Confidence<br>• Learning requirements<br>• Success opportunities<br>• Personal control | • Design instruction at appropriate level of difficulty<br>• Clearly communicate desired expectations<br>• Provide advance organizers<br>• Allow learner opportunity for choices<br>• Provide immediate feedback – success breeds success<br>• Help learner identify the effect of their effort to learning success; use standards that give evidence of individual progress<br>• Use mastery learning principles, including additional instruction, practice opportunities |
| Satisfaction<br>• Intrinsic reinforcement<br>• Extrinsic reward<br>• Equity | • Have a finished product as a result of the instruction<br>• Provide rewards for good performance or improved performance<br>• Provide practice opportunity for students to apply new knowledge<br>• Use simulation<br>• Use games with competition using new knowledge |

**Table 1 continued.** ARCS Components with Associated Motivational Strategies

## Attention

Stimulating curiosity and maintaining this interest over time is the core of the attention component of the Keller model. According to Keller (1987a) there are 3 basic ways to stimulate the learner's attention:
1. Perceptual arousal
2. Inquiry arousal
3. Variety

Perceptual arousal happens with unexpected or uncertain events and with incongruence. Inquiry arousal stimulates information seeking behavior. Not only will inquiry arousal attract the learner's attention, it may also evoke new ways of considering the material (Gagné & Driscoll, 1988). Driscoll (2005) reports that "… some level of surprise, incongruity, complexity, or discrepancy from our expectations and beliefs" (p. 125) generates interest in learning. It is important that the stimuli be novel, but not so extreme that it creates high anxiety or is ignored (Berlyne, 1966 as cited by Driscoll, 2005).

Gaining the attention of the learner and maintaining attention throughout the instruction can be accomplished through a number of strategies. Asking questions, creating a sense of mystery, or posing a problem that is of interest to the learner can stimulate an attitude of inquiry (Keller, 1987a). Using boldface type or highlighting a new word in text, using an unusual picture, providing background on the topic to be learned, comparing an example to a non-example, and telling a humorous story that relates to the topic are all strategies that can be employed by the faculty member to attract and maintain the learners' attention (Smith & Ragan, 2005). Incorporating game features in the instruction can gain and maintain attention (Brophy, 1987). Varying the instructional methods throughout the learning experience and using active learning strategies are other ways to maintain interest (Clark, 2000; Keller, 1983, 1987a).

Problem-based learning environments with authentic learning activities can generate a deeper level of inquiry throughout the instructional experience (Jonassen & Land, 2000; Keller, 1983). When learners are required to respond in some way during the learning task, they must attend to the task. For example, watching a video is a passive experience for the learner. However, responding to questions on a computer interface about the video becomes an active learning strategy. Including application, analysis, and synthesis questions stimulates attention by challenging the learner to organize the content in a new and personal way (Brophy, 1987).

## Relevance

"Relevance, in its most general sense, refers to those things which we perceive as instrumental in meeting needs and satisfying personal desires, including the accomplishment of personal goals" (Keller, 1987a, p.3). Relevance connotes meaningful context in both the cognitive and affective domains (Driscoll, 2005). If the learner perceives the task will meet a basic need, motive, or value then the task has relevance (Keller, 1983). Three sub-categories are:
1. Goal orientation (i.e., meeting needs of the learner)
2. Motive matching (i.e., matching learning style and learner interests)
3. Familiarity (i.e., connecting the instruction to learner experiences) (Keller, 1987a)

Relevance triggers increased effort, persistence, and better performance (Means, Jonassen, & Dwyer, 1997).

Strategies to promote relevance in instructional materials include the following: develop meaningful learning objectives based on a learner assessment, explicitly reinforce the intrinsic value of the current learning task to personal and/or professional goals, demonstrate how the new knowledge connects to prior learning, and give examples of the value of the instruction to the student in the present or near future (Keller, 1987a, 1987b). Relevant learning outcomes (ends-oriented) will likely be obvious to the learner. However, when relevance is primarily means-oriented, it may not be intuitively obvious to the learner and explicit statements from the faculty (or instructional program) become an important method of demonstrating relevance (Driscoll, 2005).

## Confidence

This category considers the learner's expectations, opportunities, and evidence for success, and locus of control for learning. The three sub-categories identified by Keller (1987a) include:
1. Learning requirements (i.e., creating a positive expectation for learner success)
2. Success opportunities (i.e., support and enhance learner belief in own confidence)
3. Personal control (i.e., recognition of the effect of personal effort and ability on success)

There are multiple motivational constructs that are incorporated into Keller's confidence category. These include self-efficacy, goal orientation, Expectancy Value Theory, and Attribution Theory.

To create a positive expectation for success, the instruction needs to be at an appropriate level of difficulty, challenging but not impossible; learners should be challenged to perform just above their current ability (Driscoll, 2005). This means the faculty member needs a good assessment of learner prerequisite skills and knowledge. Clear communication of the pre-requisites and the desired expectations can help to minimize the fear of the unknown as well as helping the learner recognize when these expectations are met (Keller, 1999). Learners who know the expectations can independently recognize the effect of their effort on their learning success (Driscoll, 2005).

In a qualitative study of undergraduate students with mixed efficacy levels related to the course content, Koh (2006) found that early success was important to keep both low and high self-efficacy learners motivated on mastery and performance goals. Koh found that when learners with high self-efficacy perceived they would not be successful on a complicated performance goal, they engaged in a less difficult assignment and their intrinsic motivation for learning dropped.

Feedback is a mechanism that can be used to let the learner know he or she is successful. Feedback needs to be clear, detailed, and provide information on what was done well or needs to improve (Keller, 1987a). Feedback and comments on progress are ways to facilitate learning (Bonnel, 2008). Caution with feedback must be maintained, as overwork of an external reward system has been found to actually modify the motivation of an intrinsically motivated student to value extrinsic sources of motivation (Stipek, 2002).

Whenever learning is an active process with choice, the experience becomes more relevant (Brophy, 1987; Clark, 2000; Keller, 1988; Smith & Ragan, 2005). Problem-based learning designed under a constructivist learning theory framework typically supports a learner-directed approach (Jonassen & Lund, 2000). This strategy supports personal control and contributes to confidence (Keller, 1987a, 1987b, 1987c).

## Satisfaction

Satisfaction is the measure of success occurring following completion of a learning task. Motivation is maintained when satisfaction is achieved (Rodgers & Withrow-Thorton, 2005). Keller (1987a, 1987b, 1987c) again defined three subcategories. These include:

1. Intrinsic reinforcement (i.e., meaningful opportunities for the learner to practice the new knowledge)
2. Extrinsic rewards (i.e., reinforcement for desired behaviors)
3. Equity (i.e., recognition of accomplishment as a positive attribute)

When the learner's outcome expectations are met, there is usually a corresponding increase in self-efficacy (Driscoll, 2005). However, the learner's expectations may not be the same as the designer's expectations. For example, the outcome expectations set by the designer may be for an 80% pass rate on a final simulation, yet the learner may have set a 100% expectation for self.

A logical consequence of the learning task is the demonstration of a finished product that is a result of the instruction or use of the new knowledge. Simulations or games where everyone has an opportunity to participate also meet Keller's criteria for reinforcement and equity. Authentic tasks (realistic reading materials and authentic learning environments) have great relevance to the learner and hold meaning for both the cognitive and affective domains. This relevance triggers increased effort, persistence, and better performance (Driscoll, 2005; Means, Jonassen, & Dwyer, 1997). Authentic learning is supported by constructivist theorists (i.e., Jonassen & Land, 2000). However, one of the major criticisms of constructivism is that learners can experience excess cognitive load with the amount of choice and sheer volume of information (Driscoll, 2005, Stipek, 2002). Paas, Tuovnien, van Merriënboer, and Darabi (2005) have recommended expanding research on the effect of authentic learning activities on motivation. The recommended strategies for Keller's ARCS components support the institution of authentic learning (Keller, 1987a, 1987b, 2004).

Astleitner and Hufnagl (2003) explored the effects of self-regulated learner traits on motivation level in a web-based learning environment. The treatment was a motivationally enhanced web-based learning environment (using the ARCS model); the control was the same material without the motivational enhancements. Learners with a low situation-outcome-expectancy (those who expect to actively participate in achieving outcomes) were expected to be most affected by a motivationally designed environment. Results of this study confirmed that use of embedded ARCS strategies led to higher motivation and better knowledge acquisition for students who had a low situation-outcome-expectancy.

## Summary

As nursing faculty, we can use our understanding of motivation for learning to design instructional experiences that engage our students to learn. By embracing the four components of the ARCS model, faculty members have an efficient way to incorporate motivational strategies. We should ask ourselves if we have captured the attention of our students. Have we bothered to explain why the student needs to learn the material we are teaching, or are we expecting the students to innately know the relevance of the material? Are the students building confidence by completing the instructional activities we have set before them? Are students able to demonstrate the knowledge they have gained in the assessment activities we use?

Keller synthesized motivational theories into a model that is easy to apply. This model addresses motives, values, and expectancies that influence the effort exerted by the learner. This effort coupled with the learner's abilities, skills, and knowledge influence the ultimate learning outcome. Faculty can modify the instructional environment to capitalize on the factors that influence student willingness to engage and persist in learning. Choices made by faculty in the design of instructional experiences can impact student motivation for learning and ultimately, the learning outcomes.

## Learning Activities

1. Consider a learning experience you will design for your next class. Are the elements of the ARCS model present? If so, how? If not, how can you incorporate them?
2. Discuss the ARCS Model with another faculty. How does this faculty incorporate ARCS into the teaching/learning process?
3. Talk about motivation with your students. Ask them what motivates them to do well in your class.

## Educational Philosophy

I believe that teaching/learning is an active process with faculty and students each accepting responsibility for the outcomes. The cornerstone of this collaborative venture is honesty and mutual respect. Faculty have the experience and wisdom to guide the learners experiences and must be sure that the learning activities selected are relevant to the task at hand, respect the time and effort required of the learner, as well as provide opportunities for learners to build confidence in their command of the new knowledge. The ultimate goal of learning reaches far beyond the short-term exams and papers completed in school. The real final exam is the nursing care provided for our patients. For this reason, faculty need to design instruction in such a way that it enhances the learners' ability to retain the information for the long term. — Jane M. Kirkpatrick

## References

Astleitner, H., & Hufnagl, M. (2003).The effects of situation-outcome-expectancies and of ARCS strategies on self-regulated learning with web lectures. *Journal of Educational Multimedia and Hypermedia, 12*(4), 361-376.

Atkinson, J. W. (1964). *An introduction to motivation.* Princeton, NJ: Van Nostrand.

Bandura, A. (1977). Self-efficacy: Toward a unifying theory of behavioral change. *Psychological Review, 84,* 195-215.

Bandura, A. (1982). Self-efficacy mechanism in human agency. *American Psychologist, 37,* 122-147.

Bandura, A. (1986). *Social foundations of thought and action: A social cognitive theory.* Englewood Cliffs, NJ: Prentice-Hall.

Biggs, J. (1987). *Student approaches to learning and studying; research monograph.* Melbourne, Australia: Australian Council for Educational Research.

Bonnel, W. (2008). Improving feedback to students in online courses. *Nursing Education Perspectives, 29*(5), 290-294.

Brophy, J. (1987). Synthesis of research on strategies for motivating students to learn. *Educational leadership, 45,* 40-48.

Chyung, Y., Winiecki, D., & Fenner, J.A. (2000). *Evaluation of effective interventions to solve the dropout problem in adult distance education.* Paper presented at American Educational Research Association (AERA) conference, New Orleans, LA, April 24-28, 2000. Retrieved April 6, 2006, from http://coen.boisestate.edu/ychyung/researchpaper.htm

Clark, D. (2000). Developing instruction or instructional design. Retrieved November 14, 2006 from http://www.netling.com/~donclark/hrd/learning.development.html

Deci, E., & Ryan, R. (1985). *Intrinsic motivation and self-determination in human behavior.* New York: Plenum Press.

Dembo M., & Eaton. M. (1997) School learning and motivation. In G. D. Phye (Ed.), *Handbook of academic learning: Construction of knowledge* (pp. 65-103). San Diego: Academic Press.

Driscoll, M. (2005). *Psychology of learning for instruction* (3rd ed.). Boston: Allyn and Bacon.

Dweck, C.S., & Leggett, E. L. (1988). A social-cognitive approach to motivation and personality. *Psychological Review, 95*, 256-273.

Eccles, J.S., & Wigfield, A. (2002). Motivational beliefs, values, and goals. *Annual Review of Psychology, 53*, 109-132.

Gagné, R., & Driscoll, M. (1988). *Essentials of learning for instruction* (2nd ed.) Englewood Cliffs, NJ: Prentice-Hall.

Gagné, R., Wager, W., Golas, K., & Keller, J. (2005). *Principles of instructional design* (5th ed.) Belmont, CA: Wadsworth/Thompson Learning.

Harackiewicz, J., & Linnenbrinck, E., (2005). Multiple achievement goals and multiple pathways for learning: The agenda and impact of Paul R. Pintrich. *Educational Psychologist, 40*(2), 75-84.

Hodges, C.B. (2004). Designing to motivate: Motivational techniques to incorporate in e-learning experiences. *The Journal of Interactive Online Learning, 2*(3). Retrieved Feb. 5, 2007 from http://www.ncolr.org/jiol/issues/showissue.cfm?volID=2&IssueID=8

Huang, D., Deifes-Dux, H., Imbrie, P., Daku, B., & Kallimani, J. (2004). Learning motivation evaluation for a computer-based instructional tutorial using ARCS model of motivational design. *Proceedings of 34th ASEE/IEEE Frontiers in Education Conference*, Savannah, GA, October 20-23, 2004.

Jonassen, D., & Land, S. (2000). *Theoretical foundations of learning environments*. Mahwah, NJ: Lawrence Erlbaum Associates.

Keller, J.M. (1983). Motivational design of instruction. In C.M. Reigeluth (Ed.), *Instructional design theories and models: An overview of their current status* (pp. 383-434). Hillsdale, NJ: Lawrence Earlbaum Associates.

Keller, J.M. (1987a). Strategies for stimulating the motivation to learn. *Performance and Instruction Journal, 26*(8), 1-7.

Keller, J.M. (1987b). The systematic process of motivational design. *Performance and Instruction Journal, 26*(9), 1-8.

Keller, J. M. (1987c). Development and use of the ARCS model of motivational design. *Journal of Instructional Development, 10*(3), 2-10.

Keller, J.M. (1999). Using the ARCS motivational process in computer-based instruction and distance education. In M. Theall (Ed.), *Motivation from within: Approaches for encouraging faculty and students to excel* (pp. 39-48). San Francisco, CA: Jossey-Bass.

Keller, J.M. (2004). A predictive model of motivation, volition, and multimedia learning. *Proceedings of the International Symposium & Conference: Educational Media in Schools*, Kansai University, Takatsuki-city, Osaka, Japan, August 3, 2004, 9-20.

Keller, J. M. (2007). *Motivation and performance*. In R. Reiser, R. & J. Dempsey (Eds.), *Trends and issues in instructional design and technology* (2nd ed.) (pp. 82-92). Upper Saddle River, NJ: Pearson Prentice Hall.

Koh, J.H.L. (2006) Motivating students of mixed efficacy profiles in technology skills classes: A case study. *Instructional Science, 34,* 423-449.

McKeachie, W.J., Pintrich, P.R., Lin, Y., Smith, D.S. F., & Sharma, R. (1990). *Teaching and learning in the college classroom: A review of the research literature*, Ann Arbor, MI: National Center for Research to Improve Postsecondary Teaching and Learning.

Means, T.B., Jonassen, D.H., & Dwyer, F.M. (1997). Enhancing relevance:Embedded ARCS strategies vs. purpose. *Educational Technology Research and Development, 45*(1), 5-17.

Miltiadou, M., & Savenye, W. (2003). Applying social cognitive constructs of motivation to enhance student success in online distance education. *Educational Technology Review, 11*(1). Retrieved Feb 1, 2007 from http://www.aace.org/dl/files/AACEJ/ETR11178.pdf

Moos, D. & Azevedo, R. (2006). The role of goal structure in undergraduates' use of self-regulatory processes in two hypermedia learning tasks. *Journal of Educational Multimedia and Hypermedia, 15*(1), 49-86.

Murphy, P.K., & Alexander, P.A. (2000). A motivated exploration of motivation terminology. *Contemporary Educational Psychology, 25*(1), 3-53.

Paas, F., Tuovinen, J., van Merriënboer, J., & Darabi, A. (2005). A motivational perspective on the relation between mental effort and performance: Optimizing learner involvement in instruction. *Educational Technology Research and Development, 53*(3), 25-34.

Pajares, F. (1996). Self-efficacy beliefs in academic settings. *Review of Educational Research, 66,* 543-578.

Paulsen, M., & Feldman, K. (1999). Student motivation and epistemological beliefs. In M. Theall (Ed.), *Motivation from within: Approaches for encouraging faculty and students to excel* (pp. 17 -25). San Francisco, CA: Jossey-Bass.

Phillips, J. M., & Gully, S. M. (1997). Role of goal orientation, ability, need for achievement, and locus of control in the self-efficacy and goal-setting process. *Journal of Applied Psychology, 82,* 792-802.

Pintrich, P.R. (1989). The dynamic interplay of student motivation and cognition in the college classroom. In M. Maehr and C. Ames, (Eds.), *Advances in motiva-*

*tion and achievement: Motivation enhancing environments*, Vol. 6. Greenwich, CT: JAI Press.

Pintrich, P.R., & Schunk, D. H. (2002). *Motivation in education: Theory, research, and applications* (2nd ed.). Upper Saddle River, NJ: Pearson.

Pintrich, P.R., Smith, D.A.F., Garcia, T., & McKeachie, W.J. (1991). *A manual for the use of the Motivated Strategies for Learning Questionnaire (MSLQ)*. Ann Arbor: University of Michigan, National Center for Research to Improve Post-secondary Teaching and Learning.

Radosevich, D.J., Vaidyanathan, V.T., Yeo, S., & Radosevich, D.M. (2004). Relating goal orientation to self-regulatory processes: A longitudinal field test. *Contemporary Educational Psychology, 29*, 207-229.

Rawsthorne, L.J., & Elliot, A.J. (1999). Achievement goals and intrinsic motivation: A meta-analytic review. *Personality and Social Psychology Review, 3*(4), 326-344.

Reiser, R., & Dempsey, J. (2002). *Trends and Issues in Instructional Design and Technology* (2nd ed.). Englewood Cliffs, NJ: Prentice-Hall.

Rodgers, D., & Withrow-Thorton, B. (2005). The effect of instructional media on learner motivation. *International Journal of Instructional Media, 32*(4), 333-342.

Sexton, T., & Tuckman, B. (1991). Self-beliefs and behavior: the role of self-efficacy and outcome expectations over time. *Personality and Individual Differences, 12*, 725-736.

Smith, P., & Ragan, T. (2005). *Instructional design* (3rd ed.). Hoboken, NJ: John Wiley & Sons.

Song, S.H., & Keller, J.M. (2001). Effectiveness of motivationally adaptive computer-assisted instruction on the dynamic aspects of motivation. *Educational Technology Research and Development, 49*(2), 5-22.

Stipek, D. (2006). *Motivation to learn: Integrating theory and practice* (4th ed.), Boston: Allyn and Bacon

Theall, M. & Franklin, J. (1999). What have we learned? A synthesis and some guidelines for effective motivation in higher education. In M. Theall (Ed.), *Motivation from within: Approaches for encouraging faculty and students to excel* (pp. 99-109). San Francisco: Jossey-Bass.

VandeWalle, D., Brown, S.P., Cron, W.L., & Slocum, J.W., Jr. (1999). The influence of goal orientation and self-regulation tactics on sales performance: A longitudinal field test. *Journal of Applied Psychology, 84*, 249-259.

Weiner, B. (1992). *Human motivation: Metaphors, theories, and research*. Newbury Park, CA: Sage.

Weiner, B. (2000). Intrapersonal and interpersonal theories of motivation from an attributional perspective. *Educational Psychology Review, 12*(1), 1-14.

Wlodkowski, R. (1999). Motivation and diversity: A framework for teaching. In M. Theall (Ed.), *Motivation from within: Approaches for encouraging faculty and students to excel* (pp. 7-16). San Francisco, CA: Jossey-Bass.

Zimmerman, B. (1995). Self-efficacy and educational development. In A. Bandura (Ed.), *Self-efficacy in changing societies* (pp. 202-231). New York: Cambridge University Press.

# CHAPTER 6

# INSPIRING STUDENTS

**Jeanette Rossetti, MS, EdD, RN**

---

The content of this chapter relates to the following major content areas and subconcepts on the Certified Nurse Educator Examination Detailed Test Blueprint:

**Facilitate Learning**
- Create a positive learning environment that fosters a free exchange of ideas
- Show enthusiasm for teaching, learning, and the nursing profession that inspires and motivates students

**Facilitate Learning Development and Socialization**
- Adapt teaching styles and interpersonal interactions to facilitate learner behaviors

---

## Introduction

Motivating, enlightening, inspiring students, and creating a passion for learning, are among the most important challenges for teachers. In the arena of adult higher education, much emphasis is placed on creative teaching strategies and the importance of engaging the learner. The use of instructional technology has received growing attention in the classroom, especially in the field of nursing, where it is important for the student to gain knowledge in a variety of complicated subjects. The nursing student must be competent and prepared to pass the NCLEX®. The stakes are high and nursing faculty have a heavy teaching responsibility.

However, good teaching is much more than a one-way pontification of ideas in an area of expertise. There is an important phenomenon that occurs between teacher and student that warrants serious consideration. This phenomenon has to do with inspiration. It is imperative to pass on to nursing students a love for learning, a love that will continue throughout their lifetime, a love of the profession that will enable them to be lifelong learners.

Fostering this love for learning requires a special connection to the student. This chapter focuses on that connection – a connection with students through inspiration.

# Inspiration: A Personal Reflection

It is profoundly important that those who hope to be critical educators remain in touch with their lived worlds, their pre-understandings, their perceptual landscapes (Greene, 1978, p. 102).

Being inspired by a teacher can have a positive and long-lasting effect on a student. It is important for nursing faculty to reflect on their experience as students and identify the effects of being inspired by their teachers. Personal reflection via autobiographical writing is an outlet for exploring one's connection to inspiration.

The following is the author's own reflection of being inspired, an event that took place some 20 years ago as an undergraduate nursing student.

*As a junior student in a baccalaureate nursing program in 1983, I found myself questioning the profession for which I was preparing. I had just begun my first nursing clinical in medical-surgical and pediatric nursing, and I found the patient contact unfulfilling. I seemed to handle the tasks well, but I went from patient to patient, providing care without much time to make a connection with any individual person. I found certain nursing faculty stiff, rigid, and uncaring. I remember dreading clinical days and feeling relieved when they were over. I asked myself why I had gone into nursing in the first place! I wanted to connect and build rapport with patients and educate them about health and illness. I did not want to go from task to task, rushing through the day.*

*One day, after a particularly stressful clinical experience, I just wanted to quit, leave the hospital, and drop out of the nursing program, but as I explained my feelings to my teacher, she encouraged me to "pull it together" and "go back to work." Tears were "not necessary." Thank goodness for a supportive group of peers who encouraged me to continue with the program. I still felt uncertain and depressed. How could I quit now, three years into the program?*

*I decided to continue with the hope that something would change. I knew I soon would have different clinicals with new teachers and perhaps I would find an area of nursing that I enjoyed. The next semester I was scheduled to take the psychiatric nursing clinical, the clinical everyone feared, the* One Flew over the Cuckoo's Nest *clinical. I was very nervous and did not know what to expect. My teacher was an expert in her field who truly liked psychiatric nursing and teaching. I recall that all the other students were afraid of the first day of clinical just like I was, but our teacher immediately put us all at ease and acknowledged our feelings. She seemed to know what frightened us and gave us a chance to talk about it. I was very surprised. Always positive, she exuded energy. She had a way of engendering* confidence, especially when it came to working with patients we were afraid of initially. Mental illness was new to many of us. The learning environment was challenging and rewarding, and I loved it. I felt alive. This was something I wanted to do. This was a moment of inspiration.

On the hospital units, my instructor was comfortable working with the patients. Watching her inspired me to feel that I could be a psychiatric nurse. She was available to listen and to discuss any thoughts or concerns I had about my experiences. I remember when I picked the patient I would work with one-on-one, an adolescent girl who was dealing with depression. I read as much as I could about her, the illness of depression, and the treatments scheduled. I learned a lot that semester, yet it was frightening to realize I soon would be a nurse, responsible for taking care of patients. My teacher and I had many discussions about patient care, the nursing process, and life in general. She was truly present for me and I felt I had found my place.

This teacher had a considerable effect on me personally and professionally. The effect she had on my self esteem and confidence would be difficult to overstate. I credit her with helping me get my first position in psychiatric nursing. It can be scary in nursing school when you are investing time and money and do not know what type of nursing you want to do, or for that matter, if you want to be a nurse at all. After I worked with this teacher, I knew for the first time what I wanted to be – a psychiatric nurse.

In the 1980s new nurses were told they needed medical/surgical nursing experience before entering the psychiatric nursing field. Psychiatric nursing was closed to new graduates because the managers of psychiatric units wanted to ensure that a new nurse would be competent in medical skills. My instructor gave me suggestions and advice about how to enter the field immediately after graduation. When we were finished talking I always felt that I could do whatever I wanted, that nothing could stop me. She really helped me feel confident and motivated. She also helped me look **outside the box** to see things a little differently. I felt good being around her and working and learning in my newly discovered clinical area. I felt motivated and enlightened. I was inspired, energized, and empowered.

She recommended, therefore, that I work very hard in my next critical care clinical. I was determined and earned an A. She told me not to give up, to be persistent. She gave me some concrete advice, including what to expect when I did get an interview. She asked me to let her know how my interviews went, and she told me that any hospital would be lucky to have me. Two semesters later, after many tries, I had a successful interview and got a job. I was one of the first graduates of my class to be hired.

*I enjoyed my new position and stayed at the hospital for 12 years in a variety of nursing roles. Because of my teacher, I knew that someday I would want to teach nursing students. I wanted to have the same kind of connection and rapport, be present, and inspire students the way she had inspired me. The inspirational effect of past experiences has been far reaching in my life.*

This is the author's story. What is your own personal story of inspiration? Have you had a powerful experience, one that has been long lasting? Is there someone in your history who has inspired you to be a nurse? A teacher? Explore the learning exercises at the end of the chapter to assist you in your personal reflection about inspiration.

## Defining Inspiration

If we can be a spirit-lifting presence among those with whom we work, we have begun to understand inspiration. (DePree, 2003, p. 170)

It is important to have an understanding about the phenomenon of inspiration. The word **inspiration** is used often and in many different arenas. There are inspirational works of music, inspirational quotations, and inspirational books, but what **is** inspiration? More importantly, what does it have to do with teaching and learning? The following definitions and descriptions are gleaned from literature in the areas of education, leadership, and psychology to help us understand what this phenomenon is all about.

To breathe, or blow into—these are the meanings for the Latin inspirare.

The *Oxford English Dictionary* (1989) defines **inspiration** as:

1. The action of blowing on or into.
2. The action, or an act, of breathing in or inhaling; the drawing in of the breath into the lungs in respiration. b. A drawing in of air; the absorption of air in the 'respiration of plants.'
3. The action of inspiring; the fact or condition of being inspired; a breathing or infusion into the mind or soul. a. A special immediate action or influence of the Spirit of God (or of some divinity or supernatural being) upon the human mind or soul; said esp. of that divine influence under which the books of Scripture are held to have been written. b. A breathing in or infusion of some idea, purpose, etc. into the mind; the suggestion, awakening, or creation of some feeling or impulse, esp. of an exalted kind....

4. Something inspired or infused into the mind; an inspired utterance or product. b. an inspiring principle. (p. 1036)

To "give someone the desire, enthusiasm, or confidence to do something" (2006, p. 525) is the definition of inspire by the Compact Oxford English Dictionary for Students. This definition has particular relevance for nurse educators. An integral role in the pursuit of learning is to have the desire to learn, the enthusiasm to pursue education, and the confidence to be successful in completing an educational program.

Relate the word **inspire** and the act of breathing. In a discussion of breathing techniques, Ornish (1996) illustrates how changes in one's breathing can affect the mind. Ornish demonstrates the power of language and the definition of **inspire**. "To some degree, our language reflects the importance of breathing and its influence on our mind. The term 'inspire' means both to inhale deeply and to become energized, creative, or motivated. 'Expire,' on the other hand, means to die" (p. 157). For the nurse, this connection has fascinating nuances. In patient resuscitation procedures the airway receives the highest priority; all attempts are made to first ensure a patient's airway and stimulate breathing. In education, is our first priority to ensure inspiration and stimulate energy, creativity, and motivation? This is a question that requires serious contemplation.

The word **inspiration** may mean catalyst, impetus, intuition, revelation, hope, purpose, and discovery. It is often synonymous with **motivation** (Hart, 1993), and is commonly used in artistic or problem-solving creativity. Inspiration is described as what gets one started on a project. Inspiration is related to creativity, which "swells far beyond its formal definition. It is a feeling, often of random occurrence, which produces a purely positive emotion within the inspired" (Council, 1988, p. 123). Research by Hart (1998) suggests that many people experience inspiration and that it is a significant and distinct epistemic event that cannot be willed, but, may be cultivated.

The moment of inspiration is brief but a truly inspiring event can be remembered long after the moment it occurs. From this brief point of inspiration one grows, builds, and expands. If the experience is used wisely the "inspired can become a more perceptive human" (Council, 1988, p. 123). Outcomes of inspiration are affective in nature and include a sense of joy and arousal. If one wants to preserve the reality of the experience, Council writes, one should communicate the resulting creative ideas. Of course drawing, painting, and poetry are some ways to communicate these ideas. Council powerfully writes, "… if we as a species do not inspire, it would seem that we are destined to expire" (p. 130).

## Inspiration and Leadership

Inspiration is not so much a quality in the leader (the inspirer), as it is a function of the needs of the inspired (Fairholm, 1994). Goleman, Boyatzis, and McKee (2004) state that leaders who inspire offer a sense of common purpose beyond the day-to-day tasks and they make work exciting. Leaders who inspire "create resonance and move people with a compelling vision or shared mission. Such leaders embody what they ask of others and are able to articulate a shared mission in a way that inspires others to follow" (p. 255-256).

Leadership literature is replete with examples of the ability of leaders to inspire. According to Fairholm (1994), inspiration means to "enlighten, exalt, and animate another person" (p. 161). Inspiration grows out of the interchange between leaders and followers. This interchange is similar to a relationship that offers new insight, new emotions, and/or new directions. The leader must truly appeal to the followers' emotions. A person is inspired when taken beyond routine ways of thinking and when the leader goes beyond facts by putting into words people's dreams and hopes and giving a sense of purpose and direction (Fairholm, 1991).

Charismatic or inspirational leadership has been identified as central to the transformational process (Bass, 1985). Inspirational leaders build confidence in their followers and use inspiration to increase the optimism and enthusiasm of the followers. The leader's inspirational influence on the followers is emotional and results in motivating followers to perform beyond what is expected of them. An ability to inspire is an essential characteristic of transformational leaders who are charismatic, intellectually stimulating, and individually considerate (Bass, 1998). Transformational leaders motivate others by tactics of influence (Yukl, 1994). These tactics include rational persuasion, inspirational appeals, personal appeals, and the use of symbolic behaviors.

It is essential that leaders motivate their followers and create a vision for them to follow. Giving guidance means little unless the organization's members also are inspired to reach for the new order described in the vision (Judge, 1999). To inspire others requires some knowledge and understanding of matters that are bigger and more lasting than day-to-day concerns.

It is important to note that what inspires some may not inspire others. We expect our leaders to be inspiring, enthusiastic, energetic, and positive about the future (Kouzes & Posner, 1987). "It is essential that leaders inspire our confidence in the validity of the goal" (p. 21). Leaders must have absolute and total personal belief in their dreams and be confident in their ability to make extraordinary things happen (Kouzes & Posner, 1995). Enthusiasm and passion are communicated by vivid language and expressive style: "Through their strong appeal and quiet persuasion, leaders enlist others in the dream. They breathe life into the shared vision and get people to see the exciting future possibilities" (Kouzes, et al., 1995, p. 318). Nursing faculty have the opportunity to inspire confidence in their students and help them meet their goals and dreams of becoming exceptional nurses.

## Inspiration and the Teaching/Learning Transaction in Higher Education

On the inspirational plane, I want to assert the importance, meaning, and effect of college teaching in the face of the barrage of criticicisms college teachers have endured in the last few decades. College teachers—and their students—change the world in small and sometimes, big ways (Brookfield, 2006, p. xiv).

Inspiration must be applied to higher education. It is essential for college and university teachers to reflect upon the purpose of college teaching, for "education at its best seems to both inform and to inspire" (Hart, 1993, p. 166). Education is so much more than just a presentation of facts and figures to be memorized for an examination.

The educational process that occurs between a teacher and student can be viewed as a connection, a synergy, an established rapport, or a transaction by which inspiration can occur. **Can occur** is the key. Inspiration does not occur in every teaching and learning situation. It may not be possible to **will** inspiration into being, but favorable conditions can encourage inspiration (Hart, 1993). An attitude of trust and faith, an ability to listen, and a willingness to allow events to unfold may lead to inspiration. If nurtured, inspiration can be a catalyst for learning. Inspiration will emerge naturally and regularly out of the process of learning (Hart, 1993). Inspiration should be invited into the classroom.

> Inspiration is an event of such great pleasure and power as to provide a galvanizing and sought after experience around which to organize learning. It not only provides new excitement and clarity for engaging in stimulating education but it decreases hopelessness and increases self-esteem at the same time (Hart, 1993, p. 166-167).

Inspirational teachers have a profound and long-lasting impact on their students. Students in educational programs were asked what they considered inspirational about former teachers (Burke & Nierenberg, 1998). Analysis of written narratives of more than 100 pre-service teachers revealed three dominant themes:

- Inspirational teachers were perceived to be caring toward the students.
- Teachers identified as inspirational generally had positive attitudes about life, teaching, and their students.

- These teachers inspired others because of their dedication to their jobs and their students.

Inspired teaching does not come from one particular theory, philosophy, or set of materials, but from teachers who can analyze their situation and create appropriate instruction to meet the needs of students (Duffy, 1992). Inspired teaching "originates in the creativity of teachers" (p. 444). Focusing on reading instruction, Duffy explains how direct instructional methods that are teacher-directed, sequenced, and repetitive, with the use of workbooks and frequent quizzes, can be "uninspiring, boring, dull, and essentially meaningless" (p. 442). Teachers need to be empowered and free to "create inspired instructional encounters" (p. 446) by using a variety of philosophical and theoretical approaches. Duffy describes inspired teaching as "at once conceptually coherent, responsive to students, and reflective of a broad range of professional knowledge" (p. 447).

Though it may be brief, a moment of inspiration can be remembered long afterward. For many, the moments of inspiration have long-lasting effects. "The imprint of good teachers remains long after the facts they gave us have faded" (Palmer, 1998, p. 21). Palmer also writes of the "mutual illumination that often occurs when we are willing to explore our inner dynamics with each other" (p. 23). This imprint and illumination describes the experience of inspiration.

Teaching is a complex and passionate experience comprising many different personal styles and approaches (Brookfield, 1990). Charismatic teachers are dynamic performers who "can hold audiences in the palms of their hands and in whose presence students are enthralled and inspired" (p. 8). However, charismatic teaching is but one of many teaching approaches. Teachers should be cautious about the myth of the perfect teacher (Brookfield, 1990). This point is significant because **inspiration** and **charisma** can be synonymous at times. Clarification is important because charisma is not necessary for inspiration to occur; however, the charismatic teacher is often inspirational.

"One is inspired to persevere by the presence of others" (Hooks, 1994, p. 56). Hooks shares how Paulo Freire inspired her after she witnessed him embody the practice he described in theory. "Freire's presence inspired me... it entered me in a way that writing can never touch one and it gave me courage" (p. 56). Hooks concludes by noting the need for courage as part of the formula:

Throughout my years as student and professor, I have been most inspired by those teachers who have had the courage to transgress those boundaries that would confine each pupil to a rote, assembly-line approach to learning. Such teachers approach students with the will and desire to respond to our unique beings, even if the situation does not allow the full emergence of a relationship based on mutual recognition. Yet the possibility of such recognition is always present (p. 13).

## Summary

This chapter explored the experience of inspiration via literature from the fields of education, leadership, and psychology. These definitions further the understanding of how inspiration is a factor in the educational process. Inspiration – a feeling, a spirit-lifting presence, a breathing in or infusion of some idea, a suggestion, an awakening – is an important factor when the teacher and learner interact. Results of inspiration can be increased clarity, energy, openness, and connection. In fact, inspiration **should** be nurtured and can be a catalyst for learning (Hart, 1993). In addition, the connection –viewed as a synergy and an established rapport between teacher and student – was shown to be an important component of the educational process, allowing for the opportunity for inspiration to occur.

It has been said that we teach who we are. This very well could be true. The experience of inspiration can be an important factor in a teacher's personal educational approach and can be part of the teacher's personality and approach to teaching. There is no doubt that every teacher can remember moments when they were inspired by former teachers and the illuminating effects they had. With inspiration a student can be truly energized by a teacher's presence and be motivated to seek out new knowledge. One has the opportunity to **breathe in** new ideas and feelings such as increased confidence, determination, and self-esteem.

In nursing students' education, faculty have the potential to go beyond imparting mere facts by giving their students the gifts of direction regarding career plans, increased motivation, and a sense of purpose. In the movie *Pay It Forward* (Reuther & Leder, 2000) a child's philosophy of life is that the world would be a better place if everyone tried to **pay it forward** by helping a stranger who would, in turn, help another. The results of this child's own generous gesture went far beyond his expectations. Ponder the possibilities if – instead of acts of kindness – the energy of inspiration were ignited in the classroom and passed on to students, then passed on again, and again. The effects of inspiration could become a vibrant and powerful force, reverberating to future nurses, igniting their dreams and energizing their healing touch.

## Learning Activities

"For each of us there are some moments and some teachers who were large in shaping our learning and our way of being. What they did and who they were served as catalysts for transformation and growth" (Hart, 2002, p. 6).

1. How has inspiration factored into your own transaction of learning? Reflect on your own education. Answer the following questions and make a personal connection to inspiration.
   - Think back through your own education. Don't limit yourself to just your college experience. Were any of your teachers inspirational?
   - Can you remember the names of your inspirational teachers?
   - What were the effects of being inspired?
   - Do you feel you are inspirational?
   - If yes, what are the effects of inspiration on others? Describe the effects and pay particular attention to the effect on your students.
   - Have your students write an essay on the "power of inspiration" and then engage in a discussion about it.
   - After reading this chapter, what ideas have you learned that you can use to create an inspirational environment?
2. How can you apply the above information to your teaching?

## Educational Philosophy

I believe in the importance of being able to motivate, enlighten, and inspire my students, thus creating a passion for learning. It is important to recognize that nursing students are adult, self-directed learners who excel in a nurturing, challenging, and supportive environment. Building rapport with my students is important to me and leads to increased communication during discussions in the classroom and on a one-to-one basis. This communication is vital in the teaching/learning process and in building relationships with my students. — Jeanette Rossetti

## References

Bass, B. M. (1985). *Leadership and performance beyond expectations*. New York: Free Press.

Bass. B. M. (1998). *Transformational leadership*. Mahwah, NJ: Lawrence Erlbaum Associates.

Brookfield, S. D. (2006). *The skillfull teacher*. (2nd ed.). San Francisco: Jossey-Bass.

Burke, R. W., & Nierenberg, I. (1998). In search of the inspirational in teachers and teaching. *Journal for a Just & Caring Education, 4*(3), 336-354.

Compact Oxford English Dictionary for Students. (2006). Oxford: Oxford University Press.

Council, M. (1988). Creating inspiration. *Journal of Creative Behavior, 22*(2), 123-131.

DePree, M. (2003). *Leading without power: Finding hope in serving community*. San Francisco: Jossey-Bass.

Duffy, G. G. (1992). Let's free teachers to be inspired. *Phi Delta Kappan, 73*(6), 442-447.

Fairholm, G. W. (1991). *Values leadership: Toward a new philosophy of leadership*. Westport, CT: Prager.

Fairholm, G. W. (1994). *Leadership and the culture of trust*. Westport, CT: Prager.

Goleman, D., Boyatzis, R. McKee, A. (2004). Primal leadership. Learning to lead with emotional intelligence. Boston: Harvard Business School Publishing.

Greene, M. (1978). *Landscapes of Learning*. New York: Teachers College Press.

Hart, T. R. (1993). Inspiration: An exploration of the experience and its role in healthy functioning. (Diss, University of Massachusetts, 1993). *Dissertation Abstracts International, 54*(2), 1077.

Hart, T. R. (1998). Inspiration: Exploring the experience and its meaning. *Journal of Humanistic Psychology, 38*(3), 7-35.

Hart, T. R. (2002). Little stories of large teachers. *Paths to Learning, 4*(13), 6-10.

Hooks, B. (1994). *Teaching to transgress*. New York: Routledge.

Judge, W. Q. (1999). *The leader's shadow: Exploring and developing executive character*. Thousand Oaks, CA: Sage Publications.

Kouzes, J. M., & Posner, B. Z. (1987). *The leadership challenge*. San Francisco: Jossey-Bass.

Kouzes, J. M., & Posner, B. Z. (1995). *The leadership challenge*. San Francisco: Jossey-Bass.

Ornish, D. (1996). *Dr. Dean Ornish's program for reversing heart disease*. New York: Ivy Books.

*The Oxford English Dictionary*. (2nd ed.). (1989). Oxford: Clarendon Press.

Palmer, P. J. (1998). *The courage to teach*. San Francisco: Jossey-Bass.

Reuther, S. (Producer), & Leder, M. (Director). (2000). *Pay it forward* [Motion Picture]. United States: Warner Brothers.

Yukl, G. A. (1994). *Leadership in organizations*. Engelwood Cliffs, NJ: Prentice Hall.

# CHAPTER 7

# DEFINING THE BOUNDARIES OF THE FACULTY-STUDENT RELATIONSHIP

## Christine M. Henshaw, EdD, RN, CNE

The content of this chapter relates to the following major content area and subconcepts on the Certified Nurse Educator Examination Detailed Test Blueprint:

**Pursue Continuous Quality Improvement in the Academic Nurse Educator Role**
- Engage in activities that promote one's socialization to the role
- Acquire knowledge of legal and ethical issues relevant to higher education and nursing education
- Engage in self-reflection and continued learning to improve teaching practices

## Introduction

*Professor Joan Hanson is an enthusiastic teacher who connects well with students. She is sensitive to the demands today's students face: family, work, and activities, on top of school assignments. Students appreciate that Professor Hanson is supportive and caring in her interactions with students. Student Elizabeth, who has been in several of Professor Hanson's classes, invites her professor to her wedding. Professor Hanson happily accepts, and plans to give Elizabeth, one of her favorite students, an extravagant wedding gift.*

Boundaries between nurses and patients are well-described in the nursing literature (Holder & Schenthal, 2007; Peternelj-Taylor & Yonge, 2003; Sheets, 2001). However, discussions about faculty-student boundaries have been virtually absent from the nursing literature. Many nursing faculty receive little preparation in appropriate boundaries with students. Situations arise regularly that call on faculty to make decisions about how to behave with students. When boundary situations arise, few clear guidelines exist to help faculty decide what to do.

# The Faculty-Student Relationship

## The Influence of the Teacher on the Student

Although learning is ultimately the responsibility of the learner, the teacher has significant influence on the learning process. The teacher's responsibility is to create an environment that supports and encourages learning to happen (Palmer, 1998). A large part of that environment is the relationship between the learner and the teacher. Classic research demonstrates that the connection students have with faculty outside of the classroom may be as significant as interactions during class. Staying in college, grades earned, and persistence to graduation are enhanced when students have opportunities to meet and get to know faculty beyond the classroom (Pascarella, 1980; Tinto, 1975, 1987).

In nursing, much emphasis has been placed on the student-teacher relationship. Twenty years ago, Bevis and Watson (1989) argued for a new pedagogy in nursing: a caring curriculum that addressed the needs of learners and promoted a supportive faculty role. In their view, an egalitarian relationship based on caring is essential to student learning.

This emphasis on the importance of the faculty-student relationship and on the need for a caring approach with students has the potential to raise questions about what is appropriate in teacher-student interactions. Without guidelines, faculty may be uncertain about how to approach these questions.

## A Fiduciary Relationship

Some identify the relationship between faculty and students as a fiduciary one. Although often used to describe financial relationships, the term **fiduciary** has been applied to relationships in which one party places trust in and depends on another (Gabbard & Nadelson, 1995; Plaut, 2008; Recupero, Cooney, Rayner, Heru, & Price, 2005). In addition, a power imbalance generally exists in a fiduciary relationship. The party that holds the trust of the other or who has more power in the relationship has a fiduciary responsibility to the other party.

Therapists (Strasburger, Jorgenson, & Sutherland, 1992), physicians, and social workers (Kutchins, 1991) have been identified as professionals who have a fiduciary relationship with their patients. The teacher-student relationship has also been identified as a fiduciary one (Feldman-Summers, 1989; Friedman & Boumil, 1995; Plaut, 2008). In academia, the student trusts the professor to promote a positive learning environment and to grade fairly based on the student's performance. In addition, despite efforts to equalize the power distribution between faculty and students, ultimately the professor retains the grading authority. Even if students assign their own grades, as may happen in some courses, the student may ultimately rely on the professor for a letter of recommendation that may mean getting a job or not, or getting into graduate school or not. Students rely on their professors to provide guidance, and they place their trust in their teachers to help shape their future lives and careers. These responsibilities meet the criteria of a fiduciary relationship.

## Boundaries

Boundaries differentiate one thing from another. Physical boundaries include such things as fences, walls, and skin. Invisible boundaries separate one state from another or one country from another. Psychological boundaries separate consciousness from unconsciousness. Interpersonal boundaries separate one person from another (Hartmann, 1997).

In professional relationships, boundaries help ensure the relationship remains a professional one and does not "spill over" into other types of relationships. For example, teachers have a particular role with students. The teacher role is not the same as the nursing role, even if the teacher happens to be a nurse. Teachers usually don't examine or bathe students or check students' blood sugar; those are nursing activities, not teaching activities. Although it would be highly unusual for a teacher to bathe a student, it might be appropriate for a nursing faculty member to measure the blood sugar of a student with diabetes mellitus who is experiencing signs and symptoms of hypoglycemia.

Other role distinctions may be less unambiguous. Just as the student-teacher relationship is not the same as the nurse-patient relationship, the student-teacher relationship is not the same as a financial or business relationship. Teachers typically do not sell to or buy things from students. Teachers do not usually loan money to, or borrow money from, students. Does that mean those actions never occur? Sometimes they do. Are those actions ethical or appropriate? Again, certain circumstances can be imagined when those actions might be appropriate. A teacher supervising a student at a clinical experience might loan money for lunch to the student who forgets his/her wallet. Others might argue that loaning money to a student would never be appropriate.

Perhaps the most difficult relationship to keep distinct from the student-teacher role is the social relationship. In interviews with senior nursing students, Yonge (2007) reported students recognized the need for faculty to be friendly with them, but not to be their friend. Finding that balance can be difficult. Boundaries can help teachers keep their roles straight.

Guthiel and Gabbard (1998) stated that boundaries identify "the 'edgc' of appropriate behavior" (p. 410). Appropriate behaviors fall on one side of the edge and inappropriate behaviors on the opposite side. Boundaries are necessary because of the inherent power differential in the professional-client relationship (Peterson, 1992). In addition, boundaries help separate the professional relationship from a personal or social one (Plaut, 1993). Boundaries help protect the client by defining appropriate behavior on the part of the professional (Gallop, 1998).

Boundary crossings are minor departures from normal practice. As noted above, taking the blood sugar of a student with diabetes mellitus is not a normal teacher behavior, but may be a reasonable departure from practice to meet the needs of the student. Boundary crossings typically are neutral or positive for the student. Boundary crossings do, however, often precede more serious boundary violations (Guthiel & Gabbard, 1998).

Boundary violations are more serious deviations from usual practice. Having sex with a current student is not a teacher behavior intended to benefit the student. It is a serious departure from usual teacher action that, at least in part, is designed to meet the needs of the teacher. True boundary violations usually have a negative impact on the students, and are frequently preceded by boundary crossings (Guthiel & Gabbard, 1998).

## Categories of Boundary Issues

Students are most comfortable with teacher behaviors that relate to the academic or professional role. Staying after class to answer a student's question, offering to write a letter of recommendation for a student, and even taking a group of students on a weekend trip related to a class were all seen as appropriate by introductory, undergraduate psychology students (Holmes, Rupert, Ross, & Shapera, 1999). Meeting off-campus to discuss student work, attending university events with a student, and calling a student at home about an issue related to school work were all viewed by general undergraduate students as acceptable behaviors (Owen & Zwahr-Castro, 2007).

Activities that involve groups are viewed by students as more appropriate than those that involve individual interaction with the professor outside the classroom (Ei & Bowen, 2002). Having lunch with a group of students, and even meals out that include alcohol are viewed as appropriate by some students. The issue of whether students should call professors by their first names or not got mixed reviews in studies of undergraduate students. The respondents in Ei & Bowen's survey believed that was appropriate. Those in Owen and Zwahr-Castro's study (2007) did not.

Entering into a business relationship with a student raises the potential for boundary issues. Hiring a student to babysit is seen by students as somewhat or very appropriate (Ei & Bowen, 2002; Owen & Zwahr-Castro, 2007). On the other hand, 44% of nursing faculty thought hiring a student to work for them was never appropriate (Henshaw, 2008).

Borrowing money from or loaning money to students was seen by students as problematic (Ei & Bowen, 2002). For some, borrowing from students was less acceptable than loaning to students (Owen & Zwahr-Castro, 2007). While 66.4% of nursing faculty believed that lending money to a student was appropriate at least under rare conditions (Henshaw, 2008), only 27.9% reported having done so (Henshaw, 2004).

Giving or accepting expensive gifts, talking about the professor's own personal problems, going to student parties unrelated to school activities, and inviting individual students to dinner were seen by students as inappropriate behaviors (Owen & Zwahr-Castro, 2007). These types of behaviors begin to blur the boundaries between a professional or academic relationship and a personal or social relationship.

Although undergraduate students in one study were clear that a personal friendship with a student is not appropriate (Owen & Zwahr-Castro, 2007), in qualitative written interviews of graduate students, Kolbert, Morgan, and Brendel (2002) found split views of friendships between teachers and students. Some students understood the personal relationship as a medium for learning. However, they noted that the relationship should be primarily for the student's benefit. Other students clearly disapproved of such relationships, citing issues of objectivity and fairness in evaluation, especially in regards to a potential favoritism that would result in a less positive assessment of other students. One student even noted that a personal relationship with a faculty member might result in an on-going expectation of preferred treatment on the part of the student. Students recognized the teacher-student relationship as one of unequal power and believed that it was the teacher's responsibility to avoid exploitation of the relationship. While students identified the unfair advantage they might have because of their special relationship with the teacher, faculty did not mention that effect of a relationship with one student on other students.

A different view of personal relationships between students and faculty depends on the context. In interviews with nursing students in their final nursing program clinical rotation that happened to be in a rural setting, students reported that the psychosocial process of forming a relationship with their clinical preceptor is what allowed them to take their final learning step on their way to being registered nurses (Yonge, 2007). Recognizing they would be evaluated by their preceptors prompted an understanding that the relationship needed to be a friendly one, but not one of being friends. One student noted that if the professional relationship crossed over into a friendship, the teacher's objectivity in evaluation might be jeopardized. In this setting, the author felt minor boundary crossings such as gift-giving and self-disclosure by preceptors were positive occurrences that assisted students in seeing the rural setting as a positive work environment.

The most extreme version of personal relationship is that of a dating or sexual relationship between student and teacher. Although prohibited by law for most kindergarten through twelfth-grade students, no laws exist regarding sex with most university students. As adults by law, some people believe that college students can enter into relationships with whomever they choose. While conceding that a power differential exists between teacher and student, and while acknowledging that a romantic relationship might lead to favoritism, Abramson (2007) argues that sexual relations with students are protected under the United States Constitution.

In terms of romantic or sexual relationships, graduate counseling students were mixed in their views (Kolbert et al., 2002). Some believed a sexual relationship with a professor was acceptable as long as the student would not be in a student relationship with the professor again. Others believed there would be a "residual inequitable power differential" (p. 202) that would preclude a relationship while the student was in the program, whether or not the student would be under the professor's supervision again. Faculty views were also mixed. Some believed a relationship would be equivalent to having a relationship with a patient, which would be unethical. Others believed that relationships with students were not covered by the American Counseling Association's guidelines about therapist-patient relationships, and, if consensual, were appropriate.

Most experts, however, place sex with students on a par with sex with patients and, therefore, out of bounds for professionals (Gabbard & Nadelson, 1995; Plaut, 2008; Recupero, et al., 2005). Students see sexual behaviors by teachers (flirting with students, asking students out on dates, having sexual relations with students) as significantly inappropriate (Ei & Bowen, 2002; Holmes et al., 1999; Owen & Zwahr-Castro, 2007). Teachers agree. Elementary through high school teachers found engaging in a romantic relationship with students to be a rare but serious breach of professional ethics (Barrett, Headley, Stovall, & Witte, 2006). A survey of nursing faculty revealed that 100% agreed that telling a student of a sexual attraction or becoming sexually involved with a current student was never appropriate (Henshaw, 2008). However, 36% of medical students report having had their personal space invaded to an uncomfortable extent by their supervisors and 30% report that a supervisor has dated a fellow medical student (Recupero et al., 2005). Although respondents reported supervisors were dating and having relationships with their classmates, none of them reported personally having a supervisor offer to have sex with him or her.

Even the notion of a consensual sexual relationship with a professor has been called into question. Although a student may feel at the time that a sexual relationship with a professor is not coerced, research demonstrates that perception changes with time (Hammel, Olkin, & Taube, 1996; Miller & Larrabee, 1995).

## Whose Job Is It?

The responsibility for maintaining appropriate boundaries always rests with the professional in the situation. Because of the inherent power differential in professional relationships, the students are often not in a position to advocate for themselves when boundaries are crossed. Depending on the nature of the relationship, it may be that the student does not even recognize that boundaries are an issue. It is up to the professional to safeguard the student's trust and to establish and maintain appropriate boundaries (Jacobs, 1991; Kagle & Giebelhausen, 1994; Kutchins, 1991; Peterson, 1992).

Students trust that professors will maintain the appropriate boundaries to safeguard the teacher relationship. They recognize the power differential that exists in the faculty-student relationship and rely on their faculty members to manage that power differential for them. As the party with the least power in the relationship, students are dependent on the party with the most power to protect students from harmful boundary violations. Clarifying boundaries and expectations in advance is one way to do that (Kolbert et al., 2002).

## Professional Standards

For faculty, multiple roles, such as teaching, advising, counseling, and mentoring, have the potential to make interactions with students confusing. In addition, the limits of the caring nature of the relationship between faculty and students have not been well defined. Existing professional codes of conduct provide some guidance for nursing faculty.

The American Association of University Professors' Statement on Professional Ethics (2007) provides guidelines for faculty in a variety of situations. In regards to relationships with students, the Statement notes, "As teachers, professors... respect the confidential nature of the relationship between professor and student.

They avoid any exploitation, harassment, or discriminatory treatment of students." Likewise, the National Education Association Code of Ethics (1975) states, in part, the educator, "shall not use professional relationships with students for private advantage; shall not disclose information about students obtained in the course of professional service unless disclosure serves a compelling professional purpose or is required by law; shall not accept any gratuity, gift, or favor that might impair or appear to influence professional decisions or action".

The American Nurses Association (ANA) Code of Ethics for Nurses describes the professional standards to which the nurse is held in terms of ethical behavior (ANA, 2001). The first article of the Code addresses the responsibility of the nurse to recognize the inherent dignity of every individual and to treat each individual with respect. Section 1.5 of the code extends that responsibility beyond patients to the individuals with whom the nurse interacts in whatever role the nurse is functioning. The educator role is explicitly identified as being within the scope of this code. Section 2.4 of the code notes that the nurse is responsible to establish limits and maintain boundaries in relationships nurses have with others. While recognizing the need for the nurse to be authentic and engaged with others, the code clearly places the responsibility for maintaining appropriate boundaries on the professional nurse.

Standards specifically designed to guide the actions of nurse educators are rare. The Washington State Nurse Practice Act, in the section prohibiting romantic and sexual relations between nurses and patients, includes a prohibition against such relationships between nursing students and faculty (Washington State Department of Health, 1999).

At the Nursing Education Summit of the National League for Nursing in 2008, a session proposing a code of ethics for nurse educators was held. The presenters provided an opportunity for discussion of such a code, and a draft code was offered. Although not scientific, the general consensus in the room seemed to be that such a code was needed. In a mailed survey of nurse educators in one state, 75% of respondents indicated they believed nursing faculty would support of code of conduct for nursing faculty (Henshaw, 2008).

Development of a universal code of conduct may be difficult. Many boundary issues are contextual (Yonge, 2007). As noted by students, behaviors that occur individually with a faculty member are viewed differently than those that occur in a group (Ei & Bowen, 2002). The age and level of the student, as well as the age of the faculty member may influence the appropriateness of a personal relationship (Kolbert et al., 2002). However, apart from any established code, some guidelines for faculty emerge from the literature.

# Summary

Let's look again at Professor Hanson, introduced at the beginning of the chapter. Should Professor Hanson give her student that gift? Six questions can be used to guide her decision. Depending on the situation, some or all of the questions might apply, and Professor Hanson should focus on the questions that have the most relevance in her situation.

1. **What does my profession say about this situation?** Professor Hanson should look at the existing codes of ethics for teachers and nurses, such as those published by the American Nurses Association, the American Association of University Professors, and the National Education Association. In addition, Professor Hanson should review the nurse practice act for her state. Finally, her college or university, or her department, may have some published guidelines to help her decide.

2. **Is this what teachers do?** This question can help teachers decide if they are blurring the boundaries between the academic role and other roles, such as personal or business relationships. Although boundary crossings, deviations from usual practice, may be appropriate in some situations, teachers should always stop and consider if their situation is one of those times.

3. **Am I willing to tell someone else what I'm doing?** If the teacher is uncomfortable sharing her proposed action with colleagues, there is reason to question the action. Secrecy in relationships with patients or students is often a signal that something untoward is happening. In fact, in situations where a professor is unsure what to do, asking colleagues can provide valuable insight into the decision-making process.

4. **What can go wrong and happens if something does go wrong?** What if the student's performance falters and the teacher has to assign a failing grade? Is the teacher willing to take that step, if warranted, despite development of a personal, social, or sexual relationship? In undertaking a business or financial relationship with a student, what happens if something goes wrong? Am I able to maintain objectivity if I purchase a used car from a student that quits running a week after the purchase? If, in the financial planning business I have on the side, I sell a student a stock that plummets in price, am I willing to risk the student's unhappiness?

5. **Am I aware of the power differential between the student and myself?** The power differential between faculty and students exists, regardless of our efforts to minimize it and to equalize the teacher-student relationship. Ignoring that power difference moves us toward inadvertently violating it.

6. **Whose needs are being met?** As in all fiduciary relationships, the needs of the student must be protected. As the party with the least power, the student must be guarded against inappropriate actions by the professional. Faculty who are fulfilling their own needs for social contacts, friendships, or business clients are putting their own needs ahead of the student's. It is always the professional's responsibility to ensure appropriate boundaries are set and that the student's needs are kept uppermost in the relationship. Professionals who fail to do this will move into boundary transgressions.

Professor Hanson has a choice to make. Although it might seem clear cut to some, for others, the choice is fuzzier. A nursing faculty member who lives in a small town will encounter friends or the children of friends in her classes. If this is the case with Elizabeth, a special wedding gift might be in order. If Elizabeth is a doctoral student whom Professor Hanson has been mentoring, a case might be made that this is an example of a boundary crossing, not a boundary violation. For most faculty teaching in undergraduate programs, an extravagant gift for Elizabeth changes the nature of the teacher-student relationship, putting Elizabeth at risk for unrealistic expectations from Professor Hanson, and Professor Hanson at risk for charges of unfairness from Elizabeth's classmates. Clear professional boundaries can help Professor Hanson make a wise choice in this and in every situation.

## Learning Activities

1. Meet with other nursing faculty. Consider hypothetical situations and apply the six questions listed under the Summary section of this chapter.
2. Think back over your own teaching experience or interview an experienced teacher. Have there been occasions that may be of concern relative to boundary issues? If so, how would they be handled?
3. Consider the policies at the school that you attend or in which you teach. Do any of the policies relate to teacher/student boundaries?

## Educational Philosophy

I view teaching as an opportunity to create an environment in which students are best able to learn and then to let them do the learning. Respect for students as individuals, knowledge of the field and expected competencies of graduates, and careful preparation of teaching sessions are essential foundations for teaching, along with a willingness to let the teaching and learning go where it needs to go that day to make the most of teachable moments. — Christine M. Henshaw

## References

Abramson, P. R. (2007). *Romance in the ivory tower: The rights and liberty of conscience*. Cambridge, MA: The MIT Press.

American Association of University Professors. (2007). *Statement on professional ethics*. Retrieved November 1, 2008, from http://www.aaup.org/AAUP/pubsres/policydocs/contents/statementonprofessionalethics.htm

American Nurses Association. (2001). *Code of ethics for nurses with interpretive statements*. Washington, DC: Author.

Barrett, D. E., Headley, K. N., Stovall, B., & Witte, J. C. (2006). Teachers' perceptions of the frequency and seriousness of violations of ethical standards. *Journal of Psychology, 140*(5), 421-433.

Bevis, E. O., & Watson, J. (1989). *Toward a caring curriculum: A new pedagogy for nursing*. New York: National League for Nursing.

Ei, S., & Bowen, A. (2002). College students' perceptions of student-instructor relationships. *Ethics & Behavior, 12*(2), 177-190.

Feldman-Summers, S. (1989). Sexual contact in fiduciary relationships. In G. O. Gabbard (Ed.), *Sexual exploitation in professional relationships* (pp. 193-209). Washington, DC: American Psychiatric Press.

Friedman, J., & Boumil, M. M. (1995). Betrayal of trust: Sex and power in professional relationships. Westport, CT: Praeger.

Gabbard, G. O., & Nadelson, C. (1995). Professional boundaries in the physician-patient relationship. *Journal of the American Medical Association, 273*, 1445-1449.

Gallop, R. (1998). Abuse of power in the nurse-client relationship. *Nursing Standard, 12*(37), 43-47.

Gillespie, M. (2002). Student-teacher connection in clinical nursing education. *Journal of Advanced Nursing, 37*(6), 566-576.

Gutheil, T. G., & Gabbard, G. O. (1998). Misuses and misunderstandings of boundary theory in clinical and regulatory settings. *American Journal of Psychiatry, 155*(3), 409-414.

Hammel, G. A., Olkin, R., & Taube, D. O. (1996). Student-educator sex in clinical and counseling psychology doctoral training. *Professional Psychology: Research and Practice, 27*(1), 93-97.

Hartmann, E. (1997). The concept of boundaries in counseling and psychology. *British Journal of Guidance & Counseling, 25*(2), 147-162.

Henshaw, C. M. (2004). Boundary issues between faculty and students in associate degree nursing programs (Doctoral dissertation, Seattle University, 2004). *Dissertation Abstracts International, 65*, 157.

Henshaw, C. M. (2008). Faculty-student boundaries in associate degree nursing programs. *Journal of Nursing Education, 47*(9), 409-416.

Holder, K. V., & Schenthal, S. J. (2007). Watch your step: Nursing and professional boundaries. *Nursing Management, 38*(2), 24-30.

Holmes, D. L., Rupert, P. A., Ross, S. A., & Shapera, W. E. (1999). Student perception of dual relationships between faculty and students. *Ethics & Behavior, 9*(2), 79-107.

Jacobs, C. (1991). Violations of the supervisory relationship: An ethical and educational blind spot. *Social Work, 36*(2), 130-135.

Kagle, J. D., & Giebelhausen, P. N. (1994). Dual relationships and professional boundaries. *Social Work, 39*(2), 213-220.

Kolbert, J. B., Morgan, B., & Brendel, M. M. (2002). Faculty and student perceptions of dual relationships within counselor education: A qualitative analysis. *Counselor Education & Supervision, 41*, 193-206.

Kutchins, H. (1991). The fiduciary relationship: The legal basis for social workers' responsibilities to clients. *Social Work, 36*, 106-113.

Miller, G. M., & Larrabee, M. J. (1995). Sexual intimacy in counselor education and supervision: A national survey. *Counselor Education and Supervision, 34*(4), 332-343.

National Education Association. (1975). *Code of ethics of the education profession.* Retrieved November 1, 2008, from http://www.nea.org/aboutnea/code.html

Owen, P. R., & Zwahr-Castro, J. (2007). Boundary issues in academia: Student perceptions of faculty-student boundary crossings. *Ethics & Behavior, 17*(2), 117-129.

Palmer, P. (1998). *The courage to teach.* San Francisco: Jossey-Bass

Pascarella, E. T. (1980). Student-faculty informal contact and college outcomes. *Review of Educational Research, 50*(4), 545-595.

Peternelj-Taylor, C. A., & Yonge, O. (2003). Exploring boundaries in the nurse-client relationship: Professional roles and responsibilities. *Perspectives in Psychiatric Care, 39*(2), 55-66.

Peterson, M. R. (1992). *At personal risk: Boundary violations in professional-client relationships.* New York: W. W. Norton.

Plaut, S. M. (1993). Boundary issues in teacher-student relationships. *Journal of Sex & Marital Therapy, 19*(3), 210-219.

Plaut, S. M. (2008). Sexual and nonsexual boundaries in professional relationships: Principles and teaching guidelines. *Sexual and Relationship Therapy, 23*(1), 85-94.

Recupero, P. R., Cooney, M. C., Rayner, C., Heru, A. M., & Price, M. (2005). Supervisor-trainee relationship boundaries in medical education. *Medical Teacher, 27*(6), 484-488.

Sheets, V. R. (2001). Teach nurses how to maintain professional boundaries, recognize potential problems, and make better patient care decisions. *Nursing Management, 20*(5), 36-40.

Strasburger, L. H., Jorgenson, L., & Sutherland, P. (1992). The prevention of psychotherapist sexual misconduct: Avoiding the slippery slope. *American Journal of Psychotherapy, 46,* 544-555.

Tinto, V. (1975). Dropout from higher education: A theoretical synthesis of recent research. *Review of Educational Research, 45*(1), 89-125.

Tinto, V. (1987). *Leaving college: Rethinking the causes and cures of student attrition.* Chicago: University of Chicago Press.

Washington State Department of Health. (1999). Rules update. *The Nursing Commission Newsletter, 5*(1), 6-8.

Yonge, O. (2007). Preceptorship rural boundaries: Student perspective. *Online Journal of Rural Nursing and Health Care, 7*(1), 5-12.

# CHAPTER 8

# EVIDENCE-BASED NURSING EDUCATION

## Cathleen M. Shultz, PhD, RN, CNE, FAAN

The content of this chapter relates to the following major content areas and subconcepts on the Certified Nurse Educator Examination Detailed Test Blueprint:

**Facilitate learning**
- Use teaching strategies based on: educational theory; evidence-based practices related to education
- Use knowledge of evidence-based practice to instruct learners

**Use Assessment and Evaluation Strategies**
- Incorporate current research in assessment and evaluation practices

**Pursue Continuous Quality Improvement in the Academic Nurse Educator Role**
- Demonstrate a commitment to lifelong learning

**Engage in Scholarship of Teaching**
- Exhibit a spirit of inquiry about teaching and learning, student development, and evaluation methods
- Use evidence-based resources to improve and support teaching

## Introduction

No substantial change can occur in education without a substantial change in the thinking of educators. Richard Paul, 1993

For decades, nursing education programs produced millions of nursing graduates who delivered quality nursing care. However, the delivery of health care is now quite different and there are strong national and emerging global trends that continue rapid changes. One of the strongest change proponents comes from the Institute of Medicine's (IOM) call for a major overhaul of the education of all health professionals (2003). One of IOM's goals is the preparation of graduates with the ability to engage in Evidence-based Practice (EBP). EBP includes the integration of research findings into one's clinical practice with the health beliefs and practices that the patient values to attain optimum care (p. 46).

Another national proponent is the Quality and Safety Education for Nurses (QSEN) (2008) movement for safety in clinical facilities. Also the Workforce Nursing Education Summit, held in June 2008, is a multi-sponsored 3 year project to increase faculty and student capacity; at the time of this publication, 18 states are participating. To meet these challenges, the nursing educational systems must dramatically change to accomplish the goals outlined by groups such as IOM (Finkelman & Kenner, 2007), the Magnet Program and its Forces of Magnetism (McClure & Henshaw, 2002), QSEN, Health Resources and Services Administration (HRSA), and Workforce Development efforts by the U.S. Department of Labor which lead to better health outcomes through quality nursing care. The content of these movements are essential to nursing practice and therefore require skilled nurse educators with a solid evidence-base for their work. See the CD accompanying this book for additional information on the Institute of Medicine's recommendations and how to use them in nursing education.

Nursing faculty must review what they are teaching, how they are teaching, and clearly determine relevant learning outcomes. There are national guidelines that provide direction for nursing faculty as curriculum is revised and innovations in curriculum models are explored and implemented (Halstead, 2007). The thinking of nurse educators centers on the daily practice of teaching and facilitation of learning and outcomes attainment. As a result, nurse educators are challenged to develop a science of nursing education and to engage in evidence-based teaching practices as driving forces of professional development.

Nursing education is exciting and challenging. Despite the complexities of the educator role, nursing faculty have embraced those challenges and sought methods to deepen their understanding and use of the educational process, also known as the teaching-learning process. One of those methods was use of evidence-based findings in teaching. Although nursing education studies were the majority of research publications produced by early nurse researchers, these efforts were all but abandoned as evidence-based research focusing on nursing practice, rather than education, dominated nursing's research focus. The shift from education to practice-based research began in the 1970s. Abandonment of nursing education's research roots was due to numerous reasons including researchers' limited knowledge of the research process and studies; this continued until the mid-1990s and then gained steadily in rigor, depth, design, methods, sample selection, instruments, complexity, evaluation, and funding. However much remains to be accomplished.

Today, nursing education research is stronger than ever. Several nursing organizations such as the National League for Nursing and Community Health Nurse Educators maintained and promoted the need for nursing education and nurse educator development as major missions. For example, the National League for Nursing has current nursing education priority research themes on its website (www.nln.org). More information is available on the CD accompanying this book. See Table 1.

## 1. Innovations in Nursing Education: Creating Reform
- New pedagogies
- Use of instructional technology, including new approaches to laboratory/simulated learning
- Flexible curriculum designs
- Community-driven models for curriculum development
- Processes for reforming nursing education
- Educational systems and infrastructures
- Student/teacher learning partnerships
- Community-based nursing and service learning strategies
- Clinical teaching models
- Teaching evidence-based practice
- New models for teacher preparation and faculty development, particularly as they relate to minority faculty and preparation for teaching diverse student populations

## 2. Research in Nursing Education: Evaluating Reform
- Economics of and productivity in nursing education
- Quality improvement processes
- Program evaluation models
- Student and teacher experiences in schools of nursing
- Evaluating the success of diverse student populations
- Nursing education innovations, including facilitators and barriers to innovation and reform
- Best practices in schooling, teaching, and learning
- Grading, testing and evaluation of students, faculty and curricula

## 3. Development of the Science of Nursing Education: Evidence-Based Reform
- Best practices in schooling, teaching, and learning
- Nursing education database development
- Strategies supportive of nursing education researchers
- Validation of key concepts and keywords related to evidence-based teaching practices
- Meta-analysis related to innovation or evaluation in nursing education
- Concept analysis related to innovation or evaluation in nursing education

**Table 1.** NLN's Priorities for Research in Nursing Education (2008)

# What is Evidence-Based Teaching?

There is a growing body of evidence-based information about teaching and learning. While there are gaps in what we need to know and study designs need to include larger numbers of participants, longer time, and multiple sites to strengthen the relevance of findings, there are sufficient, although weak, findings to support the practice of nurse educators (Shultz, 2009). Nurse educators are encouraged to participate in and sustain relevant nursing education research.

Evidence-based teaching (EBT) merges the best available research findings with personal teaching expertise. To develop as a nurse educator means adopting the attitude and learning activities of a lifelong learner. The nurse educator has at least two areas of development focus: the nurse educator focus and the nursing practice focus. This chapter highlights the nurse educator's focus for the development of evidence-based teaching.

Differentiating between the common term of "research utilization" and EBT is important. Although the terms are used interchangeably in the nursing literature, and there are clear similarities, the terms are not fully the same. Those involved in EBP have differentiated between the terms and their differentiation provides relevance to EBT. Research utilization is "the use of findings from a disciplined study or sets of studies in a practical application that is unrelated to the original research" (Polit & Beck, 2004). Research utilization begins with a topic or concept and seeks how to best integrate the concept into teaching practices. EBT begins with a practical problem and seeks how to solve that teaching or learning problem based upon the evidence provided by quality research (Muir-Gray, 1997).

For example a teacher wants to find and use best-practices research findings to teach students about assessing the pain of a patient with dementia (Horgas & Miller, 2008). He obtains exemplars from synthesized research findings (research utilization) and designs and conducts a four semester study to compare 2 different teaching strategies to learner success in assessing pain of patients with dementia (evidence-based teaching development).

# A Model for Building a Science of Nursing Education

In 2003, a National League for Nursing task force of nurse educators developed the Building a Science of Nursing Education Model which is available in publications (Shultz, 2009). The model depicts areas of research engagement for nurse educators and provides a comprehensive view of how a nurse educator could participate in building the nursing education science.

The central point of the model is building a science of nursing education which is an imperative. Developed by the NLN Task Group on Teaching and Learning in 2003, the task group worked seven years to synthesize and summarize published nursing education research (Shultz, 2009). Fourteen steps were identified and could be done in succession or collaboration. The nurse educator could participate in the collective building of a nursing education science at any number of steps such as "testing and applying research findings," "identifying gaps in knowledge," and "integrating and synthesizing research." The model is complex. However, it encourages the education research work of nurse educators at any point in their professional development. In addition, the task group compiled their findings into a book organized to give a foundation and guidance to emerging and seasoned nursing education researchers.

Every faculty member can contribute to the science of nursing education development by searching for evidence to support teaching strategies and evaluation methods used in their courses. Conferring with colleagues regarding knowledge gaps when evidence is not found prompts dialog and areas for potential research.

Each faculty member or group of faculty may benefit from quality discussions about the science building model and how it may be integrated into their day-to-day activities. Schools and groups could adopt a niche, or step of the model, and provide leadership within the nursing education community in a specific area.

The comprehensive work of this task group of nurse educators found many studies conducted in nursing education but the foundation for building a science remains weak. The book (Shultz, 2009) is a compendium of nurse educator research. The chapter authors and other nurse educators noted that replicated studies are lacking, one time studies dominate, most studies are descriptive or evaluative in nature, sample sizes were often small, and measurement instruments were frequently researcher-developed, used in only one study, and often lacked validity or reliability. Finally, the review found most studies were completed in one school, on one type of program and often with homogeneous populations, which limits the generalizability of findings (Shultz, 2009).

The total picture is not, however, doom and gloom. The science of nursing education is emerging. Historically, the science of nursing practice took diligence and cooperative efforts. Only after 30 years were dominant results able to significantly impact practice. Nurse educators can learn much from the development of science that occurred in the practice sector. Those insights can produce a science of nursing education more expeditiously.

## Nurse Educator Paradigm Shift

The shift from doing "what was" to supporting one's actions with evidence-based findings, represents a paradigm shift in education and practice as noted by Polit and Beck (2004). Although the EBP movement in practice follows stricter procedures and protocols, and has a larger pool of research studies, the evidence-based teaching and learning movement is entering a more mature phase. The nursing evidence-based teaching and learning movement will strengthen as the body of research grows and as interdisciplinary research concerning learning (i.e. neuroscience, brain-based learning, multiple intelligence) is integrated into the advance practice of nursing educators.

So where does the nurse educator begin? If the nurse educator is fortunate to work in an environment that embraces and supports faculty scholarship, faculty development on the role of educator, and use of evidence-based teaching and learning, then most of the infrastructure is in place to implement short and long-term career goals. If not, the nurse educator can initiate personal goals that address evidence-based teaching and learning. The important strategy is to begin.

Using evidence-based findings is often intimidating to the new nurse educator or the educator who has had no formal preparation as an educator. However, those nurse educators with research knowledge may apply that knowledge to the evidence-based aspect of their educator development. Becoming skilled at locating, critiquing, and synthesizing evidence becomes paramount for the nurse educator building a scholarly evidence-based practice.

## Synthesis of the Literature

Finding relevant published information about a chosen topic can be daunting. A comprehensive literature search is needed followed by formally critiquing publications for quality, relevance, and usefulness. Not all published research is usable. Peer reviewed journals ensure that expert colleagues have reviewed the findings prior to publication. Some findings may conflict with others and some studies are not replicable, therefore useful only to the group under study.

## Locating the Evidence

With the growth in databases and publications, the best way to find relevant literature is a search using one or more online databases. A long standing nursing database is the Cumulative Index of Nursing and Allied Health Literature (CINAHL). More databases important for nursing education research findings are on the CD accompanying this book. Most colleges have access to these databases but it does take training and time to search successfully. Librarians, especially a reference librarian, can be very helpful to maintain currency about databases.

Although electronic databases are very useful, a caution is urged. The databases are not comprehensive. In a recent 7 year study (Shultz, 2009), a further database complication was unveiled for nurse educators. Most nursing education search terms are not present in existing databases or the same search term changed over time in the database, making retrieval of nursing education studies very difficult. For example, the affective learning term "values" was searchable using the term "values" or "values clarification" in the 1970s and 1980s; the "values clarification" search term no longer exits and "values" now are most likely associated with "ethics". Search terms are chosen by authors and editors to categorize studies and a common education search-term language has not been standardized between them or between them and the database owners and mangers. Two tips are worth noting: find a reference librarian to assist in this maze of studies and always review the reference list of a published manuscript. Invaluable additional studies may be located there and they are often not categorized in the search terms. Technology has opened many sources for retrieving findings but in areas such as nursing education research, it has complicated the process.

Two findings by Shultz (2009) and colleagues may be of assistance:
1. Many educationally focused studies were located in the *Annual Review of Nursing Education* series (published by Springer) which began in 2003. These studies were not located in the electronic databases thus supporting the need to hand search the series.
2. Some of the best nursing education studies were found in nurse educators' doctoral dissertations; many results have not been published or studied further and the designs could be replicated.

There are journals which specifically publish nursing education research studies. Examples of the journals are highlighted in Table 2. Purchasing a subscription to one or more of these journals is a way to maintain currency in nursing education research knowledge and trends. Many full text articles from these journals are available through electronic databases.

| Journal |
| --- |
| International Journal of Nursing Education Scholarship |
| Journal of Nursing Education |
| Journal of Nursing Scholarship |
| Journal of Professional Nursing |
| Nurse Education in Practice |
| Nurse Educator |
| Nursing Education Perspectives |

**Table 2.** Journals Publishing Nursing Education Research*

*Note: Some interdisciplinary and other health disciplines journals publish nursing education research.

## Educational Research Studies

The quality of a research study's design and the usability of its findings are essential. Knowledge of research methodologies is foundational to scrutinizing a study. Most nursing education studies are categorized into two types labeled qualitative and quantitative.

- Qualitative research seeks meaning of events such as students' reaction to a clinical experience or a specific teaching strategy.
- Quantitative research explores cause and effect relationships such as the relationship of an active teaching strategy to the learner's academic success.

No one type is preferred, but the type must match the intent and purposes of the design.

A quantitative study is recommended to have the following components:

- A well-defined purpose with clear operational definitions.*
- A large heterogeneous sample (to prevent results being affected by race or gender) chosen by a clear sampling procedure.
- Multiple research sites to reduce the probability that an effect is due to location or culture.
- Participants who are randomly assigned to experimental or control groups to reduce the effects of confounding variables on the results and to equally distribute variances between the groups.

The asterisked (*) item is also recommended for qualitative studies which tend to have smaller samples. The study design must match the accepted research standards for the type of research; these standards may be found in any research book.

A meta-analysis is a research strategy to summarize multiple studies investigating similar interventions and outcomes. The strategy creates a larger "sample size" to indicate trends. Although common in the nursing literature, the process is complicated. The reader is referred to http://www.edres.org/meta/ for further information.

Qualitative studies have synthesis models (Noblit & Hare, 1989) which are infrequently used. Again the key is ensuring the correct research design is used to address the study's purpose and question or concern.

Lastly, nurse educators have many ways to learn teaching strategies and foster learner success. While EBT is a growing major element of the nurse educator's knowledge and professional development, experiences with students and colleagues in various contexts play a role in determining the best teaching strategy and measures of its success. It is important that student and colleague knowledge and information garnered from the setting are included with the research findings in making teaching and evaluation decisions. Cost effectiveness should also be a consideration especially during times of economic hardships on program budgets and faculty availability.

## Evaluation of Research for Usability

Explicit guidelines for determining the appropriateness of including a research study into one's teaching is beyond the purpose of this text. However, the Agency for Healthcare Research and Quality (AHRQ) reviewed existing methods to assess the strength of research evidence. The AHRQ summary found over 100 methods of review, which did find conflicting results when applied to studies. However their report (available at http://www.ahrq.gov/clinic/epcsums/strengthsum.pdf), described essential review concepts which are provided for various types of research designs.

An additional source is a research text which offers critique guidance for research studies.

Review the research articles with a research textbook or other review rubric open to the chapter on analyzing or critiquing research studies. Excellent research evaluation frameworks are Ross-Wurm and Larrabee's (1999) or a research evaluation checklist found in the *American Journal of Critical Care*, Sept. 2002 issue. The *Journal of Orthopedic Nursing* prints excellent, short briefs to assist in recognizing quality research studies.

Not including a clear question or hypothesis may have resulted from an editorial decision, but unclear operational definitions of concepts or limited descriptions of measurement methodology creates suspicion about the study's validity and ultimately limits its replicability. A serious study limitation occurs when the findings are only applicable to the study's sample and therefore have limited relevance outside a course or program. For example, a teaching strategy which demonstrates increased test scores and student satisfaction within a course, has limited generalization to other courses and programs when any of the following occurs:

- The sample's characteristics are inadequately described.
- The teaching strategy has no operational definition but it has a vague label such as "active learning strategy".
- The measurement of "student satisfaction" was unclear and the time of measurement was not included.
- The research covered one semester which raises doubts about confounding variables affecting outcomes.

## Implementing EBT in the Educational Setting

Following personal desire to utilize EBT in a nurse educator position, the most important element is administrative support. Unless this occurs, the cultural climate will not change effectively and value EBT as a vital part of nursing education. For EBT to thrive, the best work environment provides funds, recognition, support staff, and supplies for nursing education research. Time release may be needed and involved leaders create opportunities along a continuum from a partial or full course workload release to a sabbatical. Collaboration among the nursing faculty to conduct relevant educational research shares research responsibilities and potentially can strengthen the faculty's research abilities. Collegial efforts bring vitality and energy to group members who choose to work together. The strengths of each member contribute to professional development and improved research outcomes.

Recognition of nurse educator expertise is important. The National League for Nursing (NLN) developed a valid and reliable academic nurse educator examination for national certification as a Certified Nurse Educator (CNE). Certified nurse educators now number over 1,000 nurses from all fifty states. The NLN also recognizes noted nurse educators, including nursing education researchers, through the Academy of Nurse Education Fellow (ANEF). The ANEF inducted its first fellows in 2007. The newest CNEs and ANEFs are listed in *Nursing Education Perspectives* (2008, p. 257, 264-265). Visit the NLN website at www.nln.org for more information on these two initiatives.

Organizational change may include restructuring workloads to accommodate research and encouragement of faculty, staff, and students to use the new findings as well as how to find the evidence themselves. Access is crucial and quality library databases are essential. Practice strategies such as work groups, forums, and research reviews (Steller, et al. 1998); and journal clubs, research posters for local and conference presentations, and sending pertinent research articles to key personnel within a program (Rutledge & Donaldson, 1995) all have relevance to changing an education culture. Sustaining the changed culture involves initiating recognition programs such as those by the NLN mentioned earlier, adjusting rank and promotion criteria, revising committee guidelines, addressing job descriptions, and revamping the annual review process and goals to include personal development in the use of educational research. Boyer's (1990) Model of Scholarship is widely used across disciplines and offers one framework for educator related organizational change.

## Nurse Educator Competencies

Parallel to using and conducting nursing education research is attaining nurse educator competence. The nationally recognized work of the NLN's Task Group on Nurse Educator Competencies was published in 2005. The competencies stimulated a positive impact on their use for nurse educator preparation and development. They served as a test blueprint for the NLN's certification examination for nurse educators. Eight core competencies help define roles and responsibilities of nurse educators in various educational contexts thus promoting retention and recruitment efforts. Crucial to doctoral students, the competencies are being used to further determine knowledge, skills, and attitudes nurse educators need to effectively teach learners to practice in current, complex, healthcare settings (Halstead, 2007). The book is a helpful resource for scholarship development related to the nurse educator's practice. Competencies related to the content are listed on the first page of the chapter to help demonstrate application of these competencies to all the topics discussed in this book.

Two competencies, Pursue Continuous Quality Improvement in the Academic Nurse Educator Role and Engage in Scholarship, are especially relevant to evidence-based teaching. "These competencies are foundational to achieving excellence in nursing education and for building a science of nursing education. They guide faculty in designing and initiating innovations in nursing education so that transformation occurs in the way individuals are prepared for their roles and lives as nurses" (Valiga, 2007, p. 173).

## Summary

Nurse educators are faced with national challenges to update and develop relevant curriculums while creating and engaging their own professional development as scholars. Resources were presented in this chapter to assist nurse educators to contribute to building a science of nursing education and participate in their development as scholars. External resources from major organizations such as the IOM, NLN, and QSEN were discussed and samples offered to guide use of evidence-based teaching. Changing the nursing education infrastructure to support evidence-based teaching was encouraged to further sustain nurse educator development as a nurse scholar.

Competence in locating the literature, evaluating the research for usability, and implementing EBT in one's teaching and evaluation was discussed. NLN's nurse educator competencies (Halsted, 2005), Building the Science of Nursing Education Model (Shulz, 2009), and Educational Research Priorities (NLN, 2008) were reviewed to provide direction in becoming a nurse scholar who develops an evidence-based teaching practice.

EBT is essential to the scholarship role of nurse faculty. EBT is more important than ever to teach various students, engage complicated technology into teaching, and ensure the best teaching practices are engaged.

The requisite questions to ask about nursing education are limitless at this point in our science development. However, we can build on that science deliberately, systematically, and efficiently by asking relevant questions, disseminating findings of the investigations broadly, and applying the findings in our everyday teaching practices. In addition, each of us must join the journey and contribute in some way (Valiga, 2009).

## Learning Activities

1. Consider a teaching strategy of interest to you. Review the literature on that topic. Is there a best-practice guideline for this strategy? If not, can you draw on the literature to establish one?
2. Discuss how you might contribute to the science of nursing education. What topics would most interest you and how would you go about research them?
3. Visit the NCSBN.org website. Access the paper on Evidence-Based Teaching for Regulation. How does this relate to you as a nurse educator? Would you be able to use any of the guidelines contained in that paper? If so, how?

## Educational Philosophy

The most effective nurses skillfully create evidence-based nursing practices that embrace evidence-based nursing education (EBNE). The latter has reemerged as a valued, integral foundation to what we do. I believe that nurse educators are consumers and developers of evidence-based nursing education. Teachers and learners are partners in learning. We must embed the vision and demonstrate effective use of EBNE to prepare future nurses and successfully impact our nation's health issues. Our teaching heritage has depth and breadth. Our nation's health is dependent upon building the science of nursing education. — Cathleen M. Shultz

## References

Boyer, E. L. (1990). *Scholarship reconsidered: Priorities of the professoriate*. Princeton, NJ: The Carnegie Foundation for the Advancement of Teaching.

Finkelman, A., &. Kenner, C. (2007). *Teaching IOM: Implication of the IOM reports for nursing education*. Silver Spring, MD: American Nurses Association.

Halstead, J. (Ed.). (2007). *Nurse educator competencies: Creating an evidence-based practice for nurse educators*. New York: National League for Nursing.

Horgas, A., & Miller, L. (2008). Pain assessment in people with dementia. *American Journal of Nursing, 108*(7), 62-71.

Institute of Medicine, Committee on Health Professions Education Summit. (2003). *Health professions education: A bridge to quality (Quality Chasm Series)*. Washington, DC: The National Academies Press.

Muir-Gray, J. A. (1997). *Evidence based healthcare*. New York: Churchill Livingstone.

National League for Nursing. (2005). *Core competencies of nurse educators with task statements*. [Online]. Available: http://www.nln.org/facultydevelopment/pdf/corecompetencies.pdf

National League for Nursing. (2006). *Excellence in nursing education model*. New York: Author.

National League for Nursing. (2008). *Priorities for research in nursing education*. [Online]. Available: http://www.nln.org/research/priorities.htm

Noblit, G. W. & Hare, R. D. (1988). *Meta-ethnography: Synthesizing qualitative research studies*. London: Sage.

Polit, D. F., & Beck, C. T. (2004). *Nursing research: Principles and methods* (7th ed.). Philadelphia: Lippincott Williams & Wilkins.

Rutledge, D. N., & Donaldson, N. E. (1995). Building organizational capacity to engage in research utilization. *The Journal of Nursing Administration, 25*(10), 12-16.

Stetler, C. B., Brunell, M., Giuliano, K. K., Morsi, D., Prince, L., & Newell-Stokes, V. (1998). Evidence-based practice and the role of nursing leadership. *The Journal of Nursing Administration, 28*(7-8), 45-53.

Shultz, C. M. (Ed.). (2009). *Building a science of nursing education: Foundation for evidence-based teaching-learning*. New York: National League for Nursing.

Valiga, T. (2007). Creating an evidence-based practice for nurse educators. In J. Halstead, (Ed.). (2007). *Nurse educator competencies: Creating an evidence-based practice for nurse educators*. New York: National League for Nursing.

# CHAPTER 9

# ACTION RESEARCH TO DEVELOP EVIDENCE-BASED TEACHING

## Enid A. Rossi, MSN, EdD, RN

---

The content of this chapter relates to the following major content area and subconcepts on the Certified Nurse Educator Examination Detailed Test Blueprint:
**Pursue Continuous Quality Improvement in the Academic Nurse Educator Role**
- Demonstrate a commitment to lifelong learning
- Select professional development activities to continue to grow and evolve in the role
- Engage in self-reflection and continued learning to improve teaching practices

---

## Introduction

Individual, reflective action research is a method for identifying and using components of best practices that fit each unique practice situation. Nursing faculty are constantly confronted with changing role expectations and contexts. Schools' professional development programs often do not allow nurse educators to determine best practices for themselves because nurse educators' special knowledge is learned through inquiry and participation in their unique practices (Fullan, 2001; O'Toole, 1995). Action research involves a systematic study of a practice situation carried out by professionals involved in these situations so they may improve both practice and quality of understanding.

Burbules and Callister (2000), Privateer (1999), Skiba (1997), and Carnevale and Descrochers (1997) wrote that faculty are facing challenges presented by increasing class size, burgeoning financial burdens, and the changing student populations of colleges and universities. Market pressures for new communication technologies and vocational education also have changed the educational environment.

Nursing faculty in universities have described pressures associated with the multiple roles required. Professional identity issues and time constraints are identified as major contributing factors. Other factors include ever-changing role expectations, faculty restructuring, unfamiliarity with new technology, and difficulty balancing personal and professional lives. Nurse educators often perceive themselves as underprepared to fulfill all these roles (Coleman 1994; Hannah,

2000). In addition to their teaching responsibilities, nurse educators also need to maintain their clinical competence.

New faculty have an additional source of stress: Discovering the nature of teaching and making the transition from practitioner to educator. An example illustrates this: After teaching one semester, two new university nursing faculty decided to write an article about challenges with their new teaching roles. Both had been highly respected clinical experts when they became nurse educators. However, in their new setting, the teachers experienced culture shock when they found they lacked some of the knowledge and skills needed for teaching at a university. The title of the article they proposed illustrates their experience: *From Expert to Novice*.

Langemann describes teaching as a complex and intensely social art that "demands knowledge, skill, self-reflection, intuition, empathy, caring, and self confidence.... Teachers need the capacity to think about many different things all at once and must act thoughtfully under pressure, often without time to stop and ponder what to do next; they must stand apart from and assess their own teaching...." (Lagemann, 1991, p. 1). Palmer provides an analogy of good teachers as weaving "the fabric that joins them with students and subjects." The heart, defined as "the place where intellect, emotion, spirit, and will converge in the human self," is the "loom on which the threads are tied, the tension is held and the fabric is stretched" (Palmer, 1998, p. 11).

Action research provides a vehicle for faculty to stand apart from and assess the multiple dimensions of their teaching. It is a useful, contextually relevant approach for nursing faculty to learn knowledge and skills for teaching in today's climate of changing faculty roles, limited resources, and demanding workdays. This chapter presents the use of self-directed, group-supported action research to help faculty deal with these types of challenges. It discusses a program of ongoing awareness and direction for one's teaching practice through a self-study process that focuses on adjusting how faculty engage students in learning (Rossi, 2002).

## Explanation of Action Research

How can nursing faculty use action research to improve their teaching and understanding? In brief, action research is accomplished through practical actions, personal reflection on the effects of those actions, and then adjustment of practice to improve teaching effectiveness based on the results.

Educational action research is the systematic study of a teaching situation carried out by the teachers involved in that situation to improve both their practice and the quality of their understanding. This is accomplished through practical actions, personal reflection on the effects of those actions, and adjustments to practice to maximize effectiveness. The process incorporates ongoing, recursive reflection with focusing, planning, observing, acting, and revising during short-term cycles, as quickly as a single class session (Lapan, 1999; McLean, 1995; Winter & Munn-Giddings, 2001).

Key characteristics of action research include:

- Systematic. This is an ongoing approach for learning effective teaching strategies for the teacher's current students.
- Carried out by the teacher. The teacher decides the focus of inquiry (the problem to be addressed) and direction of the investigation. The action research is conducted based on individual interests and level of comfort with the process.
- Teacher-focused. With the emphasis on improving teaching practice and quality of understanding, the focus is on what the teacher does, not what the students do – athough the two are related.

A complete understanding of how to use action research requires actual participation in the process; it cannot be learned intellectually alone. Haggerson and Bowman (1992) use the metaphor of a running stream to explain the multiple viewpoints of inquiry inherent in action research. The metaphor describes one path to inquiry as analogous to sitting on the edge of the stream and making generalizations and predictions about the flow of the water. A second path is to experience the stream by being a participant-observer, investigating the mutual impact the stream and the investigator have on each other. A third path is to become the stream as a total participant. The final path of inquiry is to cross to the other side of the stream, bringing all the previous experiences along.

Ongoing reflective practice is inherent in the action research process. Such a practice involves a spiraling-cyclic, recursive process of reflecting on concrete practices in conflicted and complex situations for the purposes of enhancing understanding and changing practice. A spiraling cycle is used to designate growth and change. The focus of attention in reflective practice includes "how phenomena fit together into patterns, how events flow and unfold over time, and how patterns shift and change" (Baxter & Montgomery, 1996, p. 11; Barrell, Beloff, & Weitman, 2007).

## Steps in the Action Research Process

There are five steps in the action research process:

1. Focusing on an initial inquiry question
2. Planning
3. Implementing and observing effects
4. Re-planning and re-implementing again
5. Reflecting with revised focus

An example describes in detail how the five steps are used. (Hopkins, 1993; McLean, 1995; McNiff, Lomax, & Whitehead, 2003). The example demonstrates how action research incorporates interrelated components in mini-loop cycles that focus the teacher on the aspects of teaching practice to change and those related to the initial focus of inquiry.

## Step One: Focusing on an Initial Inquiry Question

The teacher focuses on something that is important to that teacher's situation, such as exploring a promising new approach or a skill that teacher wants to improve. Completing the following statements can help the teacher identify a focus:
- I am perplexed by...
- I have an idea I would like to try out in my class...
- I would like to change...
- I would like to improve... (Hopkins, 1993, p. 63)

**Example:** My discussion questions are disrupted by my need to keep control in class.

## Step Two: Planning

Planning involves making a decision about:
- What aspect(s) of the approach to try first
- How to obtain student feedback

Giving students a few specific questions to answer anonymously is a useful approach to obtaining feedback. Additionally, audio or video recordings of class sessions also are good ways to obtain feedback.
**Example:** I am going to audiotape questions and responses for one class session and see what is happening.

## Step Three: Implementing the Plan and Observing Effects

Implementing the plan and using students' feedback to observe its effects is the next step. The teacher reflects on student responses and attempts to determine the effectiveness of the intervention. The teacher then makes revisions based on the lessons learned.

**Example:** I learned that students think the nursing process means recalling facts rather than engaging in exploration. How can I stimulate exploration in my students? I should shift my questioning to encourage students to explore answers to their own questions.

The teacher now has identified another inquiry focus to investigate. This demonstrates the cyclical nature of action research.

## Step Four: Re-planning and Re-implementing Again

The findings from step three are used to redesign instruction. The new instruction is then implemented.

**Example:** I will try to formulate and use questions that encourage students to say what they mean and what interests them.

## Step Five: Reflecting with Revised Focus

The purpose of this step is to reflect on the revised instructional strategies implemented in step four. A focused approach is then planned and implemented.

**Example:** Based on my observations, I have noticed that my discussion questions were improving but students were still unruly. How can I keep them on track? I am going to make a greater effort to listen to students as they attempt to answer their questions.

The teacher may then decide to audiotape revised questioning and control statements.

The action research process continues through interrelated mini-cycles that facilitate ongoing growth for the teacher. Action research is a practical approach. Week-by-week action research provides specific feedback about teaching strategies and stimulates changes for improvement during the next contact with students. The nurse educator keeps refining this process until the **best practice** for the current group of students is achieved.

# Difficulties of Action Research

Rossi (2002) found that nursing faculty in a study evaluating an action research program had difficulty narrowing their initial inquiry focus. The best way to overcome this is just to start. Using the stream analogy, the teacher needs to get in the boat and become a participant-observer and a full participant in this experience. The process begins by jumping in.

Rossi (2002) also found that some faculty had difficulty knowing how to word questions that would generate the student feedback they needed, but minimize a sense of vulnerability associated with the consciousness-raising aspect of action research. Nurse educators who participate in action research need to be willing to risk seeing their teaching practice in new ways that may not support their current professional self-concepts. Rossi also found that when certain questions were asked—for example, "What in this course is working so far?" and "What is not working?"—student feedback often was a laundry list of general complaints, including aspects of the course that were not under control of the faculty. Wording the questions carefully can help minimize these issues.

The questions should be about what the teacher does, not what the students do. They must not contain evaluative words, like **best** or **worst**. Also, the questions must be focused on issues the teacher controls. The following questions can be adapted for the reader's own classroom use:

- What part of the theory content I have presented have you used in your clinical setting?
- How did the clinical conference contribute or not contribute to your understanding of what I taught in class?
- What did I do or not do in class to help you connect theory with practice?
- What is the main thing you learned by participating in the role play (or case scenario, or activity)?
- What do you still wish to learn more about?

After feedback is obtained, the nurse educator reflects on the student responses. This reflection is likely to stimulate a change. Students can be asked through another written, anonymous question whether changes are working to address the issue.

# Group Supportive Component

It may be helpful for faculty who are using action research to meet regularly in small groups to reinforce each other's commitment to the practice. Ongoing group-support meetings can encourage persistence throughout the action research process. Also, sharing the endeavor with others can be crucial for addressing teachers' concerns and satisfying their needs (Baird, 1991; Kemper & McKay, 1996).

Group support can be incorporated into the action research program to explore teachers' concerns and issues about focused-inquiry options and to encourage their persistence through the process (Rossi, 2002). Participants can schedule a series of meetings; six such meetings is a typical number used. During the meetings, participants learn the action research process and share their questions, concerns, and progress. They also explore teaching strategies and propose solutions for each other's classroom situations.

All nursing faculty in Rossi's study (2002) indicated that they greatly valued having group meetings every other week to share and discuss their common struggles, successes, and questions. The group meetings were essential for learning how to use action research and for enjoying the process. Often, one person's question would stimulate a need for clarification from others.

The same nurse educators shared they liked meeting in a social environment, such as a restaurant, away from the college or university (Rossi, 2002). They also enjoyed meeting with faculty from another college or university to discuss common issues in a supportive climate. Two of their comments follow:

- "The best aspect of this experience is working with other educators who are struggling to find the same answers."
- "I learned that my frustrations regarding teaching are real and shared by my colleagues, and that we all have a passion to do what is best for our students."

## Results of an Action Research Program in Nursing Education

Rossi (2002) reported that all nursing faculty who participated in an action research program said that the experience had been an educational eye-opener. They believed their teaching had improved and planned to continue the process. The nurse educators said the concrete feedback from students was important and useful, and provided the basis for changes. Participants reported they developed can-do attitudes and their teaching skills improved during the program. Some of their comments were:

- "It's interesting: You think you know what you're doing, and then it turns out not to be exactly what [students] need so you do an about-face. It takes the students to help update us and improve our practice."

- "We can change anything if we start listening to each other... back-and-forth listening and then modifying our innovations in the classroom."

Of particular interest to some faculty were interactive teaching approaches that engage students in learning yet do not require major time commitments from teachers and students. Another area of interest was adapting teaching approaches for diverse student profiles, aptitude levels, and expectations. Questions related to those issues included:

- "How can I encourage students to answer to their own questions instead of the faculty answering?"
- "When I see somebody putting forth a lot of extra effort [but they] can't get it, what do I do?"
- "What do you have to do to modify teaching for different generational groups?"

## Best Practices with Action Research

Sackett (2000) defines evidence-based practice as an integration of: The best research evidence with clinical expertise and patient values. A nurse's clinical judgment and consideration of patient values is analogous to a nursing faculty teaching judgment informed by the unique characteristics of the students. Action research informs teaching judgment through on-going investigations into teaching practice with students. Such investigations stimulate researching bests practice to explore options.

Best practices in nursing education often apply learning strategies from research outside of the nursing profession. Observers may believe that what works in one setting will work in another. However, Haddon and Rossi (2003) define best practices as "a careful study of teaching processes and the use of this knowledge to improve practice; an ongoing search for the best example of teaching for a particular situation."

Nurse educators in an action research program conducted by Rossi (2002) used outside best practices only as they were related to their teaching situation. At the conclusion of the action research program, these educators believed what they had learned was the best practice for their immediate situation. The impetus for learning about teaching and best practices originated from their current teaching practice issues. A comment from one participant demonstrated this: "I've learned that you can't take as gospel truth what the so-called experts tell you. I thought what I was doing was current. However, I've come to find out that for my students, it has not been helpful."

## Nursing Faculty Stories

Following are stories about four nursing faculty (Rossi, 2002). These stories are provided to enhance understanding of the action research process and demonstrate that each nurse educator's experience is unique.

### Shelly: Teacher in an Accelerated Baccalaureate Program

Shelly taught medical nursing in an accelerated baccalaureate program for students earning their second bachelor's degree. Shelly incorporated a variety of interactive learning approaches, including using case scenarios and teaching clinical skills concurrently with related theory. She particularly focused on how to incorporate her students' life and educational experiences into her teaching strategies by asking students to share their expertise during class sessions. While most of her students' feedback was positive, some made suggestions—for example, speaking slower and making copies of PowerPoint® slides to help students taking notes—that Shelly implemented.

### Theresa: First-Year Teacher at a Rural Community College

Theresa taught leadership and maternal nursing. She kept a personal diary and reflected extensively about her teaching practice as she moved through the program. She investigated two interactive approaches:
- A bingo game to review key concepts
- Complex clinical scenarios to stimulate critical thinking related to leadership issues

Her students shared very positive feedback about these strategies.

### Sally: An Experienced Medical-Surgical Teacher at a Rural Community College

Sally progressed through several mini-cycles of action research propelled by negative feedback from frustrated students. She reported: "They want me to be able to answer questions immediately and correctly in class and not refer to other students and they don't want me to contradict anything in the book. This is my life; welcome to it."

Sally said her participation in the action research program provided her with structure and support to work on these issues. She initiated changes in her teaching each week, obtaining student feedback about each change and making adjustments accordingly. Some examples are provided:

- Sally thought students preferred lectures using PowerPoint® slides, but found they did not. Sally plans to use PowerPoint® slides for her next group of students; however, because she believes each group has its own preferences.
- Sally lowered the level of her exam questions because this group of students had not been exposed to questions as difficult as the ones she used. However, she did incorporate higher-level questions for practice during lecture. Students offered much positive feedback about this change.
- Sally used a standard lecture format because this group of students seemed highly stressed and not open to changes during the last course of the program. Students requested a traditional format for lectures. She reported that students' satisfaction increased.

## Action Research with a Teaching Team

During the 2007-2008 academic year, nine didactic and clinical faculty in a nursing course at Northern Arizona University initiated a group-supportive, action research process to stimulate teaching behavior changes of team members based on student feedback. The team met every other week to discuss issues, challenges, and questions related to teaching as well as the clarity of the course. Within this framework, several anonymous action research questionnaires were given to each clinical group. The questions focus on both didactic and clinical faculty throughout the semester. Directions provided indicated that answers to these brief questions will guide clinical faculty in facilitating learning. Students are asked to only address aspects that faculty can do something about.

The first questionnaire was titled *Feedback to Your Teachers 7th Week*. The complete questionnaire is on the CD accompanying this book. The questions asked were:

- What did your didactic (or clinical) faculty do that enhanced your progress and learning?
- What is still unclear?
- What specific suggestions do you have for your didactic (or clinical) faculty?

This formative investigation provided each individual faculty validation about teaching approaches that were working well and identified areas that needed clarification or growth at this time.

Examples of feedback are:

- I learned by my clinical faculty probing for understanding and always asking questions that illicit further work and investigations.
- I appreciate being able to apply theory to my assigned family.
- I am unclear about what is expected in the discussions.
- How can I use the clinical reasoning web with the three family members?
- I need more elaboration as this material is difficult.

Faculty respond back to the students to address their concerns and make changes that can occur during the semester. In addition, possible course changes for the next semester are discussed.

A second questionnaire is administered to the students toward the end of the semester to evaluate for student growth, identify continuing issues to address, and plan for changes. The questionnaire is titled: *Take Two: Feedback to Your Teachers.* The questions are different from those of the first questionnaire and include:

- What is something significant that you have learned within the last 4-6 weeks?
- It would help me if _____
- I would like to tell my theory faculty _____
- I would like to tell my clinical faculty _____

After changes in teaching strategies based on prior action research were implemented, as well as student growth as the semester progressed, student comments changed:

- I have learned how to allocate resources for patient needs and think creatively to problem solve and advocate for families.
- I am learning what type of nurse I want to be when I'm finished. I've learned how I want to make my practice.
- I have learned how I am capable of more than I thought.
- Thanks for being great instructors! You listen to what students have to say and help us.

There was minimal feedback about areas of confusion but students did make suggestions for future courses. Copies of both questionnaires are provided in the CD accompanying this book.

## How to Begin Doing Group-Supportive Action Research

Action research focuses on identifying the area of inquiry, obtaining useful feedback from students, and using their reactions to make changes in teaching strategies and other related aspects of the course.

The learning experiences help the nurse educator discover how, where, and when to question the effectiveness of a teaching strategy. While these activities can be accomplished individually, regular meetings among faculty is an essential component to facilitate learning and commitment to the action research process. Therefore, learning experiences may be organized around group meetings to allow nurse educators sufficient time to work through the process.

### Planning for Groups

Initially, one person needs to take responsibility for arranging for the group sessions. For graduate students, the nursing faculty is the obvious choice. For practicing nurse educators, one person familiar with the group process and/or action research may serve this role. However, after sessions begin, the leadership role should be shared among members. Participants need to jointly decide the location and times of the meetings. Should they be held for two hours every other week for 12 weeks or weekly for six sessions during one academic term?

### First Group Meeting

The first group meeting should be held within the first few weeks of the term. Each participant should prepare for the session by carefully reviewing this chapter.

**Facilitator.** The group organizer should initially serve as the group facilitator. However, the facilitator's role then becomes a shared endeavor. At each session, a person is identified to initiate the session and at the end provide a summary. The facilitator for the first session explains this idea of sharing the facilitator role.

The facilitator provides a brief summary about what will occur during the meetings as each member progresses through the action research process. This process proceeds as follows:

- First meeting: Establish norms and clarify the research process
- Second meeting: Establish the focus of inquiry, plan the changes in instructional strategies, and determine how feedback will be obtained
- Third, fourth, and fifth meetings: Reflect, revise, and refocus the research

- Sixth meeting: Discuss successes and struggles and develop a plan to incorporate active research into ongoing practice

All participants are likely to go through the same general process, but they may follow slightly different sequences or have different teaching focuses.

**Members.** At the first meeting, members set standards for group sessions and agree on the norms that fit their group. The following guidelines can be used to facilitate trust among members and ensure their control over the extent of their sharing and participation (Rossi, 2002):
- During the group sessions, participants will share only at the level at which they feel comfortable
- The facilitator and participants will support each participant's choices, challenges, and discoveries at his or her own level and pace
- Each participant will have the freedom of choice in the focus and selection of teaching-related issues
- Each participant will freely make decisions about the sources of data and methods he or she wishes to use

All members initiate, seek, and provide information. Members also clarify and explore alternatives or deeper meaning to the focus queries that members seek to explore. Members encourage and support each other and harmonize to reduce tensions and assist others to explore differences. Each member helps maintain the flow of communication among the group.

## Clarifying What Action Research Is All About

The facilitator reviews and discusses with the group the definition of educational action research and its interrelated components. The facilitator emphasizes that regular meetings are held to teach and clarify the action research process and for participants to share questions, concerns, and sense-making as they progress.

## Identifying a Focus of Inquiry

The facilitator leads a discussion to facilitate development of a focus of inquiry for each participant to study. Each participant individually focuses on a question of concern related to their own practice. This becomes their **focus of inquiry**. Getting started is often the hardest step in action research, so the group members can help each other identify a personally meaningful first focus for their action research. The following statements may be used to spark ideas (Hopkins, 1993, p. 63):

- I am perplexed by...
- I have an idea I would like to try out in my class...
- I would like to change...
- I would like to improve...

For the next group meeting, participants are asked to provide one question or concern they wish to use to conduct a mini-cycle of action research. They bring printed copies of their focus and study questions to share with the other members of the group.

Each person then plans to implement a small change in their teaching, collect data for observation, reflect on the feedback, and re-plan. The feedback findings are likely to stimulate further short loops of inquiries, actions, and reflection.

## Second Meeting

A facilitator or co-facilitators is/are identified at the beginning of this session. During this meeting, participants are asked to discuss their inquiry focus and the questions they developed. Each inquiry focus should:

- Relate to what the teacher does, not what the students do
- Not contain evaluative words, such as **best** or **worst**
- Relate to something the teacher has control over

The second purpose of this meeting is planning. Participants discuss how to obtain student feedback or observations after their planned teaching strategy changes are implemented. Possible sources of student feedback are:

- Interpretive evidence or data obtained during teaching practice from students and colleagues
- Audio or videotape recordings of teaching sessions
- A report from a colleague observing students' responses
- Short questionnaires for students

Using a student questionnaire to obtain feedback is called the **class check-up**. Participants in the action research group can discuss and work together on developing these questions. Remember, the questions should be about what the teacher does and must not contain evaluative words. Also, each question should address a specific, planned change in teaching. Be careful to word questions to obtain specific information from students rather than a laundry list of general complaints.

One way to do this is to adapt the following questions to the participant's unique inquiry focus:

- What part of the theory content that I have presented have you used in your clinical setting?
- How did the clinical conference contribute or not contribute to your understanding of what I taught in class?
- What did I do or not do in class to help you connect theory with practice?
- What is the main thing you learned by participating in the role-play situation (or case scenario, or activity about setting priorities, etc.)?
- What do you still wish to learn more about?

The responses are compiled anonymously and can be shared with students at a later time to jointly make decisions about the identified teaching and student learning issues. Each participant keeps personal records of student feedback and shares aspects of that feedback with the group.

Before the next group session, participants implement one teaching change and obtain written feedback from students through the class check-up. Remember to let students know their responses will be anonymous.

## Third, Fourth, and Fifth Meetings

During the next three group meetings, participants share what they have learned about their teaching strategies from their students' feedback. These meetings should emphasize:

- Reflecting, to interpret the effects of their teaching changes
- Revising, based upon what was discovered with reflection
- Refocusing on other related issues that may become the focus of future action research mini-cycles

The participants are encouraged to move through related cyclic loops and/or two to three short mini-cycles.

## Sixth Group Meeting

The final group meeting continues with the process described. The facilitator for this session leads a focused discussion about what has been meaningful and what has been frustrating about their experiences with action research. A discussion about the steps faculty can take to continue their action research on their own may also be helpful (Rossi, 2002).

The facilitator should pose the following questions to address continued use of action research: What factors would lead you to consider making this action research process a part of your ongoing practice? Is colleague or group support needed? What kind? What reasons would guide your decision to not incorporate action research in your practice?

## Summary

Once learned, action research can be implemented naturally throughout a teacher's career. It can be a valuable tool for improvement. Consider the parallel of the action research process with the nursing process. They both represent an ongoing process for growth.

## Resources

The following Internet resources provide more information about action research. These websites are included on the CD accompanying this book.

**Action Research Resources**
http://www.scu.edu.au/schools/gcm/ar/arhome.html
Front page for a substantial action research site.

**Center for Action Research**
http://www.bath.ac.uk/carpp/
Features an approach to action research which integrates action and reflection.

**Center for Collaborative Action Research**
http://cadres.pepperdine.edu/ccar/
Resource for understanding action research.

**Web Links to Participatory Action Research Sites:**
http://www.goshen.edu/soan/soan96p.html

**Action Research**
http://www.webproject.org/action.html
Provides an action research bibliography.

University of Bath School of Management Center for Action Research in Professional Practice
www.bath.ac.uk/carpp
Includes links to doctoral and masters theses and other publications.

## Learning Activities

1. Identify an area of your teaching that you would like to investigate using action research methodology. Plan how you would conduct the research.
2. Gather four or five colleagues and establish an action research group. Share what you have learned about the effectiveness of action research with your colleagues.
3. Visit one of the websites listed in this chapter. What kind of information did you find? Was the information helpful?

## Educational Philosophy

I have a deeply held belief in an individual's abilities and potential. The individual has the ability to participate in the process of learning within an interactive learning environment and to develop personally relevant knowledge. I value self-awareness, self-efficacy, and self-choice and assume that these will contribute to learning. My role as a teacher and facilitator of learning is to stretch the learners beyond what they would learn by themselves but not so far as to cause a high level of stress. The teacher creates an environment for such learning to occur and facilitates that process. — Enid A. Rossi

## References

Baird, J. R. (1991). Individual and group reflections as a basis for teaching development. *Teachers' Professional Development* (95-113). Melbourne: ACER.

Barrell, J., Beloff, C., & Weitman, C. (2007). Action research fosters empowerment and learning communities. *Delta Kappa Gamma Bulletin, 73*(30) 36-45.

Baxter, L., & Montgomery, B. (1996). *Relating: Dialogues and dialectics.* New York: Guilford Press.

Boyden, K. M. (2000). Development of new faculty in higher education. *Journal of Professional Nursing, 16*(2), 104-111.

Burbules, N. C., & Callister, Jr., T. A. (2000). Universities in transition: The promise and the challenge of new technologies. *Teachers College Record, 102*(2), 271-293.

Carnevale, A. P., & Descrochers, D. M. (1997 April-May). The role of community colleges in the new economy. *Community College Journal,* 26-33.

Coleman, J. F. (1994). *The lived experience of veteran nurse educators teaching in selected baccalaureate or higher degree programs in nursing: A study of professional development.* Unpublished doctoral dissertation, University of North Carolina, Greensboro.

Fullan, M. G. (2001). *The new meaning of educational change* (3rd ed.). New York: Teachers College Press.

Haddon, R., & Rossi, E. (2003, July). *Developing teacher strategies that engage the learner through reflective action research.* Paper presented at the annual Nurse Educators Conference in the Rockies, Breckenridge, CO.

Haggerson, N., & Bowman A. (1992). *Informing educational policy and practice through interpretive inquiry.* Lancaster, PA: Technomic.

Hannah, C. A. (2000). *The relationship between nursing education reform factors and undergraduate nursing faculty role strain.* Unpublished doctoral dissertation.

Hopkins, D. (1993). *A teacher's guide to classroom research* (2nd ed.). Philadelphia: Open University Press.

Kember, D., & McKay, J. (1996). Action research into the quality of student learning: A paradigm for faculty development. *Journal of Higher Education, 67*(5), 528-554.

Lagemann, E. C. (1991). Talk about teaching. *Teachers College Record, 93*(1), 1-5.

Lapan, S. D. (1999). *A selected glossary of terms.* Unpublished manuscript, Flagstaff, AZ: Northern Arizona University.

McLean, J. E. (1995). *Improving education through action research: A guide for administrators and teachers.* Thousand Oaks, CA: Corwin Press.

McNiff, J., Lomax, P., & Whitehead, J. (2003). *You and your action research project.* New York: Routledge Falmer.

O'Toole, J. (1995). *Leading change: Overcoming the ideology of comfort and tyranny of custom.* San Francisco: Jossey-Bass.

Palmer, P. (1998). *The courage to teach: Exploring the inner landscape of a teacher's life.* San Francisco: Jossey-Bass.

Privateer, P. M. (1999). Academic technology and the future of higher education. *The Journal of Higher Education, 70*(1), 60-79.

Rossi, E. (2002). *Evaluation of a self-directed, group-supportive action research approach for nursing faculty teacher development*. Unpublished doctoral dissertation, Northern Arizona University.

Sackett, D. L. (2000). *Evdence-based medicine: How to practice and teach evidence-based practice*. New York: Churchill Livingston.

Skiba, D. (1997). Transforming nursing education to celebrate learning. *Nursing and Health Care Perspectives, 18*(3), 124-148.

Winter, R., & Munn-Giddings, C. (2001). *A handbook for action research in health and social care*. London: Routledge.

## Bibliography

Crow, J., Smith, L., & Keenan, I. (2006). Journeying between the education and hospital zones in a collaborative action research project. *Educational Action Research, 14*(2), 287-306.

Gay, L. R., & Airasian, P. (2000). *Educational research: Competencies for analysis and application* (6th ed.). Upper Saddle River, NJ: Merrill.

Jones, A., Sterling, H., Pollack, D., Doshier, S., Yeknic, C., Falls, D., et al. (1999). *Action research and educational practice*. Paper presented at the Arizona Educational Research Organization annual conference, Flagstaff, AZ.

Schon, D. A. (1983). *The reflective practitioner: How professionals think in action*. New York: Basic Books.

# CHAPTER 10

# WRITING FOR PUBLICATION IN NURSING:
## WHAT EVERY NURSE EDUCATOR NEEDS TO KNOW

**Marilyn H. Oermann, PhD, RN, FAAN, ANEF**

---

The content of this chapter relates to the following major content areas and subconcepts on the Certified Nurse Educator Examination Detailed Test Blueprint:

**Pursue Continuous Quality Improvement in the Academic Nurse Educator Role**
- Demonstrate a commitment to lifelong learning
- Participate in professional development opportunities that increase one's effectiveness in the role
- Select professional development activities to continue to grow and evolve in the role
- Balance the teaching, scholarship, and service demands inherent in the role of the educator and as influenced by the requirements of the institutional setting

**Engage in Scholarship of Teaching**
- Share teaching expertise with colleagues and others
- Demonstrate integrity as a scholar

---

## Introduction

As faculty prepare themselves for teaching in schools of nursing, they develop their ability to lecture, design courses, promote learning in an online environment, evaluate students' clinical performance, and construct tests, among other skills. Another competency faculty need to develop is ability to write for publication. Writing for publication is essential for faculty to disseminate their educational innovations and new initiatives to other teachers and to build evidence about educational practices in nursing. By writing for publication, teachers can share their knowledge and expertise with other faculty.

This chapter describes the process of writing for publication beginning with pre-planning and deciding what to write about, through completion of the final draft. Other content in the chapter addresses what happens once the manuscript reaches the editorial office and how to revise the manuscript to improve chances of acceptance.

## Benefits of Writing for Publication as a Nurse Educator

Through writing for publication nursing faculty share their educational innovations and new ideas about curriculum, distance education, clinical teaching, evaluation, and other topics about which faculty teaching elsewhere also are concerned. When projects and initiatives related to nursing education are published in the literature, then other groups of faculty can use that work in their own schools of nursing. Rather than everyone designing the same initiatives for their students and programs, writing for publication allows educators to share best practices.

The most effective way of communicating nursing education research is by publishing the findings. This research includes not only formal studies done by faculty but also projects that faculty planned, implemented, and then evaluated. A benefit of writing for publication is that teachers can share problems they addressed through research and what they learned, thereby guiding other faculty faced with similar problems. By disseminating the findings of studies in nursing education, faculty build evidence for practice as a teacher (Oermann, 2007). Without this evidence there is no basis for what we do and decisions we make as nurse educators. Findings of studies in nursing education can only be used widely if they are published.

Another reason to learn about writing for publication is that publishing is essential for promotion and tenure in many schools of nursing. While each school has its own criteria for promotion and tenure, including the number and types of publications required for different faculty ranks, there are some general principles that faculty should know about in terms of publishing.

- First, data-based articles published in peer-reviewed journals, also called refereed, carry more weight in promotion and tenure decisions than do descriptive articles about teaching, curriculum development, and other educational topics.
- Second, articles in peer-reviewed journals are valued more highly than non-refereed publications such as newsletters.

In peer-reviewed journals, e.g., *Nurse Educator, Journal of Nursing Education, Nursing Education Perspectives*, and *International Journal of Nursing Education Scholarship*, experts (peers) critically review each manuscript submitted to the journal, identify needed revisions, and recommend to the editor whether the paper should be accepted. Peer review of manuscripts assists the editor in ensuring that high quality articles are published in the journal (Hoyt & Poehl, 2007). Because of peer review, publishing in refereed journals, no matter what type of article, carries more weight than in non-refereed journals and writing chapters.

By writing for publication faculty gain new knowledge from the literature review they complete as part of the process. This information can then be used when developing lectures and course materials. When faculty develop new lectures and materials for teaching, they can write articles about these, gaining publications from their efforts and time.

## Why Faculty Do Not Write for Publication

Many innovations in nursing education are known only by the faculty and students in a particular school of nursing. What are barriers to writing for publication as a nurse educator?

First, writing is skill that takes practice and time to develop. The added time it takes novice writers to develop a paper may affect their motivation to write.

Second, not understanding the process of writing and how to move from ideas to submission of a manuscript may also be a barrier. Faculty may be unsure how to develop a manuscript, what to expect during the review process, and what steps to take when a manuscript is returned for revision. Writing for publication may lead to rejection of a paper and with it the faculty's own ideas; however, this is part of the process.

A third problem facing educators is finding the time to prepare a manuscript, beginning with reviewing the literature, writing the draft, editing the paper, and then revising it based on reviewers' feedback. With the busy work and personal schedules of faculty, time is often an issue.

### Strategies to Resolve Barriers to Writing

The more faculty write for publication, the easier it becomes and more quickly it can be accomplished. Every educator needs to understand the process of writing for publication beginning from how to select a journal to strategies for addressing reviewer comments. The third problem, time for writing, is more difficult to manage. There are some strategies, though, that faculty can use to build time for writing into their teaching schedule and personal lives.

Due dates can be set for completing the manuscript and each section in it (Oermann, 2002). With this strategy the author views sections of content as individual writing projects. The due dates should be recorded on the outline used for writing and should be realistic considering the faculty's teaching schedule and other responsibilities. The key to this strategy is to meet those deadlines; once a due date is moved further into the future, the manuscript may never be completed.

Faculty need to find their prime time for writing, when they are most productive, and use that time for writing (Oermann, 2002). The best time for writing varies – some authors write best early in the morning while others are most productive late at night. Some faculty may need large blocks of time for writing; others may find an hour a day works best. The prime time is unique to each author but needs to be identified and then used for writing, not for preparing classes, meeting with students and other faculty, or completing personal responsibilities. In addition to reserving this time for writing, the author should create an environment without distractions, e.g., avoid answering the telephone and checking emails.

## Process of Writing for Publication:  Planning Phase

In writing for publication there is a certain process to follow that begins with planning to write and ends with publication of the manuscript. Understanding this process facilitates writing the paper and responding to peer review in a way that improves one's chances of an acceptance decision. The unpublished document, which is submitted to the journal or publisher, is called the manuscript or paper (American Medical Association [AMA], 2007). When published, the manuscript is referred to as an article.

### Identify Purpose of Manuscript and Importance of Topic

The most important early step in writing for publication is to identify the purpose of the manuscript. The purpose may be to describe an innovation for teaching developed by faculty, a new program in the school of nursing, a research study, and other topics of interest to nurse educators. The purpose guides the literature review, to determine if the topic has already been addressed, and writing the paper to maintain its focus. Faculty should be clear about the outcomes of the manuscript for readers – what will they gain from reading it?

Related to clarifying the purpose is the need to confirm the importance of the topic for nurse educators and whether journals might be interested in publishing the paper. Faculty should ask themselves if the proposed paper will present new ideas not yet in the literature (Oermann, 2002). If others have written about the topic, for example, critical thinking, what is new and different about the proposed manuscript? The paper should make a difference in teaching, evaluation, curriculum development, working with students, and other areas of nursing education; otherwise it is not worth writing. It is best to assess the importance of the topic now rather than prepare a paper that has limited chance of publication.

## Review the Literature

Journals are interested in publishing new ideas about nursing education and innovations that have not been reported in the literature. Although faculty may think their ideas and innovations are new, a review of the literature may prove otherwise. For this reason, the next step is to review the literature on the topic. There are two objectives to this literature review: to determine if the proposed topic or slant of the manuscript has been described already in the literature and if not, to gather information that can be used in writing the paper.

There are many bibliographic databases for the author to use in reviewing the literature, but typically the two databases most useful for writing in nursing are MEDLINE, available through PubMed, and the Cumulative Index to Nursing and Allied Health Literature (CINAHL®). When searches in those databases yield limited information, faculty also should include the Education Resources Information Center (ERIC) and PsycINFO databases (Oermann, 2007).

Usually, it is sufficient to review the literature for the previous three to five years only. However, if there are limited publications on the topic within that time frame, then it is appropriate to go back further with the literature review. Faculty should record all of the information needed for preparing references no matter what reference style is used by the journal; this prevents having to recheck the information later. By keeping a list of articles, books, and other materials that were not relevant to the paper, the faculty can avoid reviewing those same sources again in a different database or at a later time.

Because of the extensive number of references retrieved in most literature searches, authors need ways of keeping track of them, storing references for future use, and retrieving them when needed. Faculty can use literature searches for lectures, development of course materials and strategies for teaching, research projects, and writing for publication. However, to do this, they need a way of storing and keeping track of those references. One way is to record the bibliographic information in a computer file. Faculty can develop their own files to store reference information or can use bibliographic management software such as EndNote®, Reference Manager®, and ProCite® (Thomson, 2008). Another product is RefWorks, an online research and bibliographic management tool. With RefWorks faculty can search bibliographic databases, store reference information, prepare citations, and format them for manuscripts using different styles (RefWorks, 2008).

## Select a Journal

All too often faculty first write their manuscript, then search for a journal interested in publishing it. Those steps, however, should be reversed. After deciding on the topic, faculty should be clear for whom they are writing the paper. For example, if the topic is about developing a portfolio, is the intended audience any nurse educator in a school of nursing or a novice teacher with limited if any knowledge about portfolios? Or, are the intended readers staff nurses who can develop a portfolio for career advancement? Knowing the intended audience is important in selecting possible journals for submission; the audience also guides how the manuscript is written in terms of depth of content, the examples used in the article, how the information is presented, and writing style.

Every manuscript is written for a defined audience and then submitted to a journal that publishes papers on that topic for those readers (Davis & Tschudin, 2007; Oermann, 2002). Thus, rather than writing a paper and then trying to find a journal interested in publishing it, the author selects possible journals for that content area and intended audience, then writes for that journal. Some journals publish only original research or only clinical practice articles; other journals publish articles on clinical practice as well as research in that clinical specialty. *Nurse Educator* publishes more non-research articles than does the *Journal of Nursing Education*. There are some journals that have short articles focusing on application of new ideas in practice without the background information and supporting rationale for those ideas, while others publish more detailed and comprehensive reviews of topics.

**Strategies for identifying possible journals.** There are literally hundreds of journals in which faculty can publish. One useful technique for identifying possible journals is to use a directory of nursing and healthcare journals available on the Internet (Table 1). The *Nurse Author & Editor Journals Directory* (www.nurseauthor.com/library.asp) is organized alphabetically and for each journal has email links to the author guidelines and editor. Faculty can search through this list for potential journals, query the editors about their interest in the topic, and gather the author guidelines, all at one Web site.

Another way of identifying possible journals is to search CINAHL® and PubMed for the topic faculty want to write about and identify journals that publish in that content area for the intended audience. A quick literature search to explore possible journals also reveals if there are articles already published on that topic.

| |
|---|
| **www.nurseauthor.com/library.asp**<br>This site provides an alphabetical list of nursing journals with email connections to editors and author information pages. |
| **www.nursingcenter.com/home/index.asp**<br>Lippincott's NursingCenter.com includes a list of journals with author guidelines and links to the editors. |
| **www.ncbi.nlm.nih.gov/sites/entrez?db=Journals**<br>Medline is the National Library of Medicine's bibliographic database covering medical, nursing, and other health related journals. You can search for possible journals in the Journals Database in PubMed. |
| **Publishers' Web pages**<br>Most nursing journals have their own Web sites that provide information about the journal. |

**Table 1.** Web Sites for Identifying Journals

**Author guidelines.** As the educator reviews possible journals, it is helpful to maintain a file of them with the author guidelines. Generally, for each manuscript the author should have a file with information about five possible journals for submission. If the query to the editor indicates there is no interest in reviewing the paper, or it is rejected by the first journal to which submitted, then the author can send the manuscript to another journal in the file.

The author guidelines provide information about the content areas and types of articles published in the journal. The manuscript cannot be written without these guidelines because they indicate how to prepare the paper such as the number of pages allowed, reference style, format for submitting the paper, and other similar details. Most journals have their author information page at their Web site. For example, all of the information needed to prepare a manuscript for submission to *Nurse Educator* can be found at http://edmgr.ovid.com/ne/accounts/ifauth.htm.

It is important to carefully read the guidelines before beginning to write because they specify formatting requirements that will influence preparing the paper.

## Write Query Letter to Editor

The next step is to write a query letter to the editors of the journals that are possible outlets for the manuscript. The intent of the query letter is to determine if the editor is interested in reviewing the paper. While faculty can prepare and submit a manuscript without first querying the editor, if the editor is not interested in reviewing it, there is time lost in preparing the paper to fit that journal and receiving the response back from the editor. If an editor is interested in reviewing the manuscript, this does not mean that it will be accepted (Davis & Tschudin, 2007).

Manuscripts can be sent to only one journal at a time. If the paper is rejected, the educator can then send it to another journal but only after being notified that it is no longer under consideration by the original journal. Query letters, in contrast, can be sent to multiple editors at a time. One advantage of using online directories is that most have email links to the editors, allowing the educator to send multiple query letters at one time. Oermann (2002) recommended that after deciding on the journal for submission, the author notify the other editors of the decision not to submit the paper to them. Query letters are short, indicating the purpose of the manuscript, if it is a research report, and the contact information and position of the author. A sample query letter is found in Figure 1.

## Decide on Authorship Credit

The standard for determining who should be listed as an author of a manuscript is specified in the *Uniform Requirements for Manuscripts Submitted to Biomedical Journals* by the International Committee of Medical Journal Editors (ICMJE) (ICMJE, 2007). Individuals can only be listed as authors if they (1) contributed substantially to "conception and design, or acquisition of data, or analysis and interpretation of data; (2) drafting the article or revising it critically for important intellectual content; and (3) final approval of the version to be published" (ICMJE, 2007). The ICMJE indicates clearly that to be listed as an author of the manuscript the individual must meet all three of these requirements. Otherwise it is inappropriate for an individual to place her or his name on a manuscript.

Individuals such as the dean, director of the program, or faculty advisor who may have supported the study and educator cannot be listed as authors of a paper unless they participated in writing it. Authorship is never assigned as a courtesy (Davidhizar, 2004). Ghost authorship is when the paper is actually written by an editor or a medical writer and not the author; this also is inappropriate.

Many readers will have heard stories about faculty who ask or demand that their names be added to a paper written by one of their students. For this to occur,

John Doe, MSN, RN, C
245 Hill Street
Pittsburgh, Pennsylvania 15228

January 1, 2009

Marilyn H. Oermann, PhD, RN, FAAN, ANEF
University of North Carolina at Chapel Hill
Editor, Journal of Nursing Care Quality
433 Carrington Hall, CB # 7460
Chapel Hill, NC 27599-7460

Dear Dr. Oermann:

I am interested in submitting a manuscript to the Journal of Nursing Care Quality. The purpose of the manuscript is to describe a teaching intervention for asthma patients that we developed and evaluated system-wide. I was the coordinator of the team that developed the intervention, and I have extensive experience in caring for patients with asthma.

We anticipate completing the manuscript by March 2009. Thank you for your consideration.

Sincerely,

*John Doe*

John Doe, MSN, RN, C
Advanced Practice Nurse
Asthma Clinic

**Figure 1.** Sample Query Letter

the faculty, similar to other authors, must meet all three conditions for authorship. Teachers cannot ask a student to write a paper and then only list the faculty's name on it, or even worse, take a student's paper written for a course and then submit that paper for publication as one's own. In situations in which the faculty and student together planned a project or study, and both of them participated in writing the manuscript, then both would be listed as co-authors.

There are times though when authors want to acknowledge the help they received with a study or project, or with writing the manuscript. In these instances, acknowledgments are used. Every person mentioned in the acknowledgment needs to give written permission to cite his or her name in the paper. Similarly, agencies, health systems, and individuals cannot be named in the text without their written permission.

An example of an acknowledgment is:

The author acknowledges the assistance of Mary Jones, EdD, RN, in developing the tool and pilot testing it with students in her program.

In this example, Mary Jones needs to provide written permission to cite her name in the acknowledgement.

## Process of Writing for Publication:  Writing Phase

The faculty has decided on the purpose of the manuscript, identified the potential readers, polled editors interested in reviewing it, gathered the author guidelines, and completed the literature review. At this point the author moves into the second phase, which is writing the paper. Gene Fowler wrote that "Writing is easy:  All you do is sit staring at a blank sheet of paper until drops of blood form on your forehead" (BrainyMedia.com, 2008). The writing phase starts with an outline, which guides the author in writing the first draft to avoid "drops of blood forming on the forehead."

Before outlining, the faculty should carefully review the author guidelines and decide how to present the content considering the readers of the journal and writing style used in it. Saver (2006) suggested reading the journal to get a sense of the articles and writing style. Some journals in nursing use more formal, academic writing styles often with passive voice. For example,

Despite extensive research on patient education, there are few studies on patients' perceptions of the role of the nurse in their education. Most research has examined the effectiveness of different teaching interventions and approaches, but few have explored the importance of nurses delivering that teaching from the point of view of the patient.

Other journals use a more informal writing style with active voice. For example, "We developed a research study in which we asked patients to rate the importance of having nurses provide their education during their hospitalization." Often in journals using an informal writing style, sentences begin with "you." For example, "*You* can best teach the patient by dividing the material into smaller content areas and using visuals to supplement your teaching."

## Develop an Outline

Once the faculty is at this stage, an outline should be developed. The outline is a general plan of the content to be included in the manuscript and its order; it serves as the blueprint for the paper (Campanelli, Feferman, Keane, Lieberman, & Roberson, 2007; Oermann, 2000). Outlines may be formal (developed using Roman numerals) or informal (a list of topics and their order). The outline is critical because it guides the faculty in what content to include in the paper and how to organize it. The outline is a working document, able to be revised as the writing proceeds, which is far easier to do than rewriting the entire manuscript.

Oermann (2000) identified advantages of outlining before beginning to write. An outline:

- Identifies the content areas to include in a manuscript
- Organizes the content in a logical order
- Facilitates identifying missing content before beginning to write
- Suggests headings and subheadings to use with the manuscript
- Keeps the author on the topic
- By assigning due dates, helps the author complete the paper on time

The goal of the outline is to group content together and decide on the best order to present it. If the organization of the content is not apparent, the faculty can record key content areas on index cards, then rearrange them until satisfied with the order (Oermann, 2000). Or, the educator can develop a concept map, similar to what students prepare as a clinical learning activity, that links content areas together. This sometimes helps the faculty decide how to present the content.

## Write the First Draft

Once the outline is done, the faculty can start writing the draft. The goal in writing the first draft is to write fast and get the content down rather than worrying about grammar and writing style (Oermann, 2002). By revising for grammar while writing, faculty shift their thinking away from the content and how to present it, often resulting in the loss of "train of thought." The outline is key in this phase because it keeps the faculty focused on the content and how to organize it. How many drafts to write depends on how clearly one can express own ideas. With practice, writing becomes easier and fewer drafts are needed.

While the title and abstract are the beginning pages of a manuscript, some faculty write the draft of the text first, then the title and abstract; others write the title and abstract first. Either way these are working documents that may need to be revised later.

In writing the draft it is important to include the citations while typing. Otherwise in later revisions the faculty will not recall the source of the information. In the draft the authors' names and dates can be listed in parentheses, which then can be easily formatted for journals using the American Psychological Association (APA) reference style (APA, 2001). When writing for journals that use a numbered system for the citations, the author's last name and publication date still should be recorded in the draft. The references can be numbered later. Otherwise every time a new reference is added somewhere in the paper, the citations would need to be renumbered.

## Revise the Draft

Once satisfied with the content, the faculty edits the draft for grammar, punctuation, spelling, and writing style. It is best to start with revising the paragraphs, then check each sentence and choice of words (Oermann, 2002). That way the author is moving from broad aspects of the paper to more specific ones.

Each paragraph should begin with an introductory sentence that captures the content in the paragraph. Faculty also should check the organization of the paragraphs to ensure the content is sequenced clearly. This is a good time to check for smooth transitions between paragraphs. After revising the paragraphs, the faculty edits the sentences and transition between them, ensures that they are grammatically correct, reviews the length and structure of the sentences within each paragraph, and checks the choice of words. At some point the faculty needs to be satisfied with the writing and submit the manuscript to avoid editing the paper beyond what is necessary to improve the writing.

## Prepare References

Not all journals to which faculty submit manuscripts use APA. Many journals use a numbered citation format such as the *Uniform Requirements* (ICMJE, 2007) and American Medical Association (AMA) *Manual of Style* (AMA, 2007). The author guidelines provide examples of the style to use when preparing references.

The name-year system, such as the APA style used in this chapter, records the author name and year of publication within the text. Another common reference style is the citation-sequence format in which Arabic numerals are used for the citations in the text, which are numbered consecutively. In some styles, the numerals are placed in parentheses while in others they are in superscripts. For example,

...developed and tested the clinical evaluation form.(1-2)
...developed and tested the clinical evaluation form.[1-2]

By numbering the citations rather than including author names and publication dates, the text is not interrupted by a list of references within a sentence. These formats may be adapted by the journal, and for this reason the faculty needs to follow the author guidelines for each journal.

Faculty must verify the accuracy of their references against the original publication. Research studies have found errors in nursing publications in the spelling of authors' names, order of names, title of the article, and journal in which published (Oermann, Cummings, & Wilmes, 2001; Oermann, Mason, & Wilmes, 2002; Oermann & Ziolkowski, 2002). Faculty also should check that the citations are placed with the correct content in the text and that they correspond to the correct reference on the reference list.

## Prepare Tables and Figures

When the faculty has detailed information to present, it is best to develop a table for those data. Tables should not be used if the information can be reported clearly in the text. The principle is to develop tables for complex and detailed information that can be displayed and understood more clearly in table form rather than narrative. Tables are used to:
- report exact values
- present detailed information
- present statistical data
- display quantitative values
- show relationships among data (Oermann, 2002)

Word or text tables also can be developed for a paper. For example, a table could be prepared listing different program evaluation models, characteristics of each, advantages and disadvantages, and nursing programs that have used each one. That information would be too detailed for the text and is better presented in a table. Table 1 in this chapter is a word or text table. Similar to tables reporting statistics, if the information can be presented as part of the text, then tables should not be used.

In the text, the faculty highlights major findings from the tables and includes summary statements about them but does not repeat information from the tables in the text (Oermann, 2002). The text should refer readers to the tables by using a phrase such as "shown in Table 1" or ...program evaluation models (Table 1).

Figures include graphs, diagrams, photographs, and other illustrations. They are valuable in showing trends in the data, changes over time, and comparisons (Oermann, 2002). Because figures are often reduced during publication, the information on the figures should be large enough that it can be seen when reduced.

## Prepare Final Copy and Submit

Before submitting the paper to the journal, the faculty should complete one final check to confirm the format is consistent with the journal requirements. For many journals, the manuscript is submitted at the journal Web site. Manuscripts are double-spaced including the title page, references, tables, and figure captions. The author information page will indicate the margins to use, but if this information is not provided, 1 to 1½ inch margins should be used on all sides. No spaces should be left between paragraphs, hard returns should not be used, and pages should be numbered as indicated in the guidelines. Some journals use running heads while others do not; once again it is the faculty's responsibility to follow these guidelines when preparing the final copy for submission.

When ready to send the manuscript to the journal, the faculty prepares a cover letter that indicates:
1. The title of the paper
2. That the paper is original and has not been published already
3. The full name and contact information for the corresponding author (Figure 2)
4. All potential conflicts of interest

If the journal has different departments, the cover letter should specify the department for which the paper was prepared. Some journals have authors sign the transfer of copyright form when submitting the manuscript. For journals that do

March 1, 2009

Marilyn H. Oermann, PhD, RN, FAAN, ANEF
University of North Carolina at Chapel Hill
Editor, *Journal of Nursing Care Quality*
433 Carrington Hall, CB # 7460
Chapel Hill, NC 27599-7460

Dear Dr. Oermann:

Attached please find the manuscript, "Evaluation of an Educational Intervention for Patients with Asthma," for your review for possible publication in the *Journal of Nursing Care Quality*. Neither the entire paper nor any part of it has been published or has been accepted for publication by another journal. The manuscript is not under review by another journal and is submitted only to the *Journal of Nursing Care Quality*.

Thank you for your consideration.

Sincerely,

*John Doe*

John Doe, MSN, RN, C
245 Hill Street
Pittsburgh, Pennsylvania 15228
412.111.2222
jdoe@aoll.com

**Figure 2.** Sample Cover Letter

not follow this procedure, the faculty should include in the cover letter a statement that the paper is original, is not under review by another journal, and has not been published elsewhere. The following statement can be used:

> "Neither the entire paper nor any part of it has been published or has been accepted for publication by another journal. The manuscript is not under review by another journal and is submitted only to [name of journal]."

## Process of Writing for Publication: Publishing Phase

After submission to the journal, the manuscript is reviewed by experts in the content area and if a research report, also by someone with expertise in research methods or statistics. This process is called peer review. Manuscripts are critiqued by peer reviewers who are experts and by the editor who makes the decision whether to publish the paper. The peer review process ensures that quality papers with accurate content and up-to-date information are accepted for publication.

Peer review is usually a blind review process. Identifying information about the author is removed from the manuscript, creating less chance of bias, and authors are unaware of who reviewed their manuscript (Oermann, 2002). With anonymity, reviewers can more honestly critique a paper than if they knew who wrote it. Reviewers complete a form to summarize their critique, which is returned to the faculty with the editor's comments. An example of a review form is in Figure 3.

A manuscript can be accepted without or with revision, the faculty can be asked to revise the manuscript and resubmit it for another review, or the paper can be rejected. When accepted for publication with revisions or if the decision is to revise and resubmit, the faculty should make the suggested changes or provide a rationale for not making them. A summary of the revisions proposed and made in the paper should accompany the manuscript. An example is provided in Table 2. By developing a summary such as this, the faculty improves chances of publication because the summary lists the proposed revisions and where they were made in the manuscript or explains why they were not done. If the manuscript is rejected, the faculty should revise it, using feedback from the peer review process, and submit it to another journal. Once accepted for publication, the faculty answer queries, carefully reads the page proofs to find any errors, and returns all materials to the publisher within the designated time frame.

## Journal of Nursing Care Quality
### Manuscript Review Form

Title:

YES   NO                                                                                    COMMENTS

____ ____   Does the paper present new findings or ideas?
____ ____   If no, does it present old material better?
____ ____   Is the content timely/relevant?
____ ____           logically and clearly developed?
____ ____           sophisticated enough for our readers?
____ ____           innovative?
____ ____   Introduction:  Is the purpose of the paper clear?
            Methods (*research paper*)
____ ____           Are the sample and sampling method adequate?
____ ____           Are the instruments reliable and valid?
____ ____           Are statistical tests appropriate?
            Methods (*other types of papers*)
____ ____           Were the objectives of the project clearly identified?
____ ____           Were the outcomes evaluated adequately?
____ ____   Do conclusions and implications go beyond what findings support?
____ ____   Are the references current?
____ ____   Is the content's application/utility made explicit to the reader's practice
            setting?
____ ____   Was the paper interesting to read?

**Recommendation:**
**( ) Accept for publication without revision**
**( ) Accept for publication after satisfactory revision**
**( ) Review again after major revision**
**( ) Reject**

Please circle the number that best indicates the overall quality of this manuscript:

| 1 | 2 | 3 | 4 | 5 | 6 |
|---|---|---|---|---|---|
| Outstanding | Excellent | Good | Acceptable | Uncertain of acceptability | Unacceptable |

Comments/Suggestions:

**Figure 3.** Sample Manuscript Review Form

| Revisions Proposed | Revisions Made |
|---|---|
| *Reviewer #1:* Where are references #5 and #11 cited in ms.? | Reference #5 on p. 4, line 19; reference #11 on p. 6, line 16 |
| Omit last line of discussion. | Omitted; last para. revised (p. 11, lines 4-7) |
| On p. 5, define criteria | Sentence rewritten with criteria for major and minor errors defined (p. 6, lines 15-23) |
| On pp. 8 and 9, clarify type of errors | Statement added on error types (p. 7, line 21) |
| *Reviewer #2:* p. 5, under design, specify criteria | Rewritten for clarity (see p. 6, section beginning on line 14) |
| Why were these particular journals selected? | Because they are widely read nursing journals; citation added for support and discussion added on p. 5 (line 21-26) |
| Why so few references from JOPAN checked compared to AJCC? | *Journal of PeriAnesthesia Nursing* had 481 citations in 31 articles. *American Journal of Critical Care* had 1181 references in 48 articles. 10% of the references from **each** journal were analyzed consistent with earlier studies. With this method the same **proportion** of references reviewed in each journal. Described on p. 6, lines 3-9 |
| Omit last sentence on p. 6 | Omitted; para. rewritten |
| Expand on why correct citation is important | Discussion (pp. 13-14) expanded and rewritten |
| Conclude in article with how to do an effective search | Discussion expanded; strategies to avoid reference errors included as new table 2 |
| Avoid redundancy in portions of text | Introduction and discussion rewritten. |
| Add implications for faculty | Discussion revised to include how faculty can teach students to avoid reference errors and its importance (see p. 13 [lines 15-18]; p. 15, lines 12-16). Strategies for searches added on p. 17, para 1. |

**Table 2.** Example of Summary to Accompany Revised Manuscript
Oermann MH MS # 111 Accuracy of References in Three Critical Care Nursing Journals

## Summary

Writing for publication is an important skill for faculty to develop. Not only is it essential in many schools of nursing for promotion and tenure decisions, but through publications faculty share their initiatives and innovations with others. Publishing ones work is the best way to contribute evidence to advance nursing education.

## Learning Activities

1. Develop an idea for a manuscript. Select three journals to which you might submit this manuscript. Obtain the author guidelines for these journals, using at least one of these directories.
2. Write a query letter to one of these journals. Review the letter to ensure that all components are included.
3. Who deserves authorship of a paper? What three criteria must be met? Think about a group with whom you have recently worked. If you decided to write a manuscript about this work, which group members would meet the criteria for authorship and who would be acknowledged instead for their contributions? Why?
4. Select an article from a nursing or healthcare journal that you read recently. Read the first paragraph of the article. Can you determine from the first paragraph what the article is about? Why or why not? Did the paragraph get your attention? Did it make you interested in reading further? Now skim the article. Was it easy to read? What did you learn about the writing style?

## Educational Philosophy

Teaching in nursing involves the assessment of student learning needs, development of experiences to meet those needs, and evaluation of student achievement. As such it is a diagnostic process beginning with knowledge of the students—their capabilities, interests, and motivations. Teaching requires involvement of the learner and a supportive environment for learning to take place. Development of this environment for learning involves not only the setting in which learning occurs, but also the interpersonal relationships between teacher and students. Teaching is an interactional process; the ability to work effectively with students in varied settings is critical in promoting their learning and developing a climate in which they can try out new ideas and approaches to care. Teaching strategies in nursing foster development of not only knowledge and skills for practice but also problem-solving and critical-thinking abilities. For this reason varied teaching methods are essential. In the clinical setting the teacher guides student learning within an environment in which the student is comfortable asking faculty for guidance. — Marilyn H. Oermann

## References

*AMA Manual of Style: A Guide for Authors and Editors* (10th ed.). (2007). New York: Oxford Press.

American Psychological Association. (2001). *Publication Manual of the American Psychological Association* (5th ed.). Washington, D.C.: Author.

BrainyMedia.com. (2008). Gene Fowler Quotes. Retrieved March 7, 2008, from http://www.brainyquote.com/quotes/authors/g/gene_fowler.html

Campanelli, P. C., Feferman, R., Keane, C., Lieberman, H. J., & Roberson, D. (2007). An advanced practice psychiatric nurse's guide to professional writing. *Perspectives in Psychiatric Care, 43,* 163-173.

Davidhizar, R. (2004). Guidelines for citing multiple authors. *Nurse Author & Editor, 14*(1), 1-4.

Davis, A.J., & Tschudin, V. (2007). Publishing in English-language journals. *Nursing Ethics, 14,* 425-430.

Hoyt, K.S., & Proehl, J.A. (2007). Peer review for professional publications. *Advanced Emergency Nursing Journal, 29,* 260-264.

International Committee of Medical Journal Editors. (2007, October). Uniform requirements for manuscripts submitted to biomedical journals: Writing and editing for biomedical publication. Retrieved March 7, 2008, from http://www.icmje.org/.

Oermann, M. H. (2000). Refining outlining skills: Part 1: The topic or sentence method. *Nurse Author & Editor, 10*(2), 4, 7-8.

Oermann, M. H. (2002). *Writing for publication in nursing.* Philadelphia: Lippincott, Williams & Wilkins.

Oermann, M. H. (2007). Approaches to gathering evidence for educational practices in nursing. *Journal of Continuing Education in Nursing, 38,* 250-257.

Oermann, M. H., Cummings, S., & Wilmes, N. (2001). Accuracy of references in four pediatric nursing journals. *Journal of Pediatric Nursing, 16,* 263-268.

Oermann, M. H., Mason, N., & Wilmes, N. A. (2002). Accuracy of references in general readership nursing journals. *Nurse Educator, 27,* 260-264.

Oermann, M. H., & Ziolkowski, L. D. (2002). Accuracy of references in three critical care nursing journals. *Journal of PeriAnesthesia Nursing, 17*(2), 78-83.

RefWorks. (2008). Home page. Retrieved March 7, 2008, from http://www.refworks.com/

Saver, C. (2006). Determining what type of article to write. *AORN Journal, 84*, 751-757.

Thomson. (2008). Home page. Retrieved March 7, 2008, from http://thomsonresearchsoft.com/compare/

# CHAPTER 11

## CAN-DO STRATEGIES FOR PUBLISHING SUCCESS:
### DARE TO SHARE, WORK SMART, ASK FOR HELP

Kathleen T. Heinrich, RN, PhD

---

The content of this chapter relates to the following major content areas and subconcepts on the Certified Nurse Educator Examination Detailed Test Blueprint:

**Pursue Continuous Quality Improvement in the Academic Nurse Educator Role**
- Demonstrate a commitment to lifelong learning
- Participate in professional development opportunities that increase one's effectiveness in the role
- Select professional development activities to continue to grow and evolve in the role
- Balance the teaching, scholarship, and service demands inherent in the role of the educator and as influenced by the requirements of the institutional setting

**Engage in Scholarship of Teaching**
- Share teaching expertise with colleagues and others
- Demonstrate integrity as a scholar

---

## Introduction

Publishing is not a luxury! For many nurse educators, it's becoming a job requirement. Which may explain why it's hard to pick up a nursing magazine or journal these days without seeing an article about writing for publication. With the number of how-to articles proliferating, why aren't more nurse educators and their students writing for publication? While know-how is crucial, 15 years of preparing nurses to publish has taught me that believing they can and asking colleagues for help are important for success (Heinrich, 2008).

Whether you want to publish or help your students or colleagues to publish, this chapter describes three can-do strategies:

1. Dare to Share
2. Work Smart
3. Ask for Help

# The Journey that Began with a Yellow Packet

## Getting the Know-How

As a 10 year old, my best friend and I whiled away summer days dreaming of writing a book about our tomboy exploits. Creative writing got left behind as I learned to write academic papers in nursing school and developed my clinical skills after graduation. It wasn't until my second year of teaching that I found a way to bridge my love of writing and my nursing career. When I took Suzanne Hall Johnson's workshop (1979), she walked us step-by-step through the publishing process as we completed the exercises in her yellow-covered packet. If we followed these steps, Suzanne promised, we'd be published. She predicted that once we felt the pleasure of seeing our name in print, we'd be hooked.

## Taking the Dare to Share

Suzanne's yellow packet would move with me every time I changed jobs over the next seven years. In the throes of writing my first manuscript (this is what articles are called before they are published), remembering Suzanne's promise helped me overcome my fears. To take the dare to share, I followed the steps in her yellow-packet:

- **Identify** the four essentials – idea, audience, vehicle and slant
- **Search** for a vehicle
- **Write** a query letter
- **Review** the literature
- **Draft** a manuscript
- **Ask** for peer editing from colleagues

When I submitted my manuscript to *Nurse Educator* (NE), it was rejected. Knowing that publishing is all about perseverance, I was disappointed but not deterred. With *NE* editor Suzanne Smith's support and feedback on revisions, my first article was published in 1985. Seeing my name in print was, as Suzanne Hall Johnson (1979) predicted, so exhilarating that writing for publication became a way of life.

## Believing You Can is the First Step

After I earned a doctoral degree in higher education in 1989, Suzanne's yellow packet accompanied me to a new faculty position on the west coast. It was there that I began to notice how scholarly writing brought out impostor fears – feelings of intellectual fraudulence (Macintosh, 1985) – in nursing students whether they were enrolled in RN to BSN, master's, or doctoral programs. Witnessing the impostor syndrome cripple the best and the brightest when left undiagnosed and treated, I wondered if Suzanne's steps might be an antidote. With her yellow packet as a guide, I designed a publication workshop for a group of doctoral students in 1994. We first dialogued about how to recognize and deal with the critical voice of the impostor, and then the rest of our time was spent on the nuts and bolts of turning academic papers into publications. By day's end, their impostor fears had morphed into a can-do sense of confidence. Participants' evaluations confirmed that integrating a *psychological* approach with Suzanne's how-to publishing steps was a winning combination. (Also see Chapter 10 by Dr. Oermann in this book.)

## Asking for Help

Having returned to the east coast, I landed my dream job as the coordinator of a master's program in nursing education in 1998. Instead of a thesis, students' graduation requirement was a publishable product. With a student to faculty ratio of 60 to 4, students reported needing more faculty support with scholarly writing to turn research projects into manuscripts. Although I published regularly, I had no idea how to teach them to write in a scholarly way. To find out, I traveled the country to attend creative writing workshops. Sharing what I was learning, I designed a two-day writing for publication workshop with a **relational** component that enabled students to practice peer editing. It worked! Instead of the one or two students a year accomplishing publication of their manuscripts after graduation, within 5 years 50% of the graduates' manuscripts were published each year (Heinrich, Neese, Facente & Rogers, 2004). These psycho-educational-relational strategies proved so effective that I began weaving them into the workshops we were conducting for faculty colleagues across campus on turning teaching into scholarship.

## Putting It All Together

Not only was I addicted to seeing my own name in print, I was becoming a scholar-mentor who enjoyed equal pleasure whenever a student or faculty mentee published. When I was granted a sabbatical in May 2002, my project for the year was to write an experiential guidebook about publishing. Intended as a portable mentor for nurses, like Suzanne's yellow packet had been for me. I had no idea that writing this book would take me 5 years and inspire a career change. In 2004, I resigned my tenured professorship to devote myself full-time to preparing nursing groups in academic and healthcare settings to present and publish. In 2008 *A Nurse's Guide to Presenting and Publishing: Dare to Share* was published.

## Three Can-Do Strategies

As I work with nurses, I am finding that presenting and publishing is not only a way for nurses to enhance their careers, it helps them to recover their passion for the profession and boost the zest in their work places (Heinrich, 2007). Grab some of the gusto for yourself. In this section, each can-do strategy – dare to share, work smart, and ask for help – will be broken down into steps (see Table 1). By applying these steps to your own practice, you'll be well on your way to writing your own publishable manuscript.

---

**Strategy 1. Dare to Share**
    A. Set a Still Point
    B. Shift Your Perspective
**Strategy 2. Work Smart**
    A. Reflect on Your Practice
        1. What's My Practice?
        2. What's My Problem/Possibility?
        3. What's the Eye-Glitter Score?
    B. Get Organized
        1. Turn Presentations into Publications
        2. Complete a Worksheet
        3. Devise a Timeline
**Strategy 3. Ask for Help**
    A. Specify Your Needs
    B. Reach Out

---

**Table 1.** Three Can-Do Strategies

## Can-Do Strategy 1: Dare To Share

Tell your stories. We say this to students; we encourage colleagues in practice and academe to share their stories. Sounds simple enough. If you've ever tried writing for publication, you'll know this dare to share is an adventuresome challenge. Just as athletes need to get in the zone, putting yourself in the proper frame of mind is essential. Two ways to get in the writing zone are: set a still point and shift your perspective.

## Set a Still Point

Each morning, before I begin writing, I pause to light a candle. Lighting this candle reminds me to set aside my everyday concerns so I can move into a receptive place where creativity blossoms. This practice is called setting a still point. Whereas a still point is a stop in the action for dancers; it can be the pause that refreshes nurse authors. A still point strategy can be as easy as walking the dog or changing from work clothes into lounge clothes. There are three principles for setting a still point:

1. Keep it simple
2. Make it quick
3. Do it every time you embark on a creative project.

Before you select your own still point, here is a short list of popular still point suggestions:

- Screen saver featuring a peaceful vacation spot
- A shell from a special beach walk
- Three cleansing breaths
- Music that inspires
- A "Do Not Disturb: Creative Nurse At Work" sign for your door knob

## Shift Your Perspective

Whether you want to, or have to, publish, what's stopping you? If you're like many nurses, you'll say it's a lack of time, credentials, and know-how (Steffel, 2007). This is only part of the story. Your impostor fears may be stalling your best efforts. Such fears manifest as a critical inner voice that appears whenever you're facing a writing challenge to tell you that you're not creative, that you have nothing new to say, that you're crazy to even try.

How do you exchange fearing you can not for believing that you **can** publish? Shift your perspective from impostor to nurse author. Start by listening to what your impostor tells you about writing and give that imposter a face and a name. Louise Marks, a writer-colleague of mine, has an impostor named Griselda (Heinrich, 2008). Griselda has frizzy hair, dyed carrot orange and fire-engine red lipstick generously outlining her wrinkled lips. Whenever Louise finds an idea for an article,

Griselda sighs and says, "Go ahead, but you're wasting your time. Why would an editor publish something that everyone already knows?" When Louise carves out an hour to write, Griselda asks when she last watered her withering plants. Pretty soon Louise finds herself cleaning her refrigerator instead of writing.

It may take some time for you to tune into your impostor's messages, to determine if your impostor is a man or woman, and to give your imposter a name. Visualizing your impostor gives form to your fears about writing, and I have yet to meet a nurse who doesn't have those fears. Once you recognize these are fears, and not reality that fuels your inner critic, you'll be eligible for our recovering impostor group. Whenever you hear that critical voice, thank your impostor for the concern and assure him/her that you do not need that kind of protection anymore. Then, instead of feeling paralyzed, you will be free to take the next step in your writing project.

## Can Do Strategy 2: Work Smart

Writing for publication is not about adding more hours to your work day; it is about working smart by building publishing into your schedule. In this section, you'll learn two ways to work smart – reflecting on your practice and getting organized.

### Reflect On Your Practice

What do nurse authors have that you don't? It's not a lack of material; just think about the amazing things that you see and do every day. Nurse authors are able to step back from the action to reflect on their practice. To become a reflective practitioner, you must know what practice you want to write about. Begin by identifying the item(s) that best describe your practice area(s) such as:

- Nursing education
  - o Clinical teaching
  - o Classroom teaching
  - o Clinical/classroom teaching
- Continuing education/staff development
- Clinical specialization
- Administration
- Research
- Consultation

Let's use Jane's practice as an example. Jane is a clinical instructor who teaches in a baccalaureate program 35 hours a week and works as a staff nurse 8 hours a week. If hours spent practicing is the deciding factor, Jane's clinical teaching is the practice to turn into publications. If passion is the deciding factor, then Jane's writing ideas may come from her clinical practice even though she only practices one day a week. When asked which aspect of her practice – clinical teaching or clinical practice – gives her the experiences and inspiration to write for publication, Jane chooses clinical teaching.

So hours spent or passion, choose your best source of inspiration by completing the following three questions:

- Where do you spend most of your time during a typical workweek?
- When it comes to your practice, what is your passion?
- Which aspect of your practice gives you the experiences and the inspiration to write?

Now that you've identified the source of your publishable ideas, you're ready to reflect on your practice. No matter how expert nurse-authors may be, they reflect on their practice with "beginner's mind." In the beginner's mind there are many possibilities, in the expert's mind there are few (Suzuki, 1982). It takes time to become a reflective practitioner. For the next week or so, keep a pad handy and whenever something in the problem or possibility realm happens, jot it down. By the end of the week, you'll have identified a problem/possibility that's intriguing enough for you to write about.

Before settling on a problem or possibility as a topic of your writing, don't forget to measure it on the eye-glitter scale. Place a star on the continuum show in Figure 1 that indicates the intrigue-factor of your problem/possibility.

EYE-GLITTER SCALE

| None | | | | | | | | | Glitter Galore | |
|---|---|---|---|---|---|---|---|---|---|---|
| 0 | 1 | 2 | 3 | 4 | 5 | 6 | 7 | 8 | 9 | 10 |

**Figure 1.** Eye-Glitter Scale

I never waste my time on an idea that rates less than a 9 on the glitter scale. The more an idea intrigues me, the more likely it is that it will intrigue my readers. So if your idea is not eye-glittering enough, keep searching.

## Get Organized

Just as educators prepare for a course by developing a syllabus, working smart involves getting organized before any writing takes place. The three organizing steps to be discussed are:

1. Complete a worksheet
2. Chunk manuscript into write-able pieces
3. Devise a time line

**Complete a worksheet.** My first step when embarking on a writing project is to complete a worksheet. According to Suzanne Hall Johnson (1979), the best publications are written around a single **idea**, for a single group, with a **slant** that entices, and made public in a single **vehicle**. The worksheet in Figure 2 expands on Suzanne's work to include all of the information I have found nurses need to prepare a writing project.

---

**Idea – The What** [Big Idea]:
    **Topic** [More focused]:
    **Focused Topic** [Narrowest]:

**Purpose – The Why** [Possibilities include: educate, motivate, advertise product, professional recognition, personal satisfaction, institutional visibility]:

**Readers – The Who:**

**Vehicle – The Where:**

**Desired Response from Readers:**

**Slant – The Wow** [Can become your title]:

**One-Sentence Description:** This article will…

---

**Figure 2.** Publication Worksheet (Adapted form Heinrich, 2008)

To demonstrate you how to use this worksheet, each item will be discussed individually and my response to the item using writing this chapter as an example will be used.

**Ideas.** Ideas are the **what** – what to write about. In my case, the topic of writing for publication is very broad, too broad for a single manuscript. My **focus** narrows writing for publication to a specific group – nurses. My **focused topic** narrows the general idea to strategies for nurses who want to write for publication.

Idea: Writing for publication

Focus: Nurses writing for publication

Focused Topic: What nurses need to know about can-do, psycho-educational-relational strategies to write for publication. Your focused topic will inform every decision you make about your publication.

**Purpose.** The purpose is the **why**. When the purpose for writing a particular piece is explicitly stated, authors are more likely to stay true to that purpose. There are at least six possibilities: educate, motivate, advertise a product, garner professional recognition, achieve personal satisfaction, and enhance institutional visibility. My purpose for writing this chapter is two-fold: to **educate** nurse educators about psycho-educational-relational strategies so they will be **motivated** to write and help their students and colleagues to write.

**Readers.** A specific group of readers are the **who**. There are two general groups of readers for who nurses write – lay and professional. Since nurse educators are my readers, my chapter is written for a professional audience. Early on, I wanted to write this chapter for nurse educators, administrators, and students. Since the rule is one group of readers per article, I narrowed my target readership to nurse educators. Knowing I am writing to nurse educators helps me decide what information, what language, and what examples to use.

If you have more than one group of readers, narrow your audience to one special group. When you've completed this manuscript, if you still want to write for another group, start a second manuscript.

**Vehicle.** Vehicles are the **where** your piece will be published. Editors call this search process "finding the best home." When you're on the look out for a home for your manuscript, there are three categories of nursing periodicals to consider. See Table 2.

| Category of Nursing Periodicals | Readership | Examples |
|---|---|---|
| 1. General interest | 1. Generalists | American Journal of Nursing |
| 2. Substantive news | 2. Nurses in specialty area, e.g. nurse educators | Journal of Professional Nursing |
| 3. Scholarly | 3. Nurse scholars and researchers | Advances in Nursing Science |

**Table 2.** Vehicles for Publication

You have a choice of formats that includes both virtual (online) and legacy (hard copy): See Table 3.

| Periodical | Format | Example |
|---|---|---|
| 1. E-zine | 1. On-line | Nurse.com |
| 2. Newsletter, Magazine | 1. On-line 2. Legacy | Reflections on Nursing Leadership<br><br>Nursing Spectrum |
| 3. Journal | 1. On-line 2. Legacy | International Journal of Nursing Education Scholarship<br><br>Nurse Educator |

**Table 3.** Choice of Formats

To help you clarify the type of vehicle to consider, here is an example using writing this chapter:

**Focused Idea:** What nurse educators need to know about psycho-educational-relational strategies to write for publication

**Readers:** Nurse educators

**Vehicle:** Book Chapter, *Teaching Nursing: The Art and Science* (2nd ed.)

The best place to begin your search for a home is with the periodicals your target group reads. An on-line search can give you the author guidelines for various nursing periodicals along with select abstracts and full-length articles. A trip to the library offers the tactile pleasure of paging through legacy magazines and journals to compare and contrast the topics and types of articles published in various vehicles.

In this case, I was invited to write this chapter. When I do have to find a home for a manuscript, I search for three good possibilities. If my manuscript is rejected by one publication, I have two back-up possibilities.

Do not be shy about publishing in online journals. When my articles appeared in Sigma Theta Tau's, on-line magazine *Reflections on Nursing Leadership* (Heinrich, 2007, 2006), I received numerous email messages from readers in response. This rarely happens when my articles are published in legacy journals. Based on reader responsiveness, I've decided to submit my next manuscript to the on-line *International Journal of Nursing Education Scholarship*. By specifying the response you hope to elicit from readers, you're more likely to write your manuscript in a way that elicits that response.

**Slant.** The slant is the wow factor. Slants become titles with a perspective that is so unique readers can't resist. There are two types of titles – descriptive (D) and emotive (E). Descriptive titles are the ones nurses typically choose for their articles. Although they tell readers about the article, descriptive titles can be a little dry. Emotive titles pluck at the heart strings. The most irresistible slants combine descriptive with emotive. To show you what I mean, I've labeled my three top choices for titles for this chapter:

1. You Can Do It (E): A Psycho-Educational-Relational Approach to Publishing (D)
2. Dare to Share, Work Smart, Hold Hands (E): A Nurse Author's Secret for Success (D)
3. Can-Do Strategies for Publishing Success (D): Dare to Share, Work Smart & Ask for Help (E)

I chose the third title. The descriptive phrase tells the reader this chapter is about publishing and the three names for strategies are short and snappy enough to pluck heart strings.

If you are concerned that titles like mine are not scholarly enough, you're not alone. This is nurse educators' most common concern about emotive slants and titles. My response? I've never had a scholarly manuscript rejected because of a

## Can Do Strategy 3: Ask for Help

When reading *Winnie-the-Pooh* recently, I was struck that the first thing Winnie and his friends do when they get into a jam is to ask themselves what kind of help they need and who can help them. If the life of children is full of asking for help, why is it so difficult for nurses to reach out and ask for help? I'm not sure. I do know that writing for publication becomes easier when you do as Pooh does. Figure out what you need and who is the best person to ask.

It is easier to ask for help when you know what you need. There are five types of helpers who can assist with writing projects.

1. **Rooters** keep authors going by reminding them how important their ideas are and how much readers will benefit from reading their publication
2. **Co-authors** assist with every step in a writing project from conceptualization to writing to signing off on the final draft
3. **Expert editors** ensure that manuscripts treat specialized information correctly when that information is outside the author's expertise
4. **Style editors** review manuscripts for proper grammar and punctuation
5. **Developmental editors** help authors new to the publishing process to learn the ropes.

See Table 6.

| Type of Help | Helper |
|---|---|
| Increased confidence | Rooter |
| Rooter | Co-author |
| Command of a subject area | Expert Editor |
| Polishing grammar and punctuation | Style Editor |
| Learning the publishing process | Developmental Editor |

**Table 6.** What Type of Help Do You Need?

Asking the question about who can assist you is clarifying. The clearer you visualize your need, the more likely it is that you will identify a colleague with exactly the right skills who is willing and eager to help. Then all you have to do is reach out. Once you see how smoothly writing projects go with the proper assistance, chances are that asking for help will come easier.

## Summary

What's the next step? Are you in search of an eye-glittering problem or possibility in your practice? Want to settle on an idea, a group of readers, a fitting vehicle or an enticing slant? Or ask for help? Whatever your next step, the psycho-educational-relational strategies presented in this chapter can make it happen:

1. Dare to Share
2. Work Smart
3. Ask for Help

Whether you want to publish, or help your students or colleagues write, for publication, practicing these steps and strategies will give you the self-confidence, the know how, and the assistance to turn ideas into publications. You can do it!

## Learning Activities

1. Jot down a still point strategy to help you move from an everyday activity to a creative-receptive frame of mind. Commit to using this strategy to signal your mind, body and spirit that it's time to step into the creativity zone.
2. Get acquainted with the impostor that prevents you from becoming a nurse author. Answer these questions: What is your impostor's favorite line or ploy to distract you from writing? What does your impostor look like (Describe or draw your impostor)? What is your impostor's name?
3. Answer this "Beginner's Mind" Questions: What's a problem or possibility from my practice that's intriguing enough to write about?
4. Think about a topic for writing an article for publication. Complete the items on the worksheet described in Figure 2.
5. Think about the audience who would read your article. Who would they be? Would you have more than one group of readers?
6. Consider the type of "helpers" presented in Table 6. Which ones may be of help to you and why?

## Educational Philosophy

At the risk of sounding contrary, I don't have a personal philosophy of teaching. Nor do I embrace the current trend toward a student-centered approach to learning. What fascinates me is how learning emerges from relationships. That's why I endeavor to co-create learning experiences that are interactive and dialogic. In interchanges that overflow with energy, we learn from one another—beginner from expert, expert from beginner; student from teacher, teacher from student. Engaged and "in the moment", our curiosity leads to questions; our disclosures flow into compassion for each other's experiences; and, our insights fire our passion for learning more. In sum, mine is a philosophy of learning that is relationship-centered. — Kathleen T. Heinrich

## References

Heinrich, K. T. (2006, Second Quarter). Joy-stealing games. *Reflections on Nursing Leadership*. Available at: http://www.nursingsociety.org

Heinrich, K. T. (2006, Third Quarter). Joy-stealing: How some nurse educators resist these faculty games. *Reflections on Nursing Leadership*. Available at: http://www.nursingsociety.org

Heinrich, K. T. (2007, Third Quarter). Full-circle moment: Recognizing the joy-stealer within. *Reflections on Nursing Leadership*. Available: http://www.nursingsociety.org

Heinrich, K. T. (2007, November/December). Dare to share: A unique approach to presenting and publishing. *Nurse Educator, 32*(6), 260-4.

Heinrich, K. T. (2008). *A nurse's guide to presenting and publishing: Dare to share*. Sudbury, MA: Jones and Bartlett Publishers

Heinrich, K. T., Neese, M. R., Facente, A., & Rogers, D. (2004). Turn accusations into affirmations: Transform nurses into published authors. *Nursing Education Perspectives, 25*(3), 139-147.

Johnson, S. H. (1979). *Publishing Workshop*. Lakewood, CO: Health Update.

MacIntosh, P. (1985). *Feeling like a fraud*. Working Paper No. 18. Wellesley, MA: Stone Center for Developmental Services and Studies.

Steefel, L. (2007, September 24) Nursing students feel the push to publish. Retrieved from *Nurse.com*. September 29, 2007.

Suzuki, S. (1982). *Zen mind, beginner's mind*. New York: Weatherhill.

# CHAPTER 12

# GETTING STARTED WITH GRANTS

## Susan Diehl, BSN, MSN, EdD, RN, FNP, APRN

The content of this chapter relates to the following major content areas and subconcepts on the Certified Nurse Educator Examination Detailed Test Blueprint:

**Pursue Continuous Quality Improvement in the Academic Nurse Educator Role**

- Participate in professional development opportunities that increase one's effectiveness in the role
- Select professional development activities to continue to grow and evolve in the role
- Balance the teaching, scholarship, and service demands inherent in the role of the educator and as influenced by the requirements of the institutional setting

**Function as a Change Agent and Leader**

- Integrate a long term, innovative, and creative perspective into the academic nurse educator role

**Engage in the Scholarship of Teaching**

- Demonstrate integrity as a scholar

**Function Effectively within the Institutional Environment and the Academic Community**

- Determine professional goals within the context of academic nursing and the mission of the nursing program and parent institution

## Introduction

Grant writing. The mere sound of the words is likely to raise fear and doubt in the mind of the nurse educator. This is a common and completely normal reaction to the topic of grant writing in higher education. It is, however, unfortunate on two counts. First, external or alternative funding is becoming increasingly important because of market pressures and resource constraints in higher education. While academics are familiar with obtaining individual research and training grants, there will be increased demand to attach funding to service and teaching activities that support both the institution's mission and individual scholarly pursuits. In fact, in some institutions revenue generation is an expected part of the faculty role (Hensen, 2003). Second, by focusing on the complaints of grantsmanship (too confusing, frustrating, time-consuming), educators often fail to see the true value of incorporating grantsmanship in their work. The obvious benefit to receiving grants is the reward of being paid for special talents and ideas. The less obvious—but equally wonderful—benefit is that the discipline of grant seeking itself can actually help shape the career of the nurse educator. Thinking like a grantseeker forces the academic to plan in organized ways that bring ideas to fruition. Many have begrudgingly admitted that being an active grantseeker has been invaluable in framing their daily activities of teaching, research, and service. It is not just a way to obtain dollars; it is a way to think.

The purpose of this chapter is to introduce nurse educators to the idea of grantsmanship so they feel confident enough to incorporate grant seeking into their professional lives. Most nurses do not realize how well positioned they are to be successful players in the grant world, so it is the intent of this chapter to provide the background that will encourage nurses to start to participate. The grant world is large. In the United States, there are more than 60,000 funding institutions from the private sector alone that constitutes more than $30 billion in grant transactions. In 2008, *Foundation Giving Trends* reports that health related programs are earning more grant funding than ever (foundationcenter.org). It is reasonable to assume that nurse educators can be highly successful in obtaining funding to support their ideas and dreams.

## The Four Elements of the Grant Process

Although the grant process is admittedly confounding at times, there are really only four elements that need to be understood to begin participating in the grant world. They are:
1. **The Great Idea:** A way to solve a problem or address a need
2. **The Grantseeker:** The person who seeks out funding to support the great idea
3. **The Grantmaker:** The organization whose purpose is to fund great ideas
4. **The Proposal:** The document that brings the first three elements together

## The Great Idea

The purpose of grants is to award money to support worthy causes. Although what is considered a worthy cause varies among grantmaking institutions, they all are interested in projects or programs that address some sort of human need. Every funded project started out with an idea.

Ideas are simply the plans and schemes that live in our heads. Whether through teaching, research, or service, nurse educators are constantly using ideas to solve problems to make things better for students, patients, and communities. It is easy to get careless with ideas, using them to serve a purpose and then letting them go. More times than one can imagine, those ideas were potential grant proposals. So, keeping track of ideas that one is interested in pursuing further is a first step to thinking like a grantseeker. Just as one keeps track of accomplishments and activities as a nurse educator, one must record potential proposal ideas as a grantseeker.

A good suggestion for storing ideas is to keep an **idea drawer**, where ideas of interest can be filed. To highlight the benefit of keeping an idea drawer, a colleague's story follows:

*As a pediatric nurse, I used to have a file drawer where I would keep things that interested me. Articles from journals and magazines, notes about things that happened at work, famous quotes, pictures, interesting programs or projects. They were in no particular order, in fact, the drawer became the place where I put things that I wasn't sure what to do with. Well, one day, I couldn't get the drawer closed, so I was forced to clean it out. A newspaper clipping about the rise in child abuse and neglect got put in a pile next to a random newsletter from a child welfare organization. Somehow, I knew that nurses needed to be involved in this issue, and I knew I might be able to do something to help. It took a lot of focusing and reframing but I kept those two pieces of paper in front of me, wrote successful grants, and began a career in developing programs to prevent child abuse and neglect. I love it. My advice? Keep an idea drawer, just clean it out more often than I did.*

This story illustrates an important principle of grantsmanship. Finding money to support ideas is a little more complex than having an idea and then finding someone to fund it. Grant cycles, current events, and changes in the nurse educator's professional life prevent the process from being this simple. This is why it is important to take track of ideas. While it is impossible to predict when an idea may become useful, there are ways to play with these ideas so they **do something**.

A way to add to the idea drawer is to keep a journal. A journal is a novice grantseeker's best friend. This is the place where brainstorming and dreaming can occur, as well as a place to practice writing skills needed to become more proficient in writing grants. How one keeps a journal is a highly personal affair, but there are many resources from the field of creative writing that can help the nurse educator become an effective dreamer on paper. Dwelling in the possibilities of passions and ideas should be an ongoing process in the life of a nurse educator. For those unfamiliar with journal writing, the book *Writing Alone and With Others* by Schneider (2003) is recommended.

Keeping a journal also helps clarify the nurse educator's passions and true interests. Grant writing experts agree the most successful projects are the ones that have a clear passion behind them. While nurse educators may claim to not have any ideas, most nurse educators have passion for their work. Having a good sense of what delights and excites the educator is critically important to the development of a professional career and finding the support for it.

The acts of defining a passion, collecting ideas, and seeing possibilities translate well when adding funding into the mix. It is just a matter of seeing the connections. When the nurse educator sees an idea that repeatedly captures his or her attention, it is time to see if the idea is a **great idea**. This is usually intuitive, but there are some qualities that separate great ideas from good ones. Ideas that are worth pursuing have some originality. This does not mean that an idea has to be wildly innovative, but it means there should be a spark to the idea that makes it different. A great idea also solves a problem. Most ideas start because of a need to change something, and a great idea shows a way to meet that need. If one has gotten this far, it is worth trying to envision the idea in practice.

Funding organizations look for opportunities to support ideas that attempt to solve worthy problems. The nurse educator should try to define the idea as a problem and then consider ways that one might solve the problem. The solutions are what funders are interested in learning more about. The time when an idea is percolating is exactly the right time to take this step. This means that when an idea is put in the idea drawer, one should immediately start to think about how this idea looks in a problem-solving context.

Several fundamental questions should be explored when thinking about putting an idea into action. There are many resources that can help the nurse educator turn ideas into fundable projects. One such book is *The Only Grant-Writing Book You Will Ever Need* (Karsh & Fox, 2006). Another fun read is *Storytelling for Grantseekers: The Guide to Creative Nonprofit Fundraising* by C. C. Clarke (2001). Consider this adapted list of fundamental questions as a beginning:

- What is the problem or need that your idea addresses? How involved or expert are you in the problem?
- Where else have you seen this problem addressed?
- How do you plan to solve the problem or meet the need?
- How would things be different or better if your idea was implemented? Locally? Globally?
- How would you know if things were better?
- What do you need to implement your idea? Money? People?

By attempting to answer these questions, ideas become more realistic and more useful in planning for grant seeking. If the answers come fairly easily, one is well on the way to a successful – and fundable – adventure. It is important to remember this is an ongoing process. One should never throw away the ideas that do not quite fit, nor should one stop adding new ones. The grantseeking process does not have an even ebb and flow. One needs to rely on being ready when opportunities present themselves, whether the ideas eventually are funded or not.

When the nurse educator believes he or she has an idea worth pursing, it is time to let colleagues review the idea or project. Before one invests the time to pursue funding, it is wise to explain the project to a selected group of three different people, and ask for their feedback.

The first person should be a colleague who knows you and understands why you are interested in this idea. This person can help evaluate and shape the nurse educator's commitment to the proposed idea.

The second person should be an experienced grantmaker or someone who has had experience with grantseeking. This person will be able to provide feedback from a funder's perspective.

The third person who should be consulted is someone who would likely oppose the idea. For example, if the idea is to design an online course, choose a person who is Internet-phobic. Although this seems odd, it is very important not to skip the third person. Nothing shapes the significance of your project more than the feedback of a dubious audience.

Explaining an idea to different people gives the nurse educator a chance to clarify and reshape the idea. One common mistake that grant writers make is assuming that everyone knows what they mean. Discussing the idea with different people is also an excellent way to perfect the organization and tone of the idea, which will be important when it is time to apply for funding. Probably the most important benefit of this exercise is that the nurse educator has begun to create a network of people who are interested in the idea. Networking is an efficient use of time, especially as the process moves to finding grants.

## The Grantseeker

The term "grantseeker" may be unfamiliar to the reader. This term is used in the grant business to describe the person who looks for funding opportunities and finds ways to obtain the funding, ie, one who actually writes grants. In short, a grantseeker is a matchmaker.

The purpose of this chapter is to blur the line between the idea person and the grantseeker, as this is the reality of the grant world today. The explosion of information technology has changed relationships and roles in the grant world. Grants have become less the domain of the professionals and more open to the people with the ideas. As recently as five years ago, professional grantseekers earned their money as matchmakers between idea people and funders. It was hard-earned money because the task was grueling. This is changing. Information about funding opportunities is available on the Internet for the person willing to invest the time to research them. While professional grantseekers continue to serve a valuable service in gatekeeping and provide assistance in writing grants, their role has become more consultative.

Above all else, funders want to support worthy causes that are likely to produce successful outcomes. To ensure success, most funders want to get as close as possible to the original source of the project or program. That means they want to deal directly with the actual person behind the idea. This means nurse educators must be accountable for their ideas, so it behooves them to become actively involved in the process of seeking out grants. This is the process nurses are least familiar with, so it should be made clear that the procedure has a bit of a learning curve. It is wise to be patient. The ability to find out about grant opportunities grows with time. As a beginner, one will need to know a little bit about the language of the grant world, adopt some behaviors of professional grantseekers, and, most importantly, decide on the type of grantseeker one wants to be.

There is no deficit of advice and guidance available on the subjects of grantseeking and grant writing. The fact that Amazon.com carries more than 60,000 titles on the subject is proof enough. Before one becomes overwhelmed with the good advice of others, it is critical for the nurse educator to know himself or herself when starting to propose projects for funding. To do this, the educator must think ahead and plan carefully what he or she truly wants to do and be. Try this short exercise:

Envision yourself five years from now. What do you see yourself doing with your passions and interests? Do you see yourself deeply involved in clinical nursing research? Will you be operating a health clinic at a homeless shelter? Will you be inventing curricula for long-distance learning in nursing?

Now do some careful soul searching about your work personality. Do you like to have a lot of things going on at once or do you prefer to focus on one project at a time? Do you prefer working alone or with others?

Whatever you see yourself doing in the future will help narrow the search for funders who will be interested in your proposals. Likewise, your work personality should define the types of grants that will be managcable for you. If you like to engage in short activities or have more than one interest, you should seek out grants that are time limited and intended for very specific purposes. If you enjoy the planning and commitment of long-term programs, your search could include larger grants that extend over longer periods of time. The real art of grantseeking lies in knowing what you want and to what you are willing to commit. It pays to be self aware from the start. Frustration with the grant process generally comes from people not taking this important step.

Although Internet searches make it easier to locate potential grantors, the sheer number of funding organizations makes it impossible to stay abreast of all of them. The beginning grantseeker should understand that time and networking will help to stay aware of opportunities down the road. One should not miss opportunities. The following is a good example:

> *Maureen has always loved technology. She was an intensive care nurse for years, and was always the first to learn the latest technology. When she became a nurse educator, she immediately became involved with instituting technology in the classroom. She designed websites and interactive electronic games for her students. Her classes were very popular with students and she continued designing teaching interventions with technology. She was enjoying her work, but it started to take a toll on her time. Someone suggested she write a grant for some release time so she could focus on a particular web project. Maureen was surprised at this suggestion. It had never occurred to her to seek help with her work.*

Maureen applied for a small grant from a technology corporation. She used the money to get release time from teaching and developed a health assessment tool that is being used by many universities on the East Coast. Maureen continued to pursue larger grants, and her work is now almost completely funded by grant awards. She admits she initially avoided grantseeking because of the investment of time it would require. "The time I gained to pursue good things clearly outweighed the time it took to apply for the grants," she says. Maureen was successful because she incorporated a grantseeking attitude into her real work. She stayed focused on matching her exact needs to grant opportunities.

New nurse educators often are surprised at the large number of grant initiatives in which they are invited to participate. Grant talk is daily discussion in higher education, and it is sometimes easy to get involved in participating even when it is not exactly the educator's cup of tea. Being flexible about opportunities, but firm about passions, is a way to avoid becoming overwhelmed or frustrated with the grant process.

## The Grantmaker

Grantmakers, also known as funders or donors, are the organizations that give money to worthy causes. In general, worthy causes are defined as activities that result in making things better for society. These organizations are set up to review, evaluate, and give money to projects or programs that fit the mission of the institution. This section provides an overview of the categories of grant institutions, types of grants, and the characteristics of grantmakers, that make the work of the grantseeker quite interesting.

There are three basic types of grantmakers. Private foundations are organizations that are created with the money of wealthy philanthropists. Large foundations like the Hearst Foundation are familiar to the public, but there are many smaller private foundations. Resources such as Foundations On-line at foundations.org compile and update grant opportunities.

Government agencies are the second major type of grantmaker. Nurses probably are somewhat familiar with some of the grant activity that takes place at government agencies such as the National Institutes of Health. Government grants can be obtained at the federal, state, and local levels. The website, www.Grants.gov, is a valuable resource for seeking out potential grants.

Private businesses and corporations are the third type of grantmaker. Their money is usually given to support needs of their local community.

The term "foundation" is also used to describe legal entities set up to meet philanthropic needs. Corporate foundations and community or public foundations are also types of funders. Nurses and their work have been funded from all of these types of institutions.

Grantmakers give away different kinds of grants, in amounts that can vary from a few thousand dollars to a few hundred thousand and more. It is important to understand the categories of grants that are available so the grantseeker can find the best fit. Brown & Brown (2008) define these categories:

- **Program grants:** These grants support the establishment of specific, targeted programs like support groups for teen mothers.
- **Start-up grants:** Also known as program development grants, these grants supply seed money for programs that are expected to become long-term and eventually be supported by other means.

- **Research grants:** These grants support the study of an issue. They are most often given to universities or nonprofit research facilities.
- **Endowment grants:** Endowment funds are invested to provide an annual flow of income to support a cause.
- **Consulting grants:** It is increasingly common for grantmakers to offer grants to hire consultants on valuable projects.
- **Training grants:** These grants support professional development and conference activities.
- **Scholarship and fellowship grants:** These grants support educational costs for individuals.

Having a sense of the type of grants an organization provides is a good start in the grantseeker's quest. However, while all funding institutions have the same goal of giving money to nonprofit organizations and their worthy causes, this is where the similarity ends.

Each institution has its own unique mission and interests. Depending on the founder's wishes, money is donated to support specific interests, such as health, education, community building, or the arts. They may also limit their funding to certain geographical locations or populations.

Each grantmaking institution has its own requirements and processes for organizations applying for grants. One institution might require query letters before the proposal is submitted; another might prefer to simply receive the proposals. Some institutions prefer individual narrative proposals; others have standard application forms. In addition, grantmaking institutions have their own timelines for distributing grants, called grant cycles.

Keeping up with each potential grantor's requirements mandates some research and accurate record keeping. The grantseeker should collect information about potential donors including a description of the institution's interest, types and amounts of grants offered in the past, and funding cycles. Also inquire about the types of institutions the grant will not support. Annual reports and histories of funded grants can help the grantseeker determine whether to pursue a foundation for funding. Information about foundations is available in on-line directories (downloadable with cost) such as, *The Foundation Directory* (http://fconline. fdncenter.org), and *The National Directory of Corporate Giving* (foundationcenter. org). These directories are also available at most libraries.

The Internet has made it much easier to collect information about prospective donors, especially in the last few years. The Foundation Center at www. foundationcenter.org is a sophisticated website that lists foundations and provides links to many foundation sites. The Foundation Center website can be easily launched from the CD accompanying this book. A subscription is required for access to detailed information about specific grants, but there is enough free information to send the grantseeker in the right direction.

Much of grantseeking is done with simple search engine searches such as Google. During online research, searches by keyword will help the grantseeker narrow the list of potential donors. Since the project should have a clear focus, and the grantseeker should know what kind of grant he or she is looking for, keywords are easily used to manage the search.

Trying to locate funders who will be excited about the project and researching their characteristics and requirements may seem like an imposing task. Instead of thinking of foundations as donors, it is helpful to think of them as partners. Brown and Brown (2001) describe the appropriate paradigm for the grantseeker.

> Grants are not free money. Foundations and other grantmakers are organizations that have missions and goals just as you do. Funders award grants because what the recipients want to do with the money fits in with the funder's own goals, initiatives and dreams, and with their founder's stated wishes. It makes sense to see a grant as a fair deal between colleagues whose interests are similar but whose resources are different (p. 5).

This explanation sets a healthy perception of grantseekers and grantmakers. This relationship should be viewed as a partnership. Partners are not givers and receivers. Partners invite each other to participate in a common venture, and partners try to understand each other. Using this concept helps the grantseeker to see the project from the grantmaker's point of view and be more attentive to matching the partners' goals and tone. This special attention will be rewarded when it is time to write the grant proposal.

## The Proposal

Writing grant proposals is not a difficult task in itself, especially if one already has thought out the idea, and knows that the funder is likely to support the project's mission. The best approach for writing grant proposals is to be clear, consistent, concise, and compelling. Most grantmakers have very specific guidelines for how grant proposals should be presented. It is the grantseeker's job to carefully review the donor's expectations and answer the questions, complete the required forms, and create a cover letter. The details of a grant proposal can be overwhelming to the nurse educator, but there are two solutions to this perceived problem. One is to remember the purpose of the proposal. The nurse educator has a great idea and has found a funder who might help make it happen. The proposal is simply a way to give the funder a logical reason to choose to support this project.

The second way is to practice with a boilerplate proposal. The boilerplate proposal is a generic outline of the project—a template—written without any particular funder in mind. Some states have a statewide form that is used by institutions in that state. The boilerplate proposal allows the writer to practice translating the great idea into the language of grantmakers.

There are many resources on writing a good grant proposal using a boilerplate. Hensen's (2003) *Grant Writing in Higher Education* has a very detailed guide to writing proposals. This author presents seven basic components of a boilerplate proposal and a short description of what each component entails.

Another useful resource is the *Proposal Writing Short Course* supplied by the FoundationCenter. (http://foundationcenter.org/getstarted/tutorials/shortcourse/need.html) This website can easily be launched from the CD accompanying this book.

Whatever boilerplate template the grantseeker uses, the point is to get the basic information on paper. Grantmakers may ask for more information or request the information in a different format, but the basics remain the same. The following components should be included:
- Introduction or summary of the project
- Statement of need and goal of the project
- Project objectives, project activities, and method of evaluation
- Budget
- Description of the grantseeker's organization and funding history
- Supporting materials
- Cover letter

## The Introduction

The introduction is a summary of the project, which grant officers will read to get a sense of what the project is about. Expert grant writers limit this section to one page. After reading the introduction, grant officers should clearly understand the need and goal of the project, the people involved, the total budget, and how much money is being requested from their institution. The introduction is where quick decisions may be made, so this section must be written in language that is clear, concise, and confident. The best advice for writing this section of the boilerplate is to write the introduction last.

## Statement of Need

The statement of need describes why the proposed project is necessary. Grantmakers look for how the specific need that is being addressed fits the larger social issue with which their institution is concerned. The funnel approach is helpful here: Start with the general problem, and then describe how it affects a specific community. Hard data that show the existence of a problem should be incorporated here, and the writer should refer to the literature thoroughly and thoughtfully. Using too many statistics is confusing, but a synthesized body of evidence provides a clear rationale for the project. Follow the statement of need with the project's overall goal and a description of the community or population it will serve.

## Work of the Project

The work of the project is described in this next section and tells exactly what the project will do. It should be written with:
- Clear objectives
- A description of the activities that will meet those objectives
- An explanation of how success will be measured

Writers often make two mistakes in this section. One is confusing **goals** with **objectives**. It is helpful to think of the goal as the endpoint, and the objectives as the intended ways to get there. Goals can be written as general statements whereas objectives are more concrete and measurable. The other mistake writers tend to make is including too many goals and objectives. One overall goal is sufficient for any grant proposal. The number of objectives may vary with the size of the project, but there rarely should be more than five.

Grantmakers prize innovation but look carefully for feasibility in grant proposals. This section is the writer's chance to demonstrate how the project can be completed successfully. Clearly defining how the activities support the objectives, how the objectives support the goal, and how the goal supports the needs statement is crucial in grant proposals.

## The Budget

Since grantmakers are financial agents, the budget is vitally important to the success of a grant proposal. Most beginning nurse grantseekers struggle with this part of the boilerplate proposal, finding it difficult to attach dollar figures to the activities and people needed for the grant. There are many print resources to assist in preparing a budget. *Storytelling for Grant Seekers: The Guide to Creative Nonprofit Fundraising* by C. C. Clarke (2001) offers straightforward and practical advice on creating budgets. The Internet is also a practical resource for obtaining information about a budget. There are two ways to obtain this information. First, a general search will reveal various templates that grantseekers have used in many different fields. A good tutorial can be found at Scholastic.com which is a teacher networking website (http://teacher.scholastic.com/professional/grants/grant.htm). The point here is that grant writing is common to many disciplines, organizations, and individuals; therefore, good guidance may come from unexpected sources. The other way to obtain information is to research the topical area of interest for organizations, forums, and individuals with similar interests. Sharing of grant opportunities and grant budget construction often comes from Internet networking with people of similar interests.

The key to grant budgets is to work through the basic budget components of revenue and expenses. By showing the difference in revenue and expenses, one is letting the funder know the amount of money that is requested. Grantmakers want to know the project is supported, so it is wise to include any in-kind donations in the revenue column.

Grant budgets are generally one or two pages long. A budget narrative, describing the use of the money, may also be requested. The narrative should include plans for future funding and a report of any other funding options the grantseeker has pursued for the project. Annual reports and a copy of the Internal Revenue Service 501(c) letter confirming nonprofit status should be attached to the budget narrative.

## The Organization's History and Funding History

The next component is a short description of the organization's history and funding activity. Grantmakers must be sure the recipients of their donations are nonprofit organizations and must ensure the person in charge of the grant is supported by an institutional structure, usually the academic institution where the nurse educator works. Universities are familiar with faculty grants and the administrative office normally has a boilerplate description of the institution's history and annual report suitable for grant submissions.

## Supporting Documents

The section for supporting documents usually includes letters of support, relevant newspaper articles or research articles, and the resumes of people involved in the project. Letters of support and endorsements are important to the grant proposal.

One should not underestimate the value of personal and professional testimonials of the person who will direct the project. Funders know that great ideas are only as good as the people who carry them out.

## Cover Letter

The cover letter is perhaps the most important part of the proposal. Grant writers will spend 90 percent of their time writing the proposal, but the cover letter can make or break the grant request. The cover letter is the best opportunity for the grantseeker to connect with the funder and highlight the uniqueness of the proposal. A good cover letter shows it was expressly written to the funder. This can be done by clearly responding to the needs and interests of the funder. When describing the project, one should present the most compelling ideas first. The letter should be visually appealing, concise, and professional, just as the rest of the proposal should be.

## Final Thoughts on the Proposal

The proposal is what brings a great idea, grantseekers, and grantmakers together. A good proposal conveys they belong together. There is no way to predict a funder's reaction to a grant proposal. If a proposal is rejected, it is important to try to get feedback from the grantmaker. Evaluating both the successes and failures in seeking grants is important learning for the nurse educator—learning that can help bring success with the next proposal.

## Summary

Nurse educators are encouraged to actively incorporate grantseeking into their professional lives. Their roles in higher education will demand it, and their work will be better because of it. The nurse educator who takes good care of ideas and develops a grantseeking attitude is well prepared to enter the world of grants. The rest comes from experience. Getting started with grants is like everything else. Getting started is the hard part.

## Learning Activities

1. Identify some of your ideas about nursing or nursing education. Describe how you might turn those ideas into grant proposals.
2. Visit the website of a professional organization such as the National League for Nursing or Sigma Theta Tau International. Find the organization's guidelines for submitting a grant proposal. Print the submission guidelines and use them to write a grant proposal. Have a colleague critique your proposal.
3. Prepare a budget proposal for a specific project or program.

## Educational Philosophy

If a teacher sets the table with energetic experiences, sound knowledge, and a welcoming spirit, learners will pull up a chair. — Susan Diehl

## References

Brown, L. G., & Brown, M. J. (2008). *Demystifying grant seeking: What you really need to do to get grants*. San Francisco: Jossey-Bass.

The Foundation Center (2008). *Foundation Giving Trends, 2008 Edition*. Retrieved February 26, 2008, from www.foundationcenter.org

Hensen, K. T. (2003). *Grant writing in higher education: A step by step guide*. Upper Saddle River, NJ: Pearson, Allyn & Bacon.

Karsh, E., & Fox, A. S. (2006). *The only grant-writing book you will ever need: Top grant writers and grant givers share their secrets*. New York: Avalon.

## Bibliography

Clarke, C. C. (2001). *Storytelling for grantseekers: The guide to creative nonprofit fundraising*. San Francisco: Jossey-Bass.

Schneider, P. (2003). *Writing alone and with others*. New York: Oxford University Press.

# CHAPTER 13

# FUTURE FORCES AFFECTING 21ST CENTURY HEALTH PROFESSIONS EDUCATION:
## MASTERING THE KNOWLEDGE, SKILLS, AND ABILITIES TO SUPPORT 21ST CENTURY LEARNING

**Daniel J. Pesut, PhD, RN, FAAN**
**Elliott Z. Pesut, BSAS**

---

The content of this chapter relates to the following major content areas and subconcepts on the Certified Nurse Educator Examination Detailed Test Blueprint:

**Pursue Continuous Quality Improvement in the Academic Nurse Educator Role**
- Demonstrate a commitment to lifelong learning

**Function as a Change Agent and Leader**
- Integrate a long term, innovative, and creative perspective into the academic nurse educator role
- Create a culture for change within the nursing program
- Promote innovative practices in educational environments
- Adapt to changes created by external factors

**Function Effectively within the Institutional Environment and the Academic Community**
- Identify how social, economic, political, and institutional forces influence nursing and higher education

---

## Introduction

The purpose of this chapter is to describe and explain future forces (2006-2016) likely to affect health professions and nursing education. These future forces are influenced and shaped by policy, politics, technology, projected scenarios, and personal and professional aspirations. Elsewhere Pesut (2000 ) has written being a futurist requires paying attention to time, learning about the future, understanding people's reactions to the future, using emotional intelligence to influence future changes, monitoring trends, and discerning consequences of trends.

Trends are used to create vision-based scenarios that stimulate strategic conversations about posited scenarios. Such conversations serve a learning function as people begin to dialogue and think about the 1st, 2nd, and 3rd order cascading-consequences of predicted futures and the consequences of those trends for students and faculty. Through analysis and interaction with scenarios people are in a better place to ask themselves if such predicted futures are desirable or not. If they are desirable, how will people rally to create the preferred future that they seek? If such futures are not desirable then how will people rally to prevent undesirable futures from unfolding?

As Bezold, Hancock, and Sullivan (1999) observe, future thinking is a tool for wiser action that stimulates the imagination, encourages creativity, identifies threats and opportunities, and allows us to align values with future choices that have consequences. As Dr. Allen Tough (1993) suggests, satisfactory futures are possible if enough people care about future generations, understand today's options, and make appropriate choices, as they learn about the problems and possibilities of future developments through time. The purposes and objectives of this chapter are to:

1. Describe educational policy statements likely to influence future health professions education and teaching and learning practices.
2. Explain some of the elements of the Knowledge Works and Institute for the Future Map of the Future Forces Affecting Education 2006-2016 and implications for future teaching-learning practices.
3. Discern consequences of technological-environmental trends and the meaning such trends have for nurse educators and students.
4. Develop personal and professional action steps to master the knowledge, skills and competencies needed to thrive in the projected future.

## 21st Century Educational Policies : Aspirations and Influence

There are a number of organizations that have put forth 21st century educational policy aspirations. For example, the Association of American Colleges and Universities (2007) has identified essential aims, learning outcomes and guiding principles to consider as educators plan, implement, and evaluate curricula. The Institute of Medicine (2002) has defined aspirational goals for a 21st century healthcare system. Achieving the identified goals depends on transforming health professions education. The American Association of Colleges of Nursing (2008) has revised its policy documents on essentials for baccalaureate, masters, and doctoral education for professional nursing practice. The TIGER (2007) initiative has proposed a healthcare future based on transforming nursing education through the use, application, and evaluation of technology in education, practice, and research contexts.

Dr. Lee Shulman (2002) suggests there is a need for a new taxonomy or table of learning that involves attention to issues of engagement, understanding, action, reflection, judgment, and commitment as people master knowledge and develop wisdom in light of social and contemporary learning challenges. Certainly the policies and perspectives of these organizations and educational leaders need to be considered as one begins to imagine how future forces will shape 21st century health professions education. Such policy suggestions take on personal and professional meaning as individuals seek to understand and develop personal and professional goals that align with professional career aspirations. Consider how the following recommendations are likely to shape the future of health professions education and teaching and learning in the discipline of nursing.

In the report, College Learning for the New Global Century, The Association of American Colleges and Universities (2007) outlines goals for future curriculum development. This report spells out the essential aims, learning outcomes, and guiding principles desirable for a 21st century college education. The report advocates future curricula include knowledge of the human culture, and the physical and natural world. Emphasis on study and mastery of science, mathematics, and the social sciences is essential, as is application of history, humanities, language, and the arts to understand and engage people with contemporary and enduring big questions. A spirit of inquiry requires intellectual and practical skills such as analysis, critical and creative thinking, reflective judgment, and written and oral communication. Such skills are enhanced and supported by quantitative literacy, information literacy, teamwork, and problem solving experiences that are transferred across contexts. Personal and professional responsibilities included in any 21st century curriculum include the need for civic knowledge and engagement sensitive to both local and global understanding and action. Such engagement requires attention and appreciation of intercultural knowledge and competence coupled with ethical reasoning and commitments to social action. Such commitments are supported by a lifelong learning mind set, intent on making a difference through solving real world problems. The report also calls for integrative learning and attention to the use of knowledge, and specialized studies and skills across general and special areas of practice to solve complex problems in a variety of disciplines and settings. While these recommendations set the stage for general education aspirations, there are more specific aspirations that have been articulated and developed for health professions education.

In June of 2002, the Institute of Medicine convened a Health Professions Education summit to develop a vision and position on the competencies needed by healthcare providers in a 21st century health care system. The results of the summit are published in a book, *Health Professions Education: A Bridge to Quality* (IOM,

2003). The vision espoused is that all health professionals should be educated to deliver patient-centered care as members of an interdisciplinary team, emphasizing evidence-based practice, quality improvement approaches, and informatics. The IOM suggests to meet the needs of a 21st century health care system all clinicians, regardless of their discipline, need to master a set of core competencies. The competencies and associated aspects of each are listed below:

1. Provide patient-centered care. This competency includes such issues as skills and abilities to identify, respect, and care about patients. Attend to differences, values, preferences, and expressed needs; relieve pain and suffering; coordinate continuous care; listen to, clearly inform, communicate with, and educate patients; share decision making and management; and continuously advocate disease prevention, wellness, and promotion of healthy lifestyles, including a focus on population health.

2. Work in interprofessional teams. This competency includes attention to skills and abilities related to cooperation, collaboration, communication, and integration of care in teams to ensure that care is continuous and reliable.

3. Employ evidence-based practice. This competency requires the integration and application of best research with a healthcare provider's clinical expertise and attention to patient values in the service of optimum care, while engaged in learning and research activities to the extent feasible.

4. Apply quality improvement. This competency requires the identification of errors and hazards in care; understanding and implementing basic safety design principles, such as standardization and simplification; continually understanding and measuring quality of care in terms of structure, process, and outcomes in relation to patient and community needs; and designing and testing interventions to change processes and systems of care, with the objective of improving quality.

5. Utilize informatics. This competency relates to skills in communicating, and managing knowledge, mitigating errors, and using information technology to support decision making.

The IOM's hope for the education of health professions is that interdisciplinarity will become a reality and core component of creating quality in the future. As Klein (1990) observes interdisciplinarity has been defined as a philosophy as well as a methodology, a concept, a process, and a way of thinking. She also notes it is a concept that represents an important attempt to define and establish common ground. Some would argue to be interdisciplinary one needs to be grounded in one's own discipline. For nurses to develop a disciplinary mind set, it is essential they be grounded in their professional nursing identities which are the intent and specific aim of the revised AACN essentials for baccalaureate, masters, and doctoral nursing education document. The authors believe that there are developmental stages associated with the acquisition of discipline specific knowledge, skills, and abilities. The American Association of Colleges of Nursing articulates the basics for the disciplinary development of nurses. AACN (2008) has outlined the essentials for baccalaureate, masters, and doctoral preparation in nursing. The Essentials of Baccalaureate Education for Professional Nursing Practice (AACN, 2007) provides the framework for the fundamental preparation and expected educational outcomes for professional nurses. Essentials documents also exist for masters and doctoral education (AACN, 2008). The essentials are based on the assumptions that a baccalaureate generalist graduate is prepared to:

1. Practice in a variety of health care settings
2. Care for patients across the health-illness continuum
3. Care for patients across the lifespan
4. Care for diverse populations
5. Use clinical/critical reasoning to address simple to complex situations
6. Engage in continuous professional development.

The nine essentials associated with this disciplinary development are summarized in the following categories:

- Integration of Liberal Education into Baccalaureate Education for Generalist Nursing Practice
- Beginning Scholarship and Analytical Methods for Evidence-Based Practice
- Information Management and Patient Care Technology within the Practice of the Baccalaureate Generalist
- Health Care Policy, Finance, and Regulatory Environments
- Interprofessional Communication and Collaboration for Improving Patient Health Outcomes
- Clinical Prevention and Population Health for Optimizing Health
- Professionalism and Professional Values
- Baccalaureate Generalist Nursing Practice

In response to the Institute of Medicine's quality series, information technology emerged as a solution to enhance quality and promote safety in the healthcare system. An invitational Summit meeting of a variety of healthcare stakeholders was held on October 30-November 1, 2006, at the Uniformed Services University of Health Services campus in Bethesda, Maryland. This meeting brought together nurse leaders to define an action plan to establish guidelines for education and practice reform in line with informatics use in nursing education and healthcare contexts. Conveners believed the summit was necessary to create plans to support the transformation of nursing practice and education given the federal initiatives to insure the deployment of the Electronic Health Record (EHR) by the year 2014.

The Technology Informatics Guiding Education Reform (TIGER) initiative supports and envisions that informatics tools, principles, theories, and practices be used by nurses to make health care safer, effective, efficient, patient-centered, timely, and equitable. The TIGER initiative released a summary report outlining a 3-year action plan to support the summit's 10-year vision. The TIGER (2007) initiative aims to enable practicing nurses and nursing students to fully engage in the unfolding digital era of healthcare. This includes educating nurses to use information technology (IT) seamlessly to provide safer, higher-quality patient care. Such an educational vision requires support from professional organizations, academic institutions, policy makers, vendors, healthcare delivery organizations, health information management professionals, and librarians. The TIGER vision was based on seven key requirements:

1. Management & Leadership: Revolutionary leadership that drives, empowers, and executes the transformation of health care.
2. Education: Collaborative learning communities that maximize the possibilities of technology toward knowledge development and dissemination, driving rapid deployment and implementation of best practices.
3. Communication and Collaboration: Standardized, person-centered, technology-enabled processes to facilitate teamwork and relationships across the continuum of care.
4. Informatics Design: Evidence-based, interoperable intelligence systems that support education and practice to foster quality care and safety.
5. Information Technology (IT): Smart, people-centered, affordable technologies that are universal, useable, useful, and standards-based.
6. Policy: Consistent, incentives-based initiatives (organizational and governmental) that support advocacy and coalition-building, achieving and resourcing an ethical culture of safety.
7. Culture: A respectful, open system that leverages technology and informatics across multiple disciplines in an environment where all stakeholders trust each other to work together toward the goal of high quality and safety.

With these seven principles as a framework, the TIGER (2007) action plan identified the following steps the nursing profession must take toward realization of the TIGER vision through 2010 and onward to reach the 10-year vision (2016) of evidence and informatics transforming nursing. The seven point action plan includes the following:

1. Promote the TIGER vision of nursing as using informatics technology to provide safer, higher quality care. Use the vision to bring one voice to the profession and increase its power, influence, and presence in the national health IT initiative.
2. Integrate informatics competencies into the nursing curriculum and the learning process. Foster faculty development through funding and incentives. Nurture collaborative partnerships with practice and industry.
3. Share the TIGER initiative at international and national meetings in health care, informatics, and nursing. Work with nursing organizations to disseminate the vision among their membership. Encourage regional and local efforts and partnerships among practice, education, research, and informatics.
4. Take an active role in the design and integration of informatics tools that are intuitive, affordable, useable, responsive, and evidence-based. Create tools that serve nurses and other professionals as members of multi-disciplinary care teams.
5. Integrate industry standards for IT interoperability with clinical standards for practice and education. Educate practice and education communities on IT standards. Establish standards, and set hard deadlines for adoption.
6. Participate visibly and vocally in the national health IT agenda. Offer congressional testimony on issues relating to the TIGER initiative. Take an active role in policy decisions at all levels to ensure ethical, safe patient care.
7. Launch a national marketing campaign to promote a culture that values health IT and supports its use to benefit patients and those who care for them.
8. Integrate technology into the strategic plans, missions, and goals of nursing organizations.

To achieve the TIGER vision, academic institutions are encouraged to:
1. Adopt informatics competencies for all levels of nursing education (undergraduate/graduate) and practice (general/specialist)
2. Encourage faculty to participate in faculty development programs in informatics
3. Develop a school task force/committee to examine the integration of informatics throughout the curriculum
4. Encourage Health Services Resources Administration Division of Nursing to continue and expand their support for informatics specialty programs and faculty development

5. Measure baseline and changes in informatics knowledge among nurse educators, nursing students, and the full range of clinicians seeking continuing education
6. Collaborate with industry and service partners to support faculty creativity in the design, acceptance, and adoption of informatics technology
7. Develop strategies to recruit, retain, and train current and future nurses in the areas of informatics education, practice, and research.

Given the national policies and perspectives of the Institute of Medicine, the Association of American Colleges of Universities, the American Association of Colleges of Nursing, and the TIGER initiative, it remains challenging to plan, implement, and deliver curricula shaped by these policy recommendations and influences. Fundamentally, nurse educators work with individual students and the relationship between and among students and faculty is where the "rubber meets the road". As nurse educators begin to develop integrative learning experiences that enable students to master the essentials, there will be a need to re-conceptualize the nature of learning and the role educators play in structuring, implementing, and evaluating the learning process.

Shulman (2002) suggests that educators need to move beyond the use and application of Bloom's taxonomy and consider at least six elements of liberal and professional learning. The elements are:

1. Engagement and motivation
2. Knowledge and understanding
3. Performance and action
4. Reflection and critique
5. Judgment and design
6. Commitment and identity.

Shulman explains it best when he writes:

"In a nutshell, the taxonomy makes the following assertion: Learning begins with student engagement, which in turn leads to knowledge and understanding. Once someone understands, he or she becomes capable of performance or action. Critical reflection on one's practice and understanding leads to higher-order thinking in the form of a capacity to exercise judgment in the face of uncertainty and to create designs in the presence of constraints and unpredictability. Ultimately, the exercise of judgment makes possible the development of commitment. In commitment, we become capable of professing our understandings and our values, our faith and our love, our skepticism and our doubts, internalizing those attributes and making them integral to our identities. These commitments, in turn, make new engagements possible—and even necessary." Shulman (2002) http://www.carnegiefoundation.org/publications/sub.asp?key=452&subkey=612

In summary, desirable futures are influenced and shaped by aspirational educational policies and practices, as well as environmental forces and developments in knowledge, technology, and self-regulation of the professions. Creating a 21st century healthcare system requires attention and adoption of essential aims and learning outcomes derived from educational policy recommendations, health professions education aspirations, discipline specific standards, and integrative learning experiences that support professional learning and formation.

There are a number of other future forces impacting and influencing the evolution of education. Nurse educators interested in the future ought to explore the Map of Future Forces developed by the Knowledge Work Foundation in collaboration with the Institute for the Future and engage in strategic learning conversations regarding the impact and influence such scenarios will have on nursing education practices and the nature of teaching and learning in the 21st century.

## Knowledge Works Foundation and the Institute for the Future Map of Future Forces Affecting Education 2006-2016

The Map of Future Forces (www.kwfdn.org/map) was developed by the Knowledge Works Foundation in collaboration with the Institute for the Future to stimulate conversations and prompt foresight, insight, and action among stakeholders concerned about the future of education. Knowledge Works commissioned the creation of the Futures Map to help people think about the future and to stimulate strategic conversations and learning among educators, consumers, policy makers, students, and individuals invested in lifelong learning. Attention to future trends enables individuals to co-create teaching and learning agendas with a variety of information and emerging technological and knowledge management tools. The map has been described as a conversation catalyst or "thinking tool" to stimulate scenario development, story-telling, and strategic conversations about possible futures in the world of education.

The Map outlines possible future developments in five areas:
1.  Family and Community
2.  Markets
3.  Institutions
4.  Education and Learning
5.  Tools and Practices.

Each of these areas is cross-referenced or cross-analyzed against six drivers of change predicted to impact developments in education. The change drivers are:

1. The evolution and expansion of a grass roots economy
2. The emergence and ongoing development of smart networking, social networking and connecting technologies
3. Positive and negative opinions played out in a global media configuration that simplifies complex issues
4. The tension and polarity between a health or illness orientation
5. The impact and influence of urban versus rural living environments
6. The merging and integration of physical and digital information through connective media and social networks.

The Map of Future Forces makes explicit trends likely to impact the future of education and consequently teaching and learning in the 21st century. The Map offers a number of scenarios based on the confluence and cross impact of projected trends in a number of areas. The Map of the future is a repository of resources and hosts an online community of people interested in exploring and creating the future of education. There are five elements of the Map of the Future:

1. Drivers
2. Impact areas
3. Trends
4. Hot spots
5. Dilemmas

Attention to these five elements requires curiosity, and a commitment to be aware of the knowledge skills and abilities needed to support 21st century learning.

Nurse educators should explore the Map of Future Forces Affecting Education developed by the Knowledge Works Foundation (www.kwfdn.org ) and the Institute for the Future (www.iftf.org). To access and explore the 2006-2016 Map of Future Forces Affecting Education, go to www.KWFDN.org/map. Nurse educators are in a position to consider how these trends will impact the future of nursing education. The next section explores some of the trends and scenarios and suggests consequences and the meaning these trends may have for students and faculty. The key environmental shifts suggested by the Knowledge Work Future Forces Map are represented in Table 1.

| Future Forces Key Environmental Shifts: Meaning for Students and Faculty | | | |
|---|---|---|---|
| Moving From | Moving Toward | Meaning for Students | Meaning for Faculty |
| Hierarchical structure | Hybrid networks and hierarchies (heterarchies) | Students will actively create networks that support their learning needs, relying on those networks for connection, resources and a sense of community, and belonging | Attention to social networks and consequences for team based learning |
| Centralized control | Empowered periphery | Successful educational outcomes depend on ownership of the learning process | Shift from a focus on control to relationship-engagement, participation, and belonging |
| Blue-ribbon panels | Context-based experience and tacit knowledge | Knowledge is no longer authority based and is derived from evidence and propositions and arguments that are contextualized | Appreciation of knowledge complexity and need to make tacit knowledge explicit through dialogue, questions, and appreciative-reflective inquiry |
| Measuring resources and assets | Mapping flows of values and benefits | Human factors and the need for emotional intelligence will surpass the inventory of available hardware and software resources | Attention to value exchange and meeting needs through the application of emotional intelligence |

**Table 1.** Future Forces Key Environmental Shifts: Meaning for Students and Faculty

| | | | |
|---|---|---|---|
| Solving discrete problems | Managing ongoing dilemmas | There is a complexity to ill-defined problems and all solutions are not self-evident. Students will need to develop reflective judgment skills | Mastery of polarity management and complexity thinking skills and principles that foster reflective practice as well as attention to student's cognitive developmental levels of understanding will be important in terms of teaching learning strategy and skill development |
| Individual computing | Participatory media | The shift from individual work to team based learning will be enhanced through the use of technologies and platforms that foster collaborative work that facilitates the exchange of ideas at an accelerated rate | Mastery and intentional use of advancements in media and technology to support learning and delivery of content |
| Proprietary knowledge and resources | Collectively generated and managed knowledge | Students will have access to more information and tools and will spend less time learning facts and more time learning how to manage newly generated knowledge. Students will need a new skill set | Appreciation and respect for intellectual property issues and development of intellectual and social capital to shared learning goals as well as development of new learning products with enhanced marketability |

**Table 1 continued.** Future Forces Key Environmental Shifts: Meaning for Students and Faculty

| Computer labs | Pervasive media rich learning | Simulations and virtual reality forums will provide multi-sensory learning opportunities | Participation in scenario development learning design teams, as architect and content experts that use evolving technology |
|---|---|---|---|
| Consumer culture | Do-it-yourself culture | Students are likely to create their own libraries with significant and meaningful web based resources | Appreciation of student knowledge and skill base in terms of learning needs and technology use |
| Acute illness | Chronic illness | Knowledge about health promotion and illness prevention will be highlighted | Attention to relationships and context of care through time and services and public health policy changes. Attention to web based resources that help people self-management and self-regulate health status |
| Service providers | Platform developers | Students will be challenged to master multiple types of learning platforms and will need flexibility and a platform mastery skill set | Collaborator and consultant on user needs and quality criteria for platform developers |

**Table 1 continued.** Future Forces Key Environmental Shifts: Meaning for Students and Faculty

| | | | |
|---|---|---|---|
| Stable professions | Dynamic | Students will have the opportunity to develop as entrepreneurs and create new types of occupations based on evolving technological and learning needs | Transformation of faculty role to one of free agent and fee for service provider, consultant and knowledge broker, as well as media learning and design expert |
| Ubiquitous, monolithic infrastructure | Lightweight, smart, ad hoc infrastructure | Students will play a greater role in defining needs and services and the administrative structures that support those services | Just in time learning and teaching that requires creative thinking and responding; bureaucratic organizations will begin to deconstruct in favor of more responsive service structures |
| One size fits all | Custom fit | Students will define their own learning goals in a context of essential knowledge and optional knowledge for successful career advancement | Individualized learning contracts based on student achievement, goals, competencies and portfolio evaluation, and skill in media and internet based learning technologies and resources |

**Table 1 continued.** Future Forces Key Environmental Shifts: Meaning for Students and Faculty

| | | | |
|---|---|---|---|
| Design for average users | Design with expert users | Students will become more sophisticated with Internet and web based technologies and may surpass faculty knowledge of what is possible | Customization of learning needs based on essential knowledge, skills, and abilities, as well as specialized need for focus and expert development, the need to stay abreast of what is technologically possible to support learning outcomes |

**Table 1 continued.** Future Forces Key Environmental Shifts: Meaning for Students and Faculty

The authors have added two additional dimensions to the suggested shifts listed in Table 1. These are what this development and transition mean for students and what the shift and transition may mean for faculty. The ideas are presented to stimulate thinking, educational planning, and skill-building into the future.

Specifically, with the evolution and development of cooperative teaching-learning technologies there will be (and perhaps already is) a shift from hierarchical structures to the evolution and development of hybrid social learning networks. Such networks shift the laws of control from a central source to an empowered periphery. People create what they want to create rather than rely on a static organizational structure to support teaching and learning efforts. At the same time there is a shift of reliance away from knowledgeable experts to context based experience and tacit knowledge shared among many individuals and used for problem solving. This shift supports just in time learning. There is also a predicted shift from static measurement of resources and assets to mapping the flow of values and intangibles in relationship exchanges. For example, what are the intangible values of nursing care in the healthcare system? People are more interested in the intangibles assets associated with learning communities, like a sense of caring, belonging, loyalty and support, and connectedness rather than the power of computing resources and technologies.

Solving disparate problems is expected to give way to management of uncertainties, polarities, and dilemmas. Ill-structured problems and uncertainties fuel reflection about complexity. Individual computing and for profit knowledge entities are yielding to open access and collectively generated knowledge. Computer laboratories are likely to give way to multimedia resource and virtual learning resource centers. Consumers will create what works for them rather than rely on packaged information defined by service providers.

Acute wellness management yields to chronic illness and quality of life management as wellness orientation and life style supersedes an emphasis on disease management. Stable professions evolve into more dynamic entrepreneurial professions. Bureaucratic structures dissolve and transform into smart-networked ad hoc infrastructures. One size fits all is overpowered and replaced by customization and friendly design. Average users evolve into more sophisticated users who are capable of harnessing the tools, social media, and practices that support their lifelong learning needs.

Given these trends and forecasts how might one prepare to master the knowledge, skills, and abilities one will need to thrive in the future? What are the consequences of some of these trends? What hot spots will they create? What are some potential dilemmas or problems that are likely to emerge that require new thinking and skill development for both students and faculty? Consider some of the consequences of the trends described below in light of what students may expect in the future and in light of what you currently know as a nurse educator and what you will need to know and master in the future.

## Scenarios about the Future: Implications for Nurse Educators and Students

### Moving from a Knowledge Economy to a Learning Market

In the future it is not so much the knowledge (content) you possess but how you can package and express that knowledge in a form that is actionable and marketable. How will you share what you know in ways to help people learn? Learning is the key filter and factor that influences decisions in the market across income categories. Public education is not the only learning resource in the future. Through story telling and the leveraging networking tools, open knowledge repositories, and peer-to-peer production methods learners and educators will increasingly experiment with sharing and exchanging learning resources. Models for organizing learning experiences over time will diversify and extend beyond those found today in private, parochial, home schooling, and charter schools. For students this means they can search out knowledge and learning opportunities that extend beyond their structured standardized curriculum based, on their personal and professional interests. For educators this means they must be creative in the ways they package, deliver, and exploit, in a positive way, their intellectual capital through the development of learning products and services beyond the traditional college or university context. Knowledgeable faculty will have opportunities to leverage what they know in a variety of ways. Partnerships with students, vendors, publishers, and colleagues that involve creating learning products may also help transform tacit knowledge into explicit opportunities to develop new learning tools that are marketable, free, and open to the commons through communities of practice and learning (Wegner, 2005).

### People Make Their own Worlds

Another significant trend is that people are becoming more active participants in creating their own worlds. Whether it means do-it-yourself (DIY) home projects, peer-to-peer media exchanges, or open-source collaboration, people more than ever have access to push button publishing to share their ideas and interact with others. The result: a much more personalized world. For students this means they are likely to develop and participate in social networks that educate them or are relevant to the world they live in. These social networks are going to become even more meaningful as the level of personalization continues to grow. Never before have people had the opportunity to see the world through so many filters. These social networks and areas of interest are driven by social services such as social book marking of Web sites, blogs, wikis, life streams, photo sharing, and the broadcast of information (also known as Real Simple Syndication or RSS – which is a just-in-time update of content of Web sites or social networks).

This means that having conversations about what is important to your students and how they want to learn becomes an important curriculum design consideration. It also means that faculty must have the flexibility and creativity to deliver learning experiences that match and challenge student preferred learning modes and styles of communication. Faculty must also master and use technological aids that will assist them in their knowledge management efforts. The use of book marking services, blogs, wikis, and other types of social media are likely to become more necessary and popular. For an example see RSS in Plain English www.commoncraft.com/rss_plain_english. As technological innovations and developments support the creation and expansion of learning communities, educators will need to stay current with technological know-how and its pedagogical applications and consequences.

## Communities Create Common-Pool Resources

Communities play a large role in our daily lives. Communities of learning and practice will be felt, seen, and heard. Driven by the connected nature of our society, online communities are fertile ground for the development of ideas and frameworks that will facilitate the discussion of our personalized world. Communities of learning and practice will be vital to the teaching learning process and educational mission. Students will become ever more comfortable using information from online communities. Some communities will have higher integrity that others – these are just the facts of the world we live in. However, that does not mean that any community is any less valuable. The value in communities is the collective knowledge they produce. Many times STRONG communities band around a common problem. Through collaboration, solutions are put forward, frameworks are developed, and polarities of unsolvable problems are managed. There is a lot to be learned from communities and the frameworks that develop within them. Communities will play a large part in the student's educational journey. They will look to communities more than ever as a resource/starting point when approaching a complex problem. In today's world, the level of complexity required in problem solving can be overwhelming to an individual and managed by a group or community. For students this means they will have more to consider when approaching problems. For faculty this means it is possible to create a sense of connectedness and ready access to a community of scholars, peers, and colleagues who can share knowledge, information, and strategies about effective teaching-learning methods.

Given the deep personalization of the Internet, communities or common pool resources will be instruments and resources that inspire and guide change. E-communities will help facilitate/conversations about solutions to wicked problems. Common pool resource communities are only as healthy as people want them to be. How would public educational and learning resources (teachers, facilities, students, funding) change if they were treated as common-pool resources? Basically this means that getting people together to solve a common problem, through individual contributions. Common pool resources is a strategy that is likely to emerge as it has value and provides access to knowledge that informs people of the possibilities for learning and action. For example see www.horsepigcow.com/2007/11/24/. Wegner (2005) discusses the importance of communities of practice and learning to support identity, commitment, meaning, and learning in disciplinary contexts. Krebs & Holley (2007) discuss the importance of network weaving to build capacity and resources in a learning community.

## Unbundled Education Supports Personalized Learning

The convergence of networks, emergent self-organization, and cooperative strategies sets the stage for a host of new education and business models that function as platforms for value creation among distributed knowledge workers, innovative users, and customers. EBay doesn't sell anything, but it provides a platform for buyers and sellers to meet, for individuals to develop careers as Power Sellers, and for third-party businesses, like Picture It Sold, to prosper. Schools and districts that become open platforms for development of innovative and diverse learning models will have a distinct advantage. For students this means they will have the opportunity to enrich their education like never before. They will have the opportunity to seek out experts and ideas that support their own creative curiosity. The personalized nature of unbundled education is going to allow for an unprecedented level of creative living and learning. Just think if you could access an idea at the time you are ready for the answer. In our hyperlinked world we will connect where we want and this is going to bring an incredible amount of value to the discussions in the classroom or work environment. For the student this also provides a much improved platform for continuing education. Students will have access to meaningful content that is customized to their skill set/experience level. Employers will be taking educational discussions back into the workplace as they look for cost effective ways to support the learning needs of their best employees. Students are likely to be more mindful of areas that need attention and development. This understanding sets the stage for more entrepreneurial activity in an education context. Unbundled education is going to speed up the rate at which we can learn and draw conclusions. Learning will become more personalized and less packaged; this will lead to engagement, motivation, and more design and discovery. For faculty this means they will be able to focus their energy on selected concepts and ideas germane to their areas of scholarship and research. Faculty may also see tremendous opportunity to translate interests and intellectual property into bundles of educational products that are marketable. Universities will likely set aside resources for their faculty members to explore and develop this niche of providing personalized content about a specific subject area. Partnerships between faculty and universities will result in development of networks of engaged students as consumers of educational innovations. Learning programs that deliver personalized content even after the student graduates are likely to be popular with alumni. Sharing learning opportunities will enable students to stay connected with their educational institutions. If you give student through time, something that is of value in their lives, they are more likely to give back to the institutions from which they graduated. This could also help keep the faculty connected to practical every day operational experiences. Keep the conversations going. Approach your star students and engage their interests to build these personalized learning (unbundled education) experiences. Think about the possibilities in the classroom to keep your content fresh and original. Connecting and sharing with students a variety of unbundled educational programs helps faculty stay on top of healthcare trends and enables them to share valuable content with students and alumni.

## Educational Careers Forge New Paths

As education is unbundled into a constellation of functions, roles, products, and services that meets the needs of the emerging learning economy, the teaching profession will experience a creative breakout. New administrative, classroom, and community roles will expand and help differentiate educational careers options. Educators in the future are likely to take on responsibilities as content experts, learning coaches, network navigators, cognitive specialists, resource managers, or community liaisons. Interactive media will link diverse groups of educators and students in ad hoc groups to perform new kinds of collective assessment and evaluation of both students and educators. For students this means they will have to alter the stereotypes and impressions they have of what is means to be a teacher. For faculty this means shedding traditional role expectations in favor of innovations. Faculty who master the emerging technologies that support teaching and learning will be in demand as consultants, advisors, and knowledge brokers. Knowledge brokers are those people who bridge the structural holes, are sought-after because they bring information between disciplines. Knowledge Workers need brokers. (www.horsepigcow.com/2008/01/12/futzing-as-the-future-of-work/). Knowledge brokers are needed to create interdisciplinarity in the health professions.

## Personalized Learning Focuses on the Craft of Teaching

Personalized learning plans will leverage new media, brain research, and school structures to create differentiated learning experiences based on individual needs. Interactive and collaborative digital spaces, such as wikis, will provide shared learning portfolios where students, educators, employers, and other stakeholders can perform assessments and real-time interventions. New classroom approaches will be controversial for many teachers because they will require "unlearning" many basic assumptions about the nature of teaching. Unions may resist the diversification of educator roles or embrace it as an opportunity to be real leaders of change.

For students this means they will be able to take charge of their educational experience. In the traditional mindset, a teacher is someone who has years of experience in a certain skill or set of ideas. The teacher seeks to bestow that knowledge on the student. The student seeks the knowledge and experience of a teacher so they might one day be a teacher to teach students.

A little confusing, but the point is this: if you are human, you are both a student and teacher. The classroom (or educational experience) needs the "traditional students" to be teachers now. (Or it's not so much that we NEED them now, but if we had them and we thought about the students we have now being the teachers we could enrich the educational experience by an infinite amount!) Today's students will be tomorrow's teachers. We are seeing the fusion of old and new school. Technology is advancing faster than most can keep up. The exchange of ideas is on a similar path. Students who are studying earnestly will get their finger on the pulse of their education faster than any students the world has previously seen. The "traditional" teaching world can embrace this (with love, support, and understanding) or fight it. The point is that students need teachers.

Education is no longer a top to bottom. It is an equal exchange of ideas, but from different perspectives. There is not much we do not know (or can not find out). What is more important is to talk about what we do know and share that perspective. Teaching is going to play an integral role in everyone's life as we move to a world where more services will be built off an independent and agile (consultant based) workforce. For teachers this means they need not be offended or frightened of the "new" student. They have much to learn. They need to love and embrace the experience students will bring to learning discussions. The fact is that to survive, the student needs the teacher, and the teacher needs the student. The educational experience is a switchboard. If you embrace new connections, your switchboard will out perform all others. The way to embrace new connections is to take a moment to learn something or realize that we are all students and teachers, and we all need each other.

## Media Becomes Personal and Collaborative

As economic identity shifts from consumer to creative producer, digital technology will turn the world of media into a very personal world. Increasingly, people will take advantage of simple tools and a worldwide platform to express themselves in everything from blogs (personal Web pages) and wikimedia (Web pages that can be edited by anyone) to podcasting (sharing audio or video files for downloading to iPods), machinima (remixed animated computer games), and mashups (video, music, or graphic media that are re-mixed). The social nature of these tools will encourage sharing, appropriating, and reinventing others' inventions in a rapid stream of collaborative innovation. The impacts of this innovation will run deep in our social and economic systems. For students this means they will have new ways to process, integrate, and present works that represent a synthesis of their understanding of materials they are required to master. For faculty this means new ways to illustrate and share discoveries, interests, and the development of scholarship.

## Life and Learning Become Serious Games

As the barriers between physical and digital spaces come down, people will move seamlessly between digital game spaces and urban neighborhoods. The intermingling of world building (alternate reality) games and real-life interactions in physical–digital space will create a culture of layered realities, where strategies from the worlds of gaming and simulation will increasingly be employed in non-game situations. For learning, this means that the cooperative, critical-thinking, and problem-solving practices encouraged in digital games will make serious games a key form of pedagogy. For students this means those simulations and three-dimensional worlds may in fact become priorities for learning. Avatars and simulated life situations provide the stimulus for developing response patterns to real world healthcare problems and issues. For faculty this means the challenge of creating scenarios and real world simulations based on carefully created and crafted learning modules that embrace the complexity of real life situations in a simulated fashion. Teaching with case based scenarios serve as the stimulus for understanding concepts, principles, and learning outcomes that serve the development of knowledge, learning, and skill acquisition in a virtual rather than real world with the subsequent challenge of helping students transfer learning across context and modes of interaction and learning.

## From Informed Citizens to Engaged Net Workers

At the intersection of traditional social-networking and connective technologies is an emerging skill set of engaged networking – the ability to form ad hoc groups and catalyze communities of action using personal interactive media. How will engaged net workers transform education? It will be important for both students and faculty to become network weavers. For students this means they will form networks that support their knowledge, learning, and skill acquisition. For faculty this means they are likely to benefit from development of network weaving skills that support the development of resource networks. This will involve the network weaving strategy of "closing the triangle" that is the catalyst for connecting people and resources that advance learning and build community. For an example of network weaving on an international scale see Pesut, Kuiper, Fesnedo Espinosa (2007) *Network Weaving: A Story About Collegial Interest in the Teaching and Learning of Clinical Reasoning in Nursing.*

## A Contemporary Conversation between an Educator and a Twenty-Something Student

Given the Map of Future Forces as a back drop, listen to a conversation between a nurse educator and his twenty-something-year-old son.

**Teacher:** Have you looked at the knowledge works Map of Future Forces Affecting Education, and if so, what do you think about it?

*Student: I think the map is awesome! I think it's awesome because it allows someone, with a little bit of time, to sit down and look at all the forces that are currently affecting the educational process. Within several minutes, people start to see patterns emerge. Certain parts of the map resonate with their ideas and perspectives. It gets them excited! The map embodies what the major future force is; change that is driven by deep personalization. Over the past twenty years, I have watched the world of ideas and interactions develop into a hyperlinked ecosystem. The Internet is quickly becoming the de facto place to find and share information, stories, and ideas. I don't think that we can possibly fathom what the Internet has done for the human race, but we will continue to see it play a large role in education. It will become a platform for every interest or every idea. The ascension of ideas will be guided by the collective intelligence of the "web mind".*

Teacher: Given the Map and what it suggests, what are your expectations of colleges, universities, and faculty of the future?

*Student: Given that the Map suggests the world is moving to a more independent learning economy; this shift will be most pronounced for the world's academic systems. To quantify things even more, I think the shift will be largely classified through expectations. In the future, students will come to expect more. Yes, this is simplistic answer, but let me explain. The expectations for a learning experience will continue to soar relative to the price of today's education. Our world is demanding more and more education to be competitive in the global marketplace. This demand is in itself devaluing the educational experience. More and more students are being forced into programs just to get "a degree." Yes, it's important to have a degree. Yes, it's important to have standards about who you hire. I argue that we are missing the point. Students expect an education that will give them something to act on. I believe there has been an awakening at many universities as they struggle with the many pressures that make it hard in academia; finances, retention, and research. The awakening is starting to ask different questions about how we should be teaching students in the classroom. The awakening is asking how can we take advantage (exploit in a positive way) the context that most students live in, whether it is through social networks, the sharing of ideas or stories.*

Teacher: What do you think teaching-learning philosophies will be like in the next 10 years?

*Student: I think that the most dramatic shift in the learning philosophies is that we will spend less time "learning" and more time will be spent building a knowledge toolset. These toolsets will help us organize and package information so that it is actionable. Learning philosophies will focus on the interactive. They will focus on the collective. They will focus on the interrelated. Learning philosophies will seek to spark the belief that learning is a value and that the effort to learn is worthwhile. I also believe that teaching and learning will be more deeply intertwined. As we all build our respective knowledge toolsets it will be important to share those with the world. Sharing knowledge toolsets with the world will continue to power the deep personalization that is powering our learning economy. Learning philosophies are going to focus on teaching people to "become empowering to their own context" (Quinn, 1996). This will change the world we live in.*

**Teacher:** What do you think teachers of the future will have to master to be successful?

**Student:** *I think the most successful teachers are those who can master the connection with their students. The best teachers are the ones who have a deep understanding of the expectations of their students. They engineer the course to satisfy and deliver. This faculty are hidden in colleges around the world. Colleges should seek out these members of their faculty and let them speak to the other members about what they observe. These observations should not be underestimated. Colleges that are smart will do their best to hire faculty who are progressive; faculty who ask unconventional questions; faculty who seek to empower their students. Faculty that seem to equip their students not just with knowledge, but with a drive to know more. I know that some of you out there think that today's students are lazy. I am here to tell you that most students have tremendous amounts of energy and they are ready to explode. It just takes a re-framing of the conversation to get the desired result. The successful teachers in the world already know this.*

**Teacher:** How will technology be utilized by teachers and students in the future?

**Student:** *I think that technology will be used to drive the learning experience to a whole new level. Teachers will use technology to engage student's interests. Students will use technology to communicate and learn. This is perhaps the most wonderful part of the education and technology discussion. The teacher and student role is going to change with regard to technology. I believe that teachers will be learning about how to use technology from their students. Faculty have a luxury that most of the world doesn't; access to minds that work with the "latest and greatest" software and communication tools. Faculty should use this resource to educate themselves about the tools available. They should become comfortable with these tools. The tools are* *enablers. There is a reason why they are so popular – they are good. Good in that they are easy to use and they provide a tremendous amount of value. The ability to learn and understand these technologies will facilitate the ability to develop knowledge platforms, produce research, or connect with those of similar interest. Technology is a currency. It can and will make the learning experience rich, but not with out a little bit of work. Students will and should demonstrate why technology is meaningful in the classroom.*

**Teacher:** As you look into the future how do you think learning will be structured?

*Student: When I look to the future I see classrooms and learning experiences that are powered by discussion or scenario based experiences. I see the world of "typical" homework being transformed into computer based learning experiences that give the essentials to students so the classroom time can become more valuable discussion points. I think that learning will be structured to incorporate more interdisciplinary study. We are all moving towards an incredibly complex world. Learning will be more about building a tool-set to deal with information; not knowing all of it. The more aptly we are able to deal with the massive amounts of information, the better we will be at filtering and making decisions.*

**Teacher:** What advice would you give today's teachers about preparing for the future?

*Student: I think the best advice I can give is that the future is going to change the way we do things. It's going to change the rate at which we learn. It's going to change who we learn from. It's going to change what we believe. These radical changes are bound to frustrate. When you are preparing for the future, first take a deep breath. Second, whenever you find yourself in a moment of frustration with your students, your lecture, your colleagues, your academic administration, or whomever may be causing you heartache; ask your self, "How am I responsible for what's happening to me?" I also encourage you to get your students and colleagues to ask the same question of them. This always helps frame the problem in the context in which you can do something about it. You can then take action. This is where the future provides so much promise; the ability to take action on small or large scales and accomplish goals is going to be facilitated by independent individuals who band together and support the communities they are part of. Know that we all play a role. We should prepare for the future first by knowing that we are all responsible for our own outcomes. Sometimes the best gift a teacher can give is to bestow that nugget of knowledge on a student.*

**Teacher:** How can tomorrow's educator best facilitate lifelong learning?

*Student: I think teachers can facilitate lifelong learning by making the learning experiences valuable and applicable to the students' contexts. During the course of my college education I came onto some really astonishing information. It was information that existed my whole life, but I wasn't ready to consume and act on it. Fortunately, a mentor passed the information along in such a way that it was valuable to my context. It was as if a lighting bolt cracked over my head. It was quite possibly the greatest learning experience I have had in my life. After that experience I strove to discover, collect, and consume more and more about the specific topics. As learning institutions move towards more personalized curriculums we are going to see an explosion of interest and effort from the students. Students are going to have access to incredible learning networks that will facilitate the story telling of experience and perspectives. This sharing is going to empower us to become lifelong learners.*

## Summary

So what do you do? What are some of the personal and professional actions steps related to future forces affecting education? There are a number of personal and professional action steps nurse educators can initiate to prepare for the future. First, active environmental scanning about future policy developments and the implications or those policies for nursing education contexts is important. Second, develop a personal and professional learning plan for mastering new technologies and discerning the application of these technologies for teaching and learning. The only way to understand technology is to use it. Third, ongoing exploration of the Map of the Future and connecting with the electronic communities and resources that are provided by this portal will provide opportunities for social networking, learning, and innovations that are likely to influence teaching learning practices. Consider making a pledge to future generations (Tough, 1993). (See Appendix.) Have a conversation with your current colleagues and students and invite them to dialogue about what they expect in terms of the future design of teaching and learning. Such dialogue sensitizes one to the issues and expectations of future generations of learners. Finally, reflect on how to create integrative learning experiences suggested by the AACN (2008) Essentials Series for baccalaureate, masters, and doctoral education using technologies of the future. Ongoing exploration, skill development and learning related to web based and other technological tools that support student learning and mastery of the knowledge, skills, and abilities will continue to be a challenge. To be a 21st century nurse educator grounded in the discipline of nursing with the ability to relate to other disciplines requires a personal and professional commitment to understand and master the future forces likely to effect education today and beyond the year 2016.

## Learning Activities

1. Explore the resources available at these futures-oriented institutions and organizations
   The World Future Society http://www.wfs.org/
   - Future Times News Letter http://www.wfs.org/futuretimeswin08.htm
   - Futures Learning Section http://www.wfs.org/futureslearning/
   Institute for Alternative Futures http://www.altfutures.com/
   - Wiser Futures Compendium http://www.altfutures.com/WF_Compendium_Web_Verision.pdf
   - Creating Health For All http://www.altfutures.com/section.asp?sec=6&nav=6
   Future Studio http://www.futurestudio.org/full-text-scenarios.htm
   - Vision 2010 Higher Education http://www.futurestudio.org/scenario%20documents/Vision%202010%20Higher%20Education%20Scenarios.pdf
   Institute for the Future http://www.iftf.org/
   - Global Health Economy Map http://www.iftf.org/features/ghe_map.html
2. Consider subscribing to Tomorrow's Professor. Visit
   https://mailman.stanford.edu/mailman/listinfo/tomorrows-professor
3. Explore the resources available through the National Center for Academic Transformation  http://www.thencat.org/whoweare.html
4. Explore the projects and information available through Educause http://www.educause.edu/content.asp?PAGE_ID=720&bhcp=1
5. Consider a subscription to Innovate – The Journal of Online Education http://www.innovateonline.info/?view=issue

6. Consider learning more about the TIGER Initiative http://www.himss.org/
   handouts/ITSolutions2007nm.pdf
   http://www.umbc.edu/tiger/index.html

## Educational Philosophy

I believe in strengths and strategy-based approaches to teaching and learning. One of the important discoveries I made early on in my teaching career was that helping students manage their own creative thinking processes is an important teaching function. As an educator I help students engage in content, process, and premise reflection. I challenge and create learning experiences that help students develop their ability to "think about their thinking". In doing so, they master the reflective, critical, creative, systems, and complexity thinking that supports their professional development and nursing care knowledge base. — Daniel J. Pesut

My educational philosophy is: (a) focus on what works and (b) take responsibility for your own outcomes. I believe that teachers and students are developing new toolsets that make expectations about learning experiences more clear, thus more powerful. I challenge faculty members to build curriculums and classes around student expectations. I challenge students to take responsibility for their educational and classroom experience. — Elliott Z. Pesut

## References

American Association of Colleges of Nursing. (2008). The essentials series http://www.aacn.nche.edu/Education/essentials.htm

Association of American Colleges and Universities. (2007). *College learning for the new global century*, Washington, DC: Author.

Bezold, C., Hancock.T., & Sullivan, E.(1999). Examining nursing from a futures perspective. In E. Sullivan (Ed.) *Creating nursing's future issues, opportunities and challenges*, pp. 3-13, St. Louis: Mosby.

Institute of Medicine. (2003). *Health professions education: A Bridge to quality*. NationalAcademy Press. Washington, DC. Accessed November 29, 2007. http://books.nap.edu/openbook.php?record_id=10681&page=R1

Institute of Medicine (2001). *Crossing the quality chasm: A new health system for the 21st century*. Washington, D.C.: National Academy Press.

Klein, J. (1990). *Interdisciplinarity, history, theory and practice*. Detroit, MI: Wayne State University Press.

Knowledge Works Foundation: Map of Future Forces Affecting Education. Accessed November 23, 2007. http://www.kwfdn.org/map/

Krebs, V., & Holley, J. (2007). Building smart communities through network weaving. Accessed February 4, 2008. http://www.orgnet.com/BuildingNetworks.pdf

Pesut, D. J. (2000). Looking forward: Being and becoming a futurist. In F. Bower. (Ed.). *Nurses Taking the Lead: Personal Qualities of Effective Leadership*. pp. 39-65, Philadelphia: W.B. Saunders.

Pesut, D. J., Kuiper, R.A., & Fesnedo Espinosa, C. (2007). Network weaving: A story about collegial interest in the teaching and learning of clinical reasoning in nursing. pp. 218-225. In S. Weinstein & A. M. Brooks (Eds.). *Nursing without borders: Values, wisdom, success markers*, Indianapolis, IN: STTI.

Quinn, R. (1996). *Deep change: Discovering the leader within*. San Francisco: Jossey Bass.

Schulman, Lee. (2002). Making differences: A table of learning, *Change, 34* (6), 346. http://carnegiefoundation.org/publications/sub.asp?key=452&subkey=612

Sullivan, E. (1999). *Creating nursing's future: Issues, opportunities, and challenges*. St. Louis: Mosby.

TIGER initiative Accessed February 8, 2008. http://www.umbc.edu/tiger/index.html Technology Informatics Guiding Education Reform (TIGER) (2007). The Tiger initiative. Evidence and informatics transforming nursing: 3 year action steps toward a 10-year vision. Accessed February 2, 2008. http://www.amia.org/inside/releases/2007/tigerinitiative_report2007_color.pdf

Tough, A. (1993). Making a pledge to future generations. *Futures, 25*(1), 90-92.

Wegner, E. (n.d.). *Quick start up guide for cultivating communities of practice*. http://www.ewenger.com/theory/start-up_guide_PDF.pdf Accessed February 8, 2008

Wegner, E. (2006). *Learning for a small planet: Research agenda*. http://www.ewenger.com/research/

## Additional Resources about the Future

World Future Society. 7910 Woodmont Avenue, Suite 450, Bethesda, MD, 20814. USA Telephone: 301-656-8274, FAX: 301-951-394.

www.wfs.org/index.htm

www.wfs.org/inter.htm
www.wfs.org/forecasts.htm

# UNIT 2: FOCUS ON STUDENTS

# CHAPTER 14

## STUDENT-FACULTY RELATIONSHIPS

### Elizabeth Stokes, EdD, RN, CNE

The content of this chapter relates to the following major content areas and subconcepts on the Certified Nurse Educator Examination Detailed Test Blueprint:

**Facilitate Learning**

- Create a positive learning environment that fosters a free exchange of ideas
- Show enthusiasm for teaching, learning, and the nursing profession that inspires and motivates students
- Demonstrate personal attributes that facilitate learning
- Respond effectively to unexpected events that affect clinical and/or classroom instruction

**Facilitate Learning Development and Socialization**

- Create learning environments that facilitate learners' self-reflection, personal goal setting, and socialization to the role of the nurse
- Assist learners to engage in thoughtful and constructive self and peer evaluation
- Encourage professional development of learners

## Introduction

In our lives we have many relationships. Examples include parent-child, spousal relationships, and friendships. The student-faculty relationship is a unique connection. The teacher may take on many roles in the student-faculty relationship. Students often view faculty as authority figures. The relationship may be somewhat parental in nature. Young school children may view the teacher as parent. Elements of other relationships such as caring, likeability, and friendliness may be a part of a student-faculty relationship. Faculty may be viewed as an advisor or mentor. In nursing education because of the type and intensity of the work and the way in which nursing carries out the majority of its clinical teaching, students and faculty work together closely.

Historically, teachers were held as role models in the community. Teachers or professors were required to adhere to strict, sometimes unwritten, moral codes. Behavior in their work and in the community was expected to be exemplary. Any hint of impropriety could result in immediate dismissal from a job. Media stories about teacher misconduct have titillated the public interest in recent years. Higher education, including professional education, has not been immune to such incidents. Nursing as a professional discipline expects faculty to be role models for students, fellow faculty, and clinical agency personnel. The Carnegie Foundation Preparation for the Professions Program (2007) in its study of nursing education identified role modeling as one of nursing's signature pedagogies. The Core Competencies of Nurse Educators with Task Statements (NLN, 2005) developed by the National League for Nursing address personal attributes of faculty such as integrity and flexibility as well as the responsibility for establishing relationships with students, faculty, colleagues, and clinical personnel to facilitate learning.

## Learning as the Goal of the Student-Faculty Relationship

The student-faculty relationship is not a social relationship. Interactions should have the flavor of a work, professional, or business relationship. Learning is the goal of the relationship. Both the faculty and the student must work toward this goal. Students view teachers as authority figures, and may feel intimidated or threatened. A threatening atmosphere may hamper learning.

An important part of the faculty's job is to set the ground rules. Course policies, rules, and expectations should be clearly delineated. Most nursing programs have general policies about course work and student conduct. Handbooks for students from the college or university and from the nursing program or school are a good source for consideration in devising policies. New faculty should discuss rules and policies with longer-employed faculty at the institution.

Although rules and policies may set the tone for class, clinical, and other course work, faculty should be aware of their approach to students. For ideal learning to occur, students should view faculty as approachable. Faculty may be friendly without establishing close social relationships. Students need to view faculty as human. "Icebreakers" at the start of class or clinical are helpful. Ask students to share their hometown or a hobby. Faculty may tell students about a hobby or favorite activity.

## Treat All Students Fairly

Faculty need to be careful to treat all students fairly. Policies and rules should be applied consistently. Students notice how other students are treated and make quick judgments if they feel the teacher has favorites. A group of students in talking with the author about an instructor had noted that she frequently called on the males in the class and talked about how she had assigned certain patients to them in clinical. This faculty did not provide similar examples with the females in the class. Becoming overly friendly with students with a particular characteristics may undermine the teacher's ability to facilitate learning for the total group.

Communication by faculty with students should convey respect. Using language that demeans the student is not acceptable. The use of sarcasm and humor at the student's expense should be avoided. Think about how your word choice and tone will be perceived. Be aware of nonverbal communication. Students should be comfortable asking questions or approaching faculty. Answer questions in class or clinical with a serious tone. Although a student's question may appear irrelevant, the student has a quandary. Such questions often arise from misunderstandings or not being able to think through the idea at the moment. You may want to follow up with the students checking their understanding of the material. Again, avoid intimidation. The fact that the teacher controls their grades (and therefore, their lives) is intimidating enough.

## Relationship with Clinical Students

Working with students in the clinical setting may require a more intense situation than the classroom. Nursing faculty work closely with their clinical groups and get to know the student's anxieties, responses to dealing with people, and work ethic. Personal events and emotions often spill over into the clinical setting. Faculty become acutely aware of student situations such as family illnesses and financial problems. Again, faculty need to set the tone for clinical learning opportunities.

Some faculty like to share meals with students as a way of showing their approachability and friendliness. Each faculty should think about these types of social situations and decide on their preferences for handling them. Be cautious about being seen with the same students repeatedly. You want to be inclusive of all students without any perception of favoritism.

In working with students in the clinical setting, faculty should develop strategies to communicate information to students without undermining student or patient confidence. Students are usually very uneasy about their clinical performance and correcting their work in the presence of patients and families is sure to increase their anxieties. Use phrases such as "let me help you," "we can get this done if we move...," or "this arrangement will facilitate your work." You may want to reinforce information provided to the patient by the student. With beginning students, the author has found it useful to talk to the patient while the student is performing the skill. In the debriefing session, reviewing the instructor's communication and asking the student to put what was said in his/her own words will help the student remember about communicating with the patient in performing future skills. Role-modeling communication skills with the patient and using the situation with the individual student or the whole clinical group is another strategy to facilitate learning therapeutic interactions.

Faculty should show respect to other nurses and staff both in the school of nursing and the clinical area. Remember that you are role-modeling working with professional colleagues. Sometimes problematic situations arise in the clinical area. An example is when a student calls attention to something that seems to be poor or unacceptable practice in the clinical environment. The situation should be discussed privately with the student or student group. Acceptable nursing practices should be reinforced with students. Faculty may need to follow through with the nurse manager or another appropriate person.

## Handling the Student Who Dominates

Students who ask questions that require an extensive answer, repeatedly ask questions, or dominate discussions are often problematic for both faculty and students. Faculty want to be careful about quashing a student's inquiry. Responding to the question is appropriate, but you may need to limit your answer. You may need to move on and check about the students' understanding of the material in question later. Using a classroom assessment (such as occasionally interspersing a sample test question on the material) to quickly determine student understanding is one useful strategy. Faculty may also plan time in the next class period to review the material, perhaps using a handout or brief visual presentation. Students who frequently ask questions or ask questions that are off topic may disrupt the flow of the class, interrupt group work, or halt the progress of discussions. If one student dominates the class with questions, you may need to limit the time given to that student. Asking or directing students to hold their questions or comments until other students have time to contribute may be necessary.

Questions or comments that are off-topic present similar problems. When faculty are aware of this pattern, talk with the student privately. Encourage the student to continue thinking, but stay focused on the work of the day. Praise the student for thinking about related topics, but indicate that others may not think in that direction. Offer the student a period of time, five to ten minutes, to discuss these questions individually.

# Incivility

Incivility has been a recent topic of discussion in nursing education. (See Chapter 15 in this book.) Luparell (2005, 2007) studied the responses of faculty to incivility by students. Incidents ranged from rudeness to open threats and violent behavior. A study by Clark and Springer (2007) looked at the perspectives of both faculty and students. Clark (2008) discussed the concept of rankism in relation to incivility by faculty directed toward students. Based on these writings, both faculty and students are guilty of incivility. Faculty need to examine their behavior and interactions with students. Demeaning and belittling remarks, pressure from unreasonable demands, and unfair and subjective treatment were identified by students as problematic behaviors. Incivility interferes with a positive learning environment. Both faculty and students are threatened by this type of situation. Open forums about incivility, promotion of collegiality and collaboration, and acknowledging dissent are ways of moving toward a healthy learning environment. Nursing faculty should lead in establishing and maintaining a civil, safe milieu (Clark, 2008).

Ideas for creating and maintaining a civil environment are reiterated by Luparell (2005). In addition to faculty examining their own behavior, setting forth expectations in course syllabi and discussing these expectations with students during course orientation are necessary. Students also need to recognize the role of feedback and constructive criticism in nursing education.

Another strategy for faculty to deal with incivility is thinking through possible responses to uncivil behavior and negative reactions to constructive criticism. Students may relate to comparing the constructive criticism given a student with the feedback that students provide on their course and instructor evaluations at the end of courses.

# The Student-Faculty Relationship Relative to Grading

Much of nursing faculty work focuses on grading and evaluation. Classroom testing, check-offs in skills laboratories, and clinical performance are all areas of concern for both faculty and students. Faculty should become adept at writing classroom tests. If the faculty has not had formal course work in test writing, taking a course or workshop may be in order. Learning about constructing tests and test questions as well as analyzing the results of a test are usually included in course work on tests, measurement, and evaluation. Books on curriculum and evaluation or measurement and evaluation include content that is useful for the nurse educator. Some programs have policies or procedures about reviewing test questions before questions are used in testing. This may be done by the team teaching the course or a committee.

Faculty should also be adept at other parts of the testing process including using test blueprints and test or item analysis data. Test blueprints facilitate covering content in a fair manner. A test blueprint correlates the course content, objectives, and the number of questions for a given test. Test analysis provides data about the reliability of the test, level of difficulty and discrimination of test items, and performance of high and low scoring students. Students often want to challenge or argue about test questions. Policies about test review should be established by the program or within courses. Some faculty have found that having the student put the challenge in writing is useful.

When students are failing in their course work, faculty should arrange a conference with the student to discuss their status. Review grades with the student. Talk about study habits and ask about difficulty with the content. Students are often at a loss about what to do except to "do better," or "study harder." The author does not view these phrases as useful problem-solvers. A specific plan for study and/or a learning contract, preferably with timelines, should be formulated. Both the student and the faculty should have copies of the plan. The plan may involve the student working with student services or other resources on study habits. Faculty should document their conferences with students. If the faculty is team teaching, the course coordinator needs to be apprised of the situation. The faculty may also need to inform the program director or other personnel.

Expectations about performance in the clinical area should be clear. Timely feedback is important for all students. Many times faculty's concern with marginal students overshadows the good work of other students. Clear expectations are essential in evaluating marginal students. Although anecdotal notes should be kept on all students, these notes are especially important in working with marginal students. When a student is marginal or failing, faculty should hold a private conference with the student to explore the possible causes for not meeting the objectives. Document the conference and any other interactions you have with the student. A learning contract may be used to delineate areas of improvement. Faculty will want to reinforce course expectations and review the evaluation criteria with the student.

## Gift Giving in the Student-Faculty Relationship

Because nursing faculty work so closely with students, students often want to express their appreciation for faculty with a celebration or gifts. Faculty need to be very cautious about both. Students should not feel obligated to include faculty in celebrations and dining in an expensive restaurant is usually out of order. Faculty may feel more comfortable paying their own way, contributing food to a party, or toning down a celebration. Faculty should never solicit gifts from students. The author recently learned of a nursing faculty who openly sought rather expensive gifts from students. Students felt obligated to comply with her wishes. Although students often want to express their appreciation for faculty individually or as a group, this should not be an obligation. A handwritten letter signed by all members of a specific class thanking faculty for their support, patience, and caring is a prized possession that can be used in place of gift giving. Classes or students may be directed to give gifts to a scholarship fund or other nursing funds.

## Advising in the Student-Faculty Relationship

Another aspect of the student-faculty relationship is advising. Faculty, in most instances, are involved in academic advising or counseling. Information or problems may arise that are not within the purview of academic advising. Students may share or start to share personal information with faculty. You may want to caution the student about personal confidences. Faculty who have training in personal or psychological counseling may be tempted to assume the role of therapist with students. However, the role of therapist may interfere with the student-faculty relationship. Although faculty should convey concern for the situation, a person outside the academic setting is better suited to deal with the problem. Provide specific resources and information about costs, if any.

In crisis situations, you may need to be more active about getting counseling for the student. Call or allow the student to call for an initial appointment. If you believe the situation is an emergency, you should not leave the student. Accompany the student to the counselor or ask someone else to be with the student. Faculty should have information about counseling and other student services readily available.

## Summary

Student-faculty relationships should be characterized by respect, integrity, and fairness. Nursing faculty need to be open and approachable. Although several areas in the student-faculty relationship can be of concern, establishing a viable work relationship with students is essential. Reflection on one's own behaviors and interactions are helpful in establishing a positive learning environment and healthy work setting for both students and faculty.

## Learning Activities

1. Consider your relationship with students. What aspects of the student-faculty relationship discussed in this chapter have you experienced? Is there anything you might change?
2. Discuss with another faculty your experience dealing with students who are failing. How did you handle this situation? How did you advise these students?
3. How do you maintain a civil environment in the classroom? How do you handle uncivil behavior? Is it working? If not, what would you change?

## Educational Philosophy

The values of dignity, integrity and caring have guided my teaching. My aim is to create a positive environment for learning. Some of my own nursing education was very negative. I remember this learning situation as stifling and demeaning. Part of my motivation in becoming a nurse educator was to change the negatives into positives. Learning is often hard, but providing support and encouragement enhances learning and builds confidence in knowledge and skill. One of my favorite teaching assignments has been to teach fundamentals students and later teach an upper level course. I am energized by what my former fundamentals students have become. I demonstrate respect for the student by coaching and guiding rather than intimidation. I continue to study and learn about what I do as a nurse educator. I try not to become complacent or stale in my teaching. I reflect on my teaching practice just as I have always done in relation to my nursing practice. My teaching has evolved over the years. I have tried to move from the "sage on the stage" to "the guide on the side." I write notes to myself about my perspective on the effectiveness of a learning activity. My focus has become how do I get students engaged in learning. I tell students that we have been researching learning for hundreds of years and we have not yet found a way to "pour" knowledge into the brain. I encourage students to assess their own learning and talk about my own assessment and reflection. My goal is to equip students for the practice of the future, the future that none of us have seen. I continually try to figure out how to foster lifelong learning and a spirit of inquiry about nursing practice. — Elizabeth Stokes

# References

Billings, D. M., & Halstead, J. A. (Eds.) (2008). *Teaching in nursing: A guide for faculty*. (3rd ed.). St. Louis: Elsevier/Saunders.

Clark, C. M., & Springer, P. J. (2007). Thoughts on incivility: Student and faculty perceptions of uncivil behavior in nursing education. *Nursing Education Perspectives, 28*(2), 93-97.

Clark, C. (2008). Student perspectives on faculty incivility in nursing education: An application of the concept of rankism. *Nursing Outlook, 56*(1), 4-8.

Luparell, S. (2005). Why and how we should address student incivility in nursing programs. In M. H. Oermann, & K. T. Heinrich, (Eds.). *Annual review of nursing education* (pp. 23-36). New York: Springer.

Luparell, S. (2007). The effects of student incivility on nursing faculty. *Journal of Nursing Education, 46*(1), 15-19.

National League for Nursing. (2005). *Core competencies of nurse educators with task statements*. New York: Author.

The Carnegie Foundation for the Advancement of Teaching. *Study of Nursing Education*. Stanford, CA: Author. http://www.carnegiefoundation.org/programs/index.asp?key=1829 Accessed October 1, 2008.

# Resources

www.nsna.org/pubs/resources/academic_clinical_conduct.
National Student Nurse Association Code of Academic and Clinical Conduct

www.nsna.org/pubs/resources/professional_conduct.asp
NSNA, Inc. Code of Professional Conduct

# CHAPTER 15

# MANAGING STUDENT INCIVILITY IN NURSING EDUCATION

## Susan Luparell, PhD, CNS-BC, CNE

The content of this chapter relates to the following major content areas and subconcepts on the Certified Nurse Educator Examination Detailed Test Blueprint:

**Facilitate Learning**

- Create a positive learning environment that fosters a free exchange of ideas
- Respond effectively to unexpected events that affect clinical and/or classroom instruction

**Facilitate Learning Development and Socialization**

- Create learning environments that facilitate learners' self-reflection, personal goal setting, and socialization to the role of the nurse
- Encourage professional development of learners

## Introduction

It's your first semester teaching and you are excited about what lies ahead in your new role as an educator. You expect your students to be full of enthusiasm, eager to hear all you have to share with them. Imagine your surprise when you discover that some students seem less than engaged in what you have to offer them. They arrive late to class, are frequently unprepared, and are often inattentive. You begin to hear stories around the lunch table about faculty experiences with students who are rude and abrasive, or even hostile. Chances are that you will eventually have your own encounter with a difficult student that leaves you with a variety of emotions from bewilderment to frustration to fear to anger. Thankfully, the large majority of time it is both delightful and fulfilling to work with nursing students. For a variety of reasons, however, an occasional interaction with a student may be less than pleasant. Dealing effectively with these difficult student situations is perhaps one of the most unexpected and challenging aspects of the faculty role.

However, research has shown that many of us enter our academic careers with unrealistically positive expectations of student behavior (Olive, 2006). Subsequently, we are almost uniformly caught off guard by uncivil encounters with students, especially when the behavior involved borders on the extreme. And, when we meet students who are challenging, either because of apathy or inappropriate behavior, we tend to respond with surprise and sometimes outrage. Why so? Perhaps because we suspect that apathetic learners will potentially become apathetic nurses. And perhaps we also suspect that uncivil students will go on to become uncivil practicing nurses, who potentially exert a toxic effect on the work environment at best and, at worst, act in a variety of unprofessional or unethical ways with patients. Unfortunately, there is a dearth of information available that definitively supports or refutes such assumptions. Similarly, there is equally little that directs nurse educators on how to respond to inappropriate behavior. The purpose of this chapter is to provide an overview of the issues related to incivility in nursing education and to offer suggestions to prevent it altogether or manage it more effectively when it occurs.

## Defining Incivility

Defining incivility and other problematic behavior in the classroom is difficult to say the least. The standard definition of incivility is "speech or action that is discourteous, rude, or impolite" (Merriam Dictionary, 2006). Andersson and Pearson (1999) described uncivil behavior as "....characteristically rude and discourteous, displaying a lack of regard for others" (p. 457). Although useful for general discussions, a drawback to this definition is that it leaves open to interpretation what discourteous, rude, or impolite behavior might actually look like. And, indeed, what is impolite to one person may not be perceived as impolite to another.

Additional difficulties arise when one tries to distinguish between incivility and other forms of inappropriate behavior, such as verbal or emotional abuse, workplace violence, or aggression. In the workplace literature, for example, violence is defined broadly as "any physical assault, threatening behavior, or verbal abuse occurring in the work setting" (NIOSH, 1996). In attempting to differentiate between incivility and aggression, some authors suggest that the intent to harm a target is overt with aggression, but the intent to harm may be quite ambiguous with incivility (Pearson, Andersson, & Wegner, 2001). Keashly (1998, 2001) described emotional abuse as the use of verbal and nonverbal hostile behaviors to negatively affect another's sense of self. Unfortunately, behaviors occasionally encountered by faculty may fall into one or more of these descriptions.

Academic incivility, as defined by Feldman (2001), occurs within the learning environment and may be so extreme that learning is altogether terminated. Feldman classified five types of classroom incivilities in higher education. Annoyances such as arriving late to class or leaving early are frequent, yet students are often unaware of their classroom impact. Classroom terrorism occurs when a student directly interferes with instruction, for example, by attempting to upstage or vocally disregard the instructor. Some incivilities include attempts to intimidate by threatening to bring to bear external power and influence, such as political pressure. Attacks on instructor psyche and threats of violence are additional types of classroom incivilities.

A common theme amongst authors is that even seemingly low level incivilities can have a significant negative impact on both the individual and the environment as a whole. For example, workplace incivility has been implicated in absenteeism, reduced organizational commitment, and decreased productivity (Pearson, Andersson, & Porath, 2000). Additionally, evidence suggests that nursing faculty can be greatly impacted even by what many might consider milder forms of incivility (Luparell, 2003), resulting in decreased morale and an inclination to resign from teaching altogether.

## Incivility in Nursing Education: Is It Really a Problem?

Some would contend that student incivility in the classroom is not at all a new phenomenon since it has been documented back to colonial times, albeit in the form of food fights and other behavior considered outlandish at the time. Even so, the apparent decline of civility in the college classroom has been a more frequent topic of discussion in recent years (Schneider, 1998) and nurse educators have also noted its apparent increase (Lashley & deMeneses, 2001). In terms of the research evidence that guides our understanding of incivility in higher education, particularly nursing education, the findings are unfortunately sparse.

Sadly, both students and faculty have reported that incivility is a moderate problem in nursing education (Clark & Springer, 2007). Tardiness, talking in class, and other inattentiveness are experienced by virtually all nursing faculty. Unfortunately, faculty also seem to be experiencing more disturbing encounters as well. In one national survey, a little over half of nursing faculty reported that they had been yelled at in the classroom, and about 43% had been yelled at in a clinical setting, where students might be assumed to be on their best behavior. Additionally, approximately 25% of the faculty reported that they had experienced objectionable physical contact by a student (Lashley & deMeneses, 2001). Moreover, nursing faculty have reported being slapped, stalked, and overtly threatened by nursing students (Luparell, 2004; Olive, 2006). At the furthest end of the spectrum, few nursing faculty are unaware of the tragic shootings at the University of Arizona College of Nursing in 2002 that left three faculty dead.

It is tempting to credit only nursing students with poor behavior in the educational environment. However, evidence suggests that nursing students have been the targets of incivility by faculty (Clark & Springer, 2007) and, anecdotally, by other students.

Additionally, faculty to faculty incivility, referred to as mean-girl games by Heinrich (2007), also contribute to a potentially unhealthy educational environment. Though beyond the scope of this chapter, when attempting to cultivate an environment of civility in nursing education, incivility in all its forms must be addressed.

## Incivility: What's the Cost?

Unfortunately, the cost of incivility in nursing education is high (Luparell, 2004; 2007a). For example, describing the effects uncivil encounters with students had on them, faculty reported loss of sleep and other physical symptoms that may or may not be short-lived. Additionally, depending on the severity of the encounter with the student, some experience a recurrent emotional response similar to post-traumatic stress response. Others reported significant damage to their confidence as a teacher and the adoption of less rigorous classroom practices. Perhaps most concerning, given the current faculty shortage, was the finding that some relinquish their faculty roles because of dissatisfying relationships with students. Interestingly, students report similar symptoms of distress when they perceive they have been treated uncivilly by faculty members (Clark, 2006).

## Incivility: Contributing Factors

There are many complex and multifaceted issues that contribute to inappropriate student behavior and full exploration of these is beyond the scope of this chapter. However, a brief examination of the role both students and faculty play in incivility is worthy of discussion.

### Student Characteristics

There is evidence that students today are quite different from past cohorts, and much has been written about the characteristics of the current generation of college students and how these characteristics influence classroom behavior. Levine and Cureton (1998) described the contemporary college student as distrustful of leadership, lacking confidence in traditional social institutions, fearful of intimacy, less prepared for the academic rigors of college, and generally overwhelmed and anxious. Societal trends have left students with a consumer's approach to higher education and they are demanding to have their expectations met in terms of convenience, quality, service, and cost.

Additionally, there may be other factors that, either individually or collectively, contribute to student misbehavior. For example, there is an increasing prevalence of physical and mental illness in the college classroom that generally mirrors society at large (Kuhlenschmidt & Layne, 1999). It recently has been suggested that today's college student is the most narcissistic in history (College students think they're so special, 2007) with a resultant penchant for responding aggressively to criticism. Lastly, the advent of the Internet and widespread availability of information on virtually any topic has resulted in the erosion of the concept of the content expert. Consequently, there may be a tendency for the contemporary college student to view the world as one large peer group (Hernandez & Fister, 2001) and perhaps this perspective influences interaction. Additionally, second degree students, who are often older and more experienced, may feel more inclined to act assertively to protect their own self interests.

## Faculty Contributions to Student Incivility

It is a difficult but necessary task for faculty to examine their role in the development of student incivility. Unfortunately, faculty can, albeit often unwittingly, contribute to student behavior. For example, Clark (2008) found that faculty attitudes of superiority contributed to student incivility. Additionally, poorly developed teaching skills can leave some students bored, angry, or resentful.

In an extensive study involving the academy in general, Boice (1996) found that classroom incivility was indeed significant and resulted in both annoyance and demoralization of faculty. Indeed, classroom incivility was a turning point in many faculty careers. Boice further found that students and faculty perceptions of the cause of incivility differed, with faculty assigning responsibility to students and students assigning responsibility to faculty. The researcher concluded that **faculty are the most crucial initiators of classroom incivility** and that, furthermore, faculty with the most awareness of incivility were least likely to experience it. Thus, it is prudent that nurse educators become well-versed on the topic.

## Incivility: What You Can Do About It

Many nursing faculty are hesitant to address inappropriate student behavior in the classroom. It has been suggested that underlying emotional issues, fear of legal or physical reprisals, fear of being blamed, and the unwillingness to inflict emotional pain on students may underlying faculty reluctance to address student incivility (Amada, 1995). Additional evidence suggests that many faculty are caught off guard when incivility occurs, and thus are unprepared and unable to act effectively (Luparell, 2004; Olive, 2006).

However, as has been noted elsewhere (Luparell, 2005), the Code of Ethics for Nurses provides the foundation needed to address uncivil behavior in nursing education. Specifically, the Code states that "the nurse, in all professional relationships, practices with compassion and respect for the inherent dignity, worth, and uniqueness of every individual...." (ANA, p.4). Furthermore, this principle of respect encompasses encounters with colleagues as well: "This standard of conduct precludes any and all prejudicial actions, any form of harassment or threatening behavior, or disregard for the effect of one's actions on others" (ANA, p.9). Lastly, the Code speaks specifically to the ethical responsibilities of faculty members, noting that "nurse educators have a responsibility to...promote a commitment to professional practice prior to entry of an individual into practice" (p.13). Additionally, prominent professional organizations, such as the American Association of Critical Care Nurses, are also recognizing the importance of healthy workplaces and are calling on all to help cultivate them (AACN, 2005).

Thus, despite the challenges that exist in dealing with uncivil or other inappropriate student behavior, there may be significant ethical ramifications if it is allowed to occur unfettered. Luhanga (2008) suggests that failing to fail the unsafe student represents a breakdown of self-regulation. It logically can be asserted that failing to fail students whose conduct is contrary to professional ethics is also a breach of self-regulation.

There are proactive, or preventative, and reactive approaches to managing classroom behavior (Feldman, 2001). In the remainder of this chapter, I offer suggestions, both synthesized from the literature and based on my own experiences, to assist faculty to cultivate a more civil learning environment.

## Share Your Values and Philosophies

Often we assume that students understand the purpose of their study and our assignments, when in fact they often do not. In the absence of such understanding, students tend to perceive assignments and faculty decision-making as arbitrary. Just as student behaviors reflect student values, faculty behaviors reflect faculty values. That is, nursing program policies generally reflect what faculty hold dear related to education, nursing, or life in general. Unfortunately, too often the connection is not clear to students, and they perceive faculty policies as nothing more than arbitrary. Thus, faculty should identify the values and philosophies that drive their teaching. For example, some faculty believe that learning is constructed socially, that is, that students can learn from each others' experiences. It is likely, then, that an instructor with this perspective creates classroom activities that allow students to dialogue with each other. It is important to provide students with the rationale for what you do in the classroom, not only regarding how you approach teaching, but why you have chosen the assignments you did for the class. These can be shared not only in the syllabus, but on the first day of class. A sample syllabus page is included in the Appendix at the end of this chapter.

## Articulate Behavioral Expectations

Because the perception of uncivil behavior varies both by individual faculty members and within the specific circumstances in which they find themselves, it is important that students have clear expectations of individual faculty preferences. Identify what classroom rules you have and why you have them. For example, some faculty are easily distracted by side conversations in the classroom. Because the distraction may disrupt the quality of the teaching and learning, the instructor may wish to expect that side conversations are kept to a minimum. Other instructors find it distracting to themselves or others when students arrive late to class and may subsequently ask students to wait until a break to enter the class to avoid disruption. However, it is wise to weigh the impact of course rules against principles of adult learning. Some students learn best when they can verbally reiterate or connect the content with a recent experience. Additionally, students arriving late may have made monumental efforts to get to class at all and may feel unfairly penalized if they are denied access. The instructor must weigh the consequences of each course expectation in light of his or her own philosophies, values, and learning. Then, this should be shared with the students to avoid the notion of arbitrariness.

## Add Behavioral Objectives to Your Course

A dilemma for nurse educators is how to capture inappropriate student behavior in terms of formal evaluation. Often challenging or disruptive students perform well in the didactic portion of the course, and their direct care with patients may also be adequate. What do you do with the student who speaks rudely to you or the staff nurses in the clinical setting or who acts out in other ways that do not directly involve patients or the classroom setting?

Adding objectives to your course or your clinical experiences that specifically address appropriate behavior is one way to 1) let students know what is expected of them, and 2) appropriately evaluate this important aspect of professional development. For example, two useful clinical objectives I have incorporated include: *Appropriately accepts and thoughtfully considers constructive feedback* and *All course-related interactions are consistent with the Code of Ethics* (ANA, 2001). These have been particularly useful objectives and, when student behavioral problems develop, provide a nice mechanism for documentation of the deficiencies as well.

## Help Students Learn to Value Feedback

It is important to establish a framework for providing feedback to the students. Too often we assume that students understand the role of constructive feedback in their professional development, yet often the students are woefully unprepared to receive such feedback. Many have been highly successful in their academic careers, thus constructive feedback is somewhat foreign to them. Here again lies a useful place to build a more trusting relationship and help students learn to value feedback in their professional development.

It is prudent to spend some time on the first day of class outlining your philosophies about the role of feedback in professional development (Luparell, 2007b). For example, I believe that trust is a prerequisite for effective feedback. That is, I need to trust that the students have a goal in mind of successful completion of my nursing course. I trust they want me to share my experienced feedback with them to help them achieve their goal. Additionally, the students must trust that, especially when I am giving constructive feedback or pointing out performance weaknesses, that my sole motivation for doing so is to help them meet their goals, as opposed to some arbitrary desire of mine to damage their psyche. This philosophy is explained in depth on the first day of class. Subsequently, any time I am giving constructive feedback during the semester, I always start by reminding the student of the role of trust and my motivations in giving them the feedback.

## Anticipate Incivility

As noted, faculty are frequently caught unprepared for uncivil student encounters (Luparell, 2004; Olive, 2006). Thus, an important proactive strategy is to anticipate incivility. Some research has shown that students are likely to act out with more extreme forms of inappropriate behavior in association with grading criteria or decisions they deem harsh, delivery of constructive feedback, and notification of failure for the clinical day or course (Luparell, 2003). Faculty should especially anticipate the potential for student misbehavior at these times. Additionally, I recommend that novice faculty practice for these situations by role playing how they might handle various potential student responses beforehand with a trusted mentor. This may minimize the likelihood of being caught unprepared.

## Take Action

I have found that attention to these proactive methods does indeed limit the incidence of challenging student interactions. However, occasionally problems still arise, even for the experienced instructor. When problems arise, it is important to act. Unfortunately, many novice faculty opt not to act to dissuade inappropriate behavior, often because they either 1) lack confidence in their skill at interpreting inappropriate behavior, 2) don't know how to respond, or 3) mistakenly believe the behavior will be self-limiting. This is rarely the case. In fact, poor behaviors will often deteriorate and come to involve greater numbers of students or worsening behavior. Additionally, many students are skilled at knowing the boundary and continually breach behavioral norms up to, but not exceeding that boundary. A later frustration occurs when other faculty attempt to address the behavior more assertively only to find an insufficient trail of documentation prohibiting their ability to take definitive action. Thus, faculty should address and document even inappropriate behavior that seems inconsequential at the time.

## Use the Disciplinary Process

I have discussed specific methods for dealing with the annoyance type of inappropriate behavior elsewhere (2005, 2007). These include strategies that are aimed at helping the student appreciate how the behavior may ultimately negatively impact him or her and enlisting the student's aid in creating a better learning environment. However, when student behavior remains consistently inappropriate or is especially egregious, faculty should take more definitive action. This includes consulting and implementing policy regarding student conduct and often results in the filing of a formal complaint. It is here that many nursing faculty seem to get entangled in the confounding emotion of potentially causing distress to a student, yet it is here that the ANA Code of Ethics can serve as the strong foundation for action.

## Campus Violence: A Contemporary Concern

Unpleasant encounters with students are relatively rare and most often can be addressed effectively in short order. Indeed, most students have the potential to experience tremendous personal and professional growth following feedback on behavior. However, as members of the larger academy, it is prudent for nursing faculty to be aware of the potential for an act of incivility to be carried to the extreme. Faculty, staff, and students are all affected by campus violence (Carr, 2005). In recent years, nursing faculty have become more acutely aware of the potential for incivility to spiral out of control and lead to tragedy. In 2003, for example, three University of Arizona nursing faculty were shot and killed on campus by a disgruntled student. Since then, tragic mass shootings at Virginia Tech in April 2007 and Northern Illinois University in February 2008 have left faculty in all disciplines feeling vulnerable. Faculty members who experience violence at the hands of their students are victims of Type 2 workplace violence (IPRC, 2001).

In its white paper on campus violence, the American College Health Association (ACHA) (Carr, 2005) analyzed campus violence patterns, types of violence, and the issues that underlie campus violence. The ACHA categorized campus violence as sexual harassment, sexual assault, stalking, dating violence, hate crimes, hazing, celebratory violence following sporting events, attempted suicide, murder/suicide, murder/non-negligent manslaughter, aggravated assault, arson, and attacks against faculty and staff. Recommendations to address campus violence include building a sense of community that strengthens the relationship between and among faculty, students, and staff, adopting zero tolerance policies for campus violence, enforcing codes of conduct, screening out students who pose a real threat, and creating classroom disruption policies that address harassment and intimidation (Carr, 2005).

Additionally, the ACHA endorses a ban on firearms on college campuses (Carr, 2005). However, in 2008 there is a movement underway, led primarily by college students, to permit legally licensed students to carry concealed weapons on college campuses. The Students for Concealed Carry on Campus (SCCC, 2007) contend that legal concealed carriers may be in the position to interrupt or halt instances of mass gun violence on campuses. It is likely that this issue will be hotly debated in the upcoming years. Nursing faculty should be prepared to weigh in on these and other topics, as well as be part of the development and implementation of campus safety policies.

## Summary

The good news is that in all likelihood, only a small percentage of your students will require your attention because of poor behavior. Two broad themes for proactively managing student behavior in the classroom are suggested in this chapter. First, it is incumbent upon faculty to be more transparent in all that we do. Secondly, we need to lay the foundations for more trusting relationships with our students. Although most faculty experience highly ambivalent emotions when forced to address student misconduct, when student behavior cannot be remediated, faculty should employ appropriate disciplinary procedures. The ANA Code of Ethics provides solid rationale for why faculty can and should address uncivil or otherwise inappropriate student behavior.

## Learning Activities

1. Review the syllabus for a nursing class. Is there a component that addresses incivility? If not, write guidelines such as those in the appendix to this chapter.
2. Discuss student incivility with a faculty teaching for 20 years and a faculty teaching for 2 years. Is there a difference in the way these two faculty handle incivility in the classroom? What did you learn from each of these faculty?
3. Talk with students in one of your classes. Ask them what they perceive to be uncivil behavior in the classroom. Are their perceptions the same as yours?
4. Identify and reflect upon the philosophies you have about teaching and learning. How do these philosophies shape your classroom and clinical teaching? How are the assignments you require influenced by these philosophies?
5. Identify and reflect upon what you value in nursing, education, and life in general. How do these values influence your expectations of students?
6. List the specific behaviors you will not permit in the classroom and why. Add these to your syllabus with the next revision.
7. Consider a real or hypothetical unpleasant encounter with a student. Visualize yourself addressing the situation in an effective manner. What are the key aspects of the scenario that lend themselves to effective management?
8. Locate and review the Student Code of Conduct at your institution paying special attention to behavioral misconduct.
9. Contact the Dean of Student Affairs Office at your institution and have a conversation about the types of student misbehavior they most often see and how they typically handle behavioral misconduct.
10. Locate and review the campus emergency plan at your institution. Consider setting up a mock emergency situation in your classroom.

## Educational Philosophy

I believe learning is most likely to occur when a relationship between student and teacher exists that is founded in trust and respect. It is incumbent upon the teacher to respect the inherent worth of the learner and to be able to demonstrate that respect outwardly. And, particularly in nursing where constructive feedback is needed to help the student develop, the student must be able to trust the instructor's intentions. Toward that end, I believe that the best educators are really coaches. They find ways to motivate their players/students to want to achieve, to believe they can achieve, and to work hard to achieve, all while giving them the tools they need to achieve. — Susan Luparell

## References

Amada, G. (1995). The disruptive college student: Some thoughts and considerations. *Journal of American College Health, 43,* 232-236.

American Association of Critical Care Nurses (AACN). (2005). *AACN standards for establishing and sustaining healthy work environments.* Available at http://www.aacn.org/WD/HWE/Docs/HWEStandards.pdf

American Nurses Association. (2001). Code of ethics for nurses with interpretive statements. Washington, DC: American Nurses Publishing.

Andersson, L. M., & Pearson, C. M. (1999). Tit for tat? The spiraling effect of incivility in the workplace. *Academy of Management Review, 24*(3), 452-471.

Boice, B. (1996). Classroom incivilities. *Research in Higher Education, 37*(4), 453-486.

Carr, J. L. (2005, February). *American College Health Association campus violence white paper.* Baltimore, MD: American College Health Association.

Clark, C. M. (2006). Incivility in nursing education: Student perceptions of uncivil faculty behavior in the academic environment. Doctoral dissertation, University of Idaho, 2006. *Dissertation Abstracts International,* AAT 3092571.

Clark, C. M., & Springer, P. (2007). Incivility in nursing education: Descriptive study on definitions and prevalence. *Journal of Nursing Education 46*(1), 7-14.

Clark, C. M. (2008). The dance of civility and incivility in nursing education. In the *Western Institute of Nursing Communicating Nursing Research Conference Proceedings, 41* (p. 249). Portland, OR: Western Institute of Nursing

*College students think they're so special.* (2007, February 27). Retrieved from November 8, 2007, from http://www.msnbc.msn.com/id/17349066

Feldmann, L. J. (2001). Classroom civility is another of our instructor responsibilities. *College Teaching, 49*(4), 137-140.

Heinrich, K.T. (2007, January/February). Joy stealing: Ten mean games faculty play and how to stop the gaming. *Nurse Educator, 32*(1), 34-8.

Hernandez, T., & Fister, D. (2001). Dealing with disruptive and emotional college students. *Journal of College Counseling, 4,* 49-62.

Injury Prevention Research Center (IPRC). (2001). *Workplace violence: A report to the nation.* Available at http://www.public-health.uiowa.edu/iprc/nation.pdf

Keashly, L. (1998). Emotional abuse in the workplace: Conceptual and empirical issues. *Journal of Emotional Abuse, 1*(1), 85-117.

Keashly, L. (2001). Interpersonal and systemic aspects of emotional abuse at work: The target's perspective. *Violence and Victims, 16*(3), 233-268.

Kuhlenschmidt, S. L. & Layne, L. E. (1999). Strategies for dealing with difficult behavior. In M.D. Svinicki & S.M. Richardson (Eds.), *New directions in teaching and learning: No. 77. Promoting civility: A teaching challenge* (pp. 45-58). San Francisco, CA: Jossey-Bass.

Lashley, F. R., & De Meneses, M. (2001). Student civility in nursing programs: A national survey. *Journal of Professional Nursing, 17*(2), 81.

Levine, A., & Cureton, J. S. (1998). What we know about today's college students. *About Campus, 3*(1), 4-9.

Luhanga, F., Yonge, O. J., & Myrick, F. (2008). "Failure to assign failing grades": Issues with grading the unsafe student. *International Journal of Nursing Education Scholarship, 5*(1), Article 8. Available at: http://www.bepress.com/ijnes/vol5/iss1/art8

Luparell, S. (2003). *Critical incidents of incivility by nursing students: How uncivil encounters with students affect nursing faculty.* Unpublished doctoral dissertation, University of Nebraska, Lincoln.

Luparell, S. (2004). Faculty encounters with uncivil nursing students: An overview. *Journal of Professional Nursing, 20*(1), 59-67.

Luparell, S. (2005). Why and how we should address student incivility in nursing programs. In M. H. Oermann & K. T. Heinrich (Eds.), *Annual review of nursing education* (Vol. 3, pp. 23-36). New York: Springer.

Luparell, S. (2007a). The effect of student incivility on nursing faculty. *Journal of Nursing Education, 46*(1), 15-19.

Luparell, S. (2007b). Addressing challenging student situations: Lessons learned. In M. H. Oermann & K. T. Heinrich (Eds.), *Annual review of nursing education* (Vol.5, pp. 101-10). New York: Springer.

Merriam-Webster. (2006). Merriam-Webster dictionary online. Retrieved April 25, 2006, from http://www.merriam-webster.com

National Institute for Occupational Safety and Health (NIOSH). (1996, July). *Violence in the workplace: Risk factors and prevention strategies.* Available at http://www.cdc.gov/NIOSH/violcont.html

Olive, D. (2006). *Nursing student incivility: The experience of nursing faculty.* Unpublished doctoral dissertation, Widener University.

Pearson, C. M., Andersson, L., & Porath, C. L. (2000). Assessing and attacking incivility. *Organizational Dynamics, 29*(2), 123-137.

Pearson, C. M., Andersson, L. M., & Wegner, J. W. (2001). When workers flout convention: A study of workplace incivility. *Human Relations, 54*(11), 1387-1419.

Schneider, A. (1998, March 27). Insubordination and intimidation signal the end of decorum in many classrooms. *The Chronicle of Higher Education*, pp. A12-A14.

Students for Concealed Carry on Campus. (2007). *Students for concealed carry on campus: About Us and FAQ*. Retrieved May 12, 2008, from http://concealed-campus.org/about.htm

## Appendix
## Sample Syllabus Page
## Course Policies and General Information

Instructor Philosophy.

Learning is a social activity. We integrate new experiences and alternative viewpoints with our previous understanding to develop new understanding and perspective. Accordingly, much emphasis is placed on active participation, sharing of ideas, and the use of critical thinking skills in this course. Attendance in class is highly encouraged. Learning activities are planned for each class period. Students who are prepared for class will gain the most benefit from lectures and discussions and will experience greater success in the course.

We are committed to facilitating the success of each student in this course. Please do not hesitate to speak with the faculty in order to have concerns addressed or questions clarified.

Academic and Behavioral Expectations

Along with the learning of theoretical concepts, development of professional behaviors is a key component of the nursing curriculum. Therefore, it is expected that the student demonstrate professional behaviors consistent with the Code of Ethics in all aspects of this course. Academic integrity and professional conduct are expected of all students. The use of another student's work or the incorporation of work not one's own without proper credit will result in sanctions at the discretion of the instructor. Similarly, inappropriate behavior or behavior judged by faculty to be disruptive to the educational environment will not be permitted and will be addressed according to the university Conduct Guidelines.

As per the university Student Academic Guidelines, it is expected that students should:
a. Be prompt and regular in attending classes,
b. Be well prepared for classes,
c. Submit required assignments in a timely manner,
d. Take exams when scheduled,
e. Meet the course and behavior standards as defined by the instructor, and
f. Make and keep appointments when necessary to meet with the instructor.

There is a large amount of content to be covered this semester and it promises to be challenging. You will be best served if you keep current with the readings and participate actively in each of your learning opportunities. It is further expected that you will:
a. Be on time to class. If you are unavoidably detained, please enter the back of the classroom and be attentive to minimizing the disruption to others.
b. Turn off your cell phone during class.
c. Keep chit-chat to a minimum in class to avoid distraction to others.
d. Treat your colleagues, the agency staff, and the faculty with respect.
e. Demonstrate ethical and professional behavior in all aspects of this course.

## Additional Suggested Readings

Amada, G. (1997). The disruptive college student: Recent trends and practical advice. *Journal of College Student Psychotherapy, 11*(4), 57-67.

Baxter, P. E., & Boblin, S. L. (2007). The moral development of baccalaureate nursing students: Understanding unethical behavior in classroom and clinical settings. *Journal of Nursing Education, 46*(1), 20.

Braxton, J. M., & Bayer, A. E. (1999). *Faculty misconduct in collegiate teaching.* Baltimore: Johns Hopkins University Press.

Carter, S. L. (1999). *Civility.* New York: HarperCollins.

Clark, C. M. (2008). Student perspectives on incivility in nursing education: An application of the concept of rankism. *Nursing Outlook, 56*(1), 4-8.

Clark, C. M., & Springer, P. J. (2007). Thoughts on incivility: Student and faculty perceptions of uncivil behavior in nursing education. *Nursing Education Perspectives, 28*(2), 93-97.

Forni, P.M. (2003). *Choosing civility: The twenty-five rules of considerate conduct.* New York: St. Martin's Press.

Heinrich, K. T. (2006, Third Quarter). Joy-stealing: How some nurse educators resist these faculty games. *Reflections on Nursing Leadership.* Available at: www.nursingsociety.org

Heinrich, K. T. (2006, Second Quarter). Joy-stealing games. *Reflections on Nursing Leadership.* Available at: www.nursingsociety.org

Hirschy, A. S., & Braxton, J. M. (2004). Effects of student classroom incivilities on students. *New Directions for Teaching & Learning, 2004*(99), 67-76

Kolanko, K. M., Clark, C. M., Heinrich, K. T., Olive, D., Serembus, J. F., & Sifford, K. S. (2006). Academic dishonesty, bullying, incivility, and violence: Difficult challenges facing nurse educators. *Nursing Education Perspectives, 27*(1), 34-43.

Thomas, S. P. (2003). Handling anger in the teacher-student relationship. *Nursing Education Perspectives, 24*(1), 17-24.

## Useful Websites

*AACN standards for establishing and sustaining healthy work environments.* Available at http://www.aacn.org/WD/HWE/Docs/HWEStandards.pdf

*ACHA campus violence white paper.* Available at http://www.acha.org/info_resources/Campus_violence.pdf

*National League for Nursing Healthful Work Environment Tool Kit* ©. Available at http://www.nln.org/facultydevelopment/HealthfulWorkEnvironment/index.htm

US Department of Education. FERPA Guidance on Emergency Management. Available at http://www.edu.gov/policy/gen/guid/fpco/ferpa/safeschools/index.html

US Department of Labor, Occupational Safety and Health Association, Workplace Violence Hazard Awareness: http://www.osha.gov/STLC/workplaceviolence/recognition.html

# CHAPTER 16

## TEACHING THE GENERATIONS:
### COPING WITH THE DIFFERENCES

**Elizabeth Stokes, EdD, RN, CNE**

---

The content of this chapter relates to the following major content areas and subconcepts on the Certified Nurse Educator Examination Detailed Test Blueprint:

**Facilitate Learning**
- Implement a variety of teaching strategies appropriate to learner needs; learning style
- Modify teaching strategies and learning experiences based on consideration of learners': past education and life experiences
- Demonstrate personal attributes that facilitate learning

**Facilitate Learning Development and Socialization**
- Provide resources for diverse learners to meet their individual learning needs
- Create learning environments that facilitate learners' self-reflection, personal goal setting, and socialization to the role of the nurse
- Adapt teaching styles and interpersonal interactions to facilitate learner behaviors

---

## Introduction

The days of predominately traditional students in nursing education programs have passed into history. Four to five decades ago nursing students were primarily 18 to 22 year olds. As associate degree programs opened, older students chose nursing as a career. Older students then began choosing baccalaureate programs as an educational path. Currently, most any type of nursing education program has students who represent a wide range of ages from several generations. Members of different generations have diverse perspectives on career, life, and learning. Nurse educators need to be aware of the differences in generations and use teaching strategies that facilitate learning for each group.

Students from as many as three or four generations can be present in any one nursing program. Faculty may also be from three or four generations. Those known as Traditionalists or the Silent Generation, born from 1925 to 1942 are faculty, either full or part-time. The Boomers, born from 1943 to 1960, are usually faculty but may have enrolled in various degree programs such as accelerated nursing options or are in graduate school at the master's or doctoral levels. Generation Xers were born between 1961 to 1981 and may be either faculty or students. The youngest generation, known as the Generation Y or the Millennials, born between 1982 and 2000 are most likely students. Each of these generations has been shaped by world events, knowledge and technology growth, and parenting practices. This chapter takes a look at these generations and how faculty address their learning needs.

## Teaching to Different Generations

The faculty and students representing the different generations view teaching and learning in diverse ways. Nurse educators need to develop instructional strategies to work with diverse generations. A comparison can be made with efforts of nurses in education and practice to become culturally aware and culturally competent. Faculty, in particular, need to become generation-competent. Stokes and Flowers (2009), after reviewing definitions of cultural competence, note that cultural competence is composed of knowledge, skills, and attitudes (p. 277). To be generation competent, faculty must become knowledgeable about the general characteristics and attitudes of different generations and understand how to design learning opportunities that will meet desired learning outcomes (Johnson & Romanello, 2006).

### Traditionalists

The Traditionalists are at retirement age. Many nurse educators in this age group are still in the workforce, either on a full or part-time basis. Born at the end of World War II, the Traditionalists were raised in a growing economy. They lived in a two parent home and may remember the wavy screens of early television. Social changes such as the civil rights movement, the Cold War, an unpopular war, and the feminist movement have been a large part of their lives. Better educated than their parents, Traditionalists are structure-oriented, loyal employees, and disciplined. They have a strong work ethic and respect authority. Traditionalists may be wary of technology and are often more comfortable with a telephone book than using the computer to find information about businesses or to shop for goods. Their first students were the Boomer generation. Boomer generation students were and are highly motivated learners who prepared for class and were concerned with assignments and grades. Learning to work with Generation X and Y as students or fellow faculty members may be a struggle for Traditionalists (Zemke, Raines, & Filipczak, 2000).

## Boomers

The Boomer generation was born into post-war prosperity. Their outlook is generally optimistic. Television replaced movies. Boomers were witnesses to celebration and tragedy as a man landed on the moon and a president was shot. Questions were raised about societal rules, and many rules and mores faded away. For many Boomers, Watergate and the Vietnam War were defining moments, and their doubts about authority were confirmed. Boomers are and have been workaholics. Their identity is associated with work, and self-sacrifice is important in job achievement. As faculty members or students, they are intense and desire rewards such as promotions or grades. Boomers usually prefer face-to-face classes with lectures; however, team learning or projects are also viewed as effective learning (Johnson & Romanello, 2005). Boomers have generally been slower in adopting and using technology than the generations following them. Whether the Boomer is a student or a faculty member, they may have difficulty working with Generations X and Y. Boomers view Generation X as having a poor work ethic and do not understand the need to be connected that is a salient characteristic of Generation Y, the Millennials (Zembe, Raines, & Filipczak, 2000).

## Generation X

Generation X might be called the generation that was forgotten until recently. With the retirement of the Boomers, Generation X is the rising workforce. Fewer in number, the Xers grew up with both parents working and were the original "latchkey kids." Many grew up with custody agreements and single parent families as the divorce rate increased. America as a country changed. The country lost a war, other industrial nations were on the scene, a president resigned from office, and the Challenger disintegrated. Many of this generation grew up with the fear of nuclear war. When their parents lost their jobs in spite of their devotion to work and company loyalty, Generation X became skeptical and looked for ways to cope. As adults they view a sense of balance between work and play as essential. As faculty or students, they tend to be casual and are not awed by authority. Their goal is to accomplish the goal or task, but not necessarily within the usual time constraints. Many Generation Xers are more comfortable working alone; they are not always good in teams (Sacks, 1996; Black, 2003; Zembe, Raines & Filipczak, 2000). Most of this generation is generally comfortable with technology and have worked at acquiring technical skills, partly because they learned these skills were needed. As workers or students, they are creative and flexible, and work independently. Generation X sometimes has little patience with the Boomers, but generally relate well to the Milliennials (Johnson & Romanello, 2005; Weston, 2006; Zemke, Raines & Filipczak, 2000).

## Generation Y, the Millennials

The Millennials are the "connected generation." Their parents, in general, have been a major part of their lives. Parents planned and managed a wide variety of activities for this generation, resulting in very structured lives. Parents have been with them during their growing years going to school activities and transporting them to shop and be with friends. A colleague of the author, who is dean of school of nursing, was stunned by the parent of a Millennial who asked if she could register for her daughter who was "just overwhelmed and could not manage this process. Could she (the mother) come and do this for her daughter?" These parents are often referred to as "helicopter parents" because they hover over the student. Even though many Millennials were raised in single parent homes, they consider this the norm and are very close to their families. Millennials tend to be confident, sociable, and optimistic as well as smart, open-minded, and achievement-oriented. They value both diversity and morality. Parents and teachers have encouraged the Millennials to participate in adult conversation both on social and political issues; they have researched information on the Internet. Well-aware of political and social issues, this generation is concerned with caring and community, and show interest in working for the betterment of society. Yet this generation seems to exhibit more stress than other groups. Violence may be a defining part of their lives. Millennials witnessed the Oklahoma City bombing and are very cognizant of the school shootings (Weston, 2006; Zembe, Raines, & Filipczak, 2000).

Even more than Generation X, the Millennials grew up in the digital mode. Skiba and Barton (2006) define members of this generation as "digital natives." For digital natives, technology has always been there. The digital native talks about the activities of technology rather than the technology **per se**. Millennials are truly the connected generation; they are connected 24/7 to the Internet and to the people in their circle of family and friends. Millennials have a global perspective and are just as likely to have a friend in the Netherlands as one across the street (Skiba, 2005; Skiba & Barton, 2006; Weston, 2006).

As students, Millennials prefer active learning. They expect learning to be fun and interactive and want to be engaged in the process. Millennials are accustomed to group projects and collaborative learning. Technology is the norm, not an enhancement or an add-on. They want frequent and instantaneous feedback. Millennials are accustomed to several sources of information with different focal points. In the classroom they want attention from authority figures and expect supervision and structure (Mangold, 2007; Skiba, 2005; Skiba & Barton, 2006).

## Faculty and the Generations

Faculty must learn to work with this generational diversity. Faculty are mostly composed of Baby Boomers and Generation X, while students tend to be Generation X or the Millennials. Faculty often teach to what they know, which includes the characteristics of the generation to which they belong. If faculty are to become generation-competent, they will need new knowledge, skills, and attitudes to work in a multigenerational setting. Learning about and reflecting on the distinctiveness of each generation helps faculty acquire knowledge about the differences in the generations. Generational differences are not right or wrong, just as cultural characteristics are not right or wrong, they vary (Johnson & Romanello, 2007). Both Generation X and Generation Y have different preferred learning modes. Each has strengths and areas that need developing to be effective in the nursing workforce. Faculty need to move outside their own comfort zone to adapt instructional strategies that fit their current student populations. Many faculty have already acquired knowledge and skills about learning styles and present information in a variety of modalities.

## Developing Instructional Strategies for Generation X and Y

### Generation X

A salient characteristic of Generation X (Xers) is survival. Xers are generally interested in new knowledge and skills, preferably directed at increasing their marketability. They expect teachers to be knowledgeable about the course material and nursing practice. The nurse educator who uses technology should be adept in its use. Generation X students are very capable of working and learning independently. Coaching works better than authoritarianism. A variety of modalities including books, audiovisual materials, and learning modules are quite acceptable for these students. Many have little patience with material they view as irrelevant. Generation Xers are interested in information that brings good grades. "Will this be on the test?" is a frequent question. Expectations should be clearly delineated. Information such as test blueprints and grading rubrics are considered important by these students. Nurse educators often need to help these students to understand the relevance of content. Using case studies in various ways is one methodology to enhance the view, or idea, that content is **useful**. Faculty may guide students to determine what knowledge and skill is needed for a nursing intervention. Case studies may also be constructed to focus on a specific aspect of a patient situation such as pharmacological therapy, healthy lifestyles, or community resources. Presentations of content should be visual and dynamic. Headers, headlines, bullets, and graphics may be used to highlight material. Reading should be relevant since Xers are most likely to read practical information. The author uses study guides with questions and directs students to specific pages in text or assigned articles. This strategy directs students specifically to pertinent content rather than assigning inclusive pages.

Generation X grew up with television and other visually appealing media, so the use of videos, film clips, streaming videos, pictures, and illustrations may promote learning. Whether teaching face-to-face or online, chunks of information rather than long presentations may enhance learning for Xers. Short sessions with breaks for questions or quick discussions with nearby students are often effective in keeping students focused. Questions or discussion should focus on essential elements of the material. The use of personal response systems (clickers) may be appropriate in some courses. Questions or discussion topics should be designed with a purpose in mind. Responses may be facts, answers to test questions, choices about prioritizing or delegating, characteristics of a patient population, or questions to assess the knowledge level of the patient. These strategies are examples of learning information that is both practical and specific.

Generation Xers do not usually function well in groups. Working in groups or teams is a needed skill for nurses who must work collaboratively intra-professionally and extra-professionally. Henry (2006) discusses setting up groups that function throughout a school term. Strategies for establishing group identity and working with group dynamics are inherent in this strategy. Faculty should serve as a resource and guide for group work. Group work assignments should be designed with specific goals. Collaborative learning may include projects, presentations or case study discussions to illustrate content. If group work involves a grade, expectations, evaluation rubrics, and grading policies should be clearly delineated. Some group work such as discussions of case studies or class content may not lend itself to grading.

## Generation Y or Millennials

Generation Y or the Millennials were raised connected to the world via technology. Their perspective tends to be global rather than parochial. They think of the world as pluralistic in culture and ethnicity. Millennials are concerned about their world and are often involved in fundraisers and community and school projects. Many in this generation have traveled widely and feel a sense of achievement from school and other activities. Millennials generally expect that education will give them the information and skills for jobs. The use of technology is expected. This generation likes interactive learning and has a desire to be engaged in the action of learning. Nurse educators may find that providing structure and using supervision and coaching works well with these students.

Pardue & Morgan (2008) indicate that college is not always a positive experience for Millennials. Many may have difficulty adjusting to being on their own, and all do not have the background for the intensity of college work. If students of this generation are to be successful in college, nursing programs may need to determine what kind of support services will enhance student success. Students may need specific help with study habits or tutoring in areas of deficiencies. Many colleges and universities have instituted more extensive orientation programs for entering classes, such as the "First Year Experiences" found on many campuses. The purpose of these programs is to provide information and skill for success in higher education.

This group is expert in technology and are willing to share with faculty and classmates their knowledge of technology. Millennials are similar to Generation X in responding to visual representations of material when appropriate. Presentations using PowerPoint® are acceptable to this group; however, they respond poorly to instructors who read their material or fill a slide with too much information. Interspersing questions, short discussions, or games with content presentations, as discussed with learning strategies for Generation X, facilitate learning for this group. Millennials tend to prefer group learning. Group projects, discussion groups, and other collaborative learning activities are useful learning strategies for this generation. Designing projects that include service learning, needs-based projects, or community-focused experiences work well with this group. Another strategy which incorporates active learning is assigning groups to develop presentations of working with different age groups of patients. A colleague of the author uses short vignettes of patient situations and asks students to role play therapeutic communication.

Many, but not all, Millennials are readers, although they may not have critical reading skills (Ahrin & Cormier, 2007). The usual mode of acquiring information is to search and use several sources, customizing the knowledge. Millennials may do well with a choice of sources for assignments. For example, students could have a choice of viewing a DVD on an ethical problem or reviewing an ethical case study presented on the Internet. Both choices could be used with a collaborative learning strategy, small group discussion, and/or a class presentation.

Ahrin and Cormier (2007) suggest using deconstruction as a teaching strategy for Millennials. Deconstruction is defined as a type of analysis. Students are encouraged to search for meaning and relationships from various information sources. This modality is applied to both reading and writing. The aim is to read critically and to articulate the meaning and application of both classroom and clinical learning. Writing helps students articulate their analysis, reflect on clinical experiences, and work with relationships of various concepts within content or patient situations.

This generation responds well to simulation activities. Simulations range from low-fidelity activities such as written case studies to high-fidelity with manikins that are capable of a variety of life-like responses. Simulations provide the opportunity to work with patient situations in a safe, non-threatening environment. Facilitation or guidance through a simulation learning experience provides knowledge and skill in problem-solving and decision-making. Although simulation with technology-enhanced manikins is new, nursing has been using a variety of simulations in its education for many years. Various stationary models and manikins have been used to teach skills in a laboratory setting. Computer programs may provide simulations to increase decision-making or delegation skills. Simulations should be carefully constructed. A debriefing session following the simulation is as important as the simulation experience itself. Debriefing should include discussion of the experience, consequences of decisions or actions, and evaluation of the learning (Bastable, 2008; Jeffries, Clochesy, & Hovancsek, 2008; Mangold, 2007).

Faculty should include clear expectations and policies in course materials. Sometimes Millennials need additional guidance about assignments. They are accustomed to "constructing" their own knowledge and may need specific information about the use of sources and documentation. Since they are always "connected," Milliennials expect immediate feedback (Skiba, 2005). The instructor may need to set rules about responses to their electronic queries; for example, replies within 48 hours.

## Summary

Generational differences in both students and faculty may present barriers to learning and understanding behaviors. Using information provided about different generations may help faculty be successful in working with a student population consisting of Generations X and Y. Faculty must become generation-aware and generation-competent to provide optimal learning opportunities for the future nursing workforce. Several books and many articles have been written about the differences in generations. In gaining knowledge about generations, a word of caution for faculty is in order. The information about generations tends to be generalities and may not be useful in some student populations or for individual students. Perspectives about events with a cohort or generation, however, may be useful in facilitating learning for a new generation of nurses.

## Learning Activities

1. Consider the characteristics of your students. How many of each generation are enrolled in your class? Do they "fit" the definition of the generations presented in this chapter? How are they the same? How are they different?
2. Consider your approach to classroom learning. Does your approach work with the generations present in your class?
3. In which generation are you a member? What characteristics about your own learning are the same as those discussed in this chapter? What characteristics are different?

## Educational Philosophy

The values of dignity, integrity and caring have guided my teaching. My aim is to create a positive environment for learning. Some of my own nursing education was very negative. I remember this learning situation as stifling and demeaning. Part of my motivation in becoming a nurse educator was to change the negatives into positives. Learning is often hard, but providing support and encouragement enhances learning and builds confidence in knowledge and skill. One of my favorite teaching assignments has been to teach fundamentals students and later teach an upper level course. I am energized by what my former fundamentals students have become. I demonstrate respect for the student by coaching and guiding rather than intimidation. I continue to study and learn about what I do as a nurse educator. I try not to become complacent or stale in my teaching. I reflect on my teaching practice just as I have always done in relation to my nursing practice. My teaching has evolved over the years. I have tried to move from the "sage on the stage" to "the guide on the side." I write notes to myself about my perspective on the effectiveness of a learning activity. My focus has become how do I get students engaged in learning. I tell students that we have been researching learning for hundreds of years and we have not yet found a way to "pour" knowledge into the brain. I encourage students to assess their own learning and talk about my own assessment and reflection. My goal is to equip students for the practice of the future, the future that none of us have seen. I continually try to figure out how to foster lifelong learning and a spirit of inquiry about nursing practice. — Elizabeth Stokes

# References

Arhin, A. O., & Cormier, E. (2007). Using deconstruction to education Generation Y nursing students. *Journal of Nursing Education, 46*(12), 562-567.

Bastable, S. B. (2008). *Nurse as educator: Principles of teaching and learning for nursing practice.* (3rd ed.). Boston: Jones and Bartlett.

Black, J. (2003). *Gen Xers Return to College.* Washington, DC: American Association of Collegiate Registrars and Admissions Officers.

Henry, P. R. (2006). Making groups work in the classroom. *Nurse Educator, 31*(1), 26-30.

Jeffries, P. R., Clochesy, J. M., & Hovancsek, M. T. (2008). Designing, implementing and evaluating simulations in nursing education. In D. M. Billings & J. A. Halstead, *Teaching in nursing: A guide for faculty* (pp. 322-334). St. Louis: Elsevier/Saunders.

Johnson, S. A., & Romanello, M. L. (2005). Generational diversity: Teaching and learning approaches. *Nurse Educator, 30*(5), 212-216.

Mangold, K. (2007). Educating a new generation: Teaching baby boomer faculty about millennial students. *Nurse Educator, 32*(1), 21-23.

Pardue, K. T., & Morgan, P. (2008). Millennials considered: A new generation, new approaches and implications for nursing education. *Nursing Education Perspectives, 29*(2), 74-79.

Sacks, P. (1996). *Generation X goes to college: An eye-opening account of teaching in post-modern America.* Peru, IL: Carus Publishing Company.

Skiba, D. J. (2005). The millennials: Have they arrived at your school of nursing? [Emerging Technologies] *Nursing Education Perspectives, 25*(6), 370-371.

Skiba, D. J. (2002). *The net generation: Implications for nursing education and practice. [Chapter 01, The book of teaching and learning, NLN Living Books].* Accessed August 2, 2008 at http://www.electronicvision.com/nln/chapter01/%20 mm_home.htm

Skiba, D. J., & Barton, A. J. (2006). Adapting your teaching to accommodate the net generation of learners. *The Online Journal of Issues in Nursing, 11*(2), Manuscript 4. Accessed August 2, 2008 at www.nursingworld.org/MainMenu-Categories/ANAMarketplace/ANAPeriodicals/OJIN/

Stokes, L. G., & Flowers, N. (2009). Multicultural education in Nursing. In D. M. Billings & J. A. Halstead, *Teaching in nursing: A guide for faculty* (pp. 268-282). St. Louis: Elsevier/Saunders.

Weston, M. (2006). Integrating generational perspective in nursing. *The Online Journal of Issues in Nursing, 11*(2), Manuscript 1. Accessed August 2, 2008 at www.nursingworld.org/MainMenuCategories/ANAMarketplace/ANAPeri-odicals/OJIN/

Zemke, R., Raines, C., & Filipczak, B. (2000). *Generations at work: Managing the clash of veterans, boomers, Xers, and nexters in your workplace.* New York: American Management Association.

# CHAPTER 17
# UNDERSTANDING AND TEACHING THE MILLENNIAL GENERATION OF NURSING STUDENTS

Marilyn McDonald, MSN, DHSc, RN

---

The content of this chapter relates to the following major content areas and subconcepts on the Certified Nurse Educator Examination Detailed Test Blueprint:

**Facilitate Learning**
- Implement a variety of teaching strategies appropriate to learner needs; learning style
- Demonstrate personal attributes that facilitate learning

**Facilitate Learning Development and Socialization**
- Provide resources for diverse learners to meet their individual learning needs
- Create learning environments that facilitate learners' self-reflection, personal goal setting, and socialization to the role of the nurse
- Adapt teaching styles and interpersonal interactions to facilitate learner behaviors

---

## Introduction

As a nurse educator of 15 years I would like to share my introduction to Millennial nursing students. After years of primarily teaching RN's in an RN to BSN program, I accepted a position teaching medical–surgical nursing to junior students in a traditional baccalaureate nursing program. I quickly learned there had been a culture change in this new generation of students.

As a self-reliant professional and a product of a rigorous seventies nursing education, I thought my years of experience had equipped me to master any challenge. After all, I was now age 50! However, my age represented a baby-boomer educator with a background and ideals much different than those of the young students I encountered. I came to know them as part of the "Millennial" generation. As I struggled to meet their needs, it was apparent, that I needed a greater understanding of what it meant to be a Millennial. By understanding my students, I could then help them to learn.

My first class with this diverse and fascinating group of students took place in a large and technologically outdated auditorium in a northeast university. Fifty-nine students whispered to each other with dissatisfaction as I slowly turned on the electronic podium for my first lecture. The answer to my inability to quickly use the technology in a new setting came when one of the students turned on the machine in a matter of seconds. But of course! These students were more technologically savvy than I was. They were Millennials.

To my surprise, there were a number of students yawning and even sleeping during my lecture. How could this happen? I was so proud to have once been nominated for teaching excellence. My linear PowerPoint® slides were no longer helpful in educating this Internet generation of students. The students were also uncomfortable with the large class size. After studying the Millennial culture I realized these students were raised in very interactive and visual classrooms where teamwork and small groups were the norm. My attempt to deliver medical-surgical lecture content in a traditional lecture style would have to evolve into something far more interesting for these students whose background and education was so different from mine.

## Who are Millennials?

The Millennials were born between 1982 and the year 2000. They have also been called generation Y, the Net Generation, and "nexters." They are preceded by the generation X'ers (born between 1960 and 1982) and the baby-boomer generation (born between 1946 and 1960) (Caputi, 2005). The term "Millennials" was coined when several thousand of them once sent suggestions about what they wanted to be called to the late news anchor Peter Jennings at abcnews.com (Raines, 2002). Although they are known by a variety of different names, this new generation of students share similar characteristics.

These students represent the largest college generation since the sixties. They are racially and ethnically diverse and 40% are children of divorced parents (Sweeney, 2007). Their diverse and technologically oriented experiences make them talented, confident, collaborative, and very creative. However, they are easily perceived as challenging and complex.

The complex nature of theses students has become a challenge for faculty from the baby boomer generation. Most of today's nurse educators are baby boomers who were raised in rigorous, authoritarian models of nursing education. "The new generation of nursing students is respectful of authority, yet they do not hesitate to challenge authority" (Walker et al., 2006, p. 372). The challenge for today's nurse educators will be to better understand the new generation of students for the purpose of creating innovative teaching/learning methods while maintaining the scientific rigor and the professional standards necessary for nursing practice.

## The Educational Theory of Paulo Freire

Theories help explain, predict, and give meaning to what we do. A theory developed by Paulo Freire can help guide educational experiences for the new generation. Paulo Freire was a Brazilian theorist who greatly impacted educators with his theory of liberatory pedagogy. The theory of liberatory education tells us "education should open minds to higher stages of consciousness rather than just deposit information for future use, for knowledge emerges only through invention and inquiry" (Cohn, 1988, p. 6). Freire's theory is based on praxis. Praxis involves analysis, discussion, and action about the world in order to change. Educators utilize praxis to transform learning. Students cannot be passive learners. They need participation, dialogue, and opportunities to think and read critically. Educators and students can be mutually engaged in the evolution and understanding of knowledge when they utilize Freire's liberatory theory.

In this theory, Freire reflects on societies in transition. Themes from his theory can give meaning to educating the new Millennial students who represent a societal culture change. Much of the theory is concerned with understanding the world-view of the learner.

> Our relationship with the learners demands that we respect them and demands equally that we be aware of the concrete conditions of their world, the conditions that shape them. To try to know the reality that our students live is a task that the educational practice imposes on us: Without this, we have no access to the way they think, so only with great difficulty can we perceive what and how they know. (Freire, 1998, p. 58)

> Educators need to know what happens in the world of the children with whom they work. They need to know the universe of their dreams, the language with which they skillfully defend themselves from the aggressiveness of their world, what they know independently of school, and how they know it. (Freire, 1998, p.74)

A curricular model that is based on Freire's principles is the Voyager Model. With this model teachers and students participate in a democratic educational environment. The Voyager curriculum is "designed to provide opportunities for teachers and students to work cooperatively in an environment of critical pedagogy" (Roulis, 2004, p. 34). Learning in this model will allow Millennial students to have an active voice through the critical dialogue, personal reflection, and action that is important to them in today's world. Nurse educators can incorporate the social themes and issues that are valued by the students while simultaneously providing nursing knowledge. Together nurse educators and Millennials can co-create meaningful educational experiences. Millennials thrive in educational environments where they can have close support and partnering with faculty.

## Generational Influences

A number of social and cultural influences from 1979 to 2000 shaped the Millennial personality. Generation X and baby boomer parents were family focused. The Federal Forum on Family Statistics reports an all time high for national attention to children in the eighties and nineties (Raines, 2002). This shift to child-centered families was very different from previous generations who may remember the old adage, "children should be seen and not heard."

The national attention on the child represented a culture change from the latchkey Generation X parents who were often products of divorce, or children of two working parents. Although this still may have been the experience for some children of the eighties and nineties, the focus by parents was clearly on "quality time" for the kids. Parents wanted experiences for their children that they did not have as latchkey children who grew up on their own. Children went everywhere with parents. The economic boom of the eighties made annual Disney type vacations the norm for many families. Children were also enrolled in as many special classes and activities that parents could schedule. Participation in sports and all types of competitive activities was encouraged and available to both male and female children. Involvement in multiple activities became the norm. Children learned to juggle a number of social activities with school and family responsibilities. Coupled with their vast exposure to various types of technology, the focus on multiple activity involvement may explain some of the strong multi–tasking tendencies of this active generation.

Strong parental involvement may also have contributed to faculty observations that these children are "hand held" and dependent. Millennial parents are known to intervene on behalf of their children with coaches, other parents, and faculty. They have high expectations of their children. They are nicknamed "helicopter parents." As the parents hover closely over the student's educational experiences, faculty may feel as though they have two students – the parent and the child.

The Millennials were raised during the economic upswing of the eighties. Many inherited the competitive nature of their dual income parents. They love challenges.

Like their parents, they demand customer satisfaction. This demand is the opposite value for faculty who are charged with preparing and mentoring students to assume responsibility and accountability as nursing professionals.

Raines (2002) states, "parents were called into service by their children who needed to be shuttled back and forth to their various activities" (p. 3). Thus, the expectation that the older generation was to be readily available, programmed them to have a sense of entitlement. Many of the Y Generation have a sense of entitlement and expect others to take care of them (Lower, 2007). Thus, generational conflicts are inherent between self-reliant "boomer" nurse educators and the new "entitled" students.

Perhaps the most startling difference between students born between 1980 and 2000 and older generations is their sense of entitlement. It is not uncommon for a Millennial to remind a faculty member that they are paying for the educational experience. Students may even view the faculty as their employee. This presents a conflict in nursing education when a professional license is at stake and nurse educators have the responsibility of determining student competence and patient safety regardless of the students expenses incurred in the education experience. The challenge for nurse educators will be to embrace the unique needs of the new students and to work together with them as they develop in their professional roles.

Faculty can avoid the intergenerational conflict by understanding the learning preferences of the new generation. Faculty can work to incorporate traits that will be perceived by the students as effective characteristics of a good teacher. Wieck (2003) found that the top six faculty traits preferred by the Millennial generation were approachability, good communication, professionalism, supportiveness, understanding, and motivating.

## Political Influences

Every baby boomer remembers the defining moment in their childhood when they witnessed the television assassination of President John F. Kennedy. The boomers were left with Kennedy's message, "Ask not what your country can do for you, ask what you can do for your country." The Generation X children of the boomers carried on this sense of patriotism, through activities like volunteering and community involvement. There was a sense of wanting to save the word.

The strong self-reliance and beliefs held by the preceding generation were shattered for many young people on September 11, 2001. This vulnerable group had already experienced media accounts of school shootings and violence in America that no other generation had known. They watched the media repeatedly air the catastrophic moments when the World Trade Center and the Pentagon were attacked. This unprecedented terrorist attack left them bonded as a generation (Raines, 2001). The Millennials became a traumatized generation.

While the results of the Viet Nam War, the draft, the protests, the deaths of American servicemen, as well as both civilian and military Vietnamese, may have bonded their Baby Boomer parents, the events on September 11th, 2001, left the Millennials with a shattered view of the world that bonded them. Their traumatic experience of terrorism may contribute to the perception by some faculty that these students are a self-oriented and "we come first" generation. Witnessing the horror of violence and trauma in America left the Millennials with a self-preservation attitude.

From a somewhat different perspective Clausing, Kurtz, Prendeville, and Walt (2003) suggest that Millennials are exceptionally altruistic, hopeful, and future-oriented as a generation. Although perceptions of them vary, the new generation of students has a world-view that has been shaped from witnessing a life-changing event unlike any other in history. They are unique.

## Understanding the Millennial Nursing Student

Although narrative reports have recently emerged in the literature, little research exists on understanding Millennial behaviors. Millennials are different from previous generations in a number of ways (See Table 1). They communicate and socialize in different ways. Much of the communication and socialization that is unique to this generation has to do with their Internet upbringing. They represent the first generation of students to be raised with the technological advances of the Internet.

According to the Pew Internet and American Life Project (2001) 82% of children are online by the seventh grade. Using the Internet for school projects both in and out of the classroom is a way of life for the majority of young students. It is not surprising that a Millennial student might find dissatisfaction with a faculty member who does not use technology in the classroom in an interesting, stimulating, and competent way.

These young students love to email and instant message while in class. This focus on "staying connected" may be perceived by a faculty member as inattentive or discourteous. However, instant messaging and email are a natural part of their communication and socialization (Oblinger, 2003).

## What to Expect from Millennial Students

Millennials:

Need to "stay connected"
Insist on customer satisfaction
Need immediacy
Use and are fascinated by multiple technologies
Learn best in small groups
Dislike reading
Prefer experiential activities
Like teamwork
Are visual-spatial learners
Are competitive
Love to be entertained
Need state of the art technology

**Table 1.** What to Expect from Millennial Students

The need for connectedness and immediacy extends beyond the classroom. Millennials expect immediate email responses from faculty as well as 24 hour availability. Although faculty need to understand this need for immediacy from their students, realistic expectations about availability must be clearly stated in all syllabi. It is ideal for syllabi to be posted online.

The use of multiple technologies in today's world may account for the short attention spans that some faculty have noticed in the new generation. Seymour Papert, a professor at MIT's media lab coined the term, "grasshopper mind" when he observed that students raised on the Internet leaped quickly from one topic to another (Olsen, 2008). According to Papert, "The presence of technology in society is a major factor in changing the entire learning environment" (Olsen, 2005, p. 3).

Millennials have distinct learning styles. Along with their fascination for technology, they learn best in small groups, prefer experiential activities, and dislike reading (Oblinger, 2003; Lower, 2007). According to Pardue and Morgan (2008), research results conducted by Levitz in 2006 found that in a sample of 97,626 college freshman, only half reported experiencing enjoyment in reading. Large traditional lecture style classrooms with linear formats do not work for the new students. They respond well to visual images. They love games that foster their competitive spirit. Class activities that promote teamwork work well.

According to Lower (2007) this is a generation that loves to be entertained. They have brought laughter and creativity into the procedure-oriented clinical laboratories of the past. Their boundless energy and need for state of the art technology has changed the landscape of nursing classroom, clinical, and laboratory experiences. Millennials are the first generation of nursing students to have sophisticated simulated learning experiences. The possibilities for utilizing simulation in fun ways to accommodate these students are endless.

## Teaching/Learning Expectations of Millennial Nursing Students

Scant research exists on teaching and learning methods for the Millennial generation (Mangold, 2007; Pardue & Morgan). Through an understanding of the Y Generation involving social, cultural, family, and political influences, we can utilize teaching and learning strategies that meet their expectations. These include:

- Use of multimedia technology
- Interactive learning
- Visual classrooms
- Fun and game playing
- Group activities and collaboration
- Innovation in teaching
- Experiential activities

## Multimedia Technology

Clearly, the new generation of nursing students needs to be "connected." The use of PDA's, laptops, iPods, videos, and CD-ROMS in innovative educational ways is an expectation of the Millennial generation. This generation has been raised with, and is accustomed to, quick and accessible ways of retrieving information. Their "grasshopper" minds respond to multiple uses of media when coupled with engaging and informative lecture content. Virtual classrooms, online labs, and computer simulation can be used alone or blended with traditional classroom and clinical experiences. Hybrid online education is a way of blending both online education with face-to-face instruction. As online educational technologies grow, there will be a great need for faculty to transform education in unique ways.

# Interactive Learning

Most nursing students and faculty have been introduced to simulated learning experiences. Human patient simulators are used in nursing laboratories to provide students with interactive clinical practice in a controlled environment. Several companies market the simulators; new and innovative models are continually being produced. Adult simulated mannequins have heartbeats, chest movements, and blood pressures. Through computer technology they can moan, talk, and even have a change in vital signs. One simulator actually simulates childbirth. Infant and pediatric models are also being used. See www.laerdal .com or www.meti.com.

Simulations in nursing education have been studied by the National League for Nursing (NLN). In 2003, after receiving a grant from the Laerdal Medical Corporation, the NLN examined the use of simulation techniques in eight schools of nursing. The study involved a case study and the comparisons of the simulated mannequin with a static mannequin. A summary of the research project can be found on the NLN's web site at www.nln.org. A guide on how to integrate simulation into nursing curriculums can be purchased at www.nln.org/publications.

Faculty can use the simulators to create patient scenarios not ordinarily found in the classroom. A number of sources report Millennials work well in groups (Oblinger, 2003; Lower, 2007; Skiba & Barton, 2006). Laboratory simulation practice provides a great opportunity for group work. Mock codes and acute and chronic scenarios can be created where it is essential for students to work together as a group. Although the simulators lack real life assessment, students have opportunities to practice and repeat skills until they are confident and competent. The software that accompanies the manikins can be programmed in ways that allow students to think critically as they analyze and synthesize information through the decisions they make with simulated case studies.

See Table 2 for a list of websites related to interactive learning.

## Utilization of Web Sites for Interactive Learning

www.laerdal.com
www.meti.com
Patient simulation manikins
www.sprojects.mmi.mcgill.ca/mvs/mvsteth.htm
A virtual stethoscope for auscultation of heart and lung sounds

www.healthsciences.merlot.org
A virtual auditory blood pressure cuff

http://us.elsevierhealth.com/
A CD-ROM virtual clinical setting

www.dupagepress.com
Interactive computer-based learning programs and games

www.dxrnursing.com
Web-based software with problem solving case studies
www.lww.com/index.html
Live tutoring to accompany texts or E-books

www.electronicvision.com/nln/.
Example of an electronic interactive chapter
www.vudat.msu.edu/jeopardygame/
On line jeopardy game

www.tegrity.com
Classroom response system software

www.secondlife.com
Three dimensional virtual lab or classroom

www.nln.org/publications
*Simulations in Nursing Education: From Conceptualization to Education*

http://us.elsevierhealth.com/
On line lab modules

**Table 2.** Utilization of Web Sites for Interactive Learning

# Visual Classrooms

Millennials are visual-spatial learners (Skiba & Barton, 2006). Technology for providing visual/virtual classrooms is rapidly evolving and Millennials will expect dynamic, new and exciting methods in lecturing. The Internet offers opportunities that are interactive and "eye-catching" for both teachers and students. Some sites are free and readily available while others are available for purchase.

McGill University offers a free virtual stethoscope that students can use to practice heart and lung assessment with both visual and audio capability. See www. sprojects.mmi.mcgill.ca/mvs/mvsteth.htm. Another free web site is available at www.healthsciences.merlot.org. Beginning nursing students can practice inflating and deflating an online blood pressure cuff. The Korotkoff blood pressure sounds are audible. Students can gain confidence before demonstrating competency with taking blood pressure.

A virtual classroom for nursing education is available from Elsevier at http:// us.elsevierhealth.com/. The virtual nursing classroom is delivered on a CD that offers an interactive experience when reading the textbook content. Elsevier (2008) states that virtual classroom education helps bridge the gap between classrooms and the real world by introducing virtual clinical settings before students enter the actual clinical setting. In the virtual hospital, students can interact with patients, practice communication, think critically, set priorities and implement care plans. Students can even select, prepare, and administer medications online. Elsevier also offers an online skills laboratory.

DxR Development Group, Inc. developed web-based software with problem solving case studies that utilize the nursing process. It is very similar to a real assessment when students work through a virtual case study. The program guides students through the nursing process by interacting with a virtual patient. There are realistic heart and lung sounds; simulated physical assessments can be performed online. Students save pertinent information to framework categories and then create nursing diagnoses and care plans. Features can be turned on or off depending on the students' skill level. For a sample CD go to www.dxrnursing.com.

Some universities have already replaced standard textbooks with E-books or online texts. Many of these textbooks have online, 24-hour tutoring available (Smeltzer, Bare, Hinkle, & Cheever, 2008). This type of tutoring is especially valuable when learning needs to be reinforced, especially for more complicated content. See www.lww.com/index.html for an example of a medical-surgical textbook that features Live Advise tutoring.

Another way to capture the attention of Internet-focused students is with dynamic and interactive web pages. These pages can be designed to allow the student to interact with the content, other students, and the instructor. As students work their way through the electronic chapters, they are directed to online activities as well as links to other web sites to find more information related to their questions (Skiba & Barton, 2006). An example of this can be found in a "Living Book," an electronic book created by the National League for Nursing. To view the online chapters, go to www.electronicvision.com/nln/.

## Fun and Game Playing

Millennials love to be entertained. There are a number of imaginative possibilities for faculty to integrate fun and games into a standard lecture format. Integrating music, animation, crossword puzzles, and humor into complex content material can be very effective. Some simple classroom games can be played that capture students' attention and enhance learning. Among the possibilities are a Drug Bee or playing the Jeopardy game.

A Drug Bee is played like a spelling bee. For example, the game can be played in a pharmacology class. Students are asked to identify the classification, action, side effects, or nursing implication for a particular drug. A wrong answer eliminates the student from continuing. Millennials are competitive and will work to win the game.

Jeopardy works well with medical-surgical lectures where students work to find answers to a wide range of topics. Students can raise hands, use bells, buzzers, or iClickers to be the first to answer a question. Prizes can be anything from candy to CDs or extra texts the faculty may have on hand. Through online quiz type game playing, students are able to determine how well they have or have not mastered key concepts. For a live example go to www.vudat.msu.edu/jeopardy_game/.

A program containing graphics and animation can be applied when teaching the renal system. Caputi (1999) developed a software program called *The PhysWhiz: The Renal System*. The visual explanations of complex subject material come to life for Millennials who love to be entertained. Many of the screens lend themselves to practice items that encourage participation. There are as many as a dozen *PhysWhiz* programs currently on the market, with the most recent ones including video portraying nurses engaged in various physical assessment techniques or patient conditions such as giving birth in *PhysWhiz II: Labor and Delivery*.

The use of an electronic classroom response system can be a fun and stimulating way to encourage student participation. Clickers facilitate rapid data gathering when playing classroom games or asking questions. Clickers are hand held audience response systems. The software is installed from a faculty's computer. The faculty poses a question to the students via a computer projector. Each student submits his or her answer with the handheld transmitter (Bruff, 2008). To view the use of clickers go to www.vanderbilt.edu/cft/resources/teaching_resources/technology/crs.htm.

## Group Activities and Collaboration

Lower (2007) states that members of the Millennial Generation like to approach projects in teams and they may resist working on individual projects. There are many ways to incorporate group work. One classic example of a group activity that is team centered with a fun and collaborative approach to learning is The Cookie Experiment (Thiel,1987). The experiment has been revised a number of times and used successfully in nursing research classes to demystify the research process. It is a creative teaching strategy that works well with students who enjoy learning in small groups. The experiment can easily be carried out in a nursing research class in a number of ways. The students are asked to examine their preferences for low fat and regular chocolate chip cookies. Students work together to decide on a conceptual model, research questions, and the format of a consent form. Students can participate both qualitatively and quantitatively and engage in discussions related to both types of research. The experience of eating the cookies while discussing the steps in the research process is a great way to dispel the myths and phobias about a subject that can be complex to young researchers. This generation is very informal and they think well when they are relaxed (Lower, 2007).

## Innovation

Nurse educators are always challenged to find new and innovative teaching/learning methods and strategies. Today's students now have the opportunity to use software applications that record lectures and slides for replay on iPods, phones, and MP3 players. If a student misses a lecture or part of a lecture, they can pipe the lecture and instructor's voice to their laptop or MP3 player and review it at another time. This may be a better alternative than writing or copying notes that do not always capture all of the teacher's presentation. To a tech-savvy Millennial, podcasting may be a natural alternative for viewing a lecture at any time or place. Software is now available that captures the words of classroom lectures then synchronizes them with digital images (Eisenberg, 2007). See www.tegrity.com.

## Experiential Activities

Nursing is an applied science. Although the use of technology and simulation are important components for the Millennial learner, the student nurse must be able to effectively apply theory to practice in real clinical scenarios. However, the unique characteristics of Millennial nursing students may pose challenges for them in the clinical settings where specific policies, rules, and regulations are the norm.

To avoid a culture shock that may occur with the first clinical experiences, faculty need to carefully orient the new students to the work culture and the specific types of patient responsibilities they will have. Clear guidelines on the use of PDAs, electronic devices, and institutional computers in classroom and clinical settings must be made available. Clinical expectations must be very clearly stated in the syllabi and in clinical handbooks. Ideally, this type of information should be posted online.

Promoting a safe environment for the students is essential. Post conferences should allow students an opportunity to safely express their feelings about the clinical experiences they encounter. Web boards, blogs, and chats can be led by students or faculty and provide students with communication tools with which they are very comfortable.

## Future Trends

The landscape for teaching in the new millennium has changed dramatically from the traditional nursing education styles of the past. What will the future bring? The possibilities for integrating technology into education and creating democratic learning models are endless.

Is the idea of a virtual campus for nursing something that we can comprehend? There are already dozens of colleges around the world that are using three dimensional online virtual worlds to teach courses. In the virtual classroom or lab students and teachers take on the identities of cartoon-like characters called avatars and interact in computer-simulated landscapes. The virtual world of learning is created by Second Life. See www.secondlife.com. According to Graves (2008), Second Life is an effective teaching tool that provides a social laboratory where role-playing, simulations, exploration, and experimentation can be tried out in a relatively risk-free environment (Graves, 2008, p.49)." The value of 3-D web sites in education is still being studied. It appears that one of the greatest benefits is that students can interact with other registered users in as many as 100 countries (Graves, 2008).

It will be essential to conduct research that studies the unique teaching and learning needs of the Millennials. What are the specific learning preferences of the Millennials? How can critical thinking be measured in simulated lab environments? Is hybrid online learning effective for entry level nursing students? All these areas need further exploration and will provide faculty with evidenced-based teaching that is essential for understanding this new generation of students.

## Retrospection

When I reflect on my first experience with Millennial nursing students I am humbled. I gained much through my realization of this group of students that came to represent a culture change. From them I realized that my years of experience and wisdom in teaching needed to be combined with their creative and innovative learning needs in a technological world. Their inattentiveness, need for self preservation, and need for immediacy are no longer alien to me as a Baby Boomer educator raised with different standards and ideals.

The Millennials have made me a better teacher. Through listening to them I grew to understand their generational needs and differences. I have found a vision and see an ongoing need for transformation in how nurse educators can shape the learning experience for the next generation of critically needed nurses. The challenges of instilling professionalism, integrity, and quality patient care have always been present for nurse educators. When we understand and meet the young students "where they are" then they too will listen and respect our values and expectations of them to become professional and caring nurses.

> It is through hearing the learners, a task unacceptable to authoritarian educators, that democratic teachers increasingly prepare themselves to be heard by learners. But by listening to and so learning to talk with learners, democratic teachers teach the learners to listen to them as well. (Freire, 1998, p.58).

## Summary

The passionate curiosity and new age talents of the Millennials is both challenging and inspiring. Social and political changes, cultural and family influences, and their Internet upbringing have shaped the Millennials into a culture with new expectations for teaching and learning. Their ability to process information quickly and to use technology in the teaching/learning process will transform the nursing education trends of the future. With the integration of technology, research, new teaching methods, and the application of democratic teaching models, students and nurse educators can learn from each other and co-create the curriculums of the future.

## Learning Activities

1. Assess your learner characteristics. Do any of your learners belong to the Millennial Generation? If so, ask them what kinds of learning experiences they believe are most helpful to their learning.
2. Review your teaching style. Which teaching/learning methods do you use that are helpful for the Millennial student to learn? Which may be less desirable for this group of students?
3. Investigate the websites listed in Table 2. Which ones contain approaches that you might use in your teaching? How would you use these approaches?

## Educational Philosophy

Education is a lifelong process. Educators need continually to acquire knowledge and find ways to deliver the knowledge to learners in energetic and dynamic ways. In order to do this, the educator must understand the learner. The developmental potential of every student should be sought and maximized by the educator. In return, students need to be actively engaged in learning in ethical and professional ways. — Marilyn McDonald

## References

Bruff, D. (2008). Classroom response systems. Retrieved February 2, 2008, from www.vanderbilt.edu/cft/resources/teaching_resources/technology/crs.htm

Caputi, L. (1999). *The phys whiz: The renal system [computer program]*. Glen Ellyn, IL: College of DuPage.

Caputi, L. (2005). *Teaching nursing: The art and science. Vol. 3*, Glen Ellyn, Illinois, College of DuPage Press.

Clark, K. (2008). New answers for e-learning. *U.S. News and World Report*. Jan. 21. p 46-49.

Clausing, S., Kurtz, D. L., Predeville, J., & Walt, J. L. (2003). Generational diversity: The nexters. *AORN Journal. 78*, p 373-379.

Cohn, S. (1988). Paulo Freire: The man and his educational theory. Retrieved March 28, 2008, from www.eric.ed.gov/ERICWebPortal/contentdelivery/servlet/ERICServlet?accno=ED307200

Eisenberg, A. (n.d.) What did the professor say? Check your ipod. Retrieved March 28, 2008, from http://www.nytimes.com/2007/12/09/business/09novel.html?_r=3&adxnnl=1&oref=slogin

Freire, P. (1998). *Teachers as cultural workers: Letters to those who teach.* Boulder, CO: Westview Press.

Graves, L. (2008). *A second life for higher ed.* U.S. News and World Report. Jan. 21, p. 49.

Lenhart, A., Simon, M., & Graziano, M. (2001). The Internet and education: Findings of the PEW Internet and American life project. Retrieved February 20, 2008, from www.pewinternet.org/

Lower, J. (2007). Brace yourself – here comes Generation Y. *American Nurse Today, 2*(8), 26-29.

Mangold, K. (2007). Educating a new generation: teaching baby boomer faculty about Millennial students. *Nurse Educator, 32*(1), 21-23.

Oblinger, D. (2003). Boomers, gen–xers & millennials: Understanding the new students. *Educause Review*, July/August, p. 37-47.

Olsen, S. (2005). *The Millennials usher in a new era.* Retrieved February 2, 2008, from www.news.com/2009_1025_3-5944666.html

Pardue, K., & Morgan, P. (2008). Millennials considered: A new generation, new approaches, and implications for nursing education. *Nursing Education Perspectives, 29*(1), 76.

Potter P., & Perry A. G. (2006). *Skills online for fundamentals of nursing.* (6th ed.). St Louis: Mosby.

Raines, C. (2002). Managing millennials. Retrieved October 30, 2007, from www.generationsatwork.com/articles/millenials.htm, www. healthscience.merlot.org

Roulis, E. (2004). *Transforming learning for the workplace of the new millennium.* Minneapolis: Scarecrow Education.

Skiba, D. J., & Barton, A. J. (2006). Adapting your teaching to accommodate the net generation of learners. *Online Journal of Issues in Nursing, 11*(2), 15.

Smeltzer, S. C., Bare, B. G., Hinkle, J. L., & Cheever, K. H. (2008). *Brunner and Suddarth's textbook of medical surgical nursing.* Philadelphia: Lippincott, Williams and Wilkins.

Sweeney, R. (2007). Millennial behaviors and higher education focus group results. *New Jersey Institute of Technology.* Retrieved December 1, 2007, from www.library/njit.edu/staff-folders/Millennials/Millenial-Summary-Handout.doc

Thiel, C. A. (1987). The cookie experiment. *Nurse Educator, 20*(3), 8-10.

Walker, J., Martin, T., White, J., Elliott, R., Norwood, A., Mangum, C., & Hayne, L. (2006). Generational (Age) differences in nursing students' preferences for teaching methods. *Journal of Nursing Education, 45*(9), 371-374.

Wieck, K. (2003). Faculty for the millennium: Changes needed to attract the emerging workforce into nursing. *Journal of Nursing Education, 42*(4), 151-158.

# CHAPTER 18

# TEACHING RN-TO-BSN STUDENTS

**Rosemarie O. Berman, PhD, RN**

---

The content of this chapter relates to the following major content areas and subconcepts on the Certified Nurse Educator Examination Detailed Test Blueprint:

**Facilitate Learning**
- Implement a variety of teaching strategies appropriate to learner needs; learning style
- Use teaching strategies based on: educational theory; evidence-based practices related to education
- Modify teaching strategies and learning experiences based on consideration of learners': past educational and life experiences
- Create opportunities for learners to develop their own critical thinking skills

**Facilitate Learning Development and Socialization**
- Identify individual learning styles and unique learning needs of learners with these characteristics: traditional vs. non-traditional
- Adapt teaching styles and interpersonal interactions to facilitate learner behaviors

---

## Introduction

Enrollment in RN-to-Baccalaureate or BSN programs has steadily increased for the past four years and may be expected to do so as clinical agencies and the general public recognizes the value of the baccalaureate prepared nurse (AACN, 2007). The diverse cohort of RN-to-BSN students offers a rich array of past clinical experiences on which to build their education and clinical practice. These students also bring a unique set of learning needs which often poses a challenge to faculty. As the stream of RNs returning to the academic arena continues, nurse educators must address these challenges to enhance student success and support the transformation process to a different level of professional nursing practice.

Nurse researchers have identified multiple concerns for both faculty and students as RNs re-enter the academic setting. Faculty in baccalaureate nursing programs are often more accustomed to traditional students with few family or work responsibilities, little or no clinical experience, and feel at ease in the classroom. RN students may be quite the opposite – clinical experts with multiple home and work responsibilities and who are less comfortable in the college or university setting. These students require a different set of teaching skills to assist them in meeting course and program objectives. The focus of this discussion is to identify teaching strategies to address the diverse experiences and the different learning needs of RN-to-BSN students.

## Learning Theory and the RN-to-BSN Student

Undergraduate baccalaureate education is often based on customary methods of pedagogy, or the art and science of teaching children. Pedagogy has strong underpinnings in authoritarianism and places the student in a dependent role. The student is expected to arrive at the classroom and be taught subject matter. Teaching methodologies are more conventional and use traditional methods of lecture and examinations. This may be the only viable option in college classrooms which have large class sizes in lecture halls, but do not necessarily work well for the returning adult student.

The RN-to-BSN student is an adult learner and teaching methodologies should be housed within the framework of adult learning theory. While there are a number of educational theories which may be applicable for adult learning, two theories – Andragogy and Transformational Theory – seem particularly relevant to working with the RN-to BSN student. These theories are presented here as a foundation for appropriate tactics for working with this distinctive group.

### Andragogy

Andragogy, or the art and science of adult learning, recognizes and values the unique needs of the adult rather than the child or adolescent student. While the historical roots of adult learning hark back to the monastic and cathedral schools of Europe, Malcolm Knowles was the contemporary learning theorist who developed the adragogical model (Knowles, Holton, & Swanson, 2005). Andragogy is based on six key assumptions:
- The need to know
- The learners' self-concept
- The role of the learners' experience
- Readiness to learn
- Orientation to learn
- Motivation

These suppositions are predicated on key behavioral, social, and psychological concepts of adulthood. Nursing has utilized these concepts in developing health education programs for adult patients, but as more and more adult students return to the academic arena for nursing, it is now necessary to extend and use these concepts in nursing education. An essential feature of the model is its flexibility, as Knowles suggests. Andragogy can be used in its entirety or by using select parts. Rather than an in-depth discussion of each principle at this point, the elements of the model are discussed later in the context of specific teaching strategies.

## Transformational Theory

A second theory that is useful in understanding adult students is Transformation Theory. The focus of Transformation Theory is on the process of how we learn to "negotiate and act on our own purposes, values, feelings, and meanings rather than those we have uncritically assimilated from others" (Mezirow, 2000, p. 8). The learning process involves a change or transformation from the learner's current frame of reference to one which is more inclusive, discriminating, and reflective. This transformation of one's behavior and/or paradigm is especially relevant to RN students, as they progress through their baccalaureate education. A number of studies on the RN student focus on this process of transformation using Transformation Theory as the conceptual framework for research (Callin, 1996; Morris & Faulk, 2007; Phillips, Palmer, Zimmerman, & Mayfield, 2002).

The process of transformation occurs in a series of phases, as adult learner alter their personal framework and assume a new paradigm. According to Mezirow (2000), transformation occurs in the following stages:

1. The presentation of a disorienting dilemma
2. A self-examination of feelings with a critical assessment of assumptions
3. A recognition that the discontent and the process of transformation are related
4. The exploration of new roles, relationships, and actions
5. A plan of a course of action
6. The acquisition of the knowledge and skills necessary for implementing the new plan
7. The testing or trying on of new roles
8. The developing of competence and confidence in the new role
9. A reintegration of the new paradigm or new perspective into their life

## Background Discussion

Current research on the RN-to-BSN student includes curricular, faculty, and student perspectives. These different perspectives all support a similar assumption that the RN student experiences a professional transformation over the course of the program (Delaney & Piscopo, 2007; Lillibridge & Fox, 2005; Phillips et al., 2002; Zuzelo, 2001). In a study focusing on program outcomes using a pre-and post-test design, graduating RN-to-BSN students scored significantly higher in five areas of professional growth: nursing practice/process, communication/collaboration, leadership, professional integration, and research and evaluation (Philips et al., 2002). In a phenomenological study exploring the experience of RN-to-BSN students, Delaney and Piscopo (2007) identified a number of themes directly related to professional transformation. Students reported formulating a new worldview with the ability to translate knowledge into empowerment and seeing the bigger picture. They also described themselves as becoming more assertive leaders and advocates, as well as being better equipped to confront and conquer challenges. Lillibridge and Fox (2007) confirmed the RN-to-BSN graduate as perceiving to have an increased knowledge base with a more global perspective on which to establish clinical practice.

However, Callin (1996) observed that not all RN students seem to experience such behavioral changes upon completion of a BSN program and postulates why some RN students experience a behavior change, while others do not. Using Mezirow's Transformation Theory as the framework for her assumptions, she suggests there are specific methods and strategies which contribute to professional transformation, while other tactics fail to stimulate professional growth. Factors to consider are related to the learning environment, peer support, a process driven curriculum and learner empowerment. In a study conducted three months post graduation, Morris and Faulk (2007) confirm the importance of the learning environment, and link the use of specific learning activities to support the development of related professional roles and values in the RN student. BSN graduates also identified both roles (advocate, educator, manager) and values (caring, altruism, autonomy, social justice) as being related to changes in specific professional behaviors.

## Curriculum

The development of critical thinking is an essential and required component of all baccalaureate nursing programs (AACN, 2008). Both faculty and students report an increase in development of critical thinking skills over the course of RN-to-BSN programs (Delaney & Piscopo, 2007; Spedic, Parsons, Hercinger, Andrews,

Parks, & Norris, 2001), as well as becoming more confident in the use of research (Lillibridge & Fox, 2005; Phillips et al., 2002).

The design and characteristics of an RN-to-BSN curriculum can either inhibit or encourage a student's progress towards the degree. A flexible curriculum design is a critical factor for RN students (Lillibridge & Fox, 2005; Nicholls & Timmins, 2005; Zuzelo, 2001). These students appreciate the flexibility of programs which accept all possible transfer credits to be used toward the degree requirements and allow for an individualized pace of study to meet their personal needs (Zuzelo, 2001).

## Students

While both faculty and RN students agree that the RN student undergoes a transformation upon completion of a RN-to-BSN program, they recognize that the students encounter a number of stressors upon return to the academic arena. Writing assignments, especially research papers, were identified as being particularly stressful for RN students (Nicholl & Timmins, 2005; Zuzelo, 2001). Often times these students have not taken a formal test for a number of years, so the prospect of preparing for and taking examinations was identified as very anxiety provoking (Nicholl & Timmins, 2005). Computer literacy is another stress-related factor that needs to be addressed with the RN student. While the RN student may be accustomed to working with computers in the clinical environment, computer literacy for research and academic use requires a different skills set. Huston, Shovein, Damazo, & Fox (2001) suggest that integrating computer technologies into the initial transition course is related to successful completion of the program. Other barriers to program completion that have been identified are financial strain, needing to be on campus, and juggling family and work with academic requirements (Huston et al., 2001; Lillilbridge & Fox, 2005; Nicholl & Timmons, 2005; Zuzelo, 2001).

Adult students have a fully formed self-concept based on meeting the role expectations and responsibilities associated with adulthood. Returning to a formal classroom setting can trigger earlier dependent behaviors associated with previous learning experiences. If a student's previous educational experiences were primarily negative, a return to the classroom setting can elicit earlier unproductive behaviors. In the traditional classroom setting, the adult learner is often forced to leave the self-directed behavior associated with work and family when they enter the classroom, creating conflict and a loss of confidence to be successful (Knowles et al., 2005).

Socialization into the academic setting and peer support throughout the program have been found to be related to success in RN-to-BSN programs (Cailin, 1996; Delaney & Piscopo, 2007; Huston et al., 2001; Lillibridge & Fox, 2005).

While workplace administration may encourage the RN student to complete the baccalaureate degree, the RN student often receives little support from workplace peers, who value experience more than education (Lillibridge & Fox, 2005; Zuzelo, 2001). The question occasionally arises whether RN students should be kept separate from the generic or pre-licensure students. Zuzelo (2002) found RN students often preferred separate from the pre-licensure student and reported that combining a mix of students in the classroom was detrimental to their experience. Other researchers reported RN students are uncomfortable in the academic role and became frustrated when asked to assimilate with the generic students (Cangelosi, 2006; Lillibridge & Fox, 2005). RN students often believed they needed to prove they were competent in the clinical area to compensate for their uneasiness with the academic role, while traditional students were more comfortable in the academic role, but lacked the clinical nursing experience. The obvious differences in age, maturity, clinical experience, as well as the additional family and work responsibilities, leave little room for a common ground between the student groups. How to use this diverse mix of student backgrounds and experiences in classroom and clinical settings poses a challenge for nursing faculty. The use of learning contracts and specialty learning competencies may address these concerns, as they validate the maturity and experience of adult learners (Foss, Janken, Langford, & Patton, 2004; Waddell & Stephens, 2000).

## Faculty

The role of the faculty-student relationship in the professional transformation of the RN-to-BSN student is not to be underestimated. Cangelosi (2004, 2006) explores qualitative components of the faculty-student relationship, as described by nursing faculty. Faculty saw themselves in the role of providing a nurturing environment for students as they move to a different level of professionalism. Astute faculty assess student needs, often without the student's knowledge or awareness, and create a context for learning and possibilities which the student does not envision. The role of faculty is to guide the student from previous patterns of knowledge and create a new paradigm for practice (Cangelosei, 2006). RN-to-BSN students value and appreciate connectivity with nursing faculty, especially when they were experiencing difficult events at home and work. They also appreciate being treated as adults, with consideration of previous life and work experiences (Cangelosi, 2004, 2006; Zuzelo, 2001).

A humanistic paradigm for nursing education emphasizes the student-teacher connection and its impact on learning and professional socialization (Gillespie, 2002, 2005). While Gillespie's (2002) work involved traditional baccalaureate students, she challenges faculty to clarify their beliefs and actions, reflecting on how they influence their connectivity with students and the transformative learning process. A connected teacher-student relationship is supportive of students who are doing well, as well as those who are at-risk (Gillespie, 2005).

## Translating Theory and Research into Practice

The nursing profession embraces the mantra to "look at the evidence" when choosing a nursing intervention. A holistic, individualized approach to patient care is now considered the norm, and nurse educators expect the students they supervise in the clinical area to address the unique needs of their patients. Likewise, faculty do not take a "one-size fits all" approach to classroom and clinical instruction for all undergraduate nursing students. Faculty are encouraged to look at the evidence when selecting instructional methods to use with a distinct cohort such as RN students returning for their baccalaureate degree. The remainder of this chapter focuses on applying current learning theory and research to specific theoretical/ evidence-based strategies to use when teaching RN-to-BSN students.

## Teaching Strategies

### Create an Environment Conducive to Learning

Learning theorists, faculty, and students agree that the environment is a key element for a positive learning experience and a successful professional transformation. Mezirow (2000) postulates that for learning transformation to occur, the student must address a disorienting dilemma, with accompanying self-examination, and a trying on of new roles, before integrating the new behavior. The classroom setting must be conducive for intellectual discourse and the free exchange of ideas for this to occur. This is a very different approach for faculty who may be more comfortable using traditional didactic techniques. Faculty focus changes from directing to facilitating learning and creating a trusting and caring milieu which allows for individual student voices to be heard (Morris & Faulk, 2007; Taylor, 2000). The andragogical model supports this emphasis on the environment and places the responsibility on the educator to create an environment "characterized by physical comfort, mutual trust and respect, mutual helpfulness, freedom of expression, and acceptance of ideas" (Knowles et al., 2005, p. 93). The classroom atmosphere should be a non-judgmental setting which allows adult students to express themselves without fear of grade repercussion or losing face. A student may be hesitant to express an opposing view if it is sensed that a faculty or fellow student will make a value judgment on the student's personal beliefs or previous actions. However, there are some behaviors that can not be tolerated. For example, if a student makes a negative comment about an ethnic group, the faculty must respond.

When working with a diverse group of students such as the RN-to-BSN cohort, faculty often find themselves in the role of moderator of opposing belief systems. While this can be uncomfortable, discomfort is a necessary element for self-examination for both faculty and students. Similar to the process of value clarification faculty expect of students in the clinical setting, faculty need to apply the process to their personal beliefs and ask themselves the following questions:

- What is it about the topic or comment that is so discomforting?
- What are the ethical principles involved?

The same questions then need to be directed to the students. As a moderator, faculty can help students identify which principle is applicable. Is it justice, autonomy, non-malfecience, fidelity, or veracity? The American Nurses' Association *Code of Ethics with Interpretive Statements* is an excellent resource for faculty and RN students.

Creating a trusting environment for students to express themselves is no easy task! However, nursing faculty have the advantage of developing a wide range of skills from working with patients in the clinical setting. These skills can be applied to the classroom setting. Just as a clinician would rather sit than stand when discussing sensitive topics with a patient, sitting among a group of students rather than standing at the front of the classroom encourages more intimacy for a free flow of ideas. Small group activities create an environment which encourages an exchange of ideas that would not happen in a large lecture hall. For example, group work such as case studies, storytelling, and role playing vignettes, have been successful in teaching cultural competency to RN student (Eshleman & Davidhizar, 2006).

With the shortage of faculty and resources, programs may not have the luxury of a separate RN-to-BSN program. Faculty may face the challenge of meeting the disparate learning and professional transformation needs of both RN and pre-licensure students in the same classroom. Faculty can turn this challenge into an opportunity to enhance learning for all student groups, by creating a cohesive environment to promote learning. While there may be obvious dissimilarities among the students, faculty need to focus on the shared commonalities. This can be achieved with small group learning activities. However, rather than allow students to self-select for group work, a heterogeneous group can benefit from the assets of one student with clinical expertise and another with a different set of academic talents. When faculty create a trusting and non-judgmental environment, welcoming of different experiences and opinions, seemingly different groups may find a common ground to learn from each other. For a summary of additional teaching strategies see Table 1.

---

### Strategies for Teaching the RN Student

- Create an environment conducive to learning
  - Develop trust

- Harness the enthusiasm
  - Build confidence

- Reveal the objectives and reveal them often
  - Inform students why they need to know

- Reduce stressors to increase success
  - Provide support services

- Design a Mentorship Program

- Flexibility with little redundancy
  - Choose assignments carefully

- Choose the right technology for the right course

**Table 1.** Strategies for Teaching the RN Student

---

## Harness the Enthusiasm

While a few students may state they have enrolled in an RN-to-BSN program for the baccalaureate degree to keep their current position, returning to school is a personal choice for most RN students. Once they have made the decision to begin a BSN program, they are anxious to begin. Often students express the sentiment that this is their time or something they have wanted to do, but family and/or work commitments had interfered until now. As a result, students begin the program exhibiting a readiness to learn (Knowles et al., 2005) and a sense of excitement and anticipation. Faculty need to take advantage of and harness that initial enthusiasm to carry the student through the program.

The initial RN to BSN bridge course is crucial to setting the stage and developing the motivational energy for the academic work to follow. The specific course content should reflect the outcomes of the program, and provide an overview of the curriculum. The course is often a sampler to whet the student's appetite for future courses. This is the time for faculty to highlight the unique aspects of their BSN program and entice the student to the next course on the academic menu. Inform students of distinct or unusual opportunities that are available during the program. This helps students anticipate what will occur along the way.

Assignments for the RN transition course can also be developed to allow a student to expand on a clinical specialty. An evidence-based practice paper allows the student to research a common intervention that is currently being used in their practice arena. (See Figure 1 through 3). The paper could focus on a nursing intervention or practice and asks the question "Is there evidence to support a current common practice on this unit?" Adults are more motivated to develop a proficiency in an area, if they perceive it will help them resolve problems or issues which they encounter on a daily basis (Knowles et al., 2005). At the end of the course the student has something concrete to take back and potentially incorporate into their practice.

Students could also be asked to develop a poster presentation for their nursing unit and bring the results to the clinical manager. If the student chooses to do so, they may continue with the topic as a project for a course in a nursing research or capstone course. Allowing students to work on a topic in their area of interest provides an immediate relevance to their clinical practice, increases confidence, and acts as a motivating factor for future learning (Knowles et al., 2005).

Previous life and work experiences are wonderful assets in a classroom of adult learners. The majority of RN students are accomplished professionals and the role of the learner's experience is a major advantage for the adult student (Knowles et al., 2005). Classroom teaching strategies should draw on the wealth of experience of the students in the classroom. RN students may have expertise in a clinical specialty which surpasses that of the faculty teaching the course. Since they are currently in the practice realm, they may be more aware of current local practice. Allowing the student the opportunity to share their knowledge and skills in the class discussion validates and expands previous learning and provides a boost in confidence. However, care needs to be taken when the information presented is not the most current or at the appropriate professional level. If that occurs, faculty will need to turn it into an opportunity for learning without compromising the self-esteem of student. This is similar to any classroom technique an educator would use

**Course Objective:**
1. Determine the value of evidence-based practice for the nursing profession and for patient care outcomes.

**Assignment Objectives:**
1. Develop an effective search strategy for a literature review.
2. Evaluate the scientific evidence for a commonly used nursing intervention.
3. Author a seven to ten page scholarly paper using APA format.

**Rationale:**
As nursing continues to develop as a theory-based profession, there is an increasing emphasis on the provision of care based on analysis of research findings. It is critical that health care and nursing are grounded in scientific evidence and not just because "it has always been done this way." This assignment provides an opportunity for the student to critically evaluate a practice or procedure routinely used in the provision of care to patients in his/her practice.

The student is to choose a topic, conduct a review of the scientific literature, and write a seven to ten page paper, following APA format. All topics are to be pre-approved by the faculty, using the attached form no later than _____ (date). Papers are to be based on a **minimum** of five current journal articles. Copies of all journal articles (online and print) must be included with the papers. Students are to submit papers in a two-pocket folder, with journal references in one pocket and the paper in the other.

**Figure 1.** Evidence-Based Practice Assignment

Proposed Topic_____

In a few short sentences, why does this topic interest you?
Please submit a minimum of three journal articles which you intend to use for this paper.

_____Topic approved
_____Topic and/or journal articles are not considered appropriate for this assignment.
        Please make appointment to meet with faculty.

Faculty Signature:_____

Faculty will return this form (and articles) to the student within one week.

**Figure 2.** Evidence-Based Practice Assignment, Topic Submission

I.   Introduction
     i.    What is the issue?
II.  Background
     i.    What is the significance of the practice issue?
III. Review of the literature
     i.    Summarize current research
           1.   Minimum of five research studies from peer-reviewed journals
IV.  Nursing and patient implications
     i.    What are the implications for patient care?
     ii.   What are the implications for nursing practice?
V.   Summary and conclusions
     i.    Summarize findings
     ii.   Implications for future research

**Figure 3.** Evidence-Based Practice Assignment, Sample Rubric

when a student gives a "wrong" answer. The students' confidence will increase as they see their contribution to classroom discussion is valued.

Successful completion of self-directed learning activities should develop competence as well as self-confidence. Since there may be wide variation in the cohort of students relative to their level of comfort and ease regarding a self-directed learning approach, faculty should anticipate some students will need more guidance. The need for further direction may be met in a variety of ways, such as in-person meetings and phone or email conferences. The beginning of each class is an excellent opportunity to discuss progress and expectations for learning activities which are taking place outside of the classroom.

As the students progress through the program and gain in self-assurance, the role of faculty changes from director to facilitator of learning. This is a crucial step for the student who is on the path to becoming a life-long learner and continuing with professional development beyond the degree completion program.

## Reveal the Objectives and Reveal Them Often

Oftentimes faculty and students review course objectives at the beginning of the semester and do not use them again until the course evaluation at the end of the semester. Contrary to the traditional pedagogy, adult students learn best when they understand the need to know (Knowles et al., 2005). The authoritarian approach of "because I said so" is an ineffective strategy for adult learners and may in fact impede learning in the formal classroom setting. The RN student needs to grasp how the content may fit into the bigger picture and its relevance to professional practice.

As the student approaches a content unit, the objectives for the unit should be readily available and reviewed. What is the student expected to learn and how does it apply to professional practice? All assignments need to have focused objectives, which are related to the course objectives, which are further related to program outcomes. Adult students are more likely to invest time in an assignment if they understand its relevance to the overall goals of the program and how they can apply their new knowledge and skills in the work environment.

Unit and course objectives are extremely helpful to students as they prepare for formal assessments. Preparing for course examinations was identified as one of the top five stressors for RN students (Nicholl & Timmins, 2005). The adult student who has recently returned to school may not have taken a written exam for a number of years and is often ill-prepared to study. Unit objectives can be quite valuable in helping the student to focus on the course content. For example, a unit on ethical issues may include the objective of "Apply ethical decision-making models in patient care situations." This tells students what they are expected to know and apply during the testing situation and directs their attention for study.

## Reduce Stressors and Increase Success

Multiple work and family responsibilities translate into multiple stressors for RN students returning for their baccalaureate degree (Nicholl & Timmins, 2005; Zuzelo, 2001). Striving to balance the demands of family, work, and school may lead students to feel frustrated and dissatisfied with their performance in all areas. Students need to learn how to balance seemingly conflicting demands, the expectations for academic work, and the resources that are available to them to ensure their success.

Time management is essential in successfully balancing the tasks and psychological obligations of multiple roles. Orientation to the academic setting should include at least one session on prioritizing activities and managing time. If there has been a significant time lapse since their previous educational experience, adult students may need to relearn how to be a student again. A university or college office of student support services might offer short seminars dealing with time and stress management, test taking, and study skills. Students should be encouraged to use those services to help ease the transition of returning to school. Faculty can support those efforts during the initial class meetings by discussing the course syllabus, class schedule, class policies regarding attendance and assignments, and ways to resolve any potential conflicts. For example, students should be informed how many hours outside of class they are expected to spend on related readings and course work. Due dates for tests and assignments should be apparent so students may arrange for additional time off from work or to plan family activities. Faculty can play a supportive role and acknowledge the work and family responsibilities of the student. However, faculty also need to emphasize the importance of academic work and the students' need to make time for study and assignments.

Support services for the adult student need to be readily accessible at a time when the student is available to make use of them. The academic support center for the university should include evening and weekend hours to accommodate the student who is employed during the day. Since writing assignments are especially stressful for many RNs returning to the academic world (Nicholl & Timmins, 2005; Zuzelo, 2001), faculty need to be very clear in providing guidelines and rubrics for grading. Many universities have writing centers and faculty should encourage students to utilize all available university resources. These resources are especially helpful for students who are not native English speakers, or who have not mastered the art of writing a research paper. There are also online resources, such as the Purdue

University Online Writing Lab (http://owl.english.purdue.edu/), that are designed for students who need a lesser degree of assistance. Many university websites allow for access to writing guidelines specific to their university or provide external links to online style guides websites from the university homepage. It is also vital that the student be aware of the university policy on academic honesty and plagiarism.

For the student who requires assistance in areas other than writing, the university may have tutors available to work with students in specific subject areas. There are also online tutorial programs such as Smarthinking.com (www.smarthinking.com) which allow the student to log on and submit work to an online tutor or "e-structors" for assistance. The university may purchase tutorial hours for their students to use, or the individual may purchase hours for personal use. While online resources lack the face-to-face connection, the availability of academic support which the student can access from home at a time that is convenient offers distinct benefits.

## Design a Mentorship Program

The use of mentoring as a successful strategy for personal and professional development is well documented in the research literature (Barker, 2006; Dorsey & Baker, 2004; Melnyk, 2007). African-American and minority undergraduate students especially appear to benefit from the mentoring relationship (Buchanan, 1999). The RN to BSN student often presents a challenge for professional development as the student must alter previously practiced behaviors in the clinical area to reflect a higher level of professional practice upon program completion. Participating in a mentorship program provides the student with an appropriate role model to emulate for integrating new behaviors and make the move to practice as a baccalaureate-prepared nurse. In addition, it is expected that the mentor relationship may continue beyond program completion, furthering both personal and professional growth.

Mentorship programs can be developed in collaboration with the clinical agencies where the student is currently employed. The nursing program could recruit and match students with Masters prepared clinicians at their clinical agency. Nursing program faculty could also support a program to develop the skills of potential mentors. The clinical agency could recruit potential mentors, assist in matching them with students, provide space for programs, and support activities that facilitate the mentor-mentee relationship. Nursing programs, students, and healthcare agencies may all benefit from this type of collaborative partnership.

## Flexibility with Little Redundancy

The characteristics of the program are critical factors for the RN student when choosing a BSN Program. Researchers suggest the RN student is seeking a "flexible, comprehensive, user friendly" academic system (Boylston, Peters, & Lacey, 2004, p. 31). The curricular design needs to allow for the maximum transfer of credits from previous college experiences, as well as include the possibility of earning college credit through non-traditional means. The National League for Nursing (NLN) offers a number of exams which the RN student may take as a substitute for an equivalent course. For example, a passing grade on the NLN Challenge exam on Health Assessment in conjunction with a practical demonstration in the skills laboratory may be considered equal to a 3-credit-hour course. The College Level Examination Program (CLEP) administered by College Board allows for students to obtain college credit for previously learned material in required liberal arts areas. University administration and college faculty may need to review transfer credit policies to provide as much credit as possible, without compromising the integrity of the degree.

Students begin an RN-to-BSN program anticipating new information and innovative teaching strategies (Cangelosi, 2006). Faculty who focus on knowledge deficits, negate the students' experiences, or re-teach information which the students have previously studied, have a negative impact on the learning experience (Cangelosi, 2004; Delaney & Piscopo, 2007). With the diverse cohort of students in the BSN program, it may be difficult for faculty to find common ground to begin a content area. It can be helpful to begin a new unit with a general discussion to gauge the familiarity with the content unit. If the students have a strong background or experience in the subject, faculty can be more flexible with the method of delivery. Lecture notes can readily be posted online and class time can be better used with discussion, or meeting the course objectives at a higher level of application, analysis, or synthesis. Faculty need to adapt the information and strategy to the individual cohort of students.

Inquiry-based learning (IBL) is a flexible teaching methodology which draws on the skills of both faculty and students to achieve the goals of professional nursing practice. In this approach, the students generate questions and content areas which need further exploration, thus decreasing the risk of redundant work. IBL changes the role of the faculty to that of a resource and facilitator, and puts more responsibility on the student for learning the content (Cleverly, 2003). IBL sets up a different type of partnership with the students and utilizes activities which support the development of critical thinking, developing skills in identifying and utilizing resources for building a theoretical base to become a life-long learner.

IBL begins with a well-authored and realistic scenario which initiates the IBL tutorial process. This interdisciplinary approach includes group discussion, reflection, and identification of learning needs. The IBL group initiates self-directed learning activities, bringing information back to the group for dialogue, with development of an action plan. Inquiry-based tactics can be used with a number of individual patient, family, and community scenarios, which promote student and faculty learning (Cleverly, 2003). Since the students identify the content areas for learning, there is active participation by the students with little redundancy. IBL also provides students with the resource skills to take with them beyond the classroom setting.

Course assignments should be designed to develop and reflect course and program outcomes. With multiple responsibilities and time a premium for most students, assignments should be chosen with much thought and consideration. How does this assignment assist the student in meeting the course and program objectives? Faculty need to ask themselves if the activity is superfluous of previously learned behaviors.

Specific learning activities and assignments have been found to be associated with development of specific roles and values in RN-to-BSN students (Morris & Faulk, 2007). Faculty choose activities which allow the student to develop competency in different areas simultaneously. For example, a family assessment assignment has the potential to foster professional behaviors as patient advocate, educator, and information manager. A preceptorship activity in management may facilitate skills as a leader and member of the healthcare team. Assignments such as these also support the development of the values of caring, altruism, and respect for autonomy and human dignity (Morris & Faulk, 2007).

## Choose the Right Technology for the Right Course

Many RN-to-BSN programs are offered in an on-line format only, and it would be unusual to find a BSN program that was not web-enhanced to some extent. In states with a large rural population and limited university level education programs, an online format may be the only viable option for RN students seeking a baccalaureate degree. These programs have been reported as successful in meeting their stated outcomes (Ouzts, Brown, & Swearingen, 2006).

For the adult RN student with multiple family and work related responsibilities, requirements to be on campus on a weekly basis may be a barrier to obtaining a baccalaureate degree (Lillibridge & Fox, 2005). An online format may be preferred. However, the variable degree of computer literacy and competency among RN students needs to be addressed for any program that expects students to use technology for meeting course objectives. For the student who has little experience with computers, email, or word processing software, the use of computer based learning can be very intimidating (Zuzelo, 2001). Many universities now require a core course in information literacy or computer science which helps to address this issue. The initial bridge course should also incorporate an introduction to the use of the information technologies that students will be expected to use throughout the program (Huston et al., 2001). Clear instruction and classroom demonstration on how to access course information online is essential for students with limited academic computer experience. Emphasizing the many advantages of using online textbook resources, web-based course management software, online library services, and Internet based professional resources provides support to the student who is computer shy.

There has been some concern regarding the use of the web-based format for the RN-to-BSN student. Socialization to the academic setting with role modeling is a crucial component for the professional transformation that is expected of the RN-to-BSN student upon graduation (Waddell & Hayes, 2000; Huston et al., 2001). Responsible use of the Internet and Internet resources may also raise some ethical concerns (Fulton & Kellinger, 2004). These issues add a cautionary note for nursing faculty and suggest the need for closer monitoring for the use of information technology in the academic setting. Faculty must continue to assess and evaluate the methodologies that are used to meet the course objectives and program outcomes.

Web-enhanced courses offer many benefits for the adult student with multiple commitments and time constraints. Course websites allow the posting of course materials, announcements, discussion forums, testing, external web links, etc. Students are able to access the course information at their own convenience and faculty are able to provide updates and information without requiring the student to be present on campus. A well-designed course website can be invaluable to the student who many only be available to do course work at odd hours of the day.

## Summary

RN-to-BSN students present a distinct set of challenges and opportunities for nursing faculty. Nurses have long recognized the need for individualized, evidence-based patient care, but now need to extend the same approach when working with students. The teaching strategies faculty use with RN-to-BSN students should respect and reflect the experiences they bring to the academic setting. Nurse educators who work with RN students have the opportunity to foster professional growth and transformation having a lasting impact on patient care.

## Learning Activities

1. Interview a faculty who teaches RN-to-BSN students. How are the teaching methods used different than a faculty who teaches generic nursing students?
2. Describe how critical thinking learning activities may be different for the RN-to-BSN student than for the generic nursing student.
3. Interview at least three RN-to-BSN students. Ask them what motivated them to return to school. Discuss with them their perceptions of the advantages to completing the BSN degree.

## Educational Philosophy

My role as educator is to provide the information, tools, and the environment to promote optimum learning. I vary my style and techniques to match the learning needs of the group of students in the classroom or clinical setting. I entered the field of nursing education with the belief that I could best promote a high standard of patient care by sharing my passion and beliefs with undergraduate nursing students. I believe each student has a unique gift to bring into the profession, and my role as educator is to assist students in developing their creative and personal art of professional nursing practice. — Rosemarie O. Berman

## References

American Association of Colleges of Nursing (AACN). (2007). *2007 Annual State of the Schools*. Washington, DC: Author.

American Association of Colleges of Nursing (AACN). (2008). *The essentials of baccalaureate education for professional nursing practice*. Washington, DC: Author.

American Nurses Association (ANA). (2001). *Code of ethics for nurses with interpretive statements*. Silver Spring, MD: American Nurses Publishing.

Barker, E. (2006). Mentoring: A complex relationship. *Journal of American Academy of Nurse Practitioners, 18*, 56-61.

Boylston, M. T., Peters, M., & Lacey, M. (2004). Adult student satisfaction in traditional and accelerated RN-to-BSN programs. *Journal of Professional Nursing, 20*(1), 23-32.

Buchanan, B. (1999). A mentoring pyramid for African American nursing students. *ABNF Journal, 10*(3), 68-70. Retrieved July 11, 2007, from the ProQuest database.

Callin, M. (1996). From RN to BSN: Seeing familiar situations in different ways. *Journal of Continuing Education in Nursing, 27*(1), 28-33.

Cangelosi, P. R. (2004). The tact of teaching RN-to-BSN students. *Journal of Professional Nursing, 20,* 167-173.

Cangelosi, P. R. (2006). RN-to-BSN education: Creating a context that uncovers new possibilities. *Journal of Nursing Education, 45,* 177-181.

Delaney, C., & Piscopo, B. (2007). There really is a difference: Nurses' experiences with transitioning from RNs to BSNs. *Journal of Professional Nursing, 23*(3), 167-173.

Dorsey, F., & Baker, C. (2004). Mentoring undergraduate students: Assessing the state of the art. *Nurse Educator, 29*(6), 260-265.

Eshleman, J., & Davidhizar, R. E. (2006). Strategies for developing cultural competency in an RN-BSN program. *Journal of Transcultural Nursing, 17*(2), 179-183.

Foss, G. F., Janken, J. K., Langford, D. R., & Patton, M. M. (2004). Using professional specialty competencies to guide course development. *Journal of Nursing Education, 43*(8), 368-375.

Fulton, J., & Kellinger, K. (2004). An ethics framework for nursing education on the internet. *Nursing Education Perspectives, 25*(2), 62-66.

Gillespie, M. (2002). Student-teacher connection in clinical nursing education. *Journal of Advanced Nursing, 37*(6), 566-576.

Gillespie, M. (2005). Student-teacher connection: A place of possibility. *Journal of Advanced Nursing, 52*(2), 211-219.

Huston, C., Shovein, J., Damazo, B., & Fox, S. (2001). The RN-BSN bridge course: Transitioning the re-entry learner. *The Journal of Continuing Education in Nursing, 32*(6), 250-253.

Knowles, M. S., Holton, E. F., & Swanson, R. A. (2005). *The adult learner: The definitive classic in adult education and human resource development* (6th ed.). Burlington, MA: Elsevier.

Lillibridge, J., & Fox, S. D. (2005). RN to BSN education: What do RNs think? *Nurse Educator, 30*(1), 12-16.

Melnyk, B. (2007). The latest evidence on the outcomes of mentoring. *Worldviews on Evidence-Based Nursing, 4*(3), 170-173.

Mezirow, J. (2000). Learning to think like an adult: Core concepts of transformation theory. In J. Mezirow (Ed.). *Learning as transformation.* (pp. 3-33). San Francisco, CA: Jossey-Bass.

Morris, A. H., & Faulk, D. (2007). Perspective transformation: Enhancing the development of professionalism in RN-to-BSN students. *Journal of Nursing Education, 46*(10), 445-451.

Nicholl, N., & Timmins, F. (2005). Programme-related stressors among part-time undergraduate nursing students. *Journal of Advanced Nursing, 50*(1), 93-100.

Phillips, C. Y., Palmer, V., Zimmerman, B. J., & Mayfield, M. (2002). Professional development: Assuring growth of RN-to-BSN students. *Journal of Nursing Education, 41*(6), 282-284.

Ouzts, K. N., Brown, J. W., & Diaz Swearingen, C. A. (2006). Developing public health competence among RN-to-BSN students in a rural community. *Public Health Nursing, 23*(2), 178-182.

Spedic, S. S., Parsons, M., Hercinger, M., Andrews, A., Parks, J., & Norris, J. (2001). Evaluation of critical thinking outcomes of a BSN program. *Holistic Nursing Practice, 15*(3), 27-34.

Taylor, K. (2000). Teaching with developmental intention. In J. Mezirow (Ed.). *Learning as transformation.* (pp. 151-180). San Francisco, CA: Jossey Bass.

U.S. Department of Health and Human Services Health Resources and Services Administration (HRSA). (2006). *The Registered Nurse Population: Findings from the March 2004 National Sample Survey of Registered Nurses.*

Waddell, D. L., & Hayes, J. M. (2000). Point/counterpoint: Does "online" nursing education short change the RN to BSN student? *Georgia Nursing, 60*(3), 38-9.

Waddell, D., L., & Stephens, S. (2000). Use of learning contracts in a RN-to-BSN leadership course. *The Journal of Continuing Education in Nursing, 31*(4), 179-184.

Zuzelo, P.R. (2001). Describing the RN-BSN learner perspective: Concerns, priorities, and practice influences. *Journal of Professional Nursing, 17*(1), 55-65.

# CHAPTER 19

## TEACHING FACULTY TO PROVIDE CULTURALLY-COMPETENT NURSING EDUCATION

### Leonie L. Sutherland, PhD, RN

The content of this chapter relates to the following major content areas and subconcepts on the Certified Nurse Educator Examination Detailed Test Blueprint:

**Facilitate Learning**
- Implement a variety of teaching strategies appropriate to learner needs; learning style
- Modify teaching strategies and learning experienced based on consideration of learners' cultural background; past educational and life experiences
- Create a positive learning environment that fosters a free exchange of ideas

**Facilitate Learner Development and Socialization**
- Identify individual learning styles and unique learning needs of learners with these characteristics: culturally diverse (including international)
- Provide resources for diverse learners to meet their individual learning needs

## Introduction

Imagine yourself as a new faculty member of a nursing department. You eagerly attend the college-sponsored faculty training seminars designed to help you improve your teaching skills. One of the seminars features active learning strategies by creating heterogeneous groups of students for small group discussions and assignments. To implement this strategy the teacher divides the class into groups, mixing up the students based on ethnic diversity and academic standing. The purpose of this mix is to provide an opportunity for students to learn from one another, using their diversity and academic strengths as skills for the group's accomplishments. After leaving the seminar you feel confident you can enhance student learning by capitalizing on these strengths.

You assign Jane, Kristine, Ann, and Tran to work together as group members. They are the perfect representation of a heterogeneous group:
- Jane, a high achiever
- Kristine, a married mother of two
- Ann, a second year college student

- Tran, a Vietnamese immigrant who has been in the United States for six years

As you move from group to group, you notice Tran sitting off to the side by himself while the three women are animatedly discussing the topic. When you approach Tran to ask him why he is not involved, he looks up and says, "They don't want me; I am too slow for them". You suddenly realize that managing a culturally diverse classroom requires more than simply implementing teaching strategies; you also must develop skills that enable you to meet the individual needs of your culturally diverse students.

As you confront your lack of cultural competence in the classroom, you can rest assured that you are not the only nurse educator experiencing this problem. Nurse educators across the country are faced with diversity issues that can present new predicaments every day. Whether your classroom has one or many ethnically diverse students, there are specific strategies you can implement to meet the learning needs of all your students (see Figure 1).

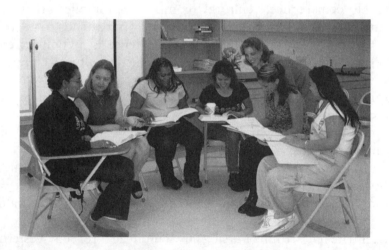

**Figure 1.** An Ethnically-Diverse Class

This chapter explores the issues of ethnic diversity in nursing education. Some of the student examples are incidents taken directly from the author's experiences in the ethnically diverse classroom. The barriers students face as members of the multicultural classroom are the foundation for pedagogical approaches. Faculty preparation to meet the challenges of diversity and strategies designed to meet the needs of individual students are discussed. Additionally, activities designed to facilitate an inclusive classroom are presented.

## Key Terms

To understand the scope of the diverse classroom, the following key terms may be helpful when applying concepts to students and educational strategies. These definitions are taken from the nursing cultural literature and adjusted for nursing education (M. Andrews & Boyle, 2008; Giger et al., 2007; Spector, 2004).

- Ethnicity: a sense of identification associated with one's common social and cultural heritage.
- Culture: non-physical traits, such as values, beliefs, attitudes, customs, and learned patterned behavior that are shared by a group of people and passed from one generation to the next.
- Cultural competence: cultural competence implies that within the educational setting, the teacher understands and attends to the total context of the student's situation. Cultural competence is a complex combination of knowledge, attitudes, and skills. Acquiring cultural competence is an ongoing process.
- Minority: a group of students, who because of cultural characteristics, receive different and sometimes unequal treatment from others in the educational system. Minority students may see themselves as recipients of collective discrimination.
- ESL/EFL: English as a second language/English as a foreign language refers to those students raised in environments where English is not the primary language. In addition to language, the environment includes values, beliefs, traditions, and the daily way of life.
- Eurocentric: refers to the nursing curriculum as it reflects Western European and American heritage.

## Ethnicity in Nursing

The Health Resources and Services Administration (HRSA) periodically conducts a national sampling survey of the registered nurse population (Health Resources and Services Administration, 2004). The results show the Registered Nurse population does not directly correlate with the U.S. census data as projected in 2006 (United States Census Bureau, 2006) (see Tables 1 and 2).

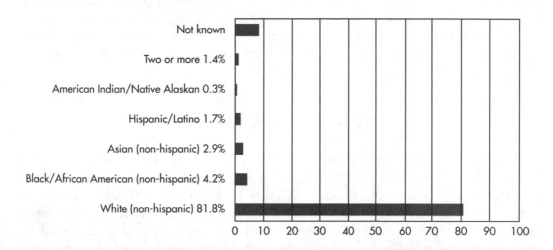

**Table 1.** Distribution of Registered Nurses

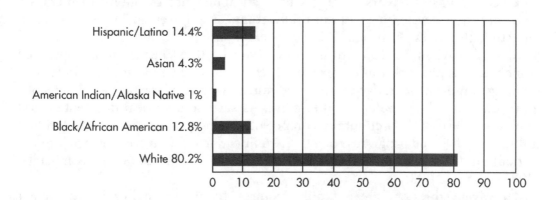

**Table 2.** Population of the US by Race

Note: Percentages do not add up to 100% due to rounding and because Hispanics may be of any race and are therefore counted under more than one category.

Similarly the nursing student population also does not reflect the predominant make-up of residents in the United States. Nursing schools throughout the country have developed programs to recruit a diverse nursing student population. While the diversity is not equally distributed along the geographic regions, nurse educators can at least expect some ethnic variations in their classrooms. Whether the classroom has few or many diverse students, specific needs have been identified that can impact the success of these students' nursing education.

## Issues Facing Nurse Educators

According to Andrews and Boyle (1999) at that time, the typical American nurse living in the United States was white, middle class, Anglo-Saxon, Protestant, and female. While this description may still apply to the majority of American nurses, a shift in the ethnic make-up can be found in nursing programs across the country as increasing numbers of Asian, Hispanic, Black, and Native American students enroll in nursing schools (Milone-Nuzzo, 2007; National League of Nursing, 2008; Symes, Tart, & Travis, 2005). Moreover, Andrews and Boyle (2008) state that the nursing workforce in the United States is very different from previous times and is now part of a multicultural workforce.

Over the past 10 years there has been an abundance of published literature concerning the development of culturally competent nurses, including practicing and student nurses. A broad CINAHL search using the terms "cultural" and "competence" yielded 3,153 returns from 1998 to 2008. When the term is changed to include "faculty cultural competence", the returns dwindle to 157. Indeed, it is vitally important that faculty prepare nurses who can practice with the skills appropriate for the populations they serve. As such, a great deal of attention has focused on developing a culturally competent nursing profession. Faculty can find multiple models and programs to help them integrate cultural competence into the curriculum (Cuellar, Walsh-Brennan, Vito, & deLeon Siantz, 2008; de Leon Siantz, 2008; Delaney, 2008).

However, educators are not only required to prepare culturally competent practitioners, they are also faced with the challenge to prepare students from ethnically diverse backgrounds who must be able to care for a variety of patients. The needs of these students necessitate that faculty critically examine their teaching methodologies and develop strategies to effectively teach in a multicultural classroom. Culturally diverse students' problems are compounded as they are required to function in the subculture of nursing that is predominantly Eurocentric, while at the same time learning to manage care for culturally diverse patients. Students who may appear to have similar backgrounds or be fluent in English can still be culturally diverse from their peers. Commitment on the part of faculty is found to be a primary factor in promoting success of students from ethnically diverse backgrounds (Wong, Seago, Keane, & Krumback, 2008). The American Academy of Nursing Expert Panel on Cultural Competence has identified the need and responsibility to find ways to help faculty to provide culturally competent health care practices (Giger et al., 2007). For faculty engaged in the nursing work of teaching, this means attempting to use teaching strategies that meet the learning needs of all students.

## Ethnically Diverse Student Profile

Cultural diversity implies a melding of people from various backgrounds. In describing the culturally diverse nursing student two terms are frequently used, minority and ESL. However, culturally diverse nursing students can represent any number of groups including African-Americans, foreign-born students, Native Americans, Asians, and Hispanics (Gilchrist & Rector, 2007). Moreover, when the teacher strives to create an inclusive classroom, one that meets the learning needs of all students, all groups must be included. Racial and ethnic differences only make up one form of diversity. Other forms of diversity include first-generation college students and economically disadvantaged students. While these students may speak fluent English, other academic barriers can place them at higher risk for failure.

### The "English as a Second Language" Student

An ESL student can experience learning barriers related to language proficiency. Nursing students who are not acculturated to the English language have lower academic achievement (Salamonson, Everett, Koch, Andrew, & Davidson, 2008). Additionally, some ESL students report that English may be their third or fourth language making language acculturation even more difficult. Recognizing the complexity of a student's language foundation, both written and verbal, can aid in identifying barriers to learning and comprehension. Students have commented that the nursing content does not give them nearly as much trouble as the "day-to day English" (Bosher & Bowles, 2008).

Regardless of the level of language skill the student possesses, the teacher needs to keep a broad view of their needs. There are nursing students who speak English fluently yet were raised in, or currently reside in, a household of diversity. These students may also exhibit some of the difficulties faced by ESL students. The daily environment for many of these students is still primarily grounded in their ethnicity.

These are environments where a hamburger is never served, where television and newspapers are in the native language, and where family life is firmly rooted in cultural traditions. The ability of the student to proficiently use the English language is an overt indicator of comprehension. Socialization that primarily includes one's own ethnic group puts students at a disadvantage in a Eurocentric curriculum. Nurse educators must remember that teaching solely from this perspective can unintentionally alienate students who are not acculturated to the American way of life.

## The Marginalized Student

Hall, Stevens, and Melies (1994) explain the characteristics of marginalization using a comprehensive concept analysis. Their definition of marginalization clearly describes the situations that ethnic minorities experience. "Marginalization is a process through which persons are peripheralized on the basis of their identities, associations, experiences, and environments" (p. 24). In essence, this means there are groups of people who are located away from the center. It means being different from those at the center or the mainstream. Additionally, those at the center are perceived to have power over those at the periphery.

A study by Diver-Stamnes and Lomascilo (2001) identified key differences in the perceived and experienced marginalization of European-American students and ethnic minority students. While all students surveyed indicated they had experienced some form of marginalization, there was a large gap in what constituted marginalization. European-American students cited discrimination in areas such as age, gender, and appearance – an individualized perspective. However, ethnic minority students cited social exclusion, discriminatory behaviors on the part of professors, stereotyping by professors and students, and lack of diversity in the faculty and curriculum – a sociological perspective. More recently, students from ethnically diverse backgrounds rated their academic institutions low in areas of diversity. They reported less interaction with faculty, decreased support for ethnically diverse faculty, and lack of sensitivity to students from diverse backgrounds (Wong, Seago, Keane, & Krumback, 2008). Clearly, the university experience is quite different for European-Americans than it is for ethnic minority students.

Teachers and faculty in all areas of education have unintentionally marginalized students. A Latino student recalled a time during grade school when she was denied a request to leave English-remediation classes even though she had mastered the content. Nursing students, too, have reported feeling and experiencing marginalization. Tran, in the chapter's opening scenario, is one example. Additionally, ethnic minority students rarely have a nursing faculty who looks like them. African-American students report they are the last to be selected for group work. Circumstances such as these can act as barriers to learning for nursing students. An awareness of these experiences and truly listening to the voices of students can be the first step in breaking down walls that may hinder learning.

## Barriers Faced by Diverse Students

The effort to overcome educational barriers for minority students has been compared to "leaping tall buildings" (Dawkins & Gilchrist, 2007). Indeed, the challenges faced by these nursing students are many and their successes are exceptional. But as nursing continues to call for a diverse workforce, faculty must take on the responsibility for helping students achieve their goal. One way teachers can assist students is to be fully cognizant of what ethnically diverse students experience on their journey to becoming a nurse.

Many characteristics set culturally diverse students apart from their Anglo counterparts. Ethnic minority students have high attrition rates and socio-demographic characteristics that interfere with success in the current educational environment. These, along with cultural values, may be barriers to success for some students. A qualitative study explored the experiences of 15 ethnic nursing students at a predominantly White nursing program. The major findings reinforce the idea that barriers exist. Students experienced loneliness and isolation, lack of understanding about cultural differences, lack of support from teachers, and even discrimination (Gardner, 2005). In another study, students reported they wanted to belong yet felt excluded. These students were very aware of their learning needs yet cultural differences prevented them from seeking assistance. ESL students found it difficult to join in conversations due to speed of speech, colloquialisms, and unfamiliar words (Rogan, San Miguel, Brown, & Kilstoff, 2006). For the teacher, this is especially important if group work is a significant part of class activities.

Yoder (1996) developed an explanatory model based on student perceptions of their nursing education. Ten years later, using the same model, researchers found that nursing students still face similar barriers. Divided into 4 categories, the barriers include personal needs, academic needs, language needs, and cultural needs (see Table 3). Moreover, the barriers exist on different levels with some students needing little assistance and the higher level where those students need a great deal of assistance (Amaro, Abriam-Yago, & Yoder, 2006). This requires additional attentiveness by the teacher to carefully assess their students' individual needs.

| Personal Needs | Academic Needs | Language Needs | Cultural Needs |
|---|---|---|---|
| • Lack of finances<br>• Insufficient time<br>• Family responsibilities<br>• Language difficulties | • Study workload<br>• Need for tutoring<br>• Need for study groups | • Translation issues<br>• Prejudice due to accents<br>• Time | • Communication<br>• Assertiveness<br>• Lack of ethnic role models |

**Table 3.** Barriers to Success

Two categories of barriers exist describing the external and internal issues facing minorities (Peter, 2005). External barriers include limited finances, poor social integration, and lack of institutional support. However, there are other external barriers, such as family responsibilities, that may affect a student's success. While not limited to ethnic minorities, the cultural tradition may command a higher priority for these types of barriers. For Hispanic students, retention and graduation rates from nursing programs were improved if students had a supportive family and received adequate financial support (Taxis, 2006). Teachers may want to be aware of the family situations that may be hindering student's progress in the classroom.

Several academic characteristics put culturally diverse students at risk for success in completing a nursing program. One study reported that due to poor primary educational preparation, African-American students have difficulty with reading comprehension, math, and test-taking skills. Instead, these students performed better using social modes for learning and demonstrated a strong preference for writing notes and studying in groups (Femea, Gaines, Brathwaite, & Abdur-Rahman, 1995). More recently, Hispanic students identified academic barriers that hinder their success in nursing school (Goetz, 2007) such as poor study habits, test-taking anxiety, poor reading comprehension, and poor test-taking skills (Peter, 2005). Ethnically diverse students frequently do not understand the nursing program's process of education. Skills such as critical thinking, problem solving, and decision making create difficulties for students as they are acculturated to respect the authority of the teacher with an unquestioning attitude (Malu, Figlear, & Figlear, 1994). To address these academic barriers programs geared towards assisting at-risk minority teens are one strategy to enhance success for minority students entering the nursing profession (Noone, Carmichael, & Carmichael, 2007; Peterson, 2002; Vint, 2008)

The literature describes many institutional obstacles faced by ethic minority students that affect retention and attrition. These institutional barriers exist since many colleges and universities are predominantly white with Euro-American values and characteristics. Moreover, the language of colleges and universities is unique. Lack of knowledge about how to navigate the educational system, both on a formal and informal basis, leads to discomfort and feelings of isolation (Dickerson, Neary, & Hyche-Johnson, 2000).

Many mainstream students never have to ask themselves "Can I really be a professional?" Yet ethnic minorities may be the first ones in their families to attend college. Gonzales (1994), a successful Mexican-American educator, eloquently describes his battle to survive his university education. Continued perseverance and the support of federally funded "special education" programs were the primary factors related to his success. Gonzales notes that minority students continue to have difficulties unless they seek out mentors who are willing to help them find their way through a higher education system that is deeply rooted in traditions. Interestingly, this same phenomenon still exists today. Interviews with Latino and American Indian nursing students revealed that many believe they are academically unprepared leading to the notion that becoming a nurse was an unreachable goal (Evans, 2004)

The description of the ethnically diverse student clearly shows that nursing faculty must be skilled in creating a classroom environment that makes it possible for all students to be successful. One method is to develop an awareness of cultural diversity that then leads to cultural competence. Cultural competence is a process requiring specific ability, openness to cultural attributes, and flexibility to adjust to those attributes, both differences and similarities (Suh, 2004). Applied to the educational milieu, it requires the educator to seek skills, practices, and attitudes that foster academic and professional achievement for all students. Leaders in nursing suggest that promoting culturally competent care is a priority (Giger, et al., 2007; Lipson & Desantis, 2008; Newell-Withrow & Slusher, 2001). For nurse educators this means using the features of the definition of cultural competence and implementing these with nursing students.

## Curriculum and Faculty Characteristics

### Eurocentric Curriculum

Historically, the nursing curriculum is based on the Anglo middle-class culture with an educational focus that is "linear, sequential, time-oriented, individualistic, competitive, dualistic" (Crow, 1993 pg. 198). The cultural bias that may present in this type of curriculum can have negative effects on students. Over the past

15 years, schools and programs of nursing have implemented many changes to address the needs of culturally diverse students (Evans, 2004; Peter, 2005; Taxis, 2006). Continued efforts in this area will help move the curriculum to one that is appropriate for all students.

Novice nurse educators may teach in the way they were taught, not intentionally, but because this is the way that is known. Combined with the heavy emphasis of successful passage of the National Council Licensing Exam (NCLEX®), it seems appropriate to focus on covering content in the nursing classroom. But just covering content does not address the specific needs students may have. Assumptions about what constitute health, nursing, family, and community may be very different for non-Anglo students. A critical examination of the way a course is organized can help identify areas that may be taught in a more inclusive manner. Faculty commitment to lessening the Eurocentric method of course development may be the first step in providing a nursing education that meets a variety of students' needs.

## Demystifying Diversity

As the classroom becomes more and more diverse, it becomes imperative for educators to increase their cultural awareness. Students are entering higher education with perspectives and views that may be drastically different from the faculty. It is time for educators to re-examine their own assumptions about students, courses, higher education, and themselves. A self-assessment can also be beneficial to determine where one's discomfort lies. A self-assessment can be conducted using one of the many tools available on the Internet. The Derek Bok Center for Teaching and Learning has focused on cultural bias in the classroom for many years and has a variety of tools available for educators (Harvard University, 2008). As a first step towards self-awareness, assessment of one's attitudes and behaviors towards ethnically diverse students can provide valuable insight into positive improvements that can be made in teaching. Developing cultural competence is a process and not an end goal and requires continued openness to new exploration.

## Patterns of Faculty Response

A study designed to discover some of the issues and problems that exist in teaching students from diverse cultures, revealed that faculty present various patterns of responding to ethnic minority students (Yoder, 1996). The researchers interviewed ethnically diverse nursing students and faculty, asking about the complex issues they face. Five patterns of responding emerged. When examined closely, the patterns of responding reflected the personal level of cultural awareness demonstrated by nursing faculty.

The researchers labeled the first pattern the **generic response**. Faculty in this category have a low level of cultural awareness. In managing curricular activities, this teacher does not make any allowances for diversity and treats every student the same. The faculty who responds in the generic pattern does not believe that ethnically diverse students have needs that are different from mainstream students.

The second pattern of response is labeled **mainstreaming**. Faculty who respond in this manner have a high level of cultural awareness and are aware of the needs of diverse students. However, instead of seeing the student as someone with unique characteristics, this faculty regards the student as having deficiencies that must be overcome. The teaching strategies are therefore geared to help the student fit into the mainstream nursing culture. The students are expected to let go of their cultural attributes and adopt the culture of the dominant group.

A third pattern identified is called the **culturally non-tolerant pattern**. Adopting this approach to teaching, the educator is unwilling to tolerate cultural differences. Indeed, culturally non-tolerant faculty may even exhibit behaviors that create barriers to learning.

The fourth pattern is labeled the **struggling pattern of response**. This pattern is displayed by faculty who are moving from a lower level of cultural awareness to a higher level. Moreover, these educators experiment with teaching strategies geared to meet the needs of culturally diverse students. While the faculty may still experience setbacks, the students' unique qualities and subsequent learning success is what drives their teaching.

The fifth and final pattern of response is labeled **bridging**. Nursing faculty who demonstrate this response possess a high level of cultural awareness and successfully adapt their teaching to meet the varied needs of culturally diverse students. An opposite of the mainstreaming response, bridging educators encourage students to maintain their ethnic identity and to function bi-culturally. This teacher's goal is to bridge the gap between the dominant world and the students' cultural world.

This study and follow-up studies demonstrates the wide variations that exist in how nursing educators approach students and implement their teaching activities for ethnically diverse students (Yoder, 1997; 2001). The findings from this research are still being used to assess student nurse perspectives of their educational experiences (Amaro, Abriam-Yago, & Yoder, 2006; Gardner, 2005). Although this research was carried out in the late 1990s the classifications can still be used to conduct a self-assessment.

## Strategies to Become a Better Teacher

So how can one become an educator who uses a bicultural response to students? How can a teacher create a safe climate that fosters learning for all students? The following strategies can help the educator develop skills that will improve the teaching-learning process. Teachers should read through these tips then implement those that fit their unique educational situation.

As educators grapple with the issues of teaching ethnically diverse students, it is important to remember to teach all students equally (Lou, 1994). The strategies an educator implements can definitely benefit students from varying cultures, but they can also help the students from the ethnic majority who struggle to achieve. Becoming a better teacher for minority students results in becoming a better teacher for all students (Wong, Seago, Keane, & Krumback, 2008).

## Learning from Ethnically Diverse Faculty

When teaching about professionalism in nursing, educators frequently look to positive role models for their students to emulate. Nurse educators as well as nursing students can learn from diversity experts in education. Look for faculty members from different cultural backgrounds. Seek them out at conferences and meetings; ask questions about how they teach. Many colleges and universities offer ethnic studies programs with experienced faculty. These educators can provide a wealth of resources relative to curriculum revision, literary resources for classroom use, and input on classroom pedagogy. If these types of programs do not exist at your institution, there may be resources available at a nearby college. Take the first step and soon a network of colleagues may emerge, willing to share their experiences.

## Student Representatives

Another source of expertise is your own students. Most courses include some form of evaluation the students complete at the end of the term. A concurrent assessment, one conducted throughout the course, is valuable for identifying the needs of students currently enrolled in the course. One educator formed a quality control team consisting of students from the class. This team met with the professor once a week to discuss the quality of the instruction. Students can provide feedback on how well a topic was explained, the quality of the handouts, and the teaching style. The professor was able to discover how well the students understood the material. Before implementing this strategy it is important to determine how the team will be selected. Some methods for selecting team members include classroom vote, random selection, and volunteers. It is important to ensure the students know they have a voice and are being heard.

## End-of-Course Survey

If a quality control team is not feasible, another way to assess one's teaching is by developing and administering a personal end-of-course survey. This survey can be designed specifically with your course in mind. Open-ended questions provide the most useful information. This personalized survey can also be implemented incrementally over the course of the term. Take a few minutes every couple weeks and ask the students to answer a question such as, "What suggestions do you have that would make the topic more interesting or easier to understand?" Their responses will provide solid feedback about what they have learned, what types of activities enhanced their learning, and any barriers that interfere with their learning.

## Helping Individual Students

Interaction with faculty and peers provides academic benefit for all students. Yet African-American student nurses have less interaction with both faculty and peers (Wong, Seago, Keane, & Krumback, 2008). Minority students may feel invisible among the larger number of white students. Many times, faculty and students will turn to the minority student as a "native informant" (Quaye & Harper, 2007 p. 37). Singling out a student to be the voice for the culture disengages the student while preventing the mainstream students from exploring their own viewpoints of diversity. This practice also sets the minority student apart from the rest of the class. It is important to enable white students to connect their own cultural views and backgrounds to the discourse.

Flinn (2004) suggests using small groups to examine the cultural aspects of disease. Each student is required to list everything they know about a certain disease, including signs, symptoms, diagnosis, and treatment. In the group, students take turns and share one fact from the list. This process continues until the students have covered everything they wrote. This inclusive approach allows for cultural differences to emerge and provides a forum for discussion. Individual students benefit because the playing field is leveled (Flinn, 2004).

## Connecting with Students

One way to get to know students is to have them complete a student profile (Davidhizar & Shearer, 2005). While some programs keep student profiles on file, an individual faculty can adopt this strategy as a way to connect with students. A student profile can include questions that will help the teacher recognize difficulties students may have with learning. Davidhizar & Shearer (2005) suggest questions relating to:

- Vital statistics
- Expectations of the course
- Learning plans
- Learning style

Furthermore, having students think about their role in learning fosters a sense of personal responsibility.

Any faculty who has interacted with foreign born students has probably struggled with name pronunciation. Students are flattered when their teachers call them by name and getting the pronunciation right is definitely a plus. For example, Nguyen is a common Vietnamese name. Many English speakers pronounce this as "Nugen". However, the correct pronunciation sounds like "Nwen". The Internet offers some useful resources providing audio recordings of name pronunciation (Inogolo, 2008). These sites are simple to navigate requiring the user to simply type the name and listen to the audio file. With some perseverance faculty can improve their skill at connecting with students on a very personal level.

## Advising

Experienced faculty know that frequent contact with students creates an environment that promotes student success. One way to accomplish this is to meet with every student at least once during the term. The face-to-face meeting provides an opportunity for the faculty and student to connect without interruption. Gentle probing questions give the educator insight into how the student is progressing. Students who connect with their professors are more likely to ask questions about difficult topics, and discuss areas of concern, and thus receive valuable assistance from the faculty. These student-faculty meetings should not be limited to ethnically diverse students. All students should be given the same opportunity.

## Making Assumption Regarding Student Comprehension

A colleague reported an incident that caused her to drastically change her method of clinical teaching. The teacher questioned a Vietnamese student about the nursing care required when administering morphine sulfate. The student, well prepared, listed the most frequent and life-threatening side effects, including respiratory depression. The teacher then asked the student what she would do to monitor respiratory depression. The student looked at the teacher blankly. She did not know what the term respiratory depression meant and, therefore, did not know what to do. Although this student could define respiratory and depression as separate words, put together these words took on a new meaning. The teacher astutely realized that common meanings might not be understandable for EFL students.

As you interact with students, in the classroom or at the clinical site, do not assume students understand. Try to use descriptions familiar to all students. For example, telling students that the urine in hepatic failure is tea-colored may not be accurate for someone who drinks green or herbal tea. Similarly, avoid jargon and witty clichés, as these can be confusing. Learn what other cultures mean when they use familiar words. When a person is poor, for some Native American groups this means the person is spiritually poor, not financially poor (Dickerson, Neary, & Hyche-Johnson, 2000). The point is not to be an expert in every culture, but to heighten your own level of awareness about how your students view the world of nursing and patient care.

## Test Review

One of the goals of pre-licensure nursing education is to prepare students to successfully pass the NCLEX®. Studies show that ELL students have higher failure rates than their mainstream counterparts (O'Neill, Marks, & Liu, 2006). Some of the lack of success is attributed directly to language and cultural values (Cunningham, Stacciarini, & Towle, 2004). Often times, exams written by nursing faculty require students to make decisions and answer questions that are grounded in a Euro-American tradition. For example, when asking students how to approach a patient who is dying, foreign-born students may say it is important to give the person hope. For these students, it would be difficult to teach about preparing for death. Therefore, it is important for all nursing students to approach these types of issues from the patient's cultural point of view and not from the nursing student's point of view. The National Council of State Boards of Nursing makes every effort to eliminate bias from questions on the NCLEX-RN®, however, it is prudent to assist students to learn to answer these questions from the patient's cultural point of view.

Faculty can help these students by conducting test study sessions. It is important that these sessions be structured to meet the needs of students who are struggling with test-taking skills. Treating all students equally means students have equal opportunity to learn. If students who excel attend the study session, their presence may be intimidating to those for whom the session is designed – the at-risk student.

To handle this issue, two separate study groups can be arranged, dividing students according to their needs. The effort put into the study groups is well worth it. Students recognize the educator's willingness to help by promoting an environment of trust and encouragement.

To organize the study sessions, prepare questions similar to the exam. Have the students answer the questions individually. Then, review each question and ask students for the correct answer. For each incorrect answer, have them explain why they chose that particular option. This approach provides valuable insight into the students' thinking and rationalizing (see Table 4).

| NCLEX® type Question & Answer | Student Response | Student Rationale |
|---|---|---|
| • A patient with metastatic cancer tells the nurse she does not know what will happen to her children when she dies. How will the nurse respond?<br><br>"Why don't we talk about the options you have for the care of your children." | "You are going to live for a long time yet, and your children will be just fine." | It is unkind to talk about a person's death with her. It is best to give her hope, which is the kind thing to do.<br><br>*In this student's culture, you never give up hope* |
| • How does the insulin make energy for the body?<br><br>Making glucose available to the cell. | Transporting glucose in the bloodstream. | Did not select the correct answer because insulin does not make glucose.<br><br>*This student used a different context for the word "making"* |

**Table 4.** Example of Student Responses and Rationales

Frequently, student answers make perfect sense when viewed from a different cultural context. An open and nonjudgmental discussion helps students understand the reasoning process required to arrive at the correct answer.

## Classroom Activities

Good classroom teaching requires a great deal of innovation and effort. The traditional lecture format frequently does not engage students in learning. Whittington (2000) found that while in lecture, 68% of student thoughts were about things other than class content, such as how difficult it is to get a parking place. Only twelve percent of thoughts were stimulated by the topic at hand and only 3% of thoughts were of a nature deep enough to analyze the subject matter. This study demonstrates that creating a classroom environment that fosters participation can positively benefit all students (Whittington, 2000).

Another factor to consider is the way in which students view the educational experience. Many Asian students believe their role is to listen to the professor, and it is the professor's role to impart information. These students may never volunteer answers in class. Indeed, they may resent any kind of active participation since this is not how they view the teaching-learning process. Conversely, the educator who wants to effectively engage students in the type of learning that fosters thinking must be cognizant that different learning preferences exist within the classroom. To successfully connect with all students, active learning must be designed in such a way that all students feel safe.

A safe classroom is one that is open to all students. Promoting a safe classroom means:

- Bringing marginalized students closer to the center.
- Setting the stage for open discussion where opinions are welcomed and all views are worthy of discussion.
- Asking students for their thoughts about a subject thereby acknowledging their views are important.

A safe classroom also demonstrates to the students that the faculty's viewpoint is only one of many.

## Active Learning

Active learning strategies can be used to engage all students in classroom participation. The overall purpose is to create an environment in which all students engage in thinking and learning. In a typical classroom, the teacher asks a question and waits for a student to respond. Most students know there are usually one or two students who always answer. The students also know that as soon as these students respond, it is safe to stop thinking. Even if the teacher asks for additional information, most students believe the answer they would have given has already been stated. Moreover, the main reason students do not participate in class is a fear of being embarrassed. This is where active learning assists the faculty to help students overcome some of these barriers.

Active learning strategies are designed so all students are comfortable participating in a safe environment. All students are required to think of a response and present it to the teacher. It is no longer acceptable to wait for the more assertive students to respond. Active learning also requires commitment on the part of the educator to prepare for lectures and include carefully designed activities that stimulate student thinking. These techniques work equally well for marginalized students, shy students, and uninvolved students. Another benefit of active learning strategies is the teacher receives immediate feedback on how well the class understands the material. Following are some examples of active learning strategies (McKeachie, 1999; McKeachie & Svinicki, 2006).

**Colored cards.** At the beginning of the term, each student is given 4 colored index cards, held together by a large paper clip or ring. The students are instructed to bring these cards to every class session. Throughout the lecture, the teacher projects multiple-choice questions onto a screen using a transparency or presentation software. Each answer to the question is color-coded, the same as the index cards. Students are required to hold up the colored index card that matches the option they believe to be the correct answer. They must hold the card directly in front of their chests (see Figure 2). When all students have selected an option the teacher provides the correct answer. This system is helpful for the following reasons:

- The teacher can immediately gauge how well the class understands the concept.
- All students are answering the question.
- No student is singled out

**Share pairs.** Not all students feel comfortable sharing their opinions in the classroom. The share pairs exercise allows for sharing of information within a small group. The teacher poses a question or thought and asks students to briefly write down their responses. After a few minutes the students pair up with another person and share their answers. This exchange provides an opportunity for students to obtain input from another student, yet they are not required to speak in front of a large group. Another variation of this exercise is to ask the pairs of students to write an answer that is acceptable to both parties. Then the pairs of students share their answers with the class. Students are all actively involved in thinking in a safe classroom environment.

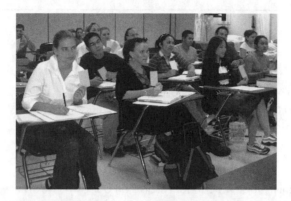

**Figure 2.** Card Response

**One-minute paper.** At times a teacher may want to gauge the students' knowledge level about a concept or topic. The one-minute paper provides a quick way to gather this information. At the beginning of the class the teacher gives the students one minute to write the answer to a question. The papers are collected. The teacher then reads the papers. Reading the papers is not time consuming since most will be a sentence or two. Valuable information can be gleaned from these papers about the students' comprehension and understanding. However, the faculty must be cognizant of the fact that EFL students may not be as articulate, especially given the short time frame.

**Group contract.** When assigning a group project there is always the risk that some students perceive the work is not divided equally. Situations such as the presence of a non-participant member or members not welcoming any work but their own can contribute to this perception. A group contract can help students develop the foundation for improved group performance. When groups are formed, either by faculty assignment or student self-selection, the first task is for the group to develop a contract. The contract contains the rules that each member agrees to follow. Each member then signs the contract and submits it to the teacher. When group conflict occurs, the faculty can pull out the contract to help with the mediation. This keeps the communication open among the students and prevents the faculty taking on the role of a judge. This technique works very well in a diverse classroom since it encourages the voices of marginalized students to be heard. Table 5 is an example of a group contract.

---

**Group Contract**

Group Name:

1. We agree to come to the meetings prepared.
2. We will start the meetings on time and end on time.
3. Every opinion will be considered.
4. We will be active participants.
5. We will take turns bringing snacks to the meetings.
6. The work will be divided equally.
7. If we have a conflict that we cannot resolve on our own, we will seek out the instructor for guidance.
8. We respect when someone is talking, we will not interrupt.
9. We will be honest in our discussions and not wait to disagree outside of the meeting.

Signed:

---

**Table 5.** Group Contract

**The group culture project.** One way to reduce marginalization of students is to design an assignment where all students begin on an equal basis. The group culture project is designed to improve students' understanding about cultures different from their own. In groups of four and five, students are asked to select an ethnic group for study; however, none of the students may be a member of the chosen ethnic group. The goal is for all students to start at the same beginning point and work together to complete the assignment. Table 6 is an example of how to design the group culture project. The final product can be a class presentation or a group paper. This project has been very successful in bridging the gap between ethnic minorities and Caucasian students in the classroom (Sutherland, 2001).

**Course Content.** Although personal and interactive learning can greatly enhance learning, at times the lecture format is best suited to the setting or topics covered. If the lecture format is the only method available, there are some strategies that can make the content delivery culturally friendly. An outline of the lecture is beneficial to students who need help organizing their thoughts. The order of the outline should

## Diversity in Nursing Practice and Care

The role of a nurse includes direct patient care activities such as teaching, advocacy, and providing support. As nurses, you will deal with patients who are unique in their needs and it will be your challenge to meet these needs. This assignment allows you to explore the various dimensions of diversity that you will experience in nursing.

The goals of the assignment are:

1. To give you an opportunity to explore the <u>current nursing literature</u> that has been written about your cultural population.
2. To give you practical experience with interaction with a cultural group that is different from your group.
3. To give you an opportunity to locate resources on the Internet.
4. To have you evaluate the information that is available to nurses who seek to learn more about your chosen group.
5. To allow you to compare the published findings with your interview findings.

### _The Research for this Cultural Diversity Project_

1. You will choose your cultural group for study.
2. You will interview 5 people who represent members of your chosen group.
   a. Read Giger and Davidhizar's cultural assessment model.
   b. Develop interview questions along the lines of the assessment model.
   c. Interview the cultural group members and be prepared to present the results in audio/visual format.
3. You will find some published literature about your cultural group.
   a. You must find 2 articles (from accepted nursing journals) that discuss your group.
   b. These articles can be found through the on-line data bases, e.g. CINAHL, Medline, and Ebsco host. Be sure the articles are from nursing journals.
      i. The articles should relate directly to your cultural group
      ii. If you find an appropriate article that is not from a nursing journal, one of the authors MUST be a nurse.
      iii. Any other deviation from selecting an article must be cleared by the instructor.
   c. Develop an annotated bibliography and turn in to instructor (abstracts from library data bases are not acceptable).
4. Find one Internet resource that can help inform nurses about the particular characteristics, values, interests, customs or beliefs of your group. Submit a print-out from your Internet source when you turn in your bibliography.
5. Consider how your diverse cultural group would be able to relate to the healthcare system and what nurses can do to improve that interaction.

**Table 6.** Sample Group Culture Project

be the same for every lecture and for an adult health lecture could include topics as:

- Overview of lecture
- Brief review of pertinent anatomy and physiology
- General signs and symptoms
- Diagnostic tests
- Specific nursing diagnoses
- Specific nursing care
- Evaluation of care

As the lecture progresses, reference to the outline helps students organize and follow along with a consistent framework (Flinn, 2004).

Another strategy that helps students connect the course content is a brief review at the beginning of the lecture. This review can be achieved as a short quiz, crossword puzzle, or brief case study. Students can quickly recognize their areas in need of improvement. By not grading the assignments, the stress level will be greatly reduced. In fact, students may enjoy these challenges as a way to measure their own learning.

If faculty have a specific course they teach every semester, the development of learning guides could be an effective tool to support student learning. Learning guides can include the outline of each lecture, the key points for the lecture or the unit, short case studies, web links, helpful tools such as acronyms, and conceptual links to clinical practice. Learning guides could also include the lay terms students may hear from their patients and contrast those with the medical terms. Students who are frequently content driven ask, "What exactly do we need to know?" can use the guides to raise their level of critical thinking. This is especially helpful for ELL students as the guides allow them to link the lecture format to a concrete visual tool that uses medical language in the correct context (Guttman, 2004).

## Evidence-Based Teaching

As the nursing profession becomes increasingly focused on evidence based practice (EBP), nursing education should also work to ensure teaching strategies are based on the best available evidence. As faculty work to develop the culturally inclusive classroom, empirical evidence will help substantiate those teaching strategies. In a letter to the editor, Ukoha (2004) eloquently describes her experiences with faculty who continue to be oblivious to the status of their classrooms. Ukoha suggests that rigorous testing of interventions would help build the base of evidence allowing faculty to confidently implement teaching and learning strategies without having to use a hit or miss approach. Just as faculty teach students to search out the best levels of evidence to guide their nursing practice, students will be well served when teachers also incorporate evidence-based pedagogies in their classes.

## Summary

Managing a diverse classroom is not always easy. The practice of teaching demands a great deal of energy and time, and the needs of students vary greatly across groups. The first step toward developing a culturally friendly classroom is self-awareness about diversity, recognition of one's beliefs and biases. Then, by slowly integrating various strategies designed to involve all students, the gap between ethnic minority and mainstream students should diminish. Not only do the ethnically diverse students benefit, the mainstream students are exposed to viewpoints that may differ from their own. A climate of respectful learning emerges, making all who participate as equal partners.

So what happened to Tran and his group? He continued to be part of the group, but the teacher made a particular effort to ensure that participation was welcomed from all students. The incident was a powerful lesson for the awareness of the effect of diversity in classroom situations.

## Learning Activities

1.  Interview a faculty member regarding his/her experiences in teaching in a multicultural classroom. Ask questions such as: What was your first experience with diversity in the classroom? Was your preparation adequate to manage diverse students? Describe what in your background prepared you for managing a diverse classroom.
2.  Observe a classroom. Are there any overt representations for various ethnic groups? What are the major classroom activities? Does the teacher make eye contact? Are differing viewpoints respected? Does the teacher create an environment where students feel safe to voice their opinions?
3.  Develop suggestions to enhance the classroom environment that you observed.

## Educational Philosophy

My teaching philosophy is to provide an environment where people can be empowered. As such, I believe the role of an educator involves the formation of a teaching-learning partnership with students. It is my responsibility to create an environment where the student is free to engage in meaningful dialogue, can apply critical thinking skills, and can feel challenged to stretch beyond the standard course content. — Leonie L. Sutherland

## References

Amaro, D. J., Abriam-Yago, K., & Yoder, M. (2006). Perceived barriers for ethnically diverse students in nursing programs. *Journal of Nursing Educaiton, 45*(7), 247-254.

Andrews, M., & Boyle, J. S. (2008). *Transcultural concepts in nursing care* (5th ed.). Philadelphia: Lippincott Williams & Wilkins.

Andrews, M. M., & Boyle, J. S. (1999). *Transcultural concepts in nursing care* (3rd ed.). Philadelphia: J. B. Lippincott Company.

Bosher, S., & Bowles, M. (2008). The effects of linguistic modification on ESL students' comprehension of nursing course test items. *Nursing Education Perspectives, 29*(3), 165-172.

Crow, K. (1993). Multiculturalism and pluralistic thought in nursing education: Native American world view and the nursing academic world view. *Journal of Nursing Educaiton, 32*(5), 198-203.

Cuellar, N. G., Walsh-Brennan, A. M., Vito, K., & De Leon Siantz, M. L. (2008). Cultural competence in the undergraduate nursing curriculum. *Journal of Professional Nursing, 24*(3), 143-149.

Cunningham, H., Stacciarini, J. R., & Towle, S. (2004). Strategies to promote success on the NCLEX-RN for students with English as a second language. *Nure Educator, 29*(1), 15-19.

Davidhizar, R. E., & Shearer, R. (2005). When your nursing student is culturally diverse. *The Health Care Manager, 4*, 356-363.

Dawkins, D., & Gilchrist, K. L. (2007). Leaping tall buildings: Barriers for minority nurse practitioners in education. *Communicating Nursing Research, 40*, 527.

de Leon Siantz, M. L. (2008). Leading change in diversity and cultural competence. *Journal of Professional Nursing, 24*(3), 167-171.

Delaney, C. (2008). Innovative learning activity. *Journal of Nursing Educaiton, 47*(5), 240.

Dickerson, S. S., Neary, M. A., & Hyche-Johnson, M. (2000). Native American graduate nursing students' learning experiences. *Journal of Nursing Scholarship, 32*(2), 189-196.

Diver-Stamnes, A. C., & Lomascolo, A. F. (2001). The marginalization of ethnic minority students: A case study of a rural university. *Equity and Excellence in Education, 34*(1), 50-57.

Evans, B. (2004). Application of the caring curriculum to education of Hispanic/ Latino and American Indian nursing students. *Journal of Nursing Educaiton, 43*(5), 219-228.

Femea, P., Gaines, C., Brathwaite, D., & Abdur-Rahman, V. (1995). Sociodemographic and academic characteristics of linguistically diverse nursing students in a baccalaureate degree nursing program. *Journal of Multicultural Nursing and Health, 1*(3), 24-29.

Flinn, J. B. (2004). Teaching strategies used with success in the multicultural classroom. *Nurse Educator, 29*(1), 10-12.

Gardner, J. (2005). Barriers influencing the success of racial and ethnic minority students in nursing programs. *Journal of Transcultural Nursing, 16*(2), 155-162.

Giger, J., Davidhizar, R. E., Purnell, L., Harden, J. T., Phillips, J., & Strickland, O. (2007). American Academy of Nursing expert panel report: Developing cultural competence to eliminate health disparities in ethnic minorities and other vulnerable populations. *Journal of Transcultural Nursing, 18*(2), 95-102.

Gilchrist, K. L., & Rector, C. (2007). Can you keep them: Strategies to attract and retain nursing students from diverse populations: Best practices in nursing education. *Journal of Transcultural Nursing, 18*(3), 277-285.

Goetz, C. R. (2007). *The process of becoming: A grounded theory study of Hispanic nursing student success.* Unpublished Doctoral Dissertation, Northern Illinois University, Dekalb.

Guttman, M. S. (2004). Increasing the linguistic competence of the nurse with limited English proficiency. *The Journal of Continuing Education in Nursing, 35*(6), 264-269.

Hall, J. M., Stevens, P. E., & Meleis, A. I. (1994). Marginalization: A guiding concept for valuing diversity in nursing knowledge developement. *Advances in Nursing Science, 16*(4), 23-41.

Harvard University. (2008). Derek Bok Center for Teaching and Learning. Accessed October 6, 2008

Health Resources and Services Administration. (2004). The Registered Nurse Population: Findings from the 2004 National Sample Survey of Registered Nurses.

Inogolo. (2008). Inogolo: English Pronunciation Guide to the Names of People, Places, and Stuff.

Lipson, J. G. & Desantis, L. A. (2008). Current approaches to integrating elements of cultural competence in nursing education. *Journal of Transcultural Nursing, 18*(1), 10-20.

Lou, R. (1994). Teaching all students equally. In P. La Bella (Ed.), *Teaching from a multicultural perspective* (Vol. 12, pp. 28-45). Thousand Oaks: Sage.

Malu, K. F., Figlear, M. R., & Figlear, E. A. (1994). The multicultural ESL nursing student: Prescription for admission. *Journal of Multicultural Nursing, 1*(2), 15-20.

McKeachie, W. J. & Svinicki, M. (2006). *McKeachie's teaching tips: Strategies, research, and theory for college and university teachers.* Boston: Houghton Mifflin.

Milone-Nuzzo, P. (2007). Diversity in nursing education: How well are we doing? *Journal of Nursing Educaiton, 46*(8), 343-344.

National League of Nursing. (2008). Headlines from the NLN. *Nurse Education Perspectives, 29*(3), 182-184.

Newell-Withrow, C., & Slusher, I. L. (2001). Diversity: An answer to the nursing shortage. *Nursing Outlook, 49*(6), 270-271.

Noone, J., Carmichael, J., & Carmichael, R. (2007). An organized pre-entry pathway to prepare a diverse nursing workforce. *Journal of Nursing Education, 46*(6), 287-291.

O'Neill, T. R., Marks, C., & Liu, W. (2006). Assessing the impact of English as a second language status on licensure examination. *CLEAR Exam Review* (Winter 2006), 14-18.

Peter, C. (2005). Learning - whose responsibility is it? *Nure Educator, 30*(4), 159-165.

Peterson, R. M. (2002). Mentoring nursing career pathways: The Maryvale High School Student Nurse Academy. *Journal of School Nursing, 18*(6), 329-335.

Quaye, S. J., & Harper, S. R. (2007). Faculty accountability for culturally inclusive pedagogy and curricula. *Liberal Education, Summer 2007*, 32-39.

Rogan, F., San Miguel, C., Brown, D., & Kilstoff, K. (2006). "You find yourself." Perceptions of nursing students from non-English speaking backgrounds of the effect of an intensive language support program on their oral clinical communication skills. *Contemporary Nurse, 23*(1), 72.

Salamonson, Y., Everett, B., Koch, J., Andrew, S., & Davidson, P. M. (2008). English language acculturation predicts academic performance in nursing students who speak English as a second language. *Research in Nursing and Health, 31*, 86-94.

Spector, R. E. (2004). *Cultural diversity in health and illness* (6th ed.). Upper Saddle River: Prentice Hall.

Suh, E. E. (2004). The model of cultural competence through an evolutionary concept analysis. *Journal of Transcultural Nursing, 15*(2), 93-102.

Sutherland, L. L. (2001). *Using a transcultural assessment model to illustrate the concept of diversity*. Paper presented as the Sigma Theta Tau Southern California Regional Conference, San Diego.

Symes, L., Tart, K., & Travis, L. (2005). An evaluation of the nursing success program: Reading comprehension, graduation rates, and diversity. *Nure Educator, 30*(5), 217-220.

Taxis, J. C. (2006). Fostering academic success of Mexican Americans in a BSN program: An educational imperative. *International Journal of Nursing Education Scholarship, 3*(1), 1-14.

United States Census Bureau. (2006). USA Quick Facts. Retrieved July, 22, 2008 from http://quickfacts.census.gov/qfd/states/00000.html

Vint, P. A. (2008). Degrees of success: Academic forum. *Minority Nurse*(4), 56-58.

Whittington, M. S. (2000). *Using think-aloud protocols to assess cognitive levels of students in college classrooms*. U. S. Department of Education. (ERIC Document Reproduction Service No. ED 450647).

Wong, S. T., Seago, J. A., Keane, D., & Krumback, K. (2008). College student's perceptions of their experiences: What do minority students think? *Journal of Nursing Educaiton, 47*(4), 190-195.

Yoder, M. (1997). The consequences of a generic approach to teaching nursing in a multicultural world. *Journal of Cultural Diversity, 4*(3), 77-82.

Yoder, M. (2001). The bridging approach; Effective strategies for teaching ethnically diverse students. *Journal of Transcultural Nursing, 12*, 319-325.

Yoder, M. K. (1996). Instructional responses to ethnically diverse nursing students. *Journal of Nursing Educaiton, 35*(7), 315-321.

# CHAPTER 20

# TEACHING NURSING STUDENTS WITH DISABILITIES

**Donna Carol Maheady, MS, EdD, RN, ARNP, CPNP**

The content of this chapter relates to the following major content areas and subconcepts on the Certified Nurse Educator Examination Detailed Test Blueprint:

**Facilitate Learning**
- Implement a variety of teaching strategies appropriate to learner needs
- Create a positive learning environment that fosters a free exchange of ideas

**Facilitate Learner Development and Socialization**
- Provide resources for diverse learners to meet their individual learning needs
- Advise learners in ways that help them meet their professional goals
- Adapt teaching styles and interpersonal interactions to facilitate learner behaviors

## Introduction

If it hasn't happened yet, it is only a matter of time before you learn that you have a student with a disability in your lecture class or clinical group. Persaud & Leedom (2002) found faculty had a significant effect on a student's ability to succeed in a nursing program. Learning and working with people with disabilities benefits nursing education and practice in many ways. Students with disabilities can bring remarkable compensatory abilities and valuable skills such as sign language and lip reading to nursing care as well as empathy and insight from their personal experiences.

A positive attitude from you, the teacher, will be the foundation to help this student achieve success in the program. Reflecting on your personal views about disability is vital prior to working with a student with a disability. An attitude that celebrates the abilities that everyone can bring to nursing will shine on your student's performance and promote harmony within the group. Keep in mind the following Chinese Proverb: The person who says it cannot be done should not interrupt the person who is doing it.

Students may be admitted with a wide range of disabilities. Some may have learning disabilities, hearing or vision loss, mobility limitations, chronic physical illness, or mental illness (Chickadonz, Beach, & Fox 1983; Creamer, 2003; Eliason,

1992; Huyer, 2003; Kolanko, 2003; Maheady, 1999, 2003, 2006; Pischke-Winn, Andreoli, & Halstead, 2003; Styrcula, 2003; Watkins, 2002; World, 2007).

This chapter presents practical information and teaching strategies that will benefit **all** students. It includes a review of admission and retention standards, people-first language, universal instructional design, and reasonable accommodations. Inclusion-building activities are presented along with learning activities for nursing educators. Case examples address accommodations that may need to be considered for a nursing student with hearing loss, learning disability, Crohn's disease, spinal cord injury, and mental illness. An example of an Individualized Nursing Education Program is included along with current and future resources for nursing students with disabilities and for faculty.

## Examples

A nursing program admitted a student born with spina bifida. The student used a wheelchair throughout the program and accommodations were made that included assigning a nursing student "buddy" to work with the student in clinical settings. The student negotiated with other nursing students when she needed help and in return she helped others when needed. She went on to graduate and now works as a registered nurse on the pediatric unit of a noted rehabilitation institute. Patients call her their "cool nurse on wheels" because she uses a wheelchair just like they do (Maheady, 2006).

Another nursing program admitted two students with significant hearing losses. The nursing students were accommodated with sign language interpreters and captioned videos. In addition, the professor's notes were provided to the sign language interpreters 2 to 3 days before the class presentation. Both students graduated and secured employment as nurses (McElyea, 2005).

A nurse born with one hand was admitted to nursing school over 20 years ago. She has practiced in a wide range of clinical areas and currently teaches nursing in Washington (Maheady, 2006). A DVD titled "Nursing with the Hand You are Given: A Message of Hope for Nursing Students with Disabilities" demonstrates nursing skills this nurse is able to perform with one hand (injections, gloves, dressing change, lifting a patient, tying a patient gown). A step by step demonstration of how the nurse dons sterile gloves is also available (Maheady & Fleming, 2005). You can order/preview the DVD at: http://nursing.wsu.edu/IAT/tv.html.

Another nursing student born with one arm was admitted to a nursing program and is working on a medical-surgical unit of an acute care hospital. Faculty and teaching assistants supported her with extended time in the nursing skills lab, and helped her identify adaptations that worked for her individual needs (Miller, 2006).

Nursing students with vision loss have also been admitted to nursing programs (Buttrell, 2007; Maheady, 2006). Accommodations included large print exams, computer screen magnification (Zoomtext), syringe magnification devices, and extra time to become familiar with new clinical sites. One nurse uses a service dog and has been working as a Diabetic Nurse Educator for many years.

A nursing student with bipolar disorder was admitted to a nursing program. During nursing school, the student gave a first–person account to her class about her life with bipolar disorder. Following her presentation, the student perceived her friends were more compassionate at clinicals and had greater understanding of mental health issues (Maheady, 2006).

## Terminology: People-First Language

Over the years, the politically correct language surrounding disability issues has changed. People with cognitive deficits have moved from being called **retarded** to being called **mentally challenged**. The word **handicapped**, acceptable in the past, is now discouraged and is often referred to as the "h" word. **Disability** is the most generally accepted term, not **handicap**. Descriptive terms change and we all have a responsibility to stay current. Referring to people with disabilities using people-first language is most important. As educators, we should refer to a student with a disability as a student first. Students with disabilities should never be referred to as the "deaf student" or the "wheelchair student." A more appropriate description would be a nursing student who is deaf (or has a hearing loss), or a student who uses a wheelchair. Above all, students are students first.

## Admission and Retention in Schools of Nursing

The exact number of students with disabilities applying to nursing programs or retained in programs is difficult to ascertain. With the passage of laws that protect the rights of persons with disabilities (Rehabilitation Act of 1973, Americans with Disabilities Act [1990]) and the general change in attitude toward people with disabilities, the numbers should continue to increase.

Magilvy and Mitchell (1995) surveyed baccalaureate nursing (BSN) and associate degree nursing (ADN) programs in an attempt to describe the extent to which nursing programs admit and graduate students with disabilities. They found that most of the schools surveyed had contact with students with visual, hearing, or mobility impairments, learning disabilities, and mental or chronic illnesses. Learning disabilities and mental impairment were cited most frequently. Schools also report having experiences with students with other disabilities including paralysis, chronic illness, back injuries, and scoliosis (Bueche & Haxton, 1983; Chickadonz, Beach & Fox, 1983; Maheady, 1999; Maheady, 2003).

Watson (1995) surveyed 247 BSN programs to determine their responses to applicants with disabilities. This survey revealed that almost half of the nursing programs studied admitted students with disabilities. The most prevalent disabilities were dyslexia and other learning disabilities.

Admission and retention policies differ among nursing programs. Decisions regarding admission of students with disabilities into nursing programs typically have been made on a case-by-case basis. Therefore, inconsistencies in admission policies are found. For example, a nursing student who uses a wheelchair was admitted to a large state university. In the same year, a nursing student with a chronic illness was denied admission to an ADN program in another state.

Sowers and Smith (2002) found that including physical attributes as admission standards results in students who cannot hear, see, or speak being excluded from nursing programs. These authors recommend that admission criteria focus on essential functions and technical standards of specific behaviors that nursing students are expected to perform. For example, an essential function may be "detecting a heart murmur." A student who is hard of hearing may be able to detect a heart murmur using an amplified stethoscope and a student who is deaf may use a stethoscope that provides visual output. These students cannot hear, but they can perform the essential function with a reasonable accommodation.

Institutions can make the adjustment from physical attributes to essential functions and technical standards. For example, the University of Oklahoma College of Nursing developed guidelines based on the technical skills necessary to perform cardiopulmonary resuscitation (CPR). These guidelines included:

- Visual acuity to identify cyanosis
- Hearing ability to understand normal speech without viewing the speaker's face
- Physical ability to perform CPR
- Speaking ability to question patients about their condition
- Manual dexterity to draw up solution in a syringe (Weatherby & Moran, 1989)

The Southern Regional Education Board Council on Collegiate Education for Nursing (2004) revised their core performance standards to assist nursing educators to develop proactive responses to support students covered by the Americans with Disabilities Act (www.sreb.org/programs/nursing/publications/adareport.asp). The core performance standards for admission and progression address the following issues:

- Critical thinking
- Interpersonal communication
- Mobility
- Motor skills
- Hearing
- Visual acuity
- Tactile ability

Educators often cite safety concerns as a reason for denying admission to a student with a disability. Sowers and Smith (2002) report there is no data to suggest that healthcare professionals with disabilities pose any greater safety risk to patients than healthcare professionals without disabilities. Good nurses, good nursing students, and good educators recognize their limitations and know when to ask for help. Knowing what you can do and what you cannot do is fundamental to nursing practice. Patient safety is fundamental to nursing practice. These facts do not change because a student has a disability; it may mean, however, that the end is reached in a nontraditional way.

## Disability Awareness Activities

Prior to the start of each academic year, it may be helpful for faculty to participate in a disability awareness in-service program. Often, the campus disability services office or counseling center may lead such a program. All colleges and universities that receive federal funds must provide equal access to the consumer of the services. Some entity on campus is responsible for providing academic accommodations for students with disabilities. It may be the disability services office, counseling center, or human resources office. Students, faculty, and staff also should be made aware of campus resources for people with disabilities. Areas covered in an in-service program might include:

- Services offered by the disability service office
- Legal entitlements of students with disabilities
- Information about incoming students with disabilities

The in-service program may also include simulation activities that allow people an opportunity to "experience" a disability. Be aware that views vary on the benefit of simulation-type activities for people without disabilities. One belief is that exercises like using a wheelchair or wearing a blindfold do little to help a person understand the disabilities. The exercises are thought to be damaging and reinforce negative stereotypes. Another view is that simulation activities can be beneficial. It is best for faculty to work in consultation with the institution's disability services staff. Simulation activities may include:

- Using a wheelchair
- Wearing dark glasses
- Wearing headphones
- Listening to a taped simulation of a person with schizophrenia hearing auditory hallucinations
- Taking an oral spelling test while wearing headphones

If deemed appropriate, faculty should consider including these types of activities for students as well as for faculty.

## Disclosure

Nursing educators need to be aware that not all students with disabilities will disclose their disability. They are scared silent. Reasons students do not disclose a disability include:

- Fear of rejection or dismissal from the program
- Students' lack of awareness that they have a disability
- Awareness that something is wrong, but lack of a formal diagnosis
- Personal reasons, such as desire for privacy
- Negative past experiences
- Naïve relative to the extent their disability will influence their work as a nursing student (Maheady, 1999)

Faculty need to be vigilant in identifying these students. Some behaviors that may indicate a disability include:

- Lip reading
- Difficulty hearing blood pressures
- Difficulty reading charts
- Incongruence between a student's performance on written examinations and application to practice

A trusting, positive relationship with a teacher can promote disclosure. Once a disability is identified, reasonable accommodations can be taken to benefit the student and – with safer nursing practice – benefit the patient.

A nursing program is under no obligation to seek out students with disabilities to determine if they need additional support. It is the student's responsibility to offer the information. Of course, an atmosphere of acceptance increases the likelihood of early disclosure of a disability.

## Promoting Self-Determination

The locus of control for a nursing student with a disability must rest with the student. Solutions to problems and issues that grant control to the student will help to promote successful outcomes. Solutions that rest primarily in the hands of faculty will reinforce co-dependency. Faculty need to work toward developing student autonomy for future clinical experiences and employment. For some new graduates, the road may be rocky; so the earlier students build confidence and coping abilities the better.

The best source for information on the impact of a disability is the person with the disability. Disability services professionals at your college or university may want third party evidence of disability and its impact to support what the student requests. But what the student reports is most important and needs to be analyzed and framed in ways that are meaningful to the accommodation process.

Structured interviews can draw out the relevant information needed to fulfill the purposes of verifying civil rights coverage and to pinpoint program modifications. If we interview students with a mind towards determining function, it's likely we will get very useful information. In fact, the information gathered directly from the student will almost certainly prove far more useful than third party evidence will. We can go beyond self-report and use professional judgment to discover relevant details. For example, ask about how the student studies, including any tools or environmental preferences or modifications involved. Consider how the student keeps track of time and conducts planning. Ask about functions such as reading, note taking, writing, and self-care. All the while, educate the student about rights and responsibilities, taking care to frame issues in terms of equality of opportunity, personal responsibility, and other disability rights and responsibilities. Expecting someone to take responsibility is a way of giving them the power they need to succeed (Marks, 2007).

# Universal Instructional Design

Originally, universal design focused on accessibility to buildings and physical spaces. Ramps were installed and handicapped parking spaces provided. The notion of universal design has broadened and is now used in the design of instruction as well as spaces. The idea is the needs of people with disabilities should encourage an instructional design that is flexible and supports diversity among learners. When instruction is designed following universal instructional design (UID) principles, it meets the needs of **all** students by providing an accessible and flexible learning environment (University of Guelph, 2003).

The Ivy Access Initiative emphasizes that UID is the "design of instructional materials and activities that allow learning goals to be achieved by individuals with wide differences in their abilities to see, hear, speak, move, read, write, understand English, attend, organize, engage, and remember" (www.brown.edu/Administration/Sheridan_Center/docs/uid.pdf, p. 1.) The University of Guelph (2003) lists seven principles of UID:

1. Be accessible and fair
2. Provide flexibility in use, participation, and presentation
3. Be straightforward and consistent
4. Be explicitly present and readily perceived
5. Provide a supportive learning environment
6. Minimize unnecessary physical effort or requirements
7. Ensure a learning space that accommodates both students and instructional methods
   www.tss.uoguelph.ca/projects/uid/UG16-implementation%20guide.pdf

Consider this example. A student with a hearing loss is attending class in a large lecture hall. The professor asks the students to form small discussion groups. This student with a hearing loss is marginalized because he cannot hear within the auditory chaos. Other marginalized students in this class include a student who uses a wheelchair who is seated in the back of the room and a student with a learning disability who works best when provided time to formulate ideas. By applying UID principles, the professor might assign questions for consideration in advance of the class, provide an asynchronous electronic forum for student contributions, use class time to debrief, and then give students time to write a reflective paper. This type of instructional design addresses the needs of this very diverse group of students.

## Accommodations

From the previous discussion it is clear that making accommodations for students with disabilities is advantageous for all students. These accommodations enhance teaching, decrease barriers, and make learning more accessible for all students in the class. Educators have long been aware that students learn and process information in different ways. There are visual, sensory, auditory, and tactile learners. This knowledge is expanded to include the fact that students can also demonstrate knowledge in different ways.

Keep in mind that an accommodation provided to a student with a disability only ensures access; it is not a guarantee of success. The Rehabilitation Act and the Americans with Disabilities Act were meant to "level the playing field" (Matt, 2003). The case law continues to evolve. Documentation from the student must indicate evidence the disability substantially limits a major life activity, such as learning. The mandate to provide reasonable accommodations does not extend to adjustments that would "fundamentally alter" the nature of the course, or course requirements. There is no law against a student asking, but asking does not automatically mean the request is a reasonable accommodation. Some schools may not have the required financial resources to accommodate the disability.

Keep in mind the laws are a floor, not a ceiling, and they do not prohibit the institution – or the faculty – from doing **more** for a student with a disability if it is appropriate. Educators can make a student's life better, even if the law does not require it. Through accommodations and extra effort, we can build relationships, foster goodwill, and provide value-added programs that exceed the norm.

## Individualized Nursing Education Programs

Students with disabilities who are educated in public schools benefit from individualized education programs under the provisions of the Individuals with Disabilities Education Act, formerly called PL 94-142 or the Education for all Handicapped Children Act of 1975. This provision can be applied to nursing students with disabilities.

Accommodations may be simple or complex and can range from an alternate examination format or time extension to a scribe or sign language interpreter. Accommodations for a disability are not "one size fits all." An effective individualized program requires teamwork and cooperation to promote the student's success. An individualized nursing education program can serve as a practical guide that describes the student's needs, identifies who is responsible for what, and promotes accountability (Maheady, 2003).

The student, faculty, and a representative from the institution's office of students with disabilities should meet as often as needed to assess the student's abilities, limitations, and needed accommodations. All information must be kept confidential, and all participants should receive a copy of the program.

Every nursing student with a disability will have different needs and circumstances. Examples of accommodations that might be included in an individualized nursing student's program are listed in Table 1.

- Amplified stethoscope to assess heart and lung sounds
- Stethoscope with visual output to visualize heart and lung sounds
- Pocket talker (device that amplifies sound in a one-on-one interaction)
- Telecommunication devices (TDDs or TTYs)
- Computer assisted real-time transcription (CART) services
- Note taker or reader
- Captioned films, videos or DVD's
- Assistive listening systems frequency modulated (FM)
- Digital blood pressure monitors
- Digital thermometers
- Face-to-face report in place of taped report
- Amplified telephone
- Lowered desk to accommodate a wheelchair
- Regularly scheduled breaks
- Sign language interpreter
- Audio taped lectures
- Extended time or a quiet room for examinations
- Visual enlarger
- Large-print books and materials, books on tape
- Scribe (person who serves as a person's hands if their disability makes it difficult for them to write, or perform tasks)
- Dragon speak (utility that turns speech into text when using a computer)

**Table 1.** Types of Accommodations

Developing an individualized program involves more than equipment and personnel. Additional information that should be included in the program includes:

- Current performance (GPA and SAT scores, letters of recommendation, observations and assessments from nursing faculty)
- Letter from the student's physician
- Annual goals and short-term objectives
- Related services (supplementary aids, services, modifications to the program eg., tutor, note taker, textbooks recorded on audiotape, computer assisted real-time transcription [CART], sign language, or oral interpreter)
- Technological devices, including voice recognition software and assistive listening devices
- Testing (additional time, oral, or alternative format, use of a calculator or computer)
- Dates and places (when services will be provided and where)
- Transition services, including preparation for the National Council Licensing Examination (NCLEX®), employment counseling, preceptorship programs
- Measuring progress through midterm and final evaluations

The following story demonstrates the importance of an individualized plan.

A nursing student had been allowed extended time for all her exams due to a documented learning disability. She is now in a clinical course learning to give injections. She is assigned a preoperative patient. She draws up the preoperative medication, walks to the patient's room, prepares the patient, inserts the needle, and freezes. The student was alarmed to discover that she did not have an extended time for performing this procedure.

This example demonstrates why it is important for an individualized plan to look at the total picture and reinforce to the student when, where, and under what circumstances specific accommodations apply.

An individualized assessment and program is imperative. Appendix 1 provides an example of an individualized nursing program focused on meeting the needs of one student with a disability.

## Case Examples

This section presents a number of short case examples. Following each example, suggestions for teaching strategies are offered.

## Case Example: Nursing Student with Hearing Loss

Maria is a junior-level student in a baccalaureate nursing program. She has a documented profound hearing loss. She reads lips and uses sign language. She has disclosed her disability and the disability services office is providing a sign language interpreter to attend classroom and clinical experiences with her. How can faculty help Maria meet the objectives of the lecture course? The following suggestions may be helpful:

- Allow the student to sit in the front of the classroom and tape lectures if desired
- Face the class, enunciate well, speak at a moderate pace, and avoid covering your mouth
- Avoid standing in front of windows or other light sources
- Provide handouts of material presented and list new vocabulary terms using a projection system
- Provide announcements, test dates, or schedule changes on paper, online, or in the classroom via a projection system
- Wear a transmitter used with an assistive listening device if needed
- Speak to the student, not the interpreter
- Provide scripts of movies or videos shown in class

During lecture classes, the student's listening can be assisted with the use of personal and group frequency modulated (FM) systems, loop systems, infrared systems, and hardwire systems. These systems use a transmitter worn by the professor and a receiver worn by the student.

It is also important to be sure all students are included in group activities. To facilitate inclusion assign students to small groups by drawing numbers from a hat. This decreases the potential the student with a disability will feel left out or be picked last by classmates.

Clinical experiences present additional challenges to a successful outcome for this student. The following are some suggestions to promote success:

- Inform the charge nurse, patients, and appropriate staff members about the student's hearing loss
- Provide the student with handouts of information presented verbally to the clinical group
- Encourage the student to purchase a special amplified and/or electronic stethoscope that best meets her individual needs
- Establish a mutually agreed upon system of communication between the faculty and the student

- Facilitate patient, staff, and peer acceptance; serve as an acceptance bridge
- Provide ongoing assessments of the student's hearing related to clinical skills – blood pressure, heart and lung sounds, monitors, alarms, patients' calls for help
- Encourage the student to practice using "99," an examination technique used to elicit vocal or tactile palpable vibrations through the bronchopulmonary system to the chest wall, as part of respiratory assessment
- Instruct the student to place all monitors in clear view to facilitate "seeing" a beeping monitor
- Assess the student's need for an amplified telephone in the clinical area
- Ask all students to speak from the front of the room instead of using a roundtable format for postconferences

There is a wide range of stethoscopes available for people with hearing loss. One is pictured in Figure 1. (More information about that specific device is available at the Cardionics website, www.cardionics.com.) There are headphone styles, amplified and electronic stethoscopes, and patch cords for people with cochlear implants. Cardionics, Welch Allyn, and 3M Littman are some of the companies that manufacture special stethoscopes. In addition, a software program called Pocket Monitor records, displays, and plays back physiologic sounds. The software, available from Cardionics can be installed on a personal digital assistant (PDA). Because of the wide range of products available, an audiologist should be consulted regarding the most appropriate stethoscope for a particular student's needs.

## Case Example: Student with a Learning Disability

John is a first-year student in an associate degree nursing program. He has a documented learning disability with difficulty reading and spelling words – particularly medical terms. Helping this student be successful may involve the following:
- Referral to the office for students with disabilities and the local association for students with learning disabilities; staff members will be able to recommend resources and learning strategies
- Recommendations for studying, such as reading charts in a particular order, highlighting in different colors, or using flashcards
- Accommodations such as the use of Franklin's eBookMan® with med-spell lookup or software such as Dragon Naturally Speaking
- Books on tape
- Permission to tape lectures

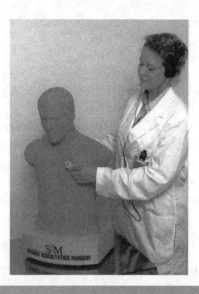

**Figure 1.** Special Stethoscopes

Butler (2000) suggests some creative devices for remembering how to spell medical terms. These suggestions may be helpful to all nursing students. For example:

- **Asthma.** Think of the first letters of the words in the sentence *Ann Seems To Have Many Attacks*. Imagine Ann having asthma attacks.
- **Coronary.** Deliberately pronounce the different parts of the word cor/on/ary. Coronary contains the letters **ron**. Think of poor Ron with coronary problems.
- **Pneumo.** Take each letter of the word and make up a silly sentence with words beginning with those letters; link the sentence to a picture in your mind. *Please Never Ever Use My Oboe*. Imagine filling your lungs to blow into an oboe.
- **Psycho.** *Please Say You Can Help Out*.

**Study buddy.** A study buddy may be helpful for this student. Some schools provide study buddies through the office of students with disabilities. A buddy may meet individually with 8 to 10 students once a week during the term, helping students adhere to a schedule for completing projects and assignments on time or with minimal extended time. They can also assist by:

- Ensuring the students allow enough study time for exams and required reading
- Helping the students schedule time during the week for leisure activities, workouts at the gym, sleep, and rest between classes
- Identifying other ways the students can make things work

The buddy keeps students on target with their weekly schedule. A WatchMinder may be helpful for a student who has problems with time management (www.watchminder.com). Using a vibration system like that of the common pager, the device privately alerts the wearer when it is time for a particular task. This device includes 75 preprogrammed messages including reminders to get to class, talk to the teacher, pay attention, turn in an assignment, relax, get help, study, or check e-mail.

## Case Example: Student with Crohn's Disease

Helen is a senior in a baccalaureate nursing program. She has documented Crohn's disease. She is receiving accommodations because of frequent clinical absences due to hospitalizations. Faculty allow her to make up the clinical time and submit papers later than other students. One day, another nursing student confronts Helen in the restroom and says, "You get away with doing so much less! No matter how much time you are absent you still end up with an A in the course. The rest of us can't miss a minute without a penalty!" Helen reports this incident to you. How might you respond to this situation?

The best way to avoid situations like this is to be proactive and institute a zero-tolerance policy for harassment of any student, including students with disabilities. With a written policy in place, this matter can be addressed as unprofessional behavior under the professional conduct code.

Nursing students and faculty need to be aware that educational institutions have a responsibility to ensure equal educational opportunities for all students, including those with disabilities. This is a legal mandate under the Rehabilitation Act of 1973 and the Americans with Disabilities Act of 1990. The laws are enforced by the Office for Civil Rights. Harassing conduct can take different forms, such as:
- Verbal, such as name calling
- Nonverbal, such as written statements
- Physical threats or humiliation

Students and faculty must recognize that students demonstrate learning in different ways or, in this case, different time frames, but that does not mean the standards have been lowered. Faculty can help students with disabilities deal with these kinds of behaviors. These students can be encouraged to role play and rehearse responses to possible negative comments or situations.

## Case Example: A Student Who Uses a Wheelchair in a Clinical Course

Michelle suffered a spinal cord injury from a skiing accident. Her lifelong passion was to become a nurse. She has been admitted to your nursing program. How can you help this student achieve success in an acute care setting?

Michelle's individual nursing education program might include many supports and accommodations. First, Michelle's abilities and limitations should be comprehensively assessed; then, the following may be recommended:

- Inform appropriate staff of the student's disability prior to the beginning of the clinical rotation
- Tour the facility with the student before the rotation starts; introduce the student to staff members
- Identify accessible hospital units with accessible patient rooms
- Assign the student to patients with adjustable IV poles
- Collaborate with staff members and the student to establish a plan of action if a patient needs CPR
- Assign student buddies or arrange for an intermediary to assist the student with patient care – lifting, turning, bathing, and treatments
- Allow the student to negotiate, barter, or trade-off tasks with assigned buddy to facilitate the student sharing the workload
- Provide a communication device, such as a cell phone or walkie-talkie, to help the student stay in touch with the teacher
- Request the student practice positioning a patient with a transfer sheet in the nursing lab
- Ask the student to use the seat belt on her wheelchair
- Request that the student practice performing wound care, catheterization, and treatments on a mannequin in a bed set at varying heights
- Encourage the student to carry extra gloves to wear after touching the wheels on the wheelchair

A student using a wheelchair must make adaptations to the way patient care is typically performed. For example, a dressing change might include these steps:

**Set up for dressing change, wash hands, glove, wheel to patient, remove gloves, and replace with a new pair. Do not touch wheelchair.**

Another example relates to emptying a bedpan. Encourage the student to practice emptying a bedpan by placing a chux on her lap and slowly carrying the bedpan to the bathroom.

Provide a diverse range of opportunities for students to demonstrate nursing skills. Diverse approaches may include hands-on whenever possible but also verbal and written assignments, developing diagrams, and completing computer simulations. Ask the student to talk through a procedure step-by-step. Let the student be the guide as someone else carries out the actions. Assign the student to direct CPR as another student in the clinical group performs the steps, or assign the student to be the recorder in a mock CPR demonstration.

To ensure inclusion of this student into the group, rotate student buddies every clinical day. Assign students to give a brief presentation during postconference. Students may choose to present a skill they feel confident in performing. Michelle may volunteer to present teaching patients transfer skills or self-catheterization. Another skill that Michelle might present is how a nurse in a wheelchair must organize and arrange equipment to be within reach when changing a dressing.

## Case Example: A Student with Mental Illness

Bianca is a junior level student in a nursing program. She has been diagnosed with a mental illness. Her physician reports she is undergoing psychotherapy and is taking medication regularly. She has difficulty taking examinations in a large classroom because she is easily distracted. Bianca also has difficulty completing examinations in the established time frame. Her physician states her reading comprehension is compromised. Accommodations suggested by her physician include a quiet room and extended time to complete exams.

How can you as faculty assist this student to be successful on examinations? Referral to the office of students with disabilities is the first step. Documentation from her physician, including multi-axial DSM-IV Diagnosis, medications, therapeutic interventions, and prognosis should be required. The following would then be suggested:

- Allow her to take her examinations in a quiet room in the office of students with disabilities or the campus testing center
- Permit the student to have additional time to complete examinations
- Recognize and anticipate periods of academic inactivity—stopouts versus dropouts
- Refer the student to the school's counseling center if indicated
- Refer the student to the local mental health organization

## The NCLEX®

Nursing students need to plan ahead if they need accommodations to take the NCLEX® examination. In compliance with the Americans with Disabilities Act (1990), state boards of nursing provide reasonable accommodation for applicants with disabilities that may affect their ability to take the NCLEX®.

Applicants need to contact their state board of nursing **early** to learn the procedure for requesting accommodations. Policies and procedures vary from state to state. In most states, the board of nursing members review applications for accommodations. Decisions are made on a case-by-case basis. Timing is important because these decisions are made during the state board of nursing meetings, which may occur monthly or less often.

In most instances, the state board of nursing asks the applicant to supply a letter verifying diagnosis from an appropriate medical professional or professional evaluator to confirm the disability and provide information about the type of accommodation required. The board usually asks for a letter from the nursing program that indicates what modifications, if any, were granted by the program.

Accommodations that might be requested by an applicant include:
- Additional time to take the test
- Adjustable-height table
- Enlarged keyboard
- Sign language interpreter
- Modifiable colors for item text and background
- Adjustable swivel arm for keyboard
- Screen magnification software

## Future Resources

The future promises to provide more and improved technology to assist people with disabilities. One product under development is a clear face mask for people who read lips (Carroll, 2002).

Some products designed for patients with disabilities may prove helpful to nurses as well.

Talking pill bottles provide audible label information. This concept may prove helpful to nurses with vision loss. (www.rxtalks.com)

Figure 2 shows a wheelchair accessible examination table currently available. Greater availability and reduction in the cost of this type of equipment will assist nurses in practice areas in the future.

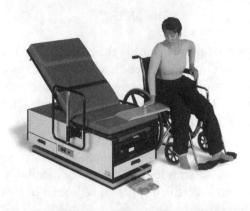

**Figure 2.** Wheelchair Accessible Exam table by Hausmann Industries, Inc.

Mandatory use of patient lifting devices and no lift or safer handling policies benefit nurses with lifting restrictions.

## Summary

Disability is part of life and part of our practice as nurses and educators. Nurses are experts in helping patients rebuild their lives following a disability, and are experienced in writing care plans, critical pathways, and care maps to direct the process. Nursing educators can do the same for students with disabilities.

Students with disabilities can enrich the nursing profession through their experience living with disabilities. They add value to health care. An open mind and positive attitude do much to dispel the myth that every nurse has to have a strong back, perfect vision, and excellent hearing. With appropriate support and reasonable accommodations, nursing students with disabilities can be successful without compromising patient safety. When you receive your next application or request for an accommodation from a student with a disability instead of thinking "No way," think "Why not?" Through your students you, other nurses, and patients will be taught!

# Resources

Following are URLs for websites that contain a wealth of information about students with disabilities. Please visit these websites for more information. These URLs are included on the CD that accompanies this book.

American Foundation for the Blind/Career Connect
http://www.afb.org/Section.asp?SectionID=7
A resource for people who want to learn about jobs performed by adults who are blind or visually impaired. Click on Explore Careers (Registered Nurses).

Association on Higher Education and Disability
www.ahead.org
An international organization of professionals committed to full participation in higher education for persons with disabilities.

Association of Medical Professionals with Hearing Losses
www.amphl.org
Information, advocacy, and network for individuals with hearing loss who are interested in working in health care.

Association of Nurses in AIDS Care (ANAC)
www.anacnet.org
ANAC has a newsletter and committee for nurses and students who are HIV-positive.

Boston University Center for Psychiatric Rehabilitation
www.bu.edu/cpr/reasaccom
This online resource offers employers and educators guidance on reasonable accommodation for people with psychiatric disabilities.

ExceptionalNurse.com
www.exceptionalnurse.com
ExceptionalNurse.com is a nonprofit resource network for nursing students and nurses with disabilities. It provides links to disability-related organizations, technology, equipment, financial aid, employment opportunities, legal resources, mentors, and research.

Job Accommodation Network
www.jan.wvu.edu/media/nurses.html
A service of the U.S. Department of Labor provides information about job accommodations and the Americans with Disabilities Act (ADA).

HEATH Resource Center, American Council on Education
www.heath.gwu.edu
HEATH is a national clearinghouse on postsecondary education for individuals with disabilities.

National Library Service for the Blind and Physically Handicapped, Library of Congress
www.loc.gov/nls
This service provides free recorded and braille reading materials to persons with visual or physical impairments that prevent the reading of standard print. Contact the reference section.

Office for Civil Rights (OCR), U.S. Department of Education
www.ed.gov/ocr
OCR can answer questions related to Section 504 of the Rehabilitation Act of 1973.

PEPNet
www.pepnet.org
PEPNet helps postsecondary institutions attract and serve individuals who are deaf or hard of hearing.

Recording for the Blind and Dyslexic
www.rfbd.org/
Provides taped educational books free on loan, books on CD, library services, and other educational and professional resources to individuals who cannot read standard print because of a visual, physical, or perceptual disability

Western University of Health Sciences
www.westernu.edu/xp/edu/cdihp/about.xml
The Center for Disabilities and the Health Professions was established in response to the concerns of the disabled community.

## Learning Activities

1. Design an individualized nursing education program with reasonable accommodations for a nursing student whose right arm is six inches long. She is having difficulty putting on sterile gloves.
2. A student with cerebral palsy affecting her left side is having difficulty starting an IV due to decreased function in her left hand. She learned to compensate by using her strongest finger, her thumb, to stabilize the IV bag against a table. How could learning about the student's ability to overcome this challenge benefit other nursing students, patients, nursing educators, and nurses?
3. Write a personal reflection paper on the following: Imagine that you become disabled and are unable to practice nursing as you did in the past. What accommodations would you expect from your employer and fellow colleagues? Put this paper in a safe place. Read it again if you ever become disabled or are confronted with making accommodations for a nursing colleague or nursing student.
4. Discuss the concept of "reasonable accommodations." What accommodations could be implemented for a student with a lifting restriction?

## Educational Philosophy

My philosophy is focused on inclusion and has evolved from my advocacy work for people with disabilities. I believe that all nursing students have the potential to learn and that nursing education programs need to provide equal access to students with disabilities. Inclusion of students with disabilities benefits patients, educators, nurses, and other students. Providing accommodations for students with disabilities enhances the teaching/learning experience for everyone. Nursing educators should welcome students with disabilities to the nursing students' table. — Donna Carol Maheady

## References

*Americans with Disabilities Act.* (1990). Public Law, No. 101-336, 42 U.S.C. 12101.

Bueche, M. N., & Haxton, D. (1983). The student with a hearing loss: Coping strategies. *Nurse Educator, 8*(4), 7-11.

Butler, S. (2000). *Common medical words with spelling tips*. Retrieved January 9, 2008, from Anglia Polytechnic University website: http://www.hcp-disability. org.uk/dyslexia/Papers/Medspelltips.doc

Buttrell, S. M. (2007, May) Nurses with Disabilities: A Phenomenological Study of Nurses Who Are Blind. Thesis, Master of Nursing, Washington State University.

Carroll, S. (2002, Winter). Progress with clear face mask project. *Journal of the Association of Medical Professionals with Hearing Losses, 1*(1). Retrieved February 2, 2004, from http://www.amphl.org/jamphl/fall2002/cordwellcarroll.html.

Carroll, S. (2004). Inclusion of people with physical disabilities in nursing education. *Journal of Nursing Education, 43*(5), 206 – 213.

Chickadoz, H. H., Beach, E. K., & Fox, J. A. (1983). Educating a deaf nursing student. *Nursing Health Care, 4*, 327-333.

Creamer, B. (2003, December). Wheelchair fails to deter paraplegic from nurse's life. *Honolulu Advertiser*. Retrieved January 9, 2008 from http://the.honoluluadvertiser.com/article/2003/Dec/28/ln/ln10a.html

*Education for All Handicapped Children Act* (1975), 20 U.S.C. 1400 et seq.

Eliason, M. (1992). Nursing students with learning disabilities: Appropriate accommodations. *Journal of Nursing Education, 31*(8), 375-376.

Fleming, S., & Maheady, D. (2004). Empowering people with disabilities. *Lifelines, 8*(6), 535-537. Retrieved February 12, 2008 from http://exceptionalnurse.com/empoweringpersons.pdf

Huyer, S. (2003, April). The gift of ADD. *Advance for Nurse Practitioners, 11*(4), 92. Retrieved December 31, 2007 from http://nurse-practitioners.advanceweb.com/Editorial/Search/AViewer.aspx?AN=NP_03apr1_npp92.html&AD=04-01-2003

*Individuals with Disabilities Education Act* (1990), 20 U.S.S. 1400 et seq.

Ivy Access Initiative *Implementing Universal Instructional Design in College Courses*. Retrieved April 4, 2009, 2008 from http://www.brown.edu/Administration/Sheridan_Center/docs/uid.pdf

Kolanko, K. (2003.) A collective case study of nursing students with learning disabilities. *Nursing Education Perspectives, 24*(5), 251–256.

Magilvy, J. L., & Mitchell, A. C. (1995). Education of nurses with special needs. *Journal of Nursing Education, 34*(1), 31-36.

Maheady, D. (1999). Jumping through hoops, walking on eggshells: The experiences of nursing students with disabilities. *Journal of Nursing Education, 38*(4), 162-170.

Maheady, D. (2003). *Nursing students with disabilities change the course.* River Edge, New Jersey: Exceptional Parent Press.

Maheady, D. & Fleming, S. (2005, Spring). Homework for future nursing students. *Minority Nurse.* Retrieved December 28, 2007, from http://www.minoritynurse.com/features/undergraduate/05-25-05a.html

Maheady, D. & Fleming, S. (2005, Summer). Nursing with the hand you are given. Minority Nurse. Retrieved January 23, 2008, from http://www.minoritynurse.com/features/undergraduate/08-02-05d.html

Maheady, D. (2006). *Leave no nurse behind: Nurses working with disAbilities.* Lincoln, NE: iUniverse.

Marks, J. (2007, October 23). ADHD documentation. Message posted to Disabled Student Services in Higher Education, archived at http://listserv.buffalo.edu/archives/dsshe-l.html

Matt, S. B. (2003, May 1). Reasonable accommodation: What does the law really require? *Journal of the Association of Medical Professional with Hearing Losses, 1.* Retrieved February 3, 2004, from http://www.amphl.org/protected/summer2003/matt2003.html

McElyea, M. (2005). *When your student is Deaf.* Retrieved January 5, 2008 from http://www.exceptionalnurse.com/DeafStudent2.pdf

Miller, K. (2006, Spring). Willing and Able: Encouragement and adaptations help nursing student overcome disability. *Medical College of Georgia Today.* Retrieved January 9, 2008 from http://www.mcg.edu/news/mcgtoday/Spr06/story11.htm

Persaud, D., & Leedom, C. L. (2002). The American with Disabilities Act: Effect on student admission and retention practices in California nursing schools. *Journal of Nursing Education, 41*(8), 349-352.

Pischke-Winn, K., Andreoli, K., & Halstead, L. (2003) *Students with disabilities: Nursing education and practice.* Retrieved January 9, 2008 from http://www.rushu.rush.edu/nursing/studisable.html

Rehabilitation Act. (1973). P.L. 93-112, Title 5, Section 504, 87 Stat.355 29 VSC Section 794.

Southern Regional Education Board Council on Collegiate Education for Nursing (2004). The Americans with Disabilities Act: Implications for Nursing Education. Retrieved February 5, 2008 from http://www.sreb.org/programs/nursing/publications/adareport.asp

Sowers, J., & Smith, M. (2002). Disability as difference. *Journal of Nursing Education, 41*(8), 331- 332.

Sowers, J., & Smith, M. (2004).Nursing faculty members' perceptions, knowledge, and concerns about students with disabilities. *Journal of Nursing Education, 43*(5), 213–218.

Styrcula, L. (2003). Disabled, not incapable: Students with disabilities can become nurses, too. *Nursing Spectrum*. Retrieved January 6, 2004, from http://www.nursingspectrum.com

University of Guelph. (2003). Universal Instructional Design Implementation Guide. Retrieved February 8, 2008 from http://www.tss.uoguelph.ca/projects/uid/UG16-implementation%20guide.pdf

Watkins, M. (2002). Disabled nursing students overcome challenges. *Nursing Spectrum*. Retrieved January. 9, 2008, from http://community.nursingspectrum.com/magazinearticles/article.cfm?AID=7550

Watson, G. (1995). Nursing students with disabilities: A survey of baccalaureate nursing programs. *Journal of Professional Nursing, 11*(3), 147-153.

Weatherby, F., & Moran, M. (1989, July/Aug.). Admission criteria for handicapped students. *Nursing Outlook, 37*(4), 179-181.

World, H. (2007). RNs in Wheelchairs Face Challenges During and After Nursing School. *Nurse.com*. Retrieved December 28, 2007, from http://news.nurse.com/apps/pbcs.dll/article?AID=/20070730/ILLINOIS09/707240303/1005/ILLINOIS

# Appendix 1
## Example of an Individualized Nursing Education Program

**Name:** Jeanne           **Date:** August, 2008

**Disability:** Student had a back injury and surgery on her spine. She has a weight lifting restriction of no more than 3 to 5 pounds per physician's order. She has no hearing in her left ear.

**Current Performance:** A junior in the baccalaureate nursing program, she is a returning student. She was admitted one year ago, and then withdrew for medical reasons. Her grade point average is 3.6. Faculty clinical evaluations of the student are excellent.

**Impact on Academic Program:** Student's back injury and physician's restriction of lifting no more than 3 to 5 pounds may impact clinical nursing courses, particularly objectives/nursing skills related to lifting patients, bathing patients, making beds, and performing cardiopulmonary resuscitation (CPR). Student's hearing loss may impact clinical nursing courses, particularly objectives related to nursing skills such as listening to blood pressures and heart sounds; auscultating lungs; hearing monitors, alarms, patients' calls for help, telephones, and taped reports.

Student's back injury and hearing loss may impact participation in lecture courses. This student may need front-row seating, permission to stand during lectures, taped lectures, handouts, note taker, and an assistive listening device. The office for students with disabilities may need to provide a remote control opener for heavy doors that are not automatic, note taker, assistive listening device. Because her last nursing course was one year ago, office of students with disabilities also might need to provide a tutor.

**Assessments:** Assessments by nursing faculty included evaluation of the student's ability to lift patients, make beds, bend down, and perform CPR. The student was found to use appropriate body mechanics, but would not be able to move heavy patients in bed given her weight lifting restrictions. It would be difficult for her to perform CPR without injuring herself.

The student's hearing was evaluated, specifically her ability to hear blood pressures and breath and heart sounds. Tapes of lung and heart sounds and a double-sided stethoscope were used. The student did not hear heart and lung sounds appropriately and was unable to hear blood pressure with a regular stethoscope. The student states she can hear material presented in lecture courses if she is allowed to sit in the front of the classroom. She states that she does not need a note taker or assistive listening device at the present time. She does not use sign language. A letter from her physician documenting her limitations and hearing loss is on file.

**Assistive Technology:** The student agrees to purchase a special stethoscope. She will consider using an assistive listening device in lectures if front row seating is ineffective.

**Short-term Goal:** Student will maintain an average grade of C or better at midterm in all nursing courses. Course work will include examinations, papers, projects, and demonstrations of clinical skills. Clinical courses will include a written evaluation by the faculty and signed by the student.

**Annual Goal:** Student will receive a final passing grade of C or better in all nursing courses. Coursework will include examinations, papers, projects, and demonstrations of clinical skills. Clinical courses will include a written evaluation by the faculty member, signed by the student. The student will meet all university requirements.

**Accommodations, Supports, and Related Services—Faculty Advisor Responsibilities**
- Refer student to campus office of students with disabilities
- Refer student to campus financial aid office
- Refer student to state vocational rehabilitation program to explore eligibility for benefits and possible funding sources for special stethoscope
- Refer student to vendors for special stethoscopes, back supports (with physician's order), and rolling suitcase for books
- Refer student to local deaf services/hearing loss organization

**Clinical Courses:** Objectives related to nursing skills: listening to heart sounds, breath sounds, blood pressures, alarms, monitors, patients' calls for help.

**Student Responsibilities (related to hearing loss)**
- Report hearing loss to clinical faculty before clinical experience begins
- Purchase special stethoscope
- Bring special stethoscope to all clinical experiences

- Report hearing loss to primary or charge nurse on unit of hospital or healthcare agency
- Request verbal report on assigned patient(s) if report is taped
- Position all patient monitors in clear view
- Inform assigned patient(s) about hearing loss
- Monitor assigned patient every 10 to 15 minutes, or more often if needed
- Assess blood pressure with special stethoscope and digital blood pressure machine when available
- Ask faculty or primary nurse to verify student assessments of patient's heart and lung sounds and blood pressure
- Schedule time with lab faculty to practice use of "99" when assessing a patient's lungs

## Student Responsibilities (related to back injury)
- Purchase back support (with physician recommendation)
- Bring back support to all clinical experiences
- Purchase rolling suitcase to transport books and equipment
- Schedule appointment with lab faculty to practice body mechanics
- Report weight lifting restriction to primary or charge nurse
- Collaborate with primary or charge nurse regarding limitations, establish a plan of action if CPR must be performed
- Work with assigned buddy or intermediary, or ask for help when indicated, eg, turning patients, bathing patients, making beds

## Faculty Responsibilities (clinical courses)
- Inform hospital/clinic charge nurse and appropriate staff members about student's hearing loss and weight lifting restriction
- Provide student with handouts of information presented verbally to the clinical group
- Assign student to work with a student "buddy" (moving patients, baths); rotate students each day
- Establish a mutually agreed upon system of communication between the faculty and the student
- Facilitate patient, staff, and peer acceptance; serve as an acceptance bridge
- Provide ongoing assessments of student's hearing related to clinical skills (blood pressures, heart and lung sounds, monitors, alarms, patients' calls for help)
- Assess student's need for an amplified telephone on hospital units, clinics or homecare agencies

- Ask students to speak from the front of the room instead of holding roundtable discussions during postconferences

**Faculty Responsibilities (lecture courses)**
- Allow student to sit in the front of the classroom
- Allow student to stand during lecture if needed
- Allow student to tape lectures
- Provide handouts of material presented
- Enunciate words carefully and talk at a moderate pace
- Face the class and use audiovisual aids
- List new vocabulary or medical terms on the chalkboard or overhead
- Provide announcements, test dates, or changes in schedule on paper, chalkboard, or overhead
- Provide scripts or captioning of films and videos
- Wear transmitter for assistive listening device if needed

**Testing Modifications**
- Student may need an adjustable height table

**Office of Students with Disabilities**
- Provide student with note taker for lecture courses for fall and spring semesters, if needed
- Provide student with remote control for heavy non-automatic door on the main campus for fall and spring semesters
- Provide student with a tutor if needed

**Transition Needs**
- A special stethoscope will be purchased by the student
- Student may need an adjustable height table when taking the NCLEX®
- Information regarding requests for NCLEX® accommodations has been given to the student.

**Evaluation of Program**
This Individualized Nursing Education Program will be reevaluated at the end of the fall semester or earlier if indicated. The student or a faculty may request a reevaluation at anytime.

Signed by:

Student_____

Faculty _____

Dean or Director _____

Office of Students with Disabilities _____

Date_____

# UNIT 3: THE NURSING CURRICULUM

# Chapter 29: Engaging Students for Affective Learning throughout the Curriculum
*Arlene H. Morris, MSN, EdD, RN*
*& Lynn Norman, BSN, MSN, EdD, RN*

# CHAPTER 21

# CURRICULUM DESIGN AND DEVELOPMENT

## Linda Caputi, MSN, EdD, RN, CNE

The content of this chapter relates to the following major content area and subconcepts on the Certified Nurse Educator Examination Detailed Test Blueprint:

**Participate in Curriculum Design and Evaluation of Program Outcomes**
- Lead in the development of designing a curriculum
- Actively participate in the design of the curriculum to reflect: institutional philosophy and mission; current nursing and health care trends; community and societal needs
- Demonstrate knowledge of curriculum development
- Revise the curriculum based on evaluation of program outcomes; societal and health care trends; stakeholder feedback
- Update courses to reflect the philosophical and theoretical framework of the curriculum
- Design courses to reflect the philosophical and theoretical framework of the curriculum
- Analyze results of program evaluation and initiate curricular changes

## Introduction

The word curriculum means many things to many people. Faculty, working together in one curriculum, should all have the same understanding and perspective of what is meant by curriculum. Otherwise, the curriculum is often delivered in a disorganized way with both students and faculty uncertain about what the expected results are and how those results will be attained.

Many faculty arrive at their positions not having any formal education on how to build a curriculum, or, they have had little experience in developing or revising a curriculum. Most schools of nursing have a curriculum committee with various charges. However, there may also be an evaluation committee, a student success committee, an admissions committee, and many other committees. From this division of labor, the faculty may see these functions as separate when in fact they are all part of the larger concept of curriculum.

This chapter looks at the curriculum, its many parts, and how to design and develop a curriculum. The goal is to make the development and revision of curriculum work that is enjoyable and exciting rather than what is more customary among faculty – a dreaded activity that sometimes is avoided until it becomes an absolute necessity.

In this chapter two terms are used to refer to the end products of curriculum. These are **program outcomes** and **student learning outcomes**. The author uses the National League for Nursing Accreditation Commission's (NLNAC) definitions of these terms which are (NLNAC, 2008, p. 102):

- Program outcomes: Performance indicators that reflect the extent to which the purposes of the nursing education unit are achieved and by which program effectiveness is documented. Program outcomes are measurable consumer-oriented indexes designed to evaluate the degree to which the program is achieving its mission and goals. Examples include but are not limited to: program completion rates, job placement rates, licensure/certification pass rates, and program satisfaction.

- Student learning outcomes: Statements of expectation written in measurable terms that express what a student will know, do, or think at the end of a learning experience; characteristics of the student at the completion of the program. Learning outcomes are measurable learner-oriented abilities that are consistent with standards of professional practice.

## Collegiality

Curriculum development is not a static, one-time event. On the contrary, curriculum is in a state of constant change. This constant change requires nursing faculty to conduct an annual review of the curriculum with possible revisions as necessary. It is essential for nurse educators to gather and discuss the development, revision, and enhancement of curriculum with a tone of collegiality (Kramer, 2005). Discussion leads to:

- A mutual understanding of the mission and philosophy of the institution and the program
- Major concepts faculty believe influence nursing practice and how these concepts are used to build student learning outcomes
- The development of student learning outcomes from which all other elements are built
- Relationships among content areas and sequencing of courses
- Collaborative development of strategies to meet the needs of the specific student population

- Selection of learning strategies and evaluation methods to ensure student learning outcomes are met

The discussions that ensue may reveal each nursing faculty has different ideas regarding what to include and exclude from the curriculum. Communication skills and problem solving are put to the test in an exchange of ideas and perspectives. Remaining focused on the program's mission, major concepts, and student learning outcomes that pull all parts of the program together is helpful in reaching mutual agreement regarding curriculum revisions. Widely divergent opinions and an inability to arrive at consensus may result in a curriculum that is fragmented and ineffective due to lack of consistent implementation.

## The Foundation: The Mission and Philosophy

Every institution has a reason to exist. Colleges and universities have affiliations, which may include government, communities, churches, or private groups. Each institution is guided by a mission, philosophy, and aims consistent with those of the affiliated groups they serve. Representatives from the affiliating groups are included on governing boards of directors and trustees of the college. The boards govern the operation of the institution. The governing boards are charged with ensuring the curricula of its various programs remain consistent with the mission and aims of their affiliated group. Changes in a curriculum must often receive the approval from these governing boards.

It is important to know and understand the institutional mission and philosophy that support the college or university. The mission and philosophy are drawn from and built upon those of the institution. Likewise, specific content within the nursing program also builds on that same framework. For example, if the mission of the institution is based on religion and spirituality, those concepts must be included in the nursing program's curriculum and all its courses.

Both the National League for Nursing Accrediting Commission (NLNAC) (2008) and the Commission on Collegiate Nursing Education (CCNE) (2008) require the nursing curriculum's mission to flow from that of the parent organization. Standard 1.1 of the NLNAC states, "The mission/philosophy and outcomes of the nursing education unit are congruent with those of the governing organization." And, Standard I-A of the CCNE states, "The mission, goals, and expected student outcomes are congruent with those of the parent institution and consistent with relevant professional nursing standards and guidelines for the preparation of nursing professionals." These statements from the accreditation bodies are extremely helpful as a reference for faculty when writing or updating the mission, philosophy, and student learning outcomes because they provide guidance and structure.

## Example Mission Statement

An example mission statement for a community college is as follows:

"To be at the forefront of higher education, serving the needs of the community. The college will be the first place residents turn to for the highest quality of educational and cultural opportunities. The college will serve as a model of distinction for community college education" (College of DuPage Catalog, 2007, p. 12).

A possible mission statement for a nursing program at that same community college is: "The mission of the Nursing Program is to serve the needs of the community. The Nursing Program supports excellence in learning and teaching, fosters an instructional climate that welcomes innovation, is open to change, and targets continual improvement and accountability."

Note that embedded in the nursing program's mission statement are the concepts of innovation, continual improvement, and accountability. As the remainder of the curriculum is developed, those concepts must be evident. That is, how is the program innovative? Program documents may explain the program continually evolves to reflect local community needs and current and emerging healthcare delivery systems in its efforts to be innovative. Also, is there a functioning systematic plan for evaluation that supports continual improvement and accountability? One step of the process builds on the next. It is important to establish a firm footing with the mission statement.

## Program Philosophy

The nursing program philosophy is next considered. This program philosophy couples the institution's philosophy with the philosophical vision of the nursing faculty. Once the nursing program philosophy is written, all areas of content and how they fit together under the program's philosophical framework are planned. Consider the following examples:

- **College Philosophy:** The college believes in the power of teaching and learning. We endorse the right of each person to access opportunities to learn and affirm the innate value of the pursuit of knowledge and its application to life. Our primary commitment is to facilitate and support student success in learning. The college is committed to excellence.

- **Nursing Program Philosophy:** The faculty is responsible for assisting individual students to become knowledgeable, demonstrate competencies, and meet the graduate learning outcomes needed for entry into beginning nursing practice. The faculty value a learning environment which:
  - Is supportive of learning
  - Fosters healthy interdependence
  - Is respectful of, and concerned about, students
  - Empowers students in their present and life-long learning

  The nursing faculty acknowledge the core competencies of *The Scope of Practice for Academic Nurse Educators* (NLN, 2005) and aspire to incorporate the eight competencies in their daily teaching activities. The faculty also acknowledge the importance of evidence-based nursing education and strive to incorporate best practices into their teaching.

The first part of the nursing program philosophy reflects the parent institution's philosophy of supporting student success. The second part reflects the parent institution's value of excellence. In addressing the core competencies of academic nurse educators, the nursing program is addressing excellence in teaching.

## Personal Philosophy of Education

Understanding the relationship between one's personal philosophy of education and the overall curriculum is essential. All teachers should think about their own philosophy of education. Does their personal philosophy support the mission of the nursing program and the overall institution? Does their approach to teaching their assigned content align with the mission of the program? Each of the content areas is a piece of the curriculum and integral to the overall plan. If a piece of the curriculum differs significantly from the other pieces because it is influenced by one person's personal philosophy influencing their teaching and is contrary to the program's philosophy, that piece will stand out and fail to support the overall plan. It is critical that all faculty are in agreement with the mission, philosophy, and all other aspects of the curriculum so the program can be implemented in the way in which it was intended. If this is not the case, the level at which students are meeting the student learning outcomes and program outcomes is difficult to attribute to the curriculum because the curriculum is not consistently applied. If program outcomes do not meet the established benchmark, faculty are at a loss for identifying causes of unacceptable outcomes if the curriculum is not consistently implemented.

## Philosophical Statements Related to the Teaching/Learning Process

Often times faculty include philosophical statements about the teaching/learning process as part of the nursing program's philosophical statements. These can be helpful if used as guides for instruction. Examples of such statements are shown in Figure 1.

There are many statements contained in Figure 1 that can be used to guide the curriculum process. For example, the statements discuss addressing the learner's knowledge level, organizing educational experiences in a logical sequence that promotes continuity, and acknowledging how faculty value the learning environment. All those statements provide guidance for structuring teaching/learning experiences in the classroom.

## Students

The philosophy of the educational institution and the philosophy of the nursing program all revolve around the central goal of teaching students to provide safe, effective nursing care. Educational institutions exist because of students, collectively and individually. The purpose of curriculum is to provide learning experiences for the students to meet the student learning outcomes.

When planning the curriculum, it is important to consider what students bring to the program. Every program has entrance criteria that, at the very least, consist of a minimum grade point average and prerequisite courses. And although meeting the same admission criteria, individual students may be highly diverse relative to ethnicity, economic background, dialect, culture, and basic values. Faculty should become familiar with the background of the student body so admission and selective criteria can be established. Additionally, as the curriculum development process proceeds, student characteristics will have a bearing on the student's ability to learn to problem solve, make decisions, and critically think as opposed to using rote memorization. Student characteristics are a major factor to consider in all stages of the curriculum design process (Caputi & Engelmann, 2008).

## Rules, Regulations, and Minimum Standards

Several groups outside the parent institution may be involved in ensuring minimum standards for nursing education are met. Standards may arise from federal laws, state regulations, or professional accreditation agencies. It is wise to understand the role these agencies play in determining curriculum. These groups may place specific constraints and limits on the curriculum or may delineate what

**Teaching and Learning**

The faculty view the teaching-learning process as a dynamic, logical interchange between the learner and the educational environment. Learning involves the acquisition of knowledge, skills, attitudes, values, and critical thinking and is evidenced by meaningful use of these acquired factors in the care of patients. The faculty believe individuals learn in a variety of ways and a diversity of resources should be available to meet individual student learning needs. The faculty believe in faculty-guided and student self-directed learning; thus, the primary roles of the faculty are those of teacher, facilitator, evaluator, advisor, and resource person. The faculty is responsible for assisting individual students to become knowledgeable, demonstrate competencies, and meet the student learning outcomes needed for entry into beginning nursing practice.

Learning is enhanced when the learner's knowledge level is identified and used to plan appropriate teaching, when educational experiences are organized in a logical sequence that promotes continuity, and when the individual student's unique needs and strengths are considered.

The faculty value a learning environment which:
- Is supportive of learning
- Fosters healthy interdependence
- Is respectful of and concerned about students
- Empowers students in their present and life-long learning

The faculty value a caring environment for students which promotes flexible, accessible educational experiences for a diverse student body. Adult learning principles are used in all interactions with students providing self-directed, purposeful learning respectful of knowledge and experience students bring to the educational environment. Adult learning theory empowers learners with mentoring and guidance allowing both autonomy and responsibility in learning experiences.

The nursing faculty acknowledge the core competencies of *The Scope of Practice for Academic Nurse Educators* (NLN, 2005) and aspire to incorporate the eight competencies in their daily teaching activities. The faculty also acknowledge the importance of evidence-based nursing education and strive to incorporate best practice into their teaching.

**Figure 1.** Philosophical Statements Related to the Teaching/Learning Process

must be included in the curriculum to achieve minimum standards. The state board of nursing is one of these influences. Some state boards of nursing are very prescriptive regarding what should be included in a nursing program. However, there is an emerging trend among boards of nursing to embrace innovation and change (Grady, 2009). Faculty should be very aware of all the state requirements prior to developing/revising a nursing curriculum and inquire about their state's vision for the future of nursing curriculum.

## Identifying Relevant Concepts

Concepts are the building blocks of student learning outcomes. It is imperative that faculty understand and agree on the major concepts that will be used as the basis for the student learning outcomes. Start by identifying the concepts faculty believe most accurately reflect the current practice and discipline of nursing. The traditional undergraduate curriculum typically uses the four concepts from the nursing metaparadigm: health, person, environment, and nursing. These four concepts have been discussed in relationship to nursing since the time of Florence Nightingale and remain the foundation for nursing practice. The graphic in Figure 2 demonstrates one possible way of visualizing the relationship of these concepts.

These four concepts relate to nursing and how nursing interacts with the other concepts within the healthcare delivery system. Faculty may use these specific terms or choose other terms to represent these components. Faculty then define each term. For example, patient can refer to an individual patient, family, community, etc. Definitions are important to inform faculty and stakeholders of the definitions that are used in the program, thus aiding clear communication of the curriculum components.

## Building a Curriculum Based on Nursing Practice

A more contemporary approach for nursing education is to identify concepts related to the practice of nursing rather than to the discipline of nursing. That is, what does the nurse do and what concepts represent the important roles the nurse fills. There is no universally accepted guideline regarding what concepts to choose with either focus – a focus on the discipline of nursing or a focus on the practice of nursing. Therefore, faculty must decide their focus and then identify concepts that make up the framework for the curriculum.

The current trend for organizing a nursing curriculum around practice is supportive of the outcomes-based curriculum discussed earlier. To determine student

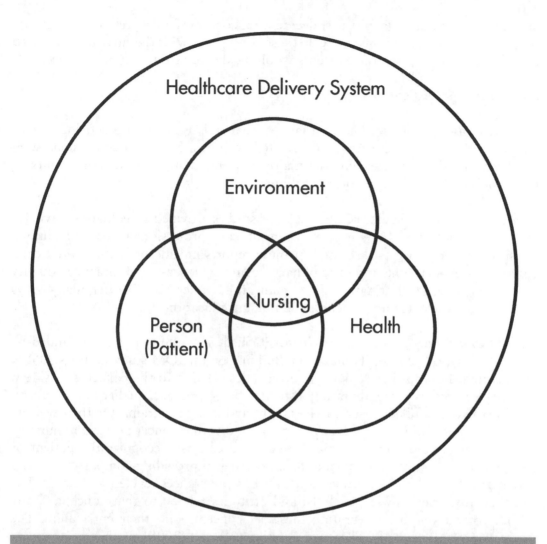

**Figure 2.** The Nursing Metaparadigm

learning outcomes, the faculty first decide what concepts best represent the graduate they are preparing. But from where do these concepts flow? If the curriculum is based on current practice, then the concepts would be derived from current practice.

## Sources for Major Concepts

There are many national initiatives that relate to the practicing nurse. Faculty review the literature, study related websites, and hold discussions with local stakeholders to determine the major concepts that relate to today's nursing professional. Some of these sources follow.

**Institute of Medicine Studies (IOM).** The IOM studies provided a wealth of knowledge that helps to frame the education of healthcare professionals today, including nursing. Major concepts discussed in these reports include patient-centered care, collaboration with the interdisciplinary team, evidence-based practice, quality improvement, and informatics. Finkelman and Kenner (2007) offer many ways these major concepts can be included in nursing education.

**Quality and Safety Education for Nurses (QSEN).** The QSEN project is funded by the Robert Wood Johnson Foundation. Building on the IOM study findings, QSEN has defined the knowledge, skills, and attitudes relating to the concepts of safety, patient-centered care, collaboration, evidence-based practice, quality improvement, and informatics and how each can be taught in nursing programs. On their website at qsen.org are definitions of the concepts and how that concept is used in nursing. For example, the definition of patient-centered care is: Recognize the patient or designee as the source of control and full partner in providing compassionate and coordinated care based on respect for patient's preferences, values, and needs. The site then lists the knowledge, skills, and attitudes related to that concept. Many schools of nursing are integrating these six concepts into their curriculum. The American Association of Colleges of Nursing (AACN) (2008) emphasizes these six concepts in the 2008 *Essentials of Baccalaureate Education*.

**National Council of State Boards of Nursing (NCSBN).** The NCSBN conducts research every three years about the activities performed by new graduates in their first six months of practice. This research is published in the *Knowledge of Newly Licensed Registered Nurses* (www.ncsbn.org). This is helpful research for determining student learning outcomes and competencies. The website also has many educational papers helpful in curriculum work. The NCSBN has recently released a document titled

*Transition to Practice Regulatory Model.* This document is thought-provoking and offers insights to changes in the workplace impacting nursing education.

**Other Health-Related Organizations.** There are several other health-related organizations that provide additional information about the work of today's nurses to inform student learning outcomes as well as appropriate content for the nursing program to teach. Such organizations are The Joint Commission, the Centers for Disease Control, and local community health agencies. These sites provide information about the health and safety of the nation as well as the people living in the community the school serves.

**The American Nurses Association.** The American Nurses Association's (2004) *Standards of Practice* and *Code of Ethics* offer additional standards directly related to the practice of nursing that should be incorporated into a nursing program curriculum.

**Nursing Education Organizations.** The various levels of education are represented by organizations. These organizations also provide information to help faculty in developing curriculum components. The National League for Nursing (NLN) is the only nursing education organization that represents all levels of nursing education. The NLN will soon release a document that levels the competencies of graduates from all programs: Practical Nursing, Association Degree, Baccalaureate Degree, and graduate level nursing education. Also for baccalaureate and higher degree programs, the AACN publishes the Essentials series. The National Association for Practical Nurse Education and Service, Inc. (NAPNES) publishes competencies for Practical Nurses. These documents are extremely helpful when developing and revising a curriculum.

**Stakeholders.** When working at this very basic level of curriculum development it is wise to talk with stakeholders such as the members of your advisory council, employers of your graduates, and your new graduates. Information gathered from these sources directly relates to the preparation of your specific student body. You must take into consideration the population you serve and that population includes your students as well as those who employ them after graduation. Education and practice must dialogue and agree on reasonable, realistic expectations for the school's graduates. Until that happens, there will continue to be a disjoint between education and practice.

## Selecting the Major Concepts and Giving them Meaning

Faculty must work together to analyze all the concepts that are derived from their search of the literature and review of relevant websites. The task is to choose concepts that reflect what faculty believe are central to student learning outcomes that represent the type of outcomes they believe best prepares their graduate for practice and is reflective of their mission and philosophy. Faculty must give careful and thoughtful consideration throughout the steps in this process. These concepts represent the foundation on which the outcomes and competencies will be built. The remaining elements of the curriculum are derived from that foundation.

## Example Concepts with Definitions

There are many concepts that can be used in formulating a curriculum. Some of those concepts with their definitions include the following:

**Caring:** In nursing, those values, attitudes, and behaviors that engender feeling cared for by recipients. "Clinical caring processes are relationship-centered and incorporate physical acts, being with (interacting), connecting, and knowing another" (Duffy, 2005, p. 61)

**Collaboration:** "Function effectively within nursing and inter-professional teams, fostering open communication, mutual respect, and shared decision-making to achieve quality patient care." (Quality and Safety Education for Nurses [QSEN], 2007). Collaboration also includes communication and partnerships with providers, patients, families, and stakeholders.

**Critical thinking:** "Purposeful, informed, outcome-focused (result-oriented) thinking." (Alfaro-LeFevre, 2009, p. 7.) Critical thinking is the process and clinical judgment is the result of that process.

**Diversity:** "The range of human variation, including age, race, gender, disability, ethnicity, nationality, religious and spiritual beliefs, sexual orientation, political beliefs, economic status, native language, and geographical background." (American Association of Colleges of Nursing [AACN], 2008, p. 37).

**Evidence-based care:** Care that integrates the best research with clinical expertise and patient values for optimum care (IOM, 2003). Evidence is used in making decisions while patient preferences and the context of the individual patient refers to the judicious use of that evidence (Von Achterberg, Schoonhoven, & Grol, 2008).

**Informatics:** Use information and technology to communicate, manage knowledge, mitigate error, and support decision making (Quality and Safety Education for Nurses [QSEN], 2007).

**Patient-centered care:** Recognize the patient or designee as the source of control and full partner in providing compassionate and coordinated care based on respect for patient's preferences, values, and needs (Quality and Safety Education for Nurses [QSEN], 2007).

**Professionalism:** "The consistent demonstration of core values evidenced by nurses working with other professionals to achieve optimal health and wellness outcomes in patients, families, and communities by wisely applying principles of altruism, excellence, caring, ethics, respect, communication, and accountability" (American Association of Colleges of Nursing [AACN], 2008, p. 26).

**Quality improvement:** "Use data to monitor the outcomes of care processes and use improvement methods to design and test changes to continuously improve the quality and safety of health care systems" (Quality and Safety Education for Nurses [QSEN], 2007). Also relates to the improvement of healthcare processes and at the local, state, and federal levels to affect positive outcomes from the impact of economics on healthcare quality.

**Safety:** Minimizes risk of harm to patients and providers though both system effectiveness and individual performance (Quality and Safety Education for Nurses [QSEN], 2007).

There are other concepts and other combinations of concepts that can be used. These are just some example concepts that are commonly used in nursing curricula.

## Putting the Concepts together in a Model

Once the concepts are selected and definitions written, the concepts are arranged into a model. A model is a visual representation of how the concepts fit together as the framework of the curriculum. A visual model is helpful for clearly and quickly communicating to stakeholders, students, and other interested parties the building blocks of the nursing curriculum. Figure 3 presents a model relating some of the concepts described previously with the addition of others. The model is helpful in demonstrating the relationship of these concepts to each other and to the other components of the curriculum.

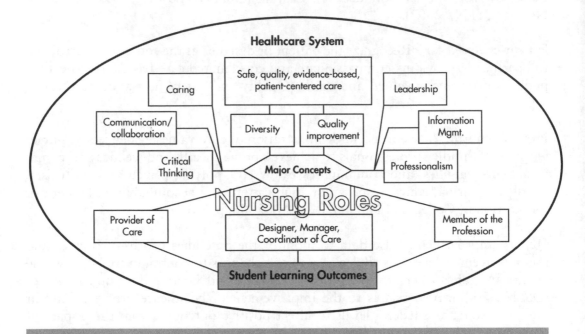

**Figure 3.** A Model of the Major Concepts of a Curriculum

Figure 4 provides another perspective on arranging the major concepts in a curriculum. This model arranges the concepts within the four major areas of the nursing metaparadigm previously discussed. Please note this is not an all-inclusive model and is presented for demonstration purposes.

Implied in this discussion is the move away from a single theory as the framework for a nursing program. In the past, nursing theories were often used as the basis for a nursing curriculum. The concepts and terms of the theory were threaded through all courses. However, single theories do not provide flexibility for updating the curriculum as issues in nursing practice change. By using a concept-based framework, faculty may change a few of the concepts without violating the principles or underlying foundation of a nursing theory. Also, some nursing

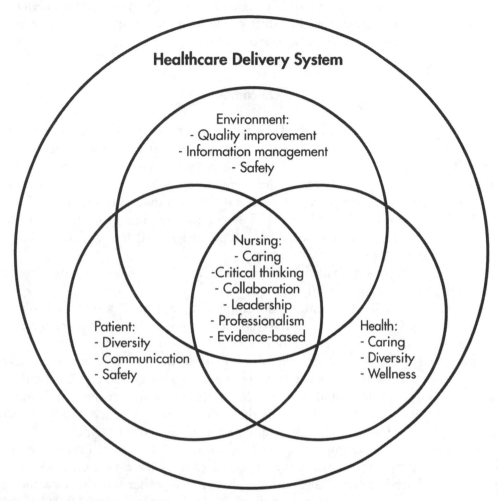

Healthcare Delivery System

Environment:
- Quality improvement
- Information management
- Safety

Nursing:
- Caring
-Critical thinking
- Collaboration
- Leadership
- Professionalism
- Evidence-based

Patient:
- Diversity
- Communication
- Safety

Health:
- Caring
- Diversity
- Wellness

**Figure 4.** Incorporating Major Concepts into the Nursing Metaparadigm

theories may not be updated in a timely manner, leaving the basis for the curriculum outdated. Therefore, the practice has shifted to a focus on what the nurse in practice does and organizing a curriculum around that practice.

## Outcomes

Once the faculty has established the value system as stated in the mission and philosophy, and have chosen important concepts, the student learning outcomes are written. The current trend in curriculum development is to focus on outcomes; it's all about outcomes. The standards from the accrediting bodies that relate to curriculum include the following and directly reference the importance of outcomes:

NLNAC (2008) Standard 4.1: The curriculum incorporates established professional standards, guidelines, and competencies, and has clearly articulated student learning and program outcomes.

CCNE (2008) standards also addresses outcomes as the basis for structuring the curriculum in their Standard III:

Standard III-A. The curriculum is developed, implemented, and revised to reflect clear statements of expected individual student learning outcomes that are congruent with the program's mission, goals, and expected student outcomes.

Standard III-B. Expected individual student learning outcomes are consistent with the roles for which the program is preparing its graduates. Curricula are developed, implemented, and revised to reflect relevant professional nursing standards and guidelines, which are clearly evident within the curriculum, expected individual student learning outcomes, and expected student outcomes.

Outcomes are important. They are what drive the curriculum. Outcomes provide information about what the expected student learning outcomes will be when the student completes the nursing program. In other words, outcomes are "those characteristics students should display at a designated time" (Boland, 2009, p. 144).

## Competencies

Competencies are more specific. Competencies are the knowledge, skills, and attitudes (values) that students develop to achieve the student learning outcomes (Boland, 2009). These outcomes address the level of the student, the level of the behavior, and the context of the behavior. For example, an outcome statement might be:

"Provides quality, safe, patient-centered nursing care through evidence-based practice."

First year competencies for that outcome might be:

- Identifies evidence-based nursing interventions for each patient that provide psychosocial and physiological integrity, and health promotion and maintenance.
- Gives examples of using therapeutic communication when interacting with patients and the patients' support network.

Second year competencies for that same outcome are written at a higher level and might be:

- Describes how information from at least one research article can be used to address nursing care for assigned patient(s) relating to psychosocial integrity, and/or health promotion and maintenance.
- Integrates principles of therapeutic communication when interacting with patients and patients' support network in the mental health environment.

## Writing Student Learning Outcomes and Related Competencies

Faculty write the student learning outcomes and competencies to be accomplished by the end of the program. The written mission and identified concepts are used to develop these outcomes and competencies. When writing outcomes faculty should ask themselves:

- "Why are we expecting this of our graduate?"
- "Why is this important?"
- "What effect will this behavior have on patient care outcomes?"

These questions help to frame your purpose for the outcomes. Using the graphic in Figure 3, a possible student learning outcome with competencies related to patient-centered care is presented in Figure 5.

Many faculty ask how many student learning outcomes are required. There are no requirements; but, the general guideline is six to ten. These are the overall outcomes that you expect students to exhibit by the end of the program. Remember that each outcome has competencies as shown in Figure 5. Outcomes are the general statements and the competencies are more specific behaviors.

Outcomes and competencies replace the older behavioral objectives used extensively in nursing education over the past forty years. Objectives were much more prescriptive and were written for students to demonstrate the knowledge and experiences needed to achieve the intended results. The debate over using behavioral objectives is found in nursing literature throughout the past decade (Bastable, 2003). Bevis and Watson (2000) noted that using intended learning outcomes delineated by learning objectives is the ultimate position of behaviorists. Although the behaviorist approach has been a tried-and-true keystone of nursing curricula for nearly four decades, some consider it a confining and restrictive paradigm for planning a nursing curriculum. From this ambivalence flow the pros and cons of using behavioral objectives.

Competencies adapted from AACN (2008) and Nursing Executive Center (2007)
Outcome: Provide safe, quality, patient-centered, evidence-based nursing care.
Sample competencies:
1. Conducts comprehensive and focused patient assessments using developmentally and culturally appropriate approaches.
2. Delivers compassionate, patient-centered, evidence-based care respectful of patient and family preferences.
3. Promotes factors that create a culture of safety and caring.
4. Delivers care within expected timeframe.
5. Etc.

**Figure 5.** A Sample Student Learning Outcome with Competencies

Those who argue against using behavioral objectives point out that behavioral objectives:
- Lead to pieces that do not reflect the sum total of the parts
- Reflect what the teacher expects precluding the students' opportunity to construct their own objectives
- Fail to capture the essence of complex cognitive processes that may not be easily observed and measured

In contrast, those who support the use of behavioral objectives put forward that behavioral objectives:
- Guide instruction and keep the teacher's thinking learner centered
- Communicate to all involved the expected measurable learning outcomes that can be used for evaluation and documentation of success or failure
- Delineate what is to be taught; thus helping both faculty and students from getting lost in the content

The debate over using learning objectives forms the basis of the broader movement toward a paradigm shift in nursing education. That paradigm shift requests, at the very least, a modification of curriculum away from a total behaviorist approach. The end result is a focus on outcomes and competencies rather than objectives.

## Leveling Outcomes throughout the Program

Once faculty have agreed on the student learning outcomes for the nursing program, those outcomes are then leveled from course to course. That is, each course addresses some or all of these outcomes but at a level expected of the student by the end of that course. The nursing courses build from one course to the next with higher leveled outcomes until they culminate in the program student learning outcomes. Blooms taxonomy for the cognitive domain is helpful in writing outcomes so they are leveled to be more complex as the student progresses through the program.

When leveling course outcomes faculty ask themselves, "What behaviors will the student demonstrate to indicate progression to the final student learning outcomes?" This is a systematic process that requires careful deliberation.

Course outcomes are leveled as they build to meet the student learning outcomes at the end of the program. Gronlund (1995) described the levels of comprehension in the cognitive domain using an adaptation of Bloom's (1956) Taxonomy. Each level represents a higher degree of complexity in thinking:

1. **Knowledge.** Knowledge is defined as remembering of previously learned materials. This may involve recall of a wide range of material, but all that is required is bringing to mind the appropriate information. Knowledge represents the lowest level of learning outcomes.

2. **Comprehension.** Comprehension is defined as the ability to grasp the meaning of material. This may be shown by translating material from one form to another. These learning outcomes go one step beyond the simple recall of material and represent the lowest level of understanding.

3. **Application.** Application refers to the ability to use learned materials in new and concrete situations. This may include the application of rules, methods, concepts, principles, laws, and theories. Learning outcomes at the application level require a higher level of understanding than the comprehension level.

4. **Analysis.** Analysis refers to the ability to break down material into its component parts so its organizational structure may be understood. This may include identification of the parts, analysis of the relationships between and among parts, and recognition of the organization principles involved. Learning outcomes at this level require an understanding of both the content and the structural form of the material.

5. **Synthesis.** Synthesis refers to the ability to put parts together to form a new whole. This may involve the production of a unique communication, such as an essay or a speech; a plan of operations, such as a research proposal; or a set of abstract relations. Learning outcomes in this area stresses creative behaviors.

6. **Evaluation.** Evaluation is concerned with the ability to judge the value of material. The judgments are based on definite criteria. These may be internal or external criteria. This is the highest level in the cognitive domain.

Before writing outcomes and their related competencies, consider the level of performance required of the students at their current educational level. Consider next the level of competence students are to obtain during the course. Are they to simply know the content, or are they expected to apply it? In teaching the fundamentals of nursing to beginning students, the lowest level of learning outcome, knowledge, may be appropriate. Table 1 lists examples of verbs that can be used when stating the outcomes at the six levels.

| Levels of Cognitive Domain | Verbs |
|---|---|
| Knowledge | List, define, match, describe, show, label, name |
| Comprehension | Estimate, defend, give examples, summarize |
| Application | Apply, demonstrate, calculate, solve, discover |
| Analysis | Analyze, diagram, illustrate, separate, break down |
| Synthesis | Combine, create, design, prepare, modify |
| Evaluation | Support, discriminate, recommend, summarize |

**Table 1.** Example Verbs for the Six Levels of the Cognitive Domain

Once outcomes are written for each course it is extremely important that faculty teach to that level and use evaluation strategies that measure if the student has achieved that level of functioning. For example, if students are expected to use critical thinking and analysis of content, faculty would select learning strategies in the classroom that put students into the role of using these thinking skills. Delivering the content through a passive methodology such as lecturing would not encourage the behaviors of critical thinking and analysis.

## Arranging Course Content

The NLNAC Standard 4.3 states, "The student learning outcomes are used to organize the curriculum, guide the delivery of instruction, direct learning activities, and evaluate student progress." The CCNE, Standard III-C states, "The curriculum is logically structured to achieve expected individual and aggregate student outcomes." These standards provide guidance and insight about structuring the curriculum.

As faculty develop the content, the student learning outcomes provide the basis for content organization and presentation. The course outcomes reflect the major concepts used to build the student learning outcomes, so should be evident when content is presented and discussed. It is important to note these concepts are applied in all facets of learning: clinical setting, skills laboratory, and classroom.

In the past, many nursing programs sequenced content from simple to complex. Faculty often worked to identify what would be considered **simple** content and what would be considered **complex** content. In today's current nursing practice it would be difficult to identify any content as **simple**. The trend is away from identifying **content** as simple or complex, and is shifting to identifying **thinking** as progressing from **simple** to **complex**. Therefore, course outcomes are leveled from simple to complex. That is, a beginning student may care for a patient with complex health problems, but would be expected to deal with those problems at a lower level of thinking than the student in an advanced nursing course. This relates to the idea that nurses are knowledge workers (Porter-O'Grady, 2010) and the use of the knowledge of nursing progresses from simple to complex. As students progress though a nursing program, they should be able to demonstrate higher levels of thinking than in earlier courses.

## Teaching/Learning Activities

Bevis (2000) operationalized curriculum in this manner: Curriculum is "those transactions and interactions that take place between students and teachers and among students with the intent that learning takes place" (p. 1). In other words, curriculum comes to life during the teaching/learning process. This is where the curriculum becomes exciting and rewarding.

Faculty must always consider the course outcomes and competencies when selecting teaching/learning activities. The classroom of today should look very different than the classroom of yesterday. Yesterday's classroom teaching methodologies predominately centered around the lecture format, a methodology that encourages rote memorization and recall of memorized information. Nursing faculty must look past content, the **what** to teach, to **how** to teach to meet program outcomes. Knowing a lot of disconnected facts is not sufficient for today's nursing professional (Tanner, 2007). The outcomes expected of today's nursing graduates require thinking skills and abilities that are not fostered by the lecture method. Again, referring to the standards of nursing's accrediting bodies, faculty must teach to the outcomes.

NLNAC's Standard 4.3 states: "The student learning outcomes are used to organize the curriculum, guide the delivery of instruction, direct learning activities, and evaluate student progress." The emphasis here is on "direct learning activities."

CCNE's Standard III-D states, "Teaching-learning practices and environments support the achievement of expected individual student learning outcomes."

The standards support the notion that teaching must be congruent with the expected outcomes. Faculty must always consider the outcomes and then plan teaching/learning strategies that encourage those behaviors in students. For example, a course outcome states students will analyze patient data to plan safe, effective nursing interventions. To teach to this outcome, faculty may be tempted to provide a lecture presenting a disease process, signs and symptoms typical of that disease process, and then a standardized care plan. When the students encounter the lecture method presenting this information, they are not encouraged to analyze the data and arrive at safe, effective nursing interventions. Rather, students are prompted to memorize the information presented by faculty. To address the course outcome of analyzing patient data, faculty might use a case study; or, present information about the disease process, typical manifestations, and medical treatments, then ask students to work in small groups to use that information to plan safe, effective nursing interventions. The small groups would then present to the class their work with rationales to support the nursing interventions selected based on their analysis of the data.

Faculty must also sort through the myriad of content presented in textbooks and select the content to be taught that supports the course outcomes. Not all content in the textbook can be, nor should be, taught in the limited amount of time provided in any nursing program. Faculty must sort through and select content that supports the outcomes. Content saturation is a term used to refer to too much content in a curriculum. This is also known as the additive curriculum – the faculty keep adding more and more content without eliminating anything. Because of the enormous volume of content the lecture method becomes the most effective way to deliver all this content and students resort to rote memorization as the best learning strategy. However, this type of teaching/learning engages the student in lower-level cognitive activity, not the kind of thinking required of today's knowledge worker nurse.

Content saturation is a problem that all faculty face. The faculty should establish guidelines that can be used for deciding what content to include and what to eliminate. One approach is to consider the information most relevant to the student learning outcomes. That is, what patient populations do the graduates serve? What are the most prevalent disease processes of the patients the graduates will care for and in the general United State population? In what depth do you want to teach? For example, when teaching physical assessment to pre-licensure nursing students, many physical assessment techniques may be too involved and not necessary for that level of practice. Faculty must understand they do not need to teach beginning students everything the faculty themselves know.

## Evaluating Student Performance and the Curriculum

A nursing program's systematic plan for evaluation includes ongoing evaluation of curriculum. The nursing accrediting bodies include evaluation in their standards:

NLNAC Standard 4.3: The student learning outcomes are used to organize the curriculum, guide the delivery of instruction, direct learning activities, and evaluate student progress. (The emphasis here is on **evaluate student progress.**)

NLNAC's Standard 4.5: Evaluation methodologies are varied, reflect established professional and practice competencies, and measure the achievement of student learning and program outcomes.

CCNE's Standard III-F: Individual student performance is evaluated by the faculty and reflects achievement of expected individual student learning outcomes. Evaluation policies and procedures for individual student performance are defined and consistently applied.

CCNE's Standard III-G: Curriculum and teaching-learning practices are evaluated at regularly scheduled intervals to foster ongoing improvement.

These standards refer to both evaluating students and evaluating the curriculum.

### Evaluating Students

Evaluating achievement of student learning outcomes requires evaluation methods that are congruent with the course outcomes. There are many methods to evaluate learning including classroom examinations, skills performance evaluations, reflective journals, clinical evaluation tools, clinical performance examinations, scholarly papers, etc. The major issue to consider is to ensure the evaluation method is valid and reliable. That is, does the evaluation method measure what it is supposed to measure and does it do so consistently over time and with all students. For example, objective exam items must be written to the level that is expected in the outcome. If the outcome states, "Recognizes...." then the test item would determine if the student can recognize. If the outcome states, "Analyzes...." then the test item must be written to determine if the student can analyze data in the manner expected as written in the outcome. All evaluation methods must adhere to this standard. The grade derived from the evaluation measure can only be used as a dependable measure if it is valid and reliable.

It is extremely important all faculty are knowledge about evaluation methods and how to use them. Faculty development may be required to assist new faculty in constructing test items that measure various levels of cognition.

Also important is how to develop evaluation techniques that measure attainment of skills and attitudes. Clinical evaluation tools must be periodically reviewed to ensure they are meeting this standard.

## Evaluating the Program and the Curriculum

The program outcomes, as defined at the beginning of this chapter, refer to "performance indicators that reflect the extent to which the purposes of the nursing education unit are achieved and by which program effectiveness is documented. Program outcomes are measurable consumer-oriented indexes designed to evaluate the degree to which the program is achieving its mission and goals" (NLNAC, 2008, p. 102). Commonly used measures of program outcomes include program completion rates, licensure/certification pass rates, job placement rates, and program satisfaction.

**Program completion rates.** The attrition rate is another measure of student performance and effectiveness of the curriculum. NLNAC (2008) refers to this as the program completion rate. NLNAC's definition is:

> Number of students who graduate within a defined period of time. Definition used by the NLNAC for the Annual Report: Program Completion = the number of students who complete the program within 150% of the time of the sated program length (the length of the program adjusted to begin with the first required nursing course). (p. 103)

Faculty should set a benchmark regarding an acceptable completion rate and measure success based on that benchmark. What percent is acceptable? Faculty must understand that not all students who enter the program will be successful. There are many variables that affect retention of nursing students beside grades. Many nursing students have full-time jobs, families to care for, and other commitments. Faculty consider the student population they serve when determining a benchmark for program completion.

It is important that faculty maintain records about why students leave a nursing program. This information is reviewed each year. Faculty may use that information to change the curriculum when it is warranted. For example, perhaps the level of outcomes for beginning nursing courses are too complex resulting in a large number of students unable to pass the course. The course may need to be revised. Or, on the contrary, perhaps the level of outcomes for nursing courses is not at the level required for preparation for the advanced nursing courses. When students enter the advanced courses they are not prepared and fail the course. Curriculum revisions may help remedy these types of situations.

**Licensure/certification pass rates.** A primary indicator of program outcomes for pre-licensure programs is the first time pass rate on the NCLEX®. All state boards of nursing use this pass rate as a measure of the quality of the nursing program. State requirements vary greatly. Some states only require a 75% pass rate while others require 85%. Still others do not establish a specific percentage but require programs to be at a certain level based on the national pass rate. For example, the Utah Board of Nursing requires schools to realize a pass rate no lower than 5% below the national average pass rate for the same time period. This requirement means the school may have a different standard to meet each period, based on the national average. The NLNAC has set the expected pass rate on national licensing exams to be at or above the national mean for all levels of programs.

Programs educating nurses for advanced roles can use certification examinations as a benchmark for meeting program outcomes as a measurable consumer-oriented index. The NLNAC requires 80% of students to pass the certification exam (NLNAC, 2008).

Faculty should set a benchmark well above that required by their states or accrediting agencies to ensure the mandated level will be reached.

**Job placement rates and employer satisfaction.** It is indeed helpful if faculty remain in contact with graduates to expedite collection of information about their post-graduation activities. Graduates should be requested to report their employers to enable faculty to conduct surveys related to the employers' satisfaction with graduates of the nursing program. The school's advisory council may also help with this task because they typically represent agencies that are used for clinical experiences, but may very well employ graduates.

Appendix A provides a sample employer survey. This survey attempts to collect data that can be used to improve the program's curriculum. The behaviors included in the table portion of the survey represent the student learning outcomes for the program. Using the student learning outcomes as part of the employer survey provides direct feedback about the usefulness of the established student learning outcomes. This information can be used to revise the curriculum accordingly.

**Program satisfaction.** It is important that graduates of a nursing program are satisfied the education they received provides what they need to perform well on the job. This data can be collected through a survey. Surveys are typically administered six to nine months after graduation to allow time for writing the licensing examination and procuring a nursing position. Appendix B provides a sample graduate survey. Again, the behaviors included in the table portion of the survey represent the program's student learning outcomes, for consistency in measuring the effectiveness of those outcomes in preparing the new graduates for their role as a nurse.

The data gathered from all these surveys are aggregated, analyzed, and trended and used as indicators of the effectiveness of the curriculum. These surveys are administered annually and provide valuable information for curriculum revision.

## Summary

This chapter has explored essential curriculum components, how they relate, how they are developed, how to implement them, and, finally, how to evaluate them. Curriculum is not static – it is a dynamic phenomenon that is considered ongoing in its maturity. This is what makes curriculum work exciting. Faculty are on a journey to make the curriculum better and better. Faculty must embrace this reality and enjoy the work of curriculum.

## Learning Activities

1. Articulate the mission and philosophy of your college or university. Relate the mission and philosophy of your college or university to those of your nursing program.

2. Interview your colleagues regarding their philosophy of education. Ask them to discuss how their philosophy influences their teaching.
3. Interview your program director regarding the program process for curriculum review and revision.
4. List and analyze the course outcomes for a specific nursing course. Identify the level of those outcomes using Bloom's Taxonomy.
5. Review your program's systematic plan for evaluation as it relates to the curriculum. Is it effective? Why or why not?

## Educational Philosophy

My educational philosophy is succinct: Give the best educational experience possible. I believe faculty should continuously challenge themselves to provide creative, interesting, and sound education – students soon learn that education doesn't have to be boring; they become self-motivated, enthusiastic, and interested... learning then follows. — Linda Caputi

## References

Alfaro-LeFevre, R. (2009). *Critical thinking and clinical judgment: A practical approach to outcome-focused thinking* (4th ed.). St. Louis: Saunders/Elsevier.

American Association of Colleges of Nursing [AACN]. (2008). *The Essentials of baccalaureate education for professional nursing practice*. Washington, D.C.: Author.

American Nurses Association [ANA]. (2004). *Nursing: Scope and standards of practice*. Silver Spring, MD: Author.

Bastable, S. (2003). Nurse as educator. Boston, MA: Jones and Bartlett. Bevis, E.O. (1982). *Curriculum building: A process* (3rd ed.). St. Louis, MO: Mosby.

Bevis, E. O., & Watson, J. (2000). *Toward a caring curriculum: A new pedagogy for nursing*. Boston, MA: Jones and Bartlett.

Bloom, B. S. (Ed.). (1956). *Taxonomy of educational objectives: Handbook I, cognitive domain*. New York: David McKay.

Boland, D. (2009). Developing curriculum: Frameworks, outcomes, and competencies. In D. Billings & J. Halstead (Ed.). *Teaching in nursing: A guide for faculty*, (3rd ed.). Saint Louis: Saunders Elsevier.

Caputi, L., & Engelmann, L. (2008). *Teaching nursing: The art and science, it's all about student success*. Glen Ellyn, IL: College of DuPage Press.

Commission on Collegiate Nursing Education (CCNE) (2008). *Standards for accreditation of baccalaureate and graduate degree nursing programs.* Washington, DC: Author.

Duffy, J. (2005). Want to graduate nurses who care? Assessing nursing students' caring competencies. In M.H. Oermann & K.T. Heinrich, (Eds.), *Annual review of nursing education*, Vol. 3, (pp. 59-76). New York: Springer.

Finkelman, A., & Kenner, C. (2007). *Teaching IOM: Implications of the IOM reports for nursing education.* Silver Spring, MD: ANA.

Grady, J. L. (2009). How can state boards of nursing encourage curricular reform? [Headlines from the NLN] *Nursing Education Perspectives, 30*(1), 59-61.

Gronlund, N. (1995). *How to write and use instructional objectives* (5th ed.). Columbus, OH: Prentice Hall.

Institute of Medicine. (2003). *Crossing the quality chasm.* Washington, DC: National Academies Press.

Kramer, N. A. (2005). Capturing the curriculum: A curriculum maturation and transformation process. *Nurse Educator, 30*(2), 80-84.

National League for Nursing Accrediting Commission (NLNAC). (2008). *NLNAC Accreditation Manual.* New York: Author.

National League for Nursing. (2005). *The scope of practice for academic nurse educators.* New York: Author.

Nursing Executive Center. (2008). *Bridging the preparation practice gap.* Washington, DC: The Advisory Board Company.

Porter-O'Grady, P. (2010, in press). Nurses as knowledge workers. In L. Caputi, (Ed.). *Teaching nursing: The art and science, Vol. 2.* Glen Ellyn, IL: College of DuPage Press.

Quality and Safety Education for Nurses [QSEN] (2007). Retrieved January 10, 2009 from http://qsen.org/competencydomains/competencies_list

Tanner, C. (2007). The curriculum revolution revisited. *Journal of Nursing Education, 46*(2), 51-52.

Von Achterberg, T. Schoonhoven, L., & Grol, R. (2008). Nursing implementation science: How evidence-based nursing requires evidence-based implementation. *Journal of Nursing Scholarship, 40*(4), 302-310.

# Appendix A
## Nursing Program
## Employer Survey

Dear Employer,

In our efforts to continue to make the Nursing Program better, we need your help in completing this survey. Would you answer the following questions? When you have finished completing the survey, please return in the self-addressed, postage-paid envelope. We appreciate and value your opinion.

1) How would you rate the overall performance of the graduates of the Nursing Program you have hired in the last year?
   a. Superior
   b. Above average
   c. Average
   d. Below average
   e. Poor

2) How would you rate the performance of the graduates of the Nursing Program when using critical thinking in patient care?
   a. Superior
   b. Above average
   c. Average
   d. Below average
   e. Poor

3) How would you rate the performance of the graduates of the Nursing Program when demonstrating caring while performing patient care?
   a. Superior
   b. Above average
   c. Average
   d. Below average
   e. Poor

4) How would you rate the performance of the graduates of the Nursing Program when performing nursing interventions?
   a. Superior
   b. Above average

c. Average
d. Below average
e. Poor

5) How would you rate the ability of the graduates of the Nursing Program to care for a diverse patient population?
   a. Superior
   b. Above average
   c. Average
   d. Below average
   e. Poor

6) In what areas are you employing graduates of the Nursing Program?
   a. Gerontology
   b. Medical/Surgical
   c. Pediatrics
   d. Obstetrics
   e. Mental Health
   f. Other: please specify _____

Please rate each of the six behaviors in the below table according to how well you believe the graduates of the Nursing Program perform. Place a check mark in the column that best represents your opinion.

| Behavior | Excellent | Good | Fair | Poor | Not Applicable |
|---|---|---|---|---|---|
| Function as a competent nurse within a legal and ethical framework to provide holistic care to patents from diverse backgrounds. | | | | | |

| | | | | |
|---|---|---|---|---|
| Effectively communicate with patients, significant support person(s), and members of the healthcare team incorporating interpersonal and therapeutic communication skills. | | | | |
| Holistically collect assessment data from multiple sources, communicate data to appropriate healthcare providers, and evaluate patient response to interventions. | | | | |
| Work with members of the healthcare team to organize and incorporate assessment and evaluation data to plan/revise patient care. | | | | |
| Demonstrate a caring and empathetic approach to the individualized care of each patient. | | | | |
| Implement patient care through skillful performance of therapeutic nursing interventions, recognizing need for changes, and collaborating with others to change the plan of care. | | | | |

Please feel free to share any comments you may have about the Nursing Program.
We welcome your comments.

_____

_____

_____

_____

_____

_____

_____

_____

_____

**Thank you for completing this survey!**

## Appendix B
## Nursing Program
## Graduate Survey

Dear Graduate:

It's been a while since you have completed the Nursing Program. Now that you've been engaged in practice, we would like to ask a few questions. Would you answer the following questions? When you have finished completing the survey, please return in the self-addressed, postage-paid envelope. We appreciate and value your opinion.

1) How would you rate the education you received?
   a. Superior
   b. Above average
   c. Average
   d. Below average
   e. Poor

2) Which instructional environment was most helpful for your learning?
   a. Classroom
   b. Nursing Laboratory
   c. Clinical
   d. All
   e. None

3) What was your experience taking the NCLEX-RN®?
   a. Passed on the first attempt.
   b. Passed on the second attempt.
   c. Passed after three or more attempts.
   d. Have not passed the exam.

4) What interventions did you use to prepare for the NCLEX-RN®?
   a. Review course
   b. Books/CD-ROM
   c. Group study
   d. Internet resources
   e. Self study

5) Are you currently employed as a Registered Nurse?
   a.  Yes
   b.  No, but I'm in school.
   c.  No

6) If currently working, in what type of facility are you employed?
   a.  Acute care
   b.  Long-term care
   c.  Community health
   d.  Physician's office
   e.  Other: please specify _____

7) What is your specialty area?
   a.  Gerontology
   b.  Medical/Surgical
   c.  Pediatrics
   d.  Obstetrics
   e.  Mental Health
   f.  Other: please specify _____

8) Do you have the job you want?
   a.  Yes
   b.  No

9) Do you believe the Nursing Program prepared you for your current nursing position?
   a.  Yes
   b.  Somewhat
   c.  No
   Please explain: _____
   _____

10) Are you currently enrolled in a nursing education program?
   a.  Yes
   b.  No, but plan to in the next two years
   c.  No

Please rate each of the six behaviors in the below table according to how well the Nursing Program prepared you to perform in your current nursing position. Place a check mark in the column of your choice.

| Behavior | Excellent | Good | Fair | Poor | Not Applicable |
|---|---|---|---|---|---|
| Function as a competent Registered Nurse within a legal and ethical framework to provide holistic care to patents from diverse backgrounds. | | | | | |
| Effectively communicate with patients, significant support person(s), and members of the healthcare team incorporating interpersonal and therapeutic communication skills. | | | | | |
| Holistically collect assessment data from multiple sources, communicate data to appropriate healthcare providers, and evaluate patient response to interventions. | | | | | |
| Work with members of the healthcare team to organize and incorporate assessment and evaluation data to plan/revise patient care. | | | | | |

| Demonstrate a caring and empathetic approach to the individualized care of each patient. | | | | |
|---|---|---|---|---|
| Implement patient care through skillful performance of therapeutic nursing interventions, recognizing need for changes, and collaborating with others to change the plan of care. | | | | |

Please feel free to share any comments you may have about the Nursing Program. We welcome your comments.

_____
_____
_____
_____
_____
_____
_____
_____
_____
_____

**Thank you for completing this survey! Best wishes for a rewarding nursing career!**

# CHAPTER 22

## DEVELOPING A CONTEMPORARY CURRICULUM FOR AN ADN PROGRAM

**Linda Caputi, MSN, EdD, RN, CNE**
**Barbara Hunt, MS, RN, APRN-CNS, AOCN®**

The content of this chapter relates to the following major content area and subconcepts on the Certified Nurse Educator Examination Detailed Test Blueprint:
**Participate in Curriculum Design and Evaluation of Program Outcomes**
- Lead in the development of designing a curriculum
- Actively participate in the design of the curriculum to reflect: institutional philosophy and mission; current nursing and health care trends; community and societal needs
- Demonstrate knowledge of curriculum development
- Revise the curriculum based on evaluation of program outcomes; societal and health care trends; stakeholder feedback
- Update courses to reflect the philosophical and theoretical framework of the curriculum
- Design courses to reflect the philosophical and theoretical framework of the curriculum

## Introduction

The Associate Degree in Nursing (ADN) program at the College of Lake County (CLC) was established approximately three decades ago. The program was based on a sound philosophy and framework utilizing a nursing theorist, adult learning principles, modular learning emphasizing student preparation prior to attending class, class participation in group discussion of case scenarios, and clinical competency testing for progression within the program and graduation. Each course was updated yearly by faculty teaching the course. For many years this program of instruction served the students and the community well as demonstrated by accreditation by the National League for Nursing Accrediting Commission (NLNAC), high NCLEX® pass rates, low attrition rates, and positive evaluations from employers of graduates from the program. Program outcomes were based on the Educational Competencies for Graduates of Associate Degree Nursing Programs developed by the National

League for Nursing (NLN) and the National Organization of Associate Degree Nursing (NOADN) (NLN, 2000).

## Factors Driving Change

In recent years there has been a turnover of faculty at CLC as a result of retirements. The turnover of faculty has reached well over 50% within just a five year time span. This trend is similar to other programs nationally which are experiencing nursing faculty shortages due to retirements (LaRocco, 2006). Also, all administrative positions for the nursing program experienced a 100% turnover. There appeared to be a disconnect between newer faculty and more experienced faculty related to a lack of understanding of the nursing curriculum, the way it was structured, and the way it was implemented.

NCLEX pass rates began to decline. Concerns about the nursing program and suggestions for improvement were voiced from a variety of sources. Listening to the voice of various stakeholders, – including students and employers of our graduates – assessing the need for an update to the curriculum, and considering the declining pass rates, the faculty analyzed this data and determined action was needed. Experienced faculty had enjoyed positive outcomes in the past, but were now disappointed in the program outcomes over recent years. New faculty believed they had some fresh ideas that may benefit the program. The dreaded words "curriculum revision" were uttered more than once. Perhaps it was time.

## Identified Areas of Concern

The faculty identified four major priorities to address. The first priority was team building and conflict resolution. Because of the various backgrounds and experience faculty brought to the task, it was important to start with team building and conflict resolution to pave the way for solid working relationships to deal with the many issues that arise with a major curriculum revision. Collaboration and collegiality are two major ingredients for successful curriculum revision (Kramer, 2005). To address these components from the onset seemed to be the smart thing to do. Although it took time initially, it actually helped move the process along.

The second priority related to clinical evaluation and competency testing. This was the primary concern voiced by students. The faculty previously had not used a clinical evaluation tool but had relied on competency testing. Students saw this as high-stakes testing. They were growing anxious with the testing performed in clinical and many were having difficulty dealing with the testing. Unsure of why competency testing worked in the past but was not working now, faculty decided to investigate another possibility for clinical evaluation.

The third priority became curriculum review and revision. Faculty strongly believed it was important to graduate nurses who were ready for today's world of nursing. Although employers always highly rated CLC graduates, faculty believed it was important to evaluate the program for currency to reflect current standards of practice.

New nursing faculty also voiced concern about the difficulty of applying the organizing framework of the nursing program, which was based on a single nursing theorist. They did not see the relationship of that organizing framework to current health care. Terminology within the program based on the nursing theory did not reflect terminology used in clinical settings. This was found to be confusing to students. It was determined to consider a curriculum revision with a broader focus rather than limited to a single nursing theorist.

## Making Time

Nursing faculty met during an 18 month period to discuss and make decisions related to the identified priority items and the concerns regarding the program. To accommodate for the large time commitment, adjustments needed to be made. These included:

- Class schedules were revised to provide time when all nursing faculty could meet over an extended period and on a regular basis throughout the academic year to work on curriculum revision.
- Nursing faculty decided to use the services of a consultant, Dr. Linda Caputi, who had expertise in nursing curriculum to assist in facilitating the curriculum review process.
- Faculty with tenure in the program voluntarily increased their teaching loads to decrease the teaching load of newly hired faculty to provide increased time for new faculty to become better oriented to the nursing program itself.

All these measures and the dedication of faculty to this cause provided the needed time and energy to tackle this work.

# First Priority: Conflict Resolution and Team Building

A consultant was hired to conduct two meetings with the nursing faculty to address conflict resolution and team building issues. The first meeting focused on conflict resolution by reviewing conflict resolution strategies and then addressing specific topics for discussion related conflicts about the current curriculum. The areas for discussion were:

- Decide on an overall shared goal for the nursing curriculum
- Identify specific needs and desires of the nursing faculty regarding curriculum review
- Identify concerns and fears of the nursing faculty regarding the curriculum review process
- Determine activities that need to occur as part of the curriculum review process

Before beginning the curriculum revision work, the nursing faculty decided on ground rules for discussion. These included:

- Participation by everyone
- Being honest
- Being tactful
- Using "I" statements
- Being respectful
- Not interrupting
- Treating all ideas as good ideas
- Confidentiality

The second meeting focused on team building within the nursing faculty. Prior to this meeting, each faculty member was to complete a computerized profile which identified the key roles each faculty member played in a group setting. During the meeting all faculty members identified what role they played. This was visually displayed on a board in the front of the room for easy viewing of where each faculty member fit in relationship to one another. The point of this exercise was to reinforce the value of every team member and the importance of having a balanced team.

Nursing faculty were then given a task to complete in which half the faculty were blindfolded and did not know the task, and the other half were to direct and coach the blindfolded faculty in performing the task. These activities were instrumental in assisting nursing faculty to value and better understand each other's perspectives and contributions. The result of these activities was an improved atmosphere of open communication and collegiality.

## Second Priority: Clinical Evaluation and Competency Testing

The issue before the nursing faculty was whether to modify the current method of clinical evaluation or change it. The nursing faculty believed it would be beneficial to dialogue with faculty from another program who use the competency testing model, but in a modified form.

A video conference was held between the nursing faculty of the two programs. The purpose was to clarify how the model was operationalized in their ADN program. Through video conferencing, nursing faculty were able to ask questions and clarify how the model was modified and applied by the other program faculty. This was a valuable step that assisted nursing faculty in thinking through the option of continuing to use competency testing with modifications.

An ad hoc committee was formed and assigned the task of bringing a recommendation to the faculty of a modified version of the current model for competency testing. The committee found it would be difficult to modify the model and stay within the time constraints given for the curriculum revision. A modified version was temporarily adopted and used with currently enrolled students. The faculty then decided the current model of competency testing for clinical evaluation should no longer be used in the program. The faculty eventually made the decision to develop a clinical evaluation tool based on graduate learning outcomes to be used when the newly revised curriculum is implemented in place of competency testing.

## Third Priority: Curriculum Evaluation and Revision

As previously mentioned, Dr. Caputi was employed as a curriculum consultant to help facilitate the curriculum revision process. The consultant asked nursing faculty to respond to questions prior to an all day meeting. The consultant then used the responses from faculty to generate and direct discussion during the meeting. Figure 1 presents these questions.

**Theoretical Beliefs**
1. What do you believe is the mission of the nursing program at CLC?
2. How do you see the following quote from Bevis and Watson (2000) operationalized: Curriculum is "those transactions and interactions that take place between students & teachers and among students with the intent that learning takes place".

**Curriculum**
3. Do you believe the current curriculum is meeting the needs of students?
   a. If so, how?
   b. If not, how would you change it?
4. Do you believe the current curriculum is meeting the needs of the community?
   a. If so, how?
   b. If not, how would you change it?
5. Are graduates leaving school with the necessary knowledge and skills for their job?
   a. If so, how?
   b. If not, how would you change it?
6. What core competencies do you identify as most important for your graduates to demonstrate?
7. What are the strengths of your graduates?
8. What are the weaknesses of your graduates?

**Delivery of the Curriculum**
9. Is your curriculum being delivered with current methods of instruction?
   a. If so, how?
   b. If not, how would you change it?
10. Are your current textbooks meeting your needs?
    a. If so, how?
    b. If not, what textbooks would you change?
    c. Suggested textbooks:
11. Do you believe the current sequencing of content is best for your program?
    a. If so, why?
    b. If not, how would you change it?

**Students**
12. What characteristics describe your students?
13. What are your beliefs about students?
14. What are your beliefs about teaching?
15. What are your beliefs about learning?
16. What strengths do your students bring to the program?

**Figure 1.** Initial Faculty Questionnaire

17. What weaknesses are common to your students?
18. What are the characteristics of students who fail nursing courses?

**NCLEX**
19. Are you happy with your latest NCLEX results?
    a. If yes, why?
    b. If not, why not?
20. What do you believe were factors that influenced your latest NCLEX results?
21. What are the characteristics of students who failed NCLEX?
22. Would you be interested in instituting an NCLEX success plan?
    a. If yes, what would the plan entail?
    b. If not, why not?

**Additional Comments**
Please add any additional comments you would like to share with me at this time.

**Figure 1 continued.** Initial Faculty Questionnaire

The questions provided a focus for discussion and opened dialogue on some of the problem areas of the curriculum. Because the questions were from a neutral person, they were not perceived as threatening or territorial.

Prior to a second meeting, the consultant again had faculty respond to a set of questions intended to help faculty think through some of the elements of a curriculum and how they individually perceived the type of curriculum they would like to develop. Figure 2 presents these questions.

1. Describe the Mission, Philosophy and Vision of the Nursing program and discuss how these items fit into the College Mission and Philosophy.
2. List the major concepts you believe should be the foundation of the nursing program and discuss how those concepts should fit into the framework for the program.
3. Describe the ideal structure and flow of the nursing program or what you believe would be the best structure and flow.

**Figure 2.** Questions Focused on the Structure of the Nursing Program Curriculum

Again, these questions were useful in guiding discussions and laying the groundwork for the detailed curriculum development that followed. Based on the faculty's answers to the questions presented in Figure 2, the decision was made to eliminate the nursing theorist as the organizing framework for the curriculum and take a more eclectic approach to developing an framework which incorporated adult learning theory as well as current recommendations for nursing education from sources such as the Institute of Medicine (IOM) reports, Quality and Safety Education in Nursing (QSEN), Healthy People 2010, the National Council of State Boards of Nursing (NCSBN) Practice Analysis, the NCLEX-RN® Test Plan, and the American Nurses Association's Standards of Practice. The faculty believed this approach would be more flexible and, therefore, more amenable to change in the future.

## Curriculum Revision

The curriculum consultant continued to work with the nursing faculty to develop the new curriculum. The nursing faculty initially attended a workshop entitled, "Curriculum Development and Implementation: A Plan for NCLEX Success." This workshop laid the groundwork for developing and implementing a new curriculum. After this workshop, the consultant led nursing faculty through a systematic process for development of the new curriculum.

### Development of a Mission and Philosophy

Nursing faculty developed an updated mission and philosophy for the nursing program. These derive from the mission and philosophy of the parent organization and include beliefs of the nursing faculty. Figure 3 presents the mission and philosophy.

**Mission of the CLC ADN Program**
The mission of the ADN Program at CLC is to provide a balanced curriculum of general and nursing education **leading to the graduate learning outcomes**. This curriculum strives to prepare qualified persons to successfully complete the NCLEX-RN, obtain licensure and practice as entry level registered nurses (RN) to contribute to the health care needs of Lake County.

**Philosophy of the CLC ADN Program**
The philosophy of the College of Lake County (CLC) Associate Degree Nursing (ADN) program represents humanistic values related to nursing and patient care as well as the purpose of developing the knowledge, attitudes, and skills necessary to meet licensure requirements as a Registered Nurse. Philosophical statements are presented that represent the enduring values and beliefs of the nursing faculty regarding the phenomenon of nursing and nursing education. These philosophical statements provide a value system upon which the curriculum components are developed. The philosophy statements of the CLC ADN program use the nursing metaparadigm in describing key components of nursing. In addition, these philosophy statements identify beliefs of the nursing faculty regarding students, faculty, learning and the process of nursing education.

**Figure 3.** Program Mission and Philosophy

The faculty then described their collective views of the concepts of nursing, people, health, environment, and nursing education. Learning was also described and is believed to be an eclectic process involving behavioral learning theory, constructivist learning theory, and principles of adult learning. The roles of student and faculty were then described and are as follows:

**Nursing Students.** Applying Adult Learning Theory, the CLC faculty believe that nursing students assume responsibility for their own learning. Students possess different learning styles. Nursing students, as adult learners, learn best when actively involved in the learning process. Nursing students learn by building upon previous knowledge and life experiences.

**Nursing Faculty.** Nursing faculty are facilitators of learning. They serve as a resource for nursing students. Their role is to guide the learning process by planning and providing learning experiences which account for a variety of student characteristics and stages of cognitive development. Nursing faculty provide feedback through formative and summative evaluations. Nursing faculty keep current in nursing knowledge and practice and update learning experiences to reflect current nursing practices.

## Core Components (CC)

Using the current initiatives in health care, the faculty identified six core components (CC) believed important for today's nursing practice which include:
1. Quality, safe, evidence-based, patient-centered care
2. Collaboration
3. Critical thinking
4. Leadership
5. Information technology
6. Professionalism

## Graduate Learning Outcomes

With the six core components identified, faculty then wrote the learning outcomes that would be expected of all their graduates to reflect these core components. Faculty believed it was important to start with describing the expected outcomes at the end of the program on which all course outcomes will be based. Using the IOM reports, QSEN, Healthy People 2010, the NCSBN Practice Analysis, the NCLEX-RN® Test Plan, and the ANA Standards of Practice as a base, the following six graduate learning outcomes were developed:
1. Quality, safe, evidence-based, patient-centered care: Provide quality, effective, and safe nursing care through evidence-based practice.
2. Collaboration: Collaborate with members of the interdisciplinary team for the purpose of providing and improving patient care.
3. Critical thinking: Analyze patient situations and apply critical thinking skills and strategies necessary to provide quality patient care.
4. Leadership: Provide leadership in a variety of healthcare settings for diverse patient populations.
5. Information technology: Communicate, manage knowledge, mitigate error, and support decision making using information technology.
6. Professionalism: Function as a competent nurse assimilating all professional, ethical, and legal principles.

## Development of a Visual Model

Nursing faculty, under the guidance of the curriculum consultant, created a visual model that represents all the factors influencing the curriculum of the ADN program. A visual model is helpful for clearly and quickly communicating to stakeholders, students, and other interested parties the basis of the nursing curriculum. To accomplish this task, the philosophy and framework were reviewed and major concepts identified.

A model was developed which illustrated the overall philosophy and organizing framework for the new curriculum. Health care was considered as being delivered within the global environment. It was felt the global environment impacted health care and influenced the agenda for healthcare (USDHHS, 2000). The healthcare setting, where health care is delivered, was viewed as containing three levels:

1. The level for patient point-of-care
2. The level within which patient care is delivered (considered the clinical microsystem)
3. The healthcare system itself

Patient-centered care, a concept of the new framework, is depicted in the model by placing the patient at the center of the healthcare system. Patients seek and receive care within the clinical microsystem, which is a subset of the overall healthcare system. Nursing functions within all three levels of the healthcare system. See Figure 4.

The six core components of professional nursing practice also interact with all three levels of the healthcare setting. Each core component (CC) has associated major concepts as well as a related graduate learning outcome (GLO). These were all added to the model to include all components into a single model. See Figure 5.

## Course Revisions

Once the faculty decided on the graduate learning outcomes as the final destination, the path to getting there involved rewriting course descriptions and identifying individual course outcomes. These outcomes would build to culminate in the final course outcomes that reflected the six graduate learning outcomes. For some courses content was moved around to better reflect a simple to complex framework. Faculty believed it was important to map the curriculum content to the NCLEX® detailed test plan and developed a tool for this task.

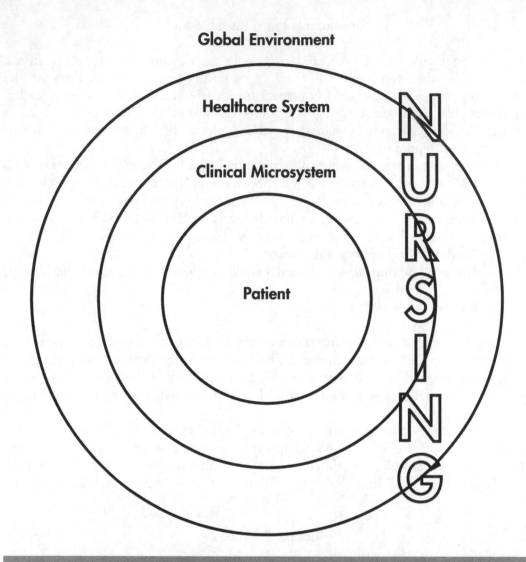

**Figure 4.** The Context for Health Care and Role of Nursing within the Global Environment

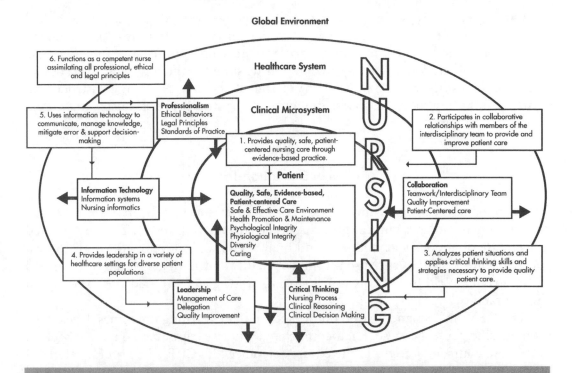

**Figure 5.** Model Depicting Organizing Framework for the New ADN Curriculum including: Core Components of Professional Nursing Practice, Major Concepts, and Graduate Learning Outcomes as they relate to the Healthcare Setting and Nursing

Once the course descriptions and course outcomes were identified the individual course syllabi were written. Faculty worked in teams to develop the revised courses. All faculty considered the use of a variety of teaching strategies to meet course outcomes. Rather than a strict approach that was used in the past where all courses were taught using case studies, faculty designed the courses to use instructional strategies that best meet the course outcomes. Case studies are still used, but are no longer the only medium.

## Clinical Evaluation Tool

Competency testing in the clinical is no longer the method used at CLC for determining a student's clinical grade. A clinical evaluation tool (CET) will be used to evaluate all students at midterm and final. CETs were developed for all clinical courses. Rubrics were written so all clinical faculty and students would be informed of the grading criteria. This is critical so all students are graded the same by all clinical faculty.

The CET was designed based on the six graduate learning outcomes, leveled for each specific clinical course. Each competency under each outcome relates back to one of the course objectives in the course reference file (CRF). The course reference file is the document that is approved by the college curriculum committees as well as the state Community College Board. Table 1 provides an example of the clinical evaluation tool used in the first clinical course.

| | |
|---|---|
| Name:<br>Date:<br>Clinical Faculty:<br>Clinical Site:<br>S = Satisfactory  NI = Needs Improvement  U = Unsatisfactory  N/A = Not applicable<br>Must earn an "S" in every competency by the end of the course. ||
| **1. Graduate Learning Outcome: Provides quality, safe, patient-centered nursing care through evidence-based practice.** ||
| Grade | Behaviors and Comments |
| | A. Performs a head-to-toe assessment. **CRF Objective(s): 2**<br>Comments: |
| | B. Identifies ways the nurse is sensitive to patient's individual needs, culture, religion, and developmental level. **CRF Objective(s): 1, 4**<br>Comments: |
| | C. Gives examples of caring behaviors of the nurse when interacting with the patient and the patient's support system. **CRF Objective(s): 1, 3**<br>Comments: |
| | D. Identifies evidence-based nursing interventions for each patient that provide psychosocial and physiological integrity, and health promotion and maintenance. **CRF Objective(s): 5**<br>Comments: |
| | E. Gives examples of using therapeutic communication when interacting with patients and the patients' support network. **CRF Objective(s): 7**<br>Comments: |
| | F. Provides information about the patient to other healthcare workers using a hand-off communication tool when appropriate. **CRF Objective(s): 7**<br>Comments: |

**Table 1.** College of Lake County, Nursing Program, Clinical Evaluation Tool, Nursing 133, Midterm & Final Evaluation

| | |
|---|---|
| | G. Safely and competently performs and documents all nursing interventions within the healthcare microsystem. **CRF Objective(s): 1, 3**<br>Comments: |
| | H. Identifies how to evaluate nursing care provided. **CRF Objective(s): 3**<br>Comments: |
| | I. Identifies patient learning needs and ways teaching can be implemented. **CRF Objective(s): 3**<br>Comments: |

**2. Graduate Learning Outcome: Participates in collaborative relationships with members of the interdisciplinary team for the purpose of providing and improving patient care.**

| Grade | Behaviors and Comments |
|---|---|
| | A. Identifies patient values, preferences, and expressed needs of patient and which members of the healthcare team is appropriate for receiving this information. **CRF Objective(s): 1**<br>Comments: |
| | B. Identifies evaluation data to collect which will provide information about progress toward achievement of outcomes and identify which member of the healthcare team with whom you would collaborate. **CRF Objective(s): 3, 9**<br>Comments: |
| | C. Gives examples of the types of decisions that need to be discussed with the patient, the patient's support network, and other members of the healthcare team. **CRF Objective(s): 9, 12**<br>Comments: |
| | D. Describes ways the nurse interacts with others to solve problems to achieve patient goals and outcomes. **CRF Objective(s): 6, 12**<br>Comments: |

**Table 1 continued.** College of Lake County, Nursing Program, Clinical Evaluation Tool, Nursing 133, Midterm & Final Evaluation

| Grade | Behaviors and Comments |
|---|---|
| | E. Summarizes own strengths, limitations, and values in functioning as a member of a team. **CRF Objective(s): 11**<br>Comments: |
| | F. Gives examples of the impact of team functioning on safety and quality of patient care. **CRF Objective(s): 9, 10**<br>Comments: |

**3. Graduate Learning Outcome: Analyzes patient situations and applies critical thinking skills and strategies necessary to provide quality patient care.**

| Grade | Behaviors and Comments |
|---|---|
| | A. Identifies clinical judgments and management decisions made by the nurse that ensure accurate and safe care when implementing all steps of the nursing process. **CRF Objective(s): 12**<br>Comments: |
| | B. Lists in order of priority nursing assessments and interventions. **CRF Objective(s): 12**<br>Comments: |
| | C. States ways the involvement of the patient and family can improve the safety and quality of health care. **CRF Objective(s): 7**<br>Comments: |
| | D. Discusses ways economic and demographic forces affect the delivery of health care to patients in the current clinical environment. **CRF Objective(s): 1**<br>Comments: |
| | E. Locates current literature about patient care and identifies difference between care provided and care described in the literature. **CRF Objective(s): 5**<br>Comments: |

**Table 1 continued.** College of Lake County, Nursing Program, Clinical Evaluation Tool, Nursing 133, Midterm & Final Evaluation

| | |
|---|---|
| | F. Identifies an actual or potential error and possible ways the error could be avoided. **CRF Objective(s): 12**<br>Comments: |

**4. Graduate Learning Outcome: Provides leadership in a variety of healthcare settings for diverse patient populations.**

| Grade | Behaviors and Comments |
|---|---|
| | A. Identifies the authority figures on the clinical unit and how they influence teamwork and patient safety. **CRF Objective(s): 10**<br>Comments: |
| | B. Describes what tasks can be delegated to an unlicensed person. **CRF Objective(s): 12**<br>Comments: |
| | C. Identifies which team members would be involved in the implementation of care for the patient. **CRF Objective(s): 9**<br>Comments: |

**5. Graduate Learning Outcome: Uses information technology to communicate, manage knowledge, mitigate error, and support decision-making.**

| Grade | Behaviors and Comments |
|---|---|
| | A. Maintains organizational and patient confidentiality. **CRF Objective(s): 1, 8**<br>Comments: |
| | B. Describes how technology and information management are related to the quality and safety of patient care. **CRF Objective(s): 8**<br>Comments: |
| | C. Identifies areas of the electronic health record pertinent to nursing care. **CRF Objective(s): 8**<br>Comments: |

**Table 1 continued.** College of Lake County, Nursing Program, Clinical Evaluation Tool, Nursing 133, Midterm & Final Evaluation

| | D. Documents patient care in an electronic health record. **CRF Objective(s): 3, 8**<br>Comments: |
|---|---|
| | E. Locates high quality electronic sources of healthcare information. **CRF Objective(s): 5, 8**<br>Comments: |

**6. Graduate Learning Outcome: Functions as a competent nurse assimilating all professional, ethical, and legal principles while implementing the roles of the professional nurse.**

| Grade | Behaviors and Comments |
|---|---|
| | A. Practices within the ethical, legal, and regulatory frameworks of nursing and standards of professional nursing practice. **CRF Objective(s): 11**<br>Comments: |
| | B. Demonstrates accountability for nursing care given by self. **CRF Objective(s): 11**<br>Comments: |
| | C. Practices within the parameters of individual knowledge and experiences. **CRF Objective(s): 11**<br>Comments: |
| | D. Employs limits and boundaries of therapeutic patient-centered care. **CRF Objective(s): 11**<br>Comments: |
| | E. Demonstrates use of appropriate institutional resources. **CRF Objective(s): 1, 11**<br>Comments: |

**Table 1 continued.** College of Lake County, Nursing Program, Clinical Evaluation Tool, Nursing 133, Midterm & Final Evaluation

The student is evaluated on each competency using a scale of S (Satisfactory), NI (Needs Improvement), or U (Unsatisfactory). All students must earn an S by midterm. Any NI would require the faculty to meet with the student to determine the appropriate interventions to improve on that behavior to earn an S by the end of the course.

## Summary

Curriculum revision typically creates much angst in nursing faculty. However, curriculum revision is an ongoing process that never ends because nursing and health care constantly change. Although CLC had made yearly changes in most courses, a look at the total program with a new, fresh approach was due. The process took approximately two years to complete and was a smoother process than originally feared. The initial team building sessions were extremely helpful in making this process a success. The faculty identified the need to change, articulated a common goal, and then set their minds to the task at hand. Implementation of the new curriculum will begin in the next school year. Faculty are excited with renewed vigor about the revised curriculum. They realize that, as with all new adventures, once implemented there will be minor changes and tweaking required. However, after undergoing a major curriculum revision, minor changes will be just that – minor.

## Learning Activities

1. Discuss with a colleague the process of curriculum revision at colleague's college. Ask how the faculty approached the task, if it appeared overwhelming, and what the results were.
2. Discuss with your colleagues lessons learned from experiences with curriculum revisions. How can those experiences be used to make future curriculum changes a less arduous task?
3. Consider a curriculum with which you are familiar. How might you revise it to make it better?

## Educational Philosophy

I believe that learning is fun and that learning is lifelong. Teachers and students share responsibility in the learning process. Teachers are facilitators of learning and serve as a resource for students. They guide the learning process by planning and providing a variety of learning experiences. Attention should be paid to providing an interactive, enjoyable environment for learning. Teaching should be student-centered by utilizing teaching strategies that take into consideration student learning styles, preferences, and previous experiences. Students, as adult learners, learn best when actively involved in the learning process. Students should take responsibility for their learning. Students learn by building upon previous knowledge and life experiences. — Barbara Hunt

My educational philosophy is succinct: Give the best educational experience possible. I believe faculty should continuously challenge themselves to provide creative, interesting, and sound education – students soon learn that education doesn't have to be boring; they become self-motivated, enthusiastic, and interested... learning then follows. — Linda Caputi

## References

Bevis, E. O., & Watson, J. (2000). *Toward a caring curriculum: A new pedagogy for nursing*. Sudbury, MA: Jones and Bartlett and the National League for Nursing.

Kramer, N. A. (2005). Capturing the curriculum: A curriculum maturation and transformation process. *Nurse Educator, 30*(2), 80-84.

LaRocco, S. (2006). Who will teach nurses? *Academe, 92*(3), 38.

National League for Nursing (NLN). (2000). *Educational competencies for graduates of associate degree nursing programs*. Sudbury, Massachusetts: Jones and Bartlett Publishers.

U.S. Department of Health and Human Services (USDHHS). (2000). *Healthy People 2010*. Washington, D.C.: U.S. Government Printing Office.

# CHAPTER 23

# CURRICULUM ALIGNMENT OF THE ESSENTIAL EDUCATIONAL COMPETENCIES IN NURSING EDUCATION

**Stephanie Holaday, DrPh, RN**

---

The content of this chapter relates to the following major content area and subconcepts on the Certified Nurse Educator Examination Detailed Test Blueprint:
**Participate in Curriculum Design and Evaluation of Program Outcomes**
- Lead in the development of designing a curriculum
- Actively participate in the design of the curriculum to reflect current nursing and healthcare trends; community and societal needs
- Demonstrate knowledge of curriculum development including identifying program outcomes, selecting appropriate evaluation strategies
- Implement program assessment models
- Analyze results of program evaluation and initiate curricular change

---

## Introduction

Nurse educators are responsible for graduating students who have demonstrated a certain level of competence that is congruent with the professional standards for entry into nursing practice. Educators must demonstrate they provide students with adequate instruction and opportunities to meet the standards that have been set (Baratz-Snowden, 1993). What students are taught and how they are taught are equally important. Assessment practices aligned with professional standards ensure educators are teaching to standards rather than what faculty perceive to be important or, worse, teaching to the test. Profesional standards send strong signals to educators about what information should be taught, assessed, and learned. Assessment and evaluation results are expected to provide accurate information to the student and the public about the student's achievement, and important feedback to nurse educators on which to base improvement efforts. For the purposes of this chapter, these educational standards will be referred to as the essential educational competencies set forth by the American Association of Colleges of Nursing (AACN) (2008), and/or the National League for Nursing (NLN) (2000).

This chapter discusses the importance of establishing full curriculum alignment in nursing education. More specifically, it addresses the importance of determining the extent to which the instructional activities, assessment practices, and evaluation methods by nurse educators adequately cover and measure the breadth, depth, and range of complexity of the essential educational competencies, as intended by the AACN and/or the NLN.

## The Problem

According to the Institute of Medicine (2000) an estimated 98,000 patients die in hospitals each year from preventable medical errors, illuminating the importance of closely assessing the progress of nursing students and ensuring a high degree of objectivity of their evaluation prior to entering the workforce. Furthermore, Lenburg (1999) noted that employers reported a widening gulf between the competencies required for practice and those that new graduates learned in their education programs. Employers are spending increasing amounts of time and resources orienting and teaching new nurses the competencies required in today's workplace. Professional nursing organizations have been calling for nurse educators to work together with service leaders to better align nursing education with practice environments (AACN, 2006; NCSBN, 2008; NLN, 2005; Lenburg, 1999). To stop the widening of the gap between education and practice, it is vital to establish full curriculum alignment with the essential educational competencies in order to prepare students for entry into nursing practice. Moreover, to ensure the achievement of the essential educational competencies, it is vital, not optional, to increase the emphasis on valid student assessments and evaluations to document the readiness of new nurses for full practice responsibilities.

A report released by the Institute of Medicine (IOM, 2003) informs us that "nurses and other health professionals are not adequately prepared to provide the highest quality and safest care possible, and there is insufficient assessment of their proficiency" (p. 1). Calls from authorities are loud and clear for healthcare disciplines to address the need for safe and competent care in our practice environments (AACN, 2007; AHRQ, 2003; IOM, 2004; Trust for America's Health, 2006). In response, there has been much attention dedicated to curricular and teaching methodology reform, but unfortunately, the degree of alignment of the essential educational competencies with the instruction, assessment, and evaluation methods by nurse educators is unknown.

## Problem #1

There is little in the nursing literature addressing curriculum alignment, especially in terms of outcome assessment or evaluation. To date, there are no studies indicating the degree of alignment between the essential educational competencies and instructional activities, assessment practices, or evaluation methods used by nurse educators.

## Problem #2

Figure 1 illustrates the four primary components of a nursing curriculum that require alignment:

1. The essential educational competencies (educational standards)
2. The instructional activities
3. The assessment practices
4. The measurement criteria or the methods used to evaluate the knowledge achieved and applied in practice.

The outcome of full alignment of these four components should be that students who graduate will be competent upon entry into practice. However, the reports indicating nurses are not competent upon entry into practice suggest that some components are not well aligned.

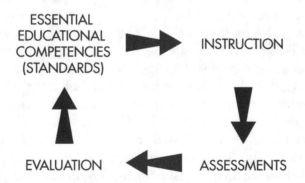

**Figure 1.** The Four Primary Components of a Nursing Curriculum

## Problem #3

If we assume that instructional delivery of theory in the classroom aligns with the essential educational competencies, and theory provides the basis for nursing practice, it seems reasonable to assume that the content studied in the classroom aligns with the content and experiences in the clinical setting. However, there is little in the literature examining the relationship between what is taught (input) and considered learned (actual outcomes) in the classroom, with what is taught (input) and considered learned (actual outcomes) in the practice setting.

Although curricular requirements are similar in nursing schools throughout the United States, there is little consistency, especially in the clinical setting, between expected outcomes and the methods used for evaluating those outcomes (Holaday & Buckley, 2008). Faculty often rely on personal perceptions and instincts about expectations in the clinical setting, resulting in much variation. A variation in expected outcomes leads to a variation in actual outcomes and proficiency. Therefore, the variations in instruction, assessment, and evaluation, especially in the clinical setting, are strongly linked to the inadequate preparation of nurses in general (Holaday & Buckley, 2008).

Content overload and fragmentation are major barriers to implementing any sort of accountability measures or education reform. Upton (1999, p. 549) asks the question, "How can we achieve evidenced-based practice if fundamental gaps and inconsistencies exist in nursing education?" These gaps, inconsistencies, and overlaps in instruction, assessment and evaluation are creating increasing stress and pressure for nurse educators and students.

## Background

According to the U. S. Department of Education (DOE) (2003), a curriculum that is aligned with educational standards is necessary for students to achieve and demonstrate proficiency. Incorporating the essential educational competencies set forth by the American Association of Colleges of Nursing (AACN) (2008), and/ or the National League for Nursing (NLN) (2000) into the curriculum is certainly necessary, but that alone is not enough to implement fully, nursing education reform, or ensure competency upon entry into nursing practice. In this time of increased public accountability, evidenced-based practice, and concern over healthcare outcomes and competency, it is imperative to have full curriculum alignment.

Full curriculum alignment requires a strong link among the following:

- Essential educational competencies (educational standards) and the instructional activities of the educators
- The instructional activities and the assessment practices of the educators
- The assessment practices and the evaluation methods used by the educators to measure achievement of the essential educational competencies (Anderson, 2002).

In other words, the concept of full curriculum alignment includes content validity, content coverage, and valid and reliable assessment and evaluation measurement practices of what is learned.

## The Essential Educational Competencies

The need to have a certain standard of competence and expertise is common to all health professions and is important to protect the public, ensure quality of care, and establish credibility of the profession (Oermann & Gaberson, 2006). Through expert consensus by a broad representation of stakeholders, both internal and external to nursing education and practice, the AACN (2008) and the NLN (2000) have identified essential educational competencies or outcomes that are expected of graduates of nursing programs upon entry into practice. Furthermore, nursing programs are accredited by either the Commission on Collegiate Nursing Education (CCNE), a subsidiary of the AACN, and/or the National League of Nursing Accrediting Commission (NLNAC), a subsidiary of the NLN. If the assumption is that nursing program outcomes should align with accreditation requirements, and the essential educational competencies are subsumed in the accreditation requirements, it should follow that the educational competencies deemed essential by the parent organization of the accrediting body align to the curriculum as outcomes for assessment and evaluation of instruction in both classroom and clinical settings. Furthermore, if the essential educational competencies transcend nursing programs, then the instruction, assessment, and evaluation of these competencies should also transcend nursing programs, enabling their use as standardized outcomes for classroom and clinical education.

The AACN and NLN essential educational competencies represent rigorously established standards for nursing education. Rigorous standards closely aligned with assessments and evaluations are major levers for high quality instruction, as well as for improving student achievement. Examining the alignment between the essential educational competencies and instruction, assessment, and evaluation practices of nurse educators in the classroom and clinical settings will shed light on (a) the appropriateness and usefulness of the instruction, assessments, and evaluations and (b) the level of preparedness of nurse educators to deliver the required curriculum to prepare students for high quality nursing care.

## History of Alignment

Webb (1997, 1999) defines alignment as the degree to which standards and assessments are in agreement, and work in conjunction with one another to guide the system toward students learning what they are expected to know and do. It is a phenomenon that has been studied in educational programs outside of nursing for a number of years (Anderson, 2002; Roach, Niebling & Kurz, 2008; Webb, 1999, 2005). Cohen (1987) and Carroll (1963) explain that objectives and assessments were analyzed as part of the mastery-learning movement during the 1960s. Analyses were performed on outcome objectives and assessment practices, and alignment was then considered achieved if the assessment practices were equivalent to the instructional activities. Content analysis by expert panels remains the primary method for determining the degree of alignment between essential educational competencies or standards and assessments. However, determining alignment today has become more complex, especially in nursing education, with the increasing amount and complexity of content that students need to learn to provide safe and effective nursing care, and the increasing pressures to transform nursing education to prepare students for today's changing healthcare system. This, of course, is in the face of an annual increase in enrollments in nursing programs since 2001 (AACN, 2008), and an ongoing nursing faculty shortage.

According to Case and Zucker (2005) the main purpose of studying and applying alignment has been to strengthen educational systems. Today, policymakers in the United States are using alignment methodologies to meet the demanding technical standards for accountability (Case & Zucker, 2005). These methodologies have become more sophisticated in response to increasingly complex goals for the education system. The No Child Left Behind (NCLB) Act of 2001 spearheaded the creation of rigorous requirements for alignment between state standards and assessments used for accountability. To be in compliance with NCLB, schools, districts, and states are required to demonstrate their assessment tools have appropriate technical adequacy and are aligned with standards. Because of this law, as well as previous reforms that promoted standards-based education, researchers have developed curriculum alignment methods that are more detailed and involved.

# Curriculum Alignment Methodologies

For there to be alignment it is essential that instructional activities, assessment practices, and evaluation methods measure the breath, depth, and range of the standards for a given level of achievement (USDOE, 2003). Assessments that devote a disproportionate number of items to a small subset of the content and skills specified in the standards, or that focus on peripheral rather than significant content, are not well aligned. Webb (1997) describes three common methods for establishing alignment among the elements of curriculum, instruction, and assessments:

1. Sequential development method
2. Expert review
3. Document analysis

These methods can be used independently or in combination with each other. The Council of Chief State School Officers (2002) later identified three preferred, more rigorous, models for designing and implementing alignment studies:

1. The Webb's Alignment Model
2. The Surveys of Enacted Curriculum Model
3. Achieve Model

Each model consists of a sequence of indices describing the general match or coherence between academic standards, large-scale assessments, and classroom instruction (Resnick, Rothman, Slattery, & Vranek 2003). A comprehensive review of these methodologies is beyond the scope of this chapter; however, some of the key aspects in these methods and models follows. These methods and models are discussed in more detail by Roach, Neibling and Kurz (2008).

## The Sequential Development Method

The Sequential Development Method is used to develop elements of the curriculum such as objectives, instruction, and assessments. It follows a logical process and is easy to understand. Standards are used to design a blueprint for the structure and content of the curriculum. The link between each standard and curriculum item is documented for evidence of alignment. This methodology ensures that each standard has an adequate number of items corresponding to it.

## The Expert Review Method

The Expert Review Method uses a panel of experts to analyze the alignment between standards and curriculum elements by comparing the two. This method is used to determine the extent of the match, providing evidence of alignment.

## The Document Analysis Method

The Document Analysis Method is used for complex alignment of standards with elements of documents within a curriculum, such as tests, assignments, etc. Standards and elements of the documents are analyzed using a system for encoding their content and structure. Elements of the documents within a curriculum are quantified and systematically compared. A panel of content experts is used to carry out the encoding and analysis. This type of methodology was used for the development of comprehensive studies such as the Third International Mathematics and Science Studies (TIMSS) and the Program for International Student Assessment (PISA).

## The Webb Alignment Model

The Webb Alignment Model (Webb, 1997; 1999; 2005) provides a series of statistics that indicate the association between content in a set of standards and content covered by assessment practices. Panels of educators and curriculum experts are trained to use an analytic process and heuristics to rate the alignment between assessment practices and standards. According to Roach, Neibling and Kurz (2008), state policy makers use the Webb alignment analyses process to modify assessments, revise standards, and verify the extent that policy elements are directed toward common expectations for learning.

## The Survey of Enacted Curriculum Model

The Survey of Enacted Curriculum Model (Porter & Smithson, 2000; 2001; 2002) involves a set of procedures for conducting content analysis and subsequent data analysis of sets of curriculum elements such as instructional content, assessment practices, and textbooks. A common language framework is used to examine the content, regardless of the elements being examined. This allows for direct comparison between elements. Roach, Neibling, and Kurz, (2008) explain the strategies that are used in this model for evaluating the emphasis of content topics in the curriculum, instruction and assessments.

## The Achieve Model

The Achieve Model uses an assessment-to-standards alignment protocol to provide a qualitative and quantitative analysis of alignment. Roach, Neibling, and Kurz (2008) explain how judgments are made about the quality and rigor of individual items and sets of items. An alignment protocol guides an expert panel to gather information about the breadth of the elements in relation to the content expressed in standards, the overall sampling of the evenness and adequateness of the content expressed in the standards, and the level of difficulty of thinking expressed by the standards (Resnick et al., 2003).

## Curriculum Alignment in the Classroom vs. Clinical Setting

Alignment of the essential educational competencies to instruction, assessment, and evaluation practices in the classroom is much less complex than alignment in the clinical setting. The major instruction activities used for assessment and evaluation in the classroom focus on cognitive skills, and include written assignments, projects, portfolios, discussion, debate, and testing. The specific instruction, assessment, and evaluation items devoted to these activities are easy to identify, manipulate, or control, and are thereby relatively easy to align to standards. In contrast, the instructional activities used for assessment and evaluation in the clinical setting must focus on cognitive, affective, and psychomotor skills, and are dependant on the type of clinical setting, the patient population, and the availability of experiences. Therefore, the specific instructional, assessment, and evaluation items devoted to these practices vary, and are somewhat difficult to predetermine, manipulate, or control, thereby making it difficult to align to standards.

In examining the numerous assessment tools available for evaluating students in the clinical setting, it appears that efforts to design tools that are more objective have resulted in instructional outcomes or competencies that are more specifically stated, narrowing their use. While reducing some of the subjectivity, Oermann and Gaberson (2006) explain that specific instructional outcomes or competencies limit the flexibility required in the clinical setting and reduce the measurement focus for evaluation to a more simple knowledge and skill level (Gronlund, 2000). It is clear that specific instructional outcomes or competencies for clinical evaluation are inappropriate for use in nursing education where critical thinking, judgments, and problem solving are vital requirements. Furthermore, since the nature of the clinical setting is unpredictable and varies with each experience, the objectives or competencies must serve as a guide, allowing instructors to develop the appropriate instruction to elicit the outcome or competency to be learned.

The use of more generally stated instructional, assessment, and evaluation items related to the clinical components of the curriculum must be used in alignment studies to allow for the necessary flexibility. This will result, however, in a looser association or limited results related to the depth of analysis between items. In other words, the results related to the emphasis and intensity with which the items are instructed and assessed may be limited and thereby reveal less meaningful data. However, results from the breadth of content analysis, or the different items covered through clinical instruction, assessment, and evaluation should reveal more accurate and meaningful data. Schmidt, McKnight, Cogan, Jakwerth, and Houang (1999) refer to these kinds of findings as "a mile wide and an inch deep". On the other hand, it must be noted that descriptions of alignment are not dichotomous (in alignment vs. out of alignment). Rather, a summary of the degree of match or alignment between the elements is revealed through a series of indices that are considered collectively (Resnick et al., 2003).

Indeed, establishing and maintaining full curriculum alignment is not easy, especially in the clinical aspects of the curriculum. Nevertheless, the need to align all instructional, assessment and evaluation practices within the curriculum of a nursing program to the essential educational competencies remains, regardless of the difficulties associated with doing so. Until we know to what extent these activities, practices, and methods align with the essential educational competencies, as intended by the AACN, the NLN, the NCSBN, the National Association for Practical Nursing Education and Service (NAPNES) and others, we cannot know which component of the curriculum requires reforming.

## Supporting Frameworks

A standards-referenced interpretive framework supports the idea of full curriculum alignment by using agreed-upon performance standards and content to hold both students and educators accountable to high levels of achievement (Young, 2004). Full curriculum alignment also draws upon signaling theory (Kirst & Venezia, 2004), which refers to communication between individuals. The concept is that if signals are unclear or contradictory they are misinterpreted or ignored by those who receive them, hindering the ability to adapt educational practices that are internally consistent or aligned to standards. This suggests, as adapted to full curriculum alignment, that students and faculty receive signals from the essential educational competencies (professional readiness standards) about what is important to teach, assess, and learn in nursing education.

The signals or essential educational competencies that are sent to nursing schools become increasingly important as nursing schools are subject to greater accountability and more students pursue an education in nursing practice.

## The Need

Serious attention needs to be devoted to reducing the variations in nursing education, in order for nurse educators to be accountable to their students, patients, and society (Holaday, 2004; Holaday & Miklancie, 2006; Holaday, Buckley & Miklancie, 2006; Holaday & Buckley, 2008). Given the importance of assuring the achievement of the essential educational competencies (AACN, 2008; NLN, 2000), we need a better understanding of the alignment between these competencies, and the instruction, assessment, and evaluation methods used by nurse educators. Establishing this alignment offers a means to reduce inconsistencies and variations, and increase equity across nursing education. Alignment is a key component in today's nursing education reform. It offers insight into a fundamental issue of great importance which is the relationship between nursing education and student readiness for professional nursing practice, an important step to ensure competency upon entry into practice.

Benner (1984) wisely pointed out that performance measures can only be as productive and accurate as the competencies selected to be measured. Much remains to be learned about the alignment of the essential educational competencies to the instructional activities, assessment practices, and evaluation methods in nursing education. There are a number of questions and issues to be examined beyond those mentioned in this chapter, such as:

- What degree of alignment is adequate to facilitate learning and improve student achievement of desired outcomes?
- How can alignment data be used for changes in the classroom and clinical settings, and to reform nursing education?
- How can aspects of student engagement be integrated into alignment studies?

## Potential Impact of Alignment Studies in Nursing Education

Alignment is an area of research and applied practice that has the potential to have a positive impact on the learning and achievement of all students. It is crucial to the validity of any assessment practice or evaluation method. The systematic and in-depth examination of the degree of alignment of the essential educational competencies to instructional activities, assessment practices, and evaluation methods will reveal a wealth of meaningful information, including:

- The applicability and usability of the AACN and NLN essential educational competencies as valid and reliable outcome indicators for instruction, assessment, and evaluation across nursing programs, classroom and clinical settings, and levels of educational preparation
- A better understanding of the validity and reliability of the assessments and evaluations given to our nursing students
- Insight into the relationship between nursing education and readiness for professional nursing practice for quality improvement
- Data for evidence-based teaching practices and faculty development
- Facilitators and barriers to education reform
- Indicators to hold faculty accountable for instruction assessment and evaluation of nursing students

Full curriculum alignment provides a mechanism for accountability by faculty and students, the momentum for institutional change, and continuous improvement. If a set of readiness standards are to be used to inform instruction, and subsequently to assess and evaluate the outcomes of that instruction, then outcomes from alignment studies should result in instruction and experiences for assessment and evaluation that align with the essential educational competencies required for entry into nursing practice. This will translate into an improvement in the quality of the nursing care delivered.

## Summary

Nurse educators must ask the following questions:
- What is the driving force behind instruction, assessment and evaluation of student outcomes in the classroom and clinical settings; is it the standards or competencies that our professional experts have deemed essential for safe and competent patient care, or is it left up to the faculty instructor to decide?

- What evidence supports the assessment practices and evaluations used by faculty (evidence-based teaching), that assures readiness for safe, competent nursing practice?

If students are not afforded opportunities to learn the knowledge, skills, and attitudes required for entry into nursing practice, they can easily become scapegoats for a nursing school's inability to adequately prepare their students. On the other hand, mere exposure to a well-aligned curriculum does not guarantee student engagement in that curriculum. Alignment data provide information about the students' opportunity to learn certain concepts and skills, but whether or not they actually take advantage of those opportunities and learn is a different matter.

Given the scope of the essential educational competencies and their cognitive complexity, it is unlikely that an alignment study will capture the full range of content knowledge and cognitive skills as intended by the AACN (2008) and NLN (2000). However, alignment represents a promising framework for analyzing the extent to which components of a nursing curriculum are coordinated. Alignment also provides empirical evidence of the influence of classroom and clinical instruction, assessment, and evaluation on student achievement.

By implementing alignment studies between the essential educational competencies and instruction activities, assessment practices, and evaluation methods, nurse educators can move nursing education from assuming that students are provided adequate opportunities to learn, to truly facilitating the opportunities to learn.

## Learning Activities

1. Review a course syllabus and the clinical evaluation tool (CET) for that course. Compare the course outcomes with the CET. Is there a relationship between the outcomes and the items on the CET?
2. Consider a course you teach or a colleague teaches. What national standards are used to determine the content and thinking taught in the course? Is there a direct alignment between these and the evaluation tools used in the clinical setting?

## Educational Philosophy

"Education is not the filling of a pail," wrote W. B. Yeats, "but the lighting of a fire." As a nurse educator, I find it vital to prepare our nursing students to think critically and act effectively, and groom them for a lifetime of learning. A curriculum structured simply to convey knowledge is not enough. I believe that learning is most effective when students are actively involved and learn in the context in which the knowledge is to be used. Grounded in constructivism, my orientation toward teaching-learning is flexible and open, integrating education and experience while drawing on the varied skills and diverse talents of my students whenever possible. I encourage students to be active creators rather than passive receptors of knowledge, with the assumption that everyone holds the responsibility for his or her own learning. — Stephanie Holaday

## References

Agency for Healthcare Research and Quality (AHRQ). (2003). *Patient safety initiative: Building foundations, reducing risk*. Interim Report to the Senate Committee on Appropriations. (AHRQ Publication No. 04-RG005). Rockville, MD: Author.

American Association of Colleges of Nursing. (2006). Hallmarks of quality and patient safety: Recommended baccalaureate competencies and curricular guidelines to assure high quality and safe patient care. *Journal of Professional Nursing, 22*(6), 329-330.

American Association of Colleges of Nursing. (2008). The Essentials of baccalaureate education for professional nursing practice. Washington, DC: Author.

Anderson, L. (2002). Curricular alignment: A re-examination. *Theory into Practice, 41*(4), 255-260.

Baratz-Snowden, J. C. (1993). Opportunity to learn: Implications for professional development. *Journal of Negro Education, 62*, 311-323.

Benner, P. (1984). *From novice to expert: Excellence and power in clinical nursing practice*. Menlo Park, CA: Addison Wesley.

Carroll, J. B. (1963). A model of school learning. *Teachers College Record, 64*, 723-733.

Case, B., & Zucker, S. (2005). *Methodologies for Alignment of Standards and Assessments*. San Antonio, TX: Harcourt.

Cohen, S. A. (1987). Instructional alignment: Searching for a magic bullet. *Educational Researcher, 16*(8), 16-20.

Council of Chief State School Officers. (2002). *Models for alignment analysis and assistance to states*. Paper prepared by the Council of Chief State School Officers. Washington, DC: Author.

Gronlund, N. (2000). *How to write and use instructional objectives* (6th ed.). Upper Saddle River, NJ: Prentice Hall.

Holaday, S. D. (2004, November). *The Clinical Performance-Based Evaluation Tool-Kit: Standardizing nursing education*. Paper presented at the annual meeting of American Association of Colleges of Nursing, The 2004 Baccalaureate Education Conference, San Antonio, TX.

Holaday, S. D., & Buckley, K. M. (2008). A standardized clinical evaluation tool-kit: Improving nursing education and practice. *Annual Review of Nursing Education, 6*(1), 123-149.

Holaday, S. D., Buckley, K. M., & Miklancie, M. A. (2006, August). *Standardizing clinical performance through a clinical evaluation tool-kit and model*. Paper presented at the meeting of the Institute for Educators in Nursing and Health Professions on Educating Nurses: Innovation to Application, Baltimore, MD.

Holaday, S. D., & Miklancie, M.A. (2006, November). *A tool-kit for advancing clinical performance evaluation*. Paper presented at the annual meeting of American Association of Colleges of Nursing, The 2006 Baccalaureate Education Conference, Orlando, FL.

Institute of Medicine (IOM). (2000). *To err is human: Building a safer health system*. Washington, DC: National Academies Press.

Institute of Medicine (IOM). (2003). *Health professions education: A bridge to quality*. Washington, DC: National Academics Press.

Institute of Medicine (IOM). (2004). *Keeping patients safe: Transforming the work environment of nurses*. Washington, DC: National Academies Press.

Kirst, M. W. & Venezia, A. (2004). *From high school to college: Improving opportunities for success in postsecondary education*. San Francisco: Jossey-Bass.

Lenburg, C. (1999, September 30). Redesigning expectations for initial and continuing competence for contemporary nursing practice. *Online Journal of Issues in Nursing, 4*(2). Retrieved February 12, 2008 from www.nursingworld.org/ojin/topic10/tpc10_1.htm

National League for Nursing. (2000). *Educational Competencies for Graduates of Associate Degree Nursing Programs*. Boston, MA: Jones and Bartlett.

National League for Nursing, Board of Governors. (2005). Position statement: Transforming Nursing Education, *Nursing Education Perspectives, 26*(3), 195-197.

National League for Nursing Accrediting Commission. (2008). *Accreditation manual with interpretive guidelines by program type for postsecondary and higher degree programs in nursing.* New York: Author.

Oermann, M. H., & Gaberson, K. (2006). *Evaluation and testing in nursing education* (2nd ed.). New York: Springer.

Porter, A. C., & Smithson, J. L. (2000, April). *Alignment of state testing programs NAEP and reports of teacher practice in mathematics and science in grades 4 and 8.* Paper presented at the annual meeting of the American Educational Research Association, New Orleans, LA.

Porter, A. C., & Smithson, J. L. (2001). Are content standards being implemented in the classroom? A methodology and some tentative answers. In S. Fuhrman (Ed.), *From the Capitol to the classroom: Standards-based reform in the states.* One Hundredth Yearbook of the National Society for the Study of Education (pp. 60-80). Chicago: University of Chicago Press.

Porter, A. C., & Smithson, J. L. (2002). *Alignment of assessments, standards, and instruction using curriculum indicator data.* Paper presented at the annual meeting of the American Educational Research Association, New Orleans, LA.

Resnick, L. B., Rothman, R., Slattery, J. B., & Vranek, J. L. (2003). Benchmarking and alignment of standards and testing. *Educational Assessment, 9,* 1-27.

Roach, A., Niebling, B., & Kurz, A. (2008). Evaluating the alignment among curriculum, instruction, and assessments: Implications and applications for research and practice. *Psychology in the Schools, 45*(2) 158-176.

Schmidt, W. H., McKnight, C. S., Cogan, L. S., Jakwerth, P. M., & Houang, R. T. (1999). *Facing the consequences: Using TIMSS for a closer look at U.S. mathematics and science education.* Boston: Kluwer.

Trust for America's Health (TFAH). (2006). *Ready or not? Protecting the public's health from diseases, disasters and bioterrorism.* Washington, D.C.: Author. Retrieved February 12, 2007 from www.rwjf.org/files/publications/other/TFAH2006Revised.pdf

Upton, D. J. (1999). How can we achieve evidenced-based practice if we have a theory-practice gap in nursing today? *Journal of Advanced Nursing, 29*(3) 549-555.

U.S. Department of Education (DOE). (2003). Standards and assessments: Non-regulatory guidance. Retrieved February 28, 2008, from www.ed.gov/policy/elsec/guid/saaguidance03.doc.

Webb, N. L. (1997). *Criteria for alignment of expectations and assessments in mathematics and science education.* Council of Chief State School Officers and National Institute for Science Education Research Monograph No. 6, Madison: University of Wisconsin, Wisconsin Center for Education Research.

Webb, N. L. (1999). Alignment of science and mathematics standards and assessments in four states. Washington, DC: Council of Chief State School Officers.

Webb, N. L. (2005). *Web Alignment Tool (WAT) Training Manual.* Madison, WI: Wisconsin Center for Education. Retrieved March 3, 2008 from www.wcer.wisc.edu/wat/index.aspx

Young, M. (2004). *The standards-referenced interpretive framework: Using assessments for multiple purposes.* San Antonio, TX: Harcourt.

# CHAPTER 24

# THE CONCEPT-BASED CURRICULUM FOR NURSING EDUCATION

**Jean Giddens, PhD, RN**

---

The content of this chapter relates to the following major content area and subconcepts on the Certified Nurse Educator Examination Detailed Test Blueprint:

**Participate in Curriculum Design and Evaluation of Program Outcomes**

- Lead in the development of designing a curriculum
- Actively participate in the design of the curriculum to reflect current nursing and healthcare trends; community and societal needs
- Demonstrate knowledge of curriculum development including identifying program outcomes, developing competency statements, writing course objectives, selecting appropriate learning activities; selecting appropriate evaluation strategies
- Analyze results of program evaluation and initiate curricular change

---

## Introduction

The term **curriculum** includes the arrangement of subject matter in the context of a learning environment. In academic settings, curriculum refers to the organizational structure of a program of study. The goal of a curriculum is for learners to gain the knowledge, skills, attitudes, and values associated with a discipline. Because faculty are responsible for curriculum development, implementation, and revision, it is critical that all faculty members understand the curriculum in which they teach. It is almost inevitable that nurse educators will experience a major curriculum revision process one or more times during their teaching careers.

Regardless of the academic setting or program of study, a curriculum should reflect current trends within the discipline; nursing education is no exception. Given the rapid and continuous changes experienced in health care, nurse educators must be able to respond accordingly. Contemporary changes in health care and nursing practice, along with changes in today's college-bound learners, have resulted in the need for nurse educators to rethink educational approaches and curricular design. An emerging educational trend seen across multiple disciplines is conceptual learning. This chapter presents conceptual learning approaches for nursing education in the context of curriculum development.

## Background: The Emergence of Content Saturation

Several trends have impacted nursing education curricula immensely over the past 2 decades. The rapid expansion of healthcare information (such as in the fields of genetics, immunology, and biomedical therapies) has resulted in the incorporation of this information into curricula. Changes in population demographics have required an enhancement or addition of content in many areas, such as geriatrics, cultural diversity, and medical conditions (e.g., obesity, diabetes, and metabolic syndrome), to name a few. Additionally, the increased complexity of health care and medical technologies has resulted in ever-increasing specialization in nursing practice. With good intentions, nurse educators have attempted to address these trends by incorporating specialty content within nursing curricula. Although this may seem like a logical response, the end result has been the addition of content to the point of saturation. Few educators would argue the volume of curricular content in nursing education is excessive. As Ironside (2004) aptly points out, "The dilemma nurse educators are increasingly facing is not what to include in a course, but what to leave out" (p. 5). This is not a problem unique to nursing education; all health-related disciplines are also experiencing similar issues. The Institute of Medicine (2003) cites an "overly crowded curricula" (p. 38) as one of many challenges in health education reform. Failure to address these issues contributes to an academic–practice gap that afflicts the efficiency of health care today.

Content saturation is a shared challenge among nursing faculty and students. Faculty are often frustrated with the amount of content that needs to be taught in the allotted time frame. Nursing faculty feel responsible to cover all content, believing if they do not, students will never learn it. Because of the excessive content to deliver in a given course or class period, the predominant teaching strategy continues to be fast-paced, PowerPoint®-enhanced lectures. On the receiving end, students feel overwhelmed by excessive reading assignments and are expected to learn in passive learning environments. The large volume of content delivered often translates to little more than students memorizing information just to pass exams. The student experience is further illustrated by Diekelmann (2002), who wrote "...textbooks are thicker and course content more complex. Students complain of 'too much content' as they appear to have reached their limits with memorization" (p. 469).

These issues have far-reaching effects related to long-term student achievement and the nursing profession. The emphasis on content and memorization does little to foster critical thinking and the lifelong learning skills required of nurses. Additionally, content saturation makes it difficult for faculty to move away from the lecture podium and adopt student-centered learning strategies. Although lecture is considered an effective method to deliver a large amount of content in a short period of time, it does little to meet the diverse learning needs among today's students. Many ethnic minority students have high-context learning preferences, which are best met through student-centered approaches and social learning. The success of ethnically diverse students is potentially jeopardized by a continuation of one mode of educational delivery to the exclusion of others (Giddens, 2008).

Given these challenges, nurse educators must seek alternatives to curriculum design complemented by changes in teaching approaches. Leaders in nursing education have been calling for change in curriculum design and pedagogical approaches for decades, and the need for change has never been greater (Diekelmann & Scheckel, 2004; Ironside, 2004; Long, 2004; National League for Nursing, 2005; Tanner, 2002). A concept-based curriculum addresses many of these issues.

## The Conceptual Approach: Foundations for Curriculum Design and Teaching

The application of a conceptual approach within nursing has been visible in the literature for a number of years. The steady increase in published concept analysis articles in the nursing literature speaks to the increased interest in this trend. What exactly is a concept, and what is meant by a conceptual approach? Concepts are classifications or unifying structures in which knowledge can be organized. Another way to think about concepts is they are similar to categories of information supporting a common theme; in nursing, they can be compared to categories of nursing knowledge.

There is an important relationship between knowledge, concepts, and theory; knowledge is represented through concepts, and concepts are the building blocks of theory. Carrieri-Kohlman, Lindsey, and West (2003) describe the conceptual approach as "a process that deliberately attempts to examine the nature and substance of nursing from a conceptual perspective" (p. 1). This may seem complex and confusing, but actually, just the opposite is true. Humans begin the process of categorizing information at a young age, which represents an early form of conceptualization. For example, when preschool children learn colors, the process requires they learn that various objects can be blue. As they gain more experience, they understand there is variability in shades of blue (light blue, navy blue, royal blue, etc.). This understanding allows children to recognize the color blue among objects or shades not previously encountered. In other words, it is not necessary to teach a child every example of blue for them to recognize and understand this.

If we translate this rather simple example to nursing education, the same process potentially applies. In nursing, a concept is an overarching idea, theme, or category that represents information or knowledge associated with nursing practice. Students who attain a deep understanding of concepts associated with nursing practice will be able to recognize the concept and will generally know what to do when presented with it. For example, students who understand the concept of infection should be able to recognize when an individual with diabetes has developed an infection within the nail bed on the great toe and generally know what interventions to initiate, even if they had not previously studied it or had experience with that specific infection in the past. Their level of understanding is further deepened with exposure to additional examples of infections as they encounter them in practice. Following this line of reasoning, it is easy to understand how the conceptual approach can potentially aid content management in a curriculum and advance thinking and learning among students.

## General Steps for Concept-Based Curriculum Development

The decision to develop a new curriculum is usually based on a perceived need for change by administration or by faculty. Often, external forces (such as professional or regulatory mandates, accreditation requirements, or practice issues) are driving forces for curriculum change. Regardless of the impetus for curriculum change, it is the faculty who are ultimately responsible for the process (Dillard & Siktberg, 2009).

Although often lumped together for purposes of discussion, it is important to consider the differences between developing a new curriculum and curriculum revision. Developing a new curriculum is an extensive process that often takes a year or more to complete. This process essentially involves starting with a clean slate and building a curriculum based on what is hopefully a shared vision among faculty members. On the other hand, curriculum revision is a process whereby faculty make changes (minor or extensive) to an existing curriculum, often based on program feedback and/or perceived issues among faculty. Although a curriculum revision is not as time consuming as developing a new curriculum, in some ways, the work can be more difficult because of the impact of changes on other existing courses, much like a domino effect. In other words, it can be a challenge to keep track of changes in courses and ensure these changes are tracked over time.

Curriculum development is traditionally accomplished under the direction of a curriculum committee. In small nursing programs, this might include all full-time faculty members. Larger nursing programs may designate a group of faculty to carry out this process. Because of the complexity, a faculty member with curriculum expertise should lead the process. It is also ideal for the committee to be composed of individuals with diverse clinical backgrounds who are energetic and committed to completing the work. The committee should develop a work plan that outlines a time frame for the accomplishment of major milestones, but it is essential that time frames be realistic, especially considering the fact that faculty are doing this work in addition to other faculty obligations (Iwasiw, Goldenberg, & Andrusyszyn, 2005). When a group of individuals is working on a curriculum on behalf of a larger faculty group, communication between the committee and the faculty is vital so all faculty members feel they are kept informed and have an opportunity to provide input. Transparency is essential. The process of developing and initiating a concept-based curriculum follows traditional steps of curriculum development, but with an emphasis on the selection and organization of concepts as foundational for curriculum content.

## Initial Phase: Groundwork

The initial steps of curriculum development involve considering what currently is and what could be. This phase is foundationally crucial to curriculum development and includes several steps. These steps may not necessarily be accomplished in the order presented, and in fact, may be completed simultaneously.

**Mission statement.** A common starting point for curriculum work is to review and potentially revise the program mission statement. All academic organizations have a mission that describes the overall charge of the academic unit that sets the direction, scope, and parameters of the institution. The mission statement of a nursing program is congruent with the mission statement of the parent institution.

**Philosophy.** Philosophy acts as general guiding principles related to operation of the program and the curriculum it represents; ideally, the philosophy provides consistency and integrity to all curriculum components (Csokasy, 2002). Nursing programs may have their own philosophy statement or may defer to the philosophy of the parent institution. Components of a nursing program philosophy may include general beliefs about nursing, theory, teaching, and learning; roles of faculty; roles of students, and beliefs about critical thinking, diversity, and culture. Although it is desirable for faculty to agree on a program philosophy, in reality, this is often difficult, just as it would be difficult to obtain faculty consensus on a religion or a political candidate. Regardless, the philosophy of the nursing program and/or institution must be considered during curriculum development.

**Consideration of contextual parameters.** Additional issues that impact curricular decisions are internal and external contextual factors or parameters. In other words, developing or revising a curriculum must be within the context of reality for the program itself. Internal factors originate from within the nursing program and parent institution. These include, but are not limited to, type of program (associate, baccalaureate, registered nurse (RN)-to-Bachelor of Science in Nursing, graduate, etc.), institutional policies, institutional culture, human resources (number of faculty, number of staff), physical resources (classroom space, technology), student characteristics, and financial resources.

There are also multiple external factors to consider. The characteristics of the community served, such as population demographics, culture, available healthcare systems, and social, political, and economic influences, must be addressed. Nursing education standards from state boards of nursing and nursing education organizations (American Association of Colleges of Nursing, 2008); nursing accrediting agencies, such as the Commission on Collegiate Nursing Education (CCNE, 2008) and National League for Nursing Accrediting Commission (NLNAC, 2008); Department of Education standards; and professional nursing practice standards (American Nurses Association [ANA], 2004) must also be addressed. Inclusion of these factors may seem intuitive, but they are important considerations for all decisions that are made.

**Collecting and analyzing information.** Another initial step in curriculum development or revision is the collection and analysis of information on which to base decisions. Evaluating the literature and hiring consultants are important ways to learn about current trends and strategies related to the profession and nursing education; this also provides a mechanism to gain outside perspectives. Collecting information from key stakeholders, such as faculty, current students, alumni, local healthcare agencies, and community leaders (Keating, 2006), is another vital component. Although time consuming, this process is essential for sound decision making and to achieve a curriculum that reflects contemporary nursing practice.

### Setting Course: A Conceptual Approach for Curriculum Design

Based on the previously described steps, the curriculum committee should next focus on specific aspects of the curriculum, including the goals, organization or framework, and instructional delivery.

**Program student learning outcomes.** Program student learning outcomes serve as the overarching intent of the curriculum and collectively serve as a beacon for the curriculum development that follows; these should be congruent with the mission statement and philosophy of the nursing program and academic organization

(Figure 1). Student learning outcomes are written or revised from the context of the desired traits of the graduate, and ideally, these are used as targets for program evaluation.

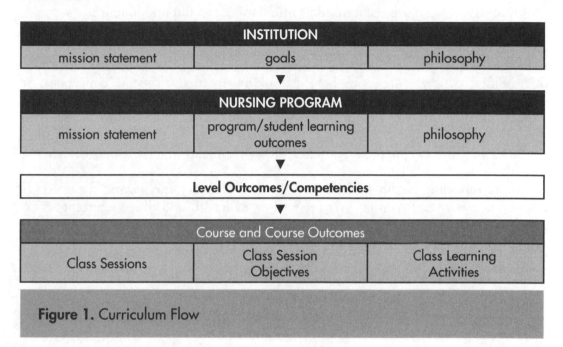

**Figure 1.** Curriculum Flow

**Identification of level objectives, competencies, or outcomes.** Another component of curriculum design is the identification of learner goals at various points associated with curricular progression that lead to the program student learning outcomes. These may be in the form of outcomes and their related competencies for each course, semester, and level of the curriculum and should be congruent with or link to the overall program objectives (see Figure 1). Level outcomes become parameters to guide decisions about the type and number of courses offered but should be flexible enough to allow revisions to and refinement of courses over time.

**Concepts as an organizing framework.** Over the course of nursing education history, several organizing frameworks either individually or in combination have been used, including the medical model, nursing theories, the complexity approach, the health stages approach, and competency-based curriculum. Each of these organizational frameworks have benefits and limitations.

As previously discussed, a concept-based curriculum uses concepts associated with nursing practice as an organizing framework. Although concepts are components of theory, a concept-based curriculum is eclectic in that the concepts may come from multiple sources, but are recognized as foundational to nursing practice.

There is no one set of concepts that is the "correct list" to use for a concept-based curriculum. The number and types of concepts to be used are decisions that must be made by the curriculum committee. It might be useful for faculty to first think about overarching concept categories before thinking about the specific concepts. For example, concept categories might be identified by categories based on the National Council for Licensure Examination for Registered Nurses (NCLEX-RN®) test plan or based on the *Scope and Standards of Nursing Practice* (ANA, 2004). Another classification of concepts focuses on healthcare recipients and providers of care.

**Concepts reflecting health and illness.** A useful category for organizing concepts impacting healthcare recipients is referred to as **health and illness concepts**. This group of concepts represents the core knowledge and skills of patient-centered nursing care on three continuums:

1. Age (life-span)
2. Health (wellness, health promotion, acute illness, and chronic illness)
3. Environment (representing nursing care in a variety of environmental contexts, such as inpatient and community settings)

Table 1 presents examples of health- and illness-related concepts.

**Professional nursing concepts.** A category of concepts that focuses on nurses as providers of care reflects professional attributes, core roles, and the context in which nurses practice. Concepts in this category, known as **professional nursing concepts**, may target the individual nurse, a group of nurses, organizations, or system-level contexts. Table 1 lists examples of concepts associated with professional nursing practice.

| Heath & Illness Concepts | Professional Nursing Concepts |
|---|---|
| • Oxygenation<br>• Perfusion<br>• Infection<br>• Pain<br>• Anxiety<br>• Substance Abuse<br>• Cognition<br>• Sexuality | • Communication<br>• Critical Thinking<br>• Advocacy<br>• Leadership<br>• Ethics<br>• Clinical Judgment<br>• Patient Teaching<br>• Safety |

**Table 1.** Examples of Health and Illness and Professional Nursing Concepts

**Selecting and defining concepts.** The selection of concepts follows decisions about categories. When concepts are used as a basis for teaching and curriculum design, it is critical the concepts are well defined and mutually understood by faculty and students. The concepts selected must not only be clear but also useful for teaching and learning (Giddens & Brady, 2007). The actual process of generating a list of concepts varies, but concepts should be easily identifiable or reflected in the nursing literature. They can be found in any nursing textbook.

Other ideas to generate concepts may include reviewing nursing taxonomies, such as Nursing Diagnosis or Functional Health Patterns (Gordon, 1994), or using the Delphi technique, in which faculty or other experts complete a series of questionnaires that ask for their opinions or judgments about which concepts to include. The process of concept selection is difficult work, requiring deep thought and reflection (Giddens, 2008). Faculty must avoid the temptation to select an excessive number of concepts, or they will potentially suffer the consequences of concept saturation.

It is critical to have complete understanding by faculty and students related to the concepts selected for the curriculum. Consider, for example, the confusion that might arise among faculty and students if a concept such as power was used in the curriculum, without a clear articulation of the meaning and focus. Because concepts selected should be reflective of nursing care and practice, definitions should be verified in the literature.

**Selecting exemplars as content.** An important feature of a concept-based curriculum is the potential to manage excessive curricular content. This is based on the premise that students gain a deep understanding of a concept and what the concept represents, and can make connections to examples of that concept. In the context of nursing concepts, clinical exemplars are specific examples or cases used to connect common problems to the representing concept. Students should be able to recognize other clinical problems that also represent the concept and should have a general idea of what to do, even if the situation is not specifically presented in the curriculum. Ideally, exemplars are based on state, national, and global health incidence and prevalence statistics for population groups through the life-span or importance within practice. Basing decisions about exemplars on these factors helps faculty to make good decisions about the clinical conditions to select as exemplars and ensures that students will be exposed to the most common conditions seen in clinical practice across population groups.

Most exemplars link to more than one concept. For example, stroke links to the concepts of perfusion and intracranial regulation; pneumonia links to infection and oxygenation. Because of this, decisions must be made regarding the exemplars used to illustrate a concept, and interrelated concepts should be purposefully acknowledged. This planning is essential to prevent content repetition, which could result if the exemplar is used for several concepts.

**Arrangement of courses.** Another important decision that must be made as part of curriculum design is the general arrangement of courses.

**Traditional approach.** One option is to maintain the traditional population-based and content-based course arrangement (adult, maternal-child, geriatrics, mental health, community, leadership, etc). When this is done, concepts serve as a common link across the courses. In some cases it may be best to designate concepts as core, that is, those that are foundational to each course, and to designate others as **secondary** or **interrelated** but not specifically used to guide content. If this approach is taken, faculty must be very purposeful in linking the content to the concepts. A perceived benefit of this approach is the familiarity of faculty with teaching within specialty areas, and an opportunity for students to learn concentrated information about a population or content areas within a specific time frame. Drawbacks to this approach include the tendency for faculty to continue teaching as they always have, without really changing anything. Furthermore, there may be the temptation to re-teach the concept over and over in each course in which it appears, as opposed to focusing on linking exemplars to the concept. There is also the risk of students not making conceptual links across population or content areas when exemplars are presented within standard courses.

**Integrated approach.** Another option is to abandon the traditional course arrangement in favor of concept courses that integrate population-specific information around each concept. When this is done, concepts are divided into and featured in designated courses. The benefit of this is students learn about the concept and featured exemplars within the same course so a deep understanding about the concept is gained through exemplar reinforcement. Concepts are presented as foundational to nursing practice and are emphasized more than excessive content details. Conceptual links across problems, population groups, and settings are made. Known challenges of an integrated curriculum include concerns related to faculty expertise in teaching across specialties and tracking and organizing content. There is also the risk that students' understanding of specialty knowledge is limited. For this reason, faculty must be purposeful in providing enough content detail through exemplars to minimize these concerns.

If an integrated approach is desired, concept sequencing, or the order in which concepts will be presented within the curriculum, must be determined. Concepts can be arranged in a number of ways, including from simple to complex, in concept categories (i.e., health and illness concepts, and professional nursing concepts), or in groupings based on logical, interrelated connections. For example, the concepts of pain, nausea, vomiting, and fatigue are clearly different, but they are also closely interrelated; therefore, it would be logical to place them together within a course.

## Course Design and Course Development

**Prerequisite courses.** As part of the initial evaluation described previously, the curriculum committee evaluates the prerequisite courses (those required to enter the nursing program) and considers the appropriateness of these for achieving the goals of the nursing program. Some prerequisite courses are required by the parent institution and are not negotiable. Faculty should not only look at the type of courses, but also the total credit hours required. Changes in courses required for program entry are often made as part of a curriculum revision or new curriculum development process.

**Nursing courses.** The curriculum design selected and the level outcomes (see Figure 1) provide the basis for decisions about didactic and clinical courses within the curriculum. Curriculum committee members must make decisions not only about the course focus and content, but also about the number of credit hours, delivery method (clinical course, classroom, online, etc.), expertise available, and type of assignments that might be expected. It is important to balance the amount of work students are expected to complete across all semesters or terms.

As with any other curriculum development, course development typically includes a course description, course outcomes, credit hours, a general content outline with unit objectives, learning activities, and a plan for student evaluation. Each class session is planned accordingly. Generally, the individual faculty chooses teaching strategies, although the course content is determined by the curriculum committee. The number of class sessions, teaching strategies, and assignments should be appropriate for the type of course, content, credit hours, course delivery, level of student, and number of students expected in the course. Objectives for individual class sessions should link to course outcomes (Figure 1).

**Conceptual teaching approaches.** As nursing courses are developed, faculty should also consider teaching approaches that facilitate conceptual learning. Creating and adopting a concept-based curriculum does not automatically translate to conceptual learning – faculty must also adopt conceptual approaches to their teaching. A learning activity that first focuses on the concept (concept overview) is conducted prior to exemplar presentations. Exemplar learning activities should present content information about the exemplar in enough depth for students to have a deep understanding of the exemplar and, just as importantly, can understand how it connects to the concept and interrelated concepts. Faculty should resist the temptation to simply develop concept and exemplar lectures. Ideally, faculty will practice integrative pedagogy; learning activities should focus on a clinical situation, be student-centered, and be purposeful; in other words, the learner should clearly realize the benefit of the activity. It is important to note there is not a list of teaching strategies that are specific to conceptual learning; it is the focus and links to the concepts that are critical. Common teaching strategies used to promote conceptual learning include case study, role play, concept maps, debate, simulation, jigsaw, and games.

## Managing Resistance

One of the universal frustrations of curriculum revision is resistance from faculty. Members of the curriculum committee should expect this, as it is a normal response to change. Resistance derives from many sources. Faculty may not perceive a need to change, or there may be a lack of understanding about the changes that are proposed. Faculty may feel threatened their expertise or favorite course may no longer exist. The resistance may be associated with faculty fatigue, or it may represent an underlying power struggle between faculty and administration or within the faculty group. The source of the resistance may be difficult to identify and may be a combination of factors. Regardless of the source, it is to be expected and cannot be avoided. However, the committee should be aware of any identified sources and respond appropriately. Forcing something on resistant faculty rarely works; acknowledging concerns and working through the change process is needed for success to follow.

**Communication.** Open communication among members of the curriculum committee, and between members of the committee and faculty, is essential. The curriculum committee members must keep channels of communication open and listen to various points of view. There is no one individual who has all the answers, and everyone potentially has something valuable to contribute. Likewise, when the faculty group is large and a select group of faculty form the curriculum committee, it is imperative for the larger faculty group to be informed of the process and decisions along the way. Often, resistance is lessened over time as faculty have an opportunity to think about the plans and become accustomed to the idea of change.

**Faculty engagement.** Faculty who are included in the process – even in a small role – are more likely to take ownership of the work. This typically translates to engagement and commitment to the process. Ways to engage faculty include asking for assistance in a literature search, asking for assistance with interpretation of focus group data, and asking for participation on a task force for one specific assignment related to curriculum development/revision.

**Faculty development.** Changing from a traditional to a conceptual curriculum approach generally requires extensive faculty development to include understanding the need and rationale for the approach, gaining an understanding of the curriculum development process, and gaining an understanding of how to teach in a concept-based curriculum. Faculty development can occur through mentorship within the faculty and through outside consultation. Faculty development should be seen as an ongoing process occurring over time. It is best to commit to regularly scheduled faculty development activities that begin during curriculum development and continue through the implementation phase (Iwasiw et al., 2005).

## Curriculum Implementation

The process of implementing a concept-based curriculum poses several challenges because it usually represents a deviation from traditional curricular design. It is advisable that all stakeholders (students, the parent institution, and the healthcare agencies) be well informed during the development phase so the change is not a surprise.

## Overlapping Curricula

One challenge that frequently exists is the process of phasing out an old curriculum while beginning a new one. The overlap in old and new approaches can create confusion for everyone involved, particularly for faculty and administrators who must plan academic schedules for two simultaneously running curricula. Nurse preceptors in clinical agencies may also be confused with changes to clinical requirements or assignments.

## Faculty Challenges

A noteworthy challenge faced by faculty is adopting conceptual teaching strategies. Designing learning activities that link exemplars to the concepts in a meaningful way represents a significant amount of work. Faculty may find this process not only difficult but threatening, particularly when teaching strategies do not go as well as planned. Faculty who do not feel supported may become frustrated and lose faith in the direction taken. Positive reinforcement, collegial support, and ongoing faculty development are necessary for successful transition to this new approach.

## Student Challenges

Students who are enrolled during the time of curriculum change may verbalize a wide range of comments about the process. Some students feel victimized by curriculum changes. Students in the last class of an outgoing curriculum may feel cheated because they perceive that what they received was less than optimal; they also may believe faculty attention is focused primarily on the work involving the new curriculum. By contrast, it is not uncommon for students in the first class of a new curriculum to feel angry about being "guinea pigs," citing that faculty are disorganized as they learn to adjust to the new curriculum. These feelings may be further aggravated initially by a conceptual approach because the role of the student changes from that of passive recipient to active learner.

Several strategies can minimize student concerns. First, involving students in the curriculum development and implementation process provides a mechanism to gain student perspectives (Keating, 2006). Students can serve as appointed representatives on the curriculum committee and as ambassadors or mentors to incoming students. Second, faculty should be clear and consistent about student expectations, particularly about student participation in conceptually based learning activities. Third, faculty should regularly elicit student feedback as the new curriculum is implemented. Input from the student perspective may reveal issues that faculty had not anticipated or were unaware of. This allows faculty to make necessary adjustments and gives students a voice in the process.

## Managing the Curriculum and Planning Program Evaluation

A common experience among faculty after a new curriculum is developed is to breathe a sigh of relief when work is done. In truth, curriculum work is ongoing because of the need to manage what has been developed, evaluate the program, and plan for periodic curriculum revision.

### Maintaining Curriculum Integrity

**Curriculum drift** refers to inadvertent changes to the curriculum plan and is a common problem with even the best-designed curriculum. One of the most common causes of curriculum drift is that faculty either intentionally or unintentionally alter the curriculum plan through changes within a course. This is particularly problematic among faculty who resist curriculum change and among new or part-time faculty who have not received adequate orientation to the curriculum. Curriculum drift can also occur with planned changes to the curriculum. What may seem as minor adjustments or changes can result in unexpected consequences because of the impact of that change across one or more courses.

To maintain integrity, ongoing curriculum oversight must be planned. The curriculum committee should include strategies for this oversight in each regularly scheduled meeting. Yearly curriculum retreats allow faculty to discuss the courses they teach, share concerns, and revisit the curriculum plan. Regular course reports submitted by faculty may be beneficial in detecting modifications made. The mapping of concepts and exemplars also helps to maintain an understanding of the curriculum plan.

### Program Evaluation

Evaluation of the curriculum is foundational to overall program assessment and incorporates the collection and analysis of various types of data. As mentioned previously, revisions to the curriculum are based on evaluation data; furthermore, these data are used for nursing program self-assessment reports needed for accreditation. Ongoing evaluation of the curriculum is an accreditation standard for both the NLNAC (2008) and the CCNE (2008). For these reasons, a comprehensive plan for program evaluation is needed. A full discussion about program evaluation is beyond the scope of this chapter, but a few key points are mentioned here. The primary types of data collected include evaluation of student performance (such as standardized test performance, student progression rates, graduation rates, NCLEX® performance, etc.), student evaluation of faculty and courses, student evaluation of the program (formative surveys, focus groups, exit interviews), alumni evaluation, faculty evaluation of the program, and graduate/employer evaluation (Keating, 2006).

## Summary

There is a well-established need for new models of nursing education curricula to address the issues of content saturation and a rapidly changing healthcare environment. A concept-based curriculum provides a mechanism for content management by focusing on concepts and selected exemplars. Because concepts tend to be long-lasting, a concept-based curriculum has the potential to be flexible enough to adjust to rapid changes within the health sciences.

Nursing faculty adopting a concept-based curriculum follow the same general steps as with any curriculum development process, with the major differences occurring within the curriculum design stage. Concepts provide the foundation for teaching and learning; exemplars represent the specific content that links to concepts. Selection of concepts and exemplars requires tremendous discussion and negotiation among curriculum committee members. Because a concept-based curriculum represents a significant deviation from traditional curricula, an organized approach with adequate faculty support mechanisms is essential to ensure success.

## Learning Activities

1. Using a popular search engine and search for "Concept-Based Nursing Curriculum". Choose one of the top ten sites listed. How did the content relate to this chapter?
2. Consider revising the curriculum of a nursing program in which you or a colleague teaches. Using a concept-based model, what concepts would you select? How

would those concepts be related to demonstrate the overall approach to your curriculum?
3. For the curriculum you revised in activity #2, how would the teaching strategies change from the approach currently being used?

## Educational Philosophy

As a nurse educator, I view the role of teaching as a guide to learning. I advocate student-centered learning utilizing an array of teaching strategies that are meaningful for students. My ability to incorporate such approaches in teaching has resulted from talking with, reading, and interpreting the work of many leaders in nursing education and the education discipline over the past 20 years—coupled with an intuitive approach to the learning process. My collective experiences have led me to different ways of thinking and challenging the notion of "business as usual" in nursing education. A true measure of success for nursing education will occur when nursing schools are perceived as inviting to potential students and can meet the needs of diverse learners. — Jean Giddens

## References

American Association of Colleges of Nursing. (2008). *Essentials of baccalaureate education for professional nursing practice.* Washington DC: Author.

American Nurses Association. (2004). *Nursing scope and standards of practice.* Washington DC: Author.

Carrieri-Kohlman, V., Lindsey, A. M., & West, C. M. (2003). *Pathophysiological phenomena in nursing: Human responses to illness* (3rd ed.). Philadelphia: Saunders.

Commission on Collegiate Nursing Education. (2008). Standards for accreditation of baccalaureate and graduate nursing education programs. Retrieved February 12, 2008, from www.aacn.nche.edu/accreditation/NEW_STANDARDS.htm

Csokasy, J. (2002). A congruent curriculum: Philosophical integrity from philosophy to outcomes. *Journal of Nursing Education, 41*(1), 32-33.

Diekelmann, N. (2002). "Too much content...." Epistemologies' grasp and nursing education. *Journal of Nursing Education, 41,* 469-470.

Diekelmann, N., & Scheckel, M. (2004). Leaving the safe harbor of competency-based and outcomes education: Rethinking practice education. *Journal of Nursing Education, 43*(9), 385-388.

Dillard, N., & Siktberg, L. (2009). Curriculum development. In D. Billings & J. Halstead (Eds.), *Teaching in nursing* (3rd ed., pp. 75-90). Philadelphia: Saunders.

Giddens, J. (2008). Achieving diversity in nursing through multicontextual learning environments. *Nursing Outlook, 56*(2), 78-83.

Giddens, J., Brady, D., Welborn-Brown, P., Wright, M., Smith, D., & Harris, J. (2008). A new curriculum for a new era of nursing education. *Nursing Education Perspectives, 29*(4), 200-204.

Giddens, J., & Brady, D. (2007). Rescuing nursing from content saturation: The case for a concept-based curriculum. *Journal of Nursing Education, 46,* 65-69.

Gordon, M. J. (1994). *Nursing diagnosis: Process and application* (3rd ed.), St. Louis, MO: Mosby.

Institute of Medicine. (2003). *Health professions education: A bridge to quality.* Washington DC: National Academies Press.

Ironside, P. M. (2004). "Covering content" and teaching thinking: Deconstructing the additive curriculum. *Journal of Nursing Education, 43,* 5-12.

Iwasiw, C., Goldenberg, D., & Andrusyszyn, M. (2005). *Curriculum development in nursing education.* Boston: Jones and Bartlett.

Keating, S. B. (2006). *Curriculum development and evaluation in nursing.* Philadelphia: Lippincott Williams & Wilkins.

Long, K. A. (2004). Preparing nurses for the 21st century: Reenvisioning nursing education and practice. *Journal of Professional Nursing, 20*(2), 82-88.

National League for Nursing. (2005). *Transforming nursing education.* Retrieved March 29, 2009 from http://www.nln.org/aboutnln/PositionStatements/transforming052005.pdf

National League for Nursing Accrediting Commission. (2008). *Standards and criteria.* Retrieved February 21, 2008, from www.nlnac.org/manuals/SC2008.htm

Tanner, C. A. (2002). Clinical education, circa 2010. *Journal of Nursing Education, 41,* 51-52.

# CHAPTER 25

# ACCELERATED NURSING PROGRAMS AND SECOND DEGREE NURSING STUDENTS

Stephanie D. Holaday, DrPH, RN
Kathleen M. Buckley, PhD, RN, IBCLC
Margaret A. Miklancie, PhD, RN

The content of this chapter relates to the following major content areas and subconcepts on the Certified Nurse Educator Examination Detailed Test Blueprint:

**Facilitate Learning**

- Implement a variety of teaching strategies appropriate to: content; setting; learner needs
- Modify teaching strategies and learning experiences based on consideration of learners' past educational and life experiences
- Create a positive learning environment that fosters a free exchange of ideas

**Facilitate Learner Development and Socialization**

- Identify individual learning styles and unique learning needs of learners with these characteristics: traditional vs. non-traditional
- Adapt teaching styles and interpersonal interactions to facilitate learner behaviors

## Introduction

A variety of accelerated baccalaureate nursing (BSN) programs are now available in the United States. Although there are variations in admission requirements, curriculum, and program length, most of these programs are designed for adult learners who already hold a degree in another field. According to the American Association of Colleges of Nursing (AACN, 2007) the initiation of accelerated programs is quickly outpacing any other entry-level type of programs for undergraduates. As a result, nursing schools around the country face the challenge of fulfilling the requirements for a BSN in a shorter time frame than the traditional four-year program. As nurse educators, we must ensure that while designing and teaching in these programs, we maintain the quality and integrity of our nursing education without compromising health care to the public. Are we, in fact, ready to accelerate our BSN programs?

This chapter discusses the challenges of educating students who already hold non-nursing baccalaureate degrees (second-degree students) in accelerated baccalaureate nursing programs. The challenges are posed by a dual set of special needs and requirements:

1. The needs of the second-degree students
2. The requirements of accelerated nursing programs

Suggestions and recommendations are presented to nurse educators and administrators who offer accelerated programs to second-degree students. These recommendations are based on the literature and the experiences of faculty from two nursing schools with accelerated programs in the Washington, DC metropolitan area. Faculty and students from these two schools have experienced setbacks, challenges, and successes over the years. Yet, as students have progressed to graduation each year, the many lessons learned have provided considerable insight and contributed greatly to professional and personal growth for all. As Oscar Wilde phrased it, "experience is simply the name we give our mistakes".

## A Comprehensive Screening Process

Nurses and other healthcare professionals have been identified as being ill prepared for the demands of patient care in our healthcare system today (Institute of Medicine, 2004, 2003; Lewis & Lewis, 2000). In response, much attention has been dedicated to transforming the healthcare system and education programs within the system. One of the many responses has been a re-examination of admission requirements, and rethinking eligibility for admission to nursing programs, as well as methods to determine that eligibility. Admission requirements and student eligibility take on an increased importance in accelerated programs.

The pace of an accelerated nursing program is taxing and difficult for students to assimilate and manage. It is important to identify students who will flourish with an accelerated curriculum and to screen out others better suited for a more traditional pathway. We must take care not to set students on a track for failure by accepting applicants who merely meet the admission criteria on paper. Major setbacks occur when students believe they have the ability to succeed in an accelerated nursing program while continuing to maintain their previous activities, such as working full-time or managing their family and personal responsibilities as usual. These setbacks can be psychologically damaging and costly to the student, distressing to faculty, and costly to the nursing school.

It is clear that pre-admission grade point average (GPA) is a predictor of academic performance in healthcare education; however the relationship between pre-admission GPA and clinical performance is less clear (Byrd, Garza, & Nieswiadomy, 1999; Ferguson, 2002; Salvatori, 2006). In addition to GPA, we found the two most useful measures for predicting success in the accelerated nursing programs to be

1. Standardized pre-admission testing, especially in science and math
2. A comprehensive interview

Although science and math grades of C are the minimum entry standard for nursing, this standard does not ensure competence in the clinical setting. There is no time to teach or even review basic science or math concepts in an accelerated program, but a firm foundation in the sciences and mathematics is an essential pre-requisite for nursing courses to build upon. Knowledge of various sciences, humanities, and mathematics is necessary to make important decisions about critical and complex situations in the clinical setting. Furthermore, basic principles of mathematics are fundamental to safe practice and necessary to master calculations of medication dosages. Passing scores, especially in science and math, on standardized tests such as the National League for Nursing (NLN, 2007) Pre-Admission Examination have provided a way to objectively examine applicants' readiness for entry into the accelerated nursing program, as well as provided a tool for counseling students on the likelihood of their success.

There is general agreement in the literature that the admission screening process should include assessment of both cognitive and non-cognitive characteristics of applicants (Agho, Mosley & Smith-Paul, 1998; Scott, 1995). A personal interview incorporated into the screening process is strongly recommended as an effective way of assessing non-cognitive characteristics prior to acceptance into the accelerated nursing program. It is also recommended that the people conducting the interview be trained and provided with explicit rating guidelines, as this is critical to the reliability and validity of the interview process (Salvatori, 2006).

The interview process needs to include an open discussion about the many demands of the nursing program caused by the fast timeframe of an accelerated pathway. Throughout the interview applicants should be evaluated for their understanding of the compactness of the program, their ability to handle the stress of the fast pace, their coping strategies, their support systems, and their overall readiness for the accelerated program. Applicants should also be evaluated regarding their computer skills, capabilities, and previous exposure to independent, online instruction, especially if web-based education is a significant teaching strategy in the program. Seldomridge and DiBartolo (2005) recommend encouraging students to develop a budget that does not depend on regular employment. Based on their study of outcomes of an accelerated nursing program on the East coast, they also recommend that prospective applicants meet with current students to discuss the demands of the weekly class and clinical schedules. With appropriate counseling, straight-forward advisement, and open discussion, the student and the interviewer can jointly evaluate the student's readiness for an accelerated program.

## Ongoing Advisement

While identifying appropriate students for entry into an accelerated program is crucial, equally important is providing a mechanism to support and nurture their success through each step of the program. A built-in guidance and advisement process is recommended, with regular scheduled meetings between the student and an assigned advisor, not just at the milestones in the program but between the milestones as well. It is vital to provide close and individual attention to the changing needs of this fast-paced group, as there is no time for even the smallest of concerns to slip through the cracks. It is also important to have options available to accommodate students who encounter unanticipated problems after entering the accelerated pathway. One option is to construct a bridge to the more traditionally paced program, allowing students to move to a slower pace if needed. Other options would be to offer evening and/or weekend classes, or to set up an evening or weekend program, providing more flexibility.

## Use of Screening Data

Data from the screening process can be used to develop a profile of students' educational and experiential backgrounds. These profiles can be a valuable resource for educators in any program, and are especially valuable for educators working with second-degree students who are experienced in other parts of their lives. Faculty can draw from this reservoir of talent to enhance the teaching-learning process. For example, students in our programs who were former managers were noted to emerge quickly as leaders when an organizational task needed to be accomplished. A student who had worked in a viral/bacterial laboratory was able to explain to other students in very simple terms the meaning of a "shift to the left" and a "shift to the right". Another student who had been a massage therapist shared alternative relaxation techniques with faculty, staff, and peers for patients with pain and anxiety issues. Other students with a background in library science and computer technology have been valuable assets in assisting other students to access resources and information, and expanding methods of communication through development and maintenance of list-serves. Students holding degrees in biology, chemistry, or nutrition made excellent contributions to pathophysiology and pharmacology classes.

## A Core Group of Experienced Faculty

The typical second-degree nursing student is older than the traditional undergraduate student, very motivated and competitive with high academic expectations (AACN, 2005). Many of these students have backgrounds and experiences that go well beyond those of the faculty. They are experienced at "working the system", have a high level of inquiry, and often challenge the "usual", as well as their instructors (Anderson, 2002). To address the challenges presented by these students, assist their transition, facilitate their success, and allow them to flourish, Anderson explains that it is essential to have a consistent group of seasoned faculty who are comfortable teaching adult learners and secure in their own role as an educator and as a nurse.

As the nursing faculty shortage intensifies it is becoming increasingly more difficult to find faculty with the credentials needed to teach the accelerated courses to this special group of students. It is especially difficult to find and consistently employ experienced part-time clinical instructors who are trained in specialty areas such as pediatrics, obstetrics, and psychiatric nursing. However, in our experience, the more we rely on nursing instructors with little or no teaching experience, or those with no formal education in teaching methods, assessment, evaluation, or curriculum development, the weaker the accelerated program becomes. A successful accelerated program must remain committed to a core group of experienced faculty who are dedicated to the special needs of the second degree student.

## Multiple Modes of Communication

It is difficult to transition from a life in a respected career position to a life as an undergraduate student again. To ease this transition for the second-degree students, provide satisfaction and facilitate program planning, it is vital that communication among administrators, faculty, and students is structured, timely, and clear. Electronic communication tools, such as listservs, or online course software (e.g., WebCT or Blackboard) that incorporate discussion groups are very helpful. These mechanisms provide the opportunity for open and asynchronous communication, and can be used for simple announcements and/or for more open discussions at the convenience of the participants.

Open communication is critical. Student exit surveys from our programs have revealed that students want to know their concerns were heard and they mattered, even if immediate action was impossible. Representation "at the table" on student affairs or curriculum committees and at Student Nurses Association board meetings are mechanisms that not only provide students with opportunities for their voice to be heard, but also foster engagement into the nursing profession.

Another mechanism for students to voice concerns is to establish regular forums such as "town hall" meetings. This type of venue provides students, administrators, and faculty the opportunity for open, face-to-face discussions to share, clarify, verify and amplify information. It is important to keep in mind, however, that some issues and concerns can be addressed promptly, and others are not so easily tackled. But most importantly, this type of forum provides the opportunity for mutual understanding, with a positive regard for each other as adults. Experience has suggested that second-degree students can be quite reasonable, if they understand the rationale behind the decisions.

Posting communication notices related to schedules and requirements as far in advance as possible, with as little change as possible is a necessity. Second-degree students have carefully structured their lives to meet the requirements of accelerated programs and there is little room in their schedule for surprises or sudden changes. If possible, a one-year calendar with all scheduled classes, clinical sites and times should be posted at the beginning of the program. Our student exit surveys revealed this type of calendar helped provide the structure needed to balance both personal and academic lives.

## Engaging Students into the Nursing Profession

Haring-Smith (2004) discusses the importance of establishing an environment that allows students, faculty, and staff to contribute actively and thoughtfully to the life and learning of the profession of nursing. According to the National Survey of Student Engagement report (2004), engagement is related to:

- The time and the quality of effort students devote to purposeful activities
- The available educational practices that channel student's energy toward those activities

To promote engagement and not simply endorse service learning, Spiezio (2002) explains that faculty must explicitly and directly embed educational practices related to the art of political participation into the curriculum. For example, networking activities with politically active nurse professionals and organizations is a teaching strategy that channels students to deal directly with policy issues, engaging them into the nursing profession. Students in an accelerated program have little time for extracurricular activities. However, by integrating professional activities into the curriculum and providing the necessary blocks of time to participate in such activities, we are facilitating a broader view of nursing while channeling students to become engaged into the profession of nursing.

Kuh (2003) identified the characteristics of an academic culture that engaged students. These characteristics are educational practices that:

- Offer a high level of academic challenge, (high expectations)
- Respect diverse talents
- Integrate education and experience
- Foster an ongoing practice of learned skills
- Offer active and collaborative learning
- Encourage out-of-class contact and strong interactions between students and faculty
- Provide adequate time on tasks with prompt feedback

An important message emphasized in the literature on motivation to learn is that controlling environments have been consistently shown to reduce students' interest in whatever they are doing, even when they are doing things that would be highly motivating in other contexts (Singham, 2007). It is important to not mandate rules that force students to obey, thinking they will learn as a result of these rules. Consistent with adult learning theory, it is vital to provide second-degree students as much control, flexibility and choice as possible over what, how, when, and where learning occurs, with a goal of moving away from an authoritarian education (Speck, 1996). Haring-Smith (2004) discusses the importance of establishing an environment that allows students and faculty to contribute actively and thoughtfully to the life and learning of the discipline. By viewing the curriculum with the needs and characteristics of the second-degree students in mind, and incorporating student input when and where we can, we are forming meaningful connections between students and faculty and sending the message that together we are embarking on an exciting learning adventure.

To engage students in learning, Tinto (1993) stresses the importance of connecting with them. To facilitate this we must communicate with them, including communicating our expectations for learning as well as our concern for students and their learning. Consistent with adult learning theory, second-degree students need, appreciate, and demand organized and clear explanations of how each class will help them attain their goal, to justify learning the content. According to Speck (1996) students will commit to learning when the goals and objectives are considered realistic and important to them. By providing information such as why the content is important to learn and therefore worth studying, along with the assignments and required readings, we are communicating and connecting with our students. We also communicate, connect, and engage with our students when we ask them how they are experiencing a course or the program in general, or when we ask for feedback after a test or a project.

Haring-Smith (2004) proposes that a key to engaging students in learning is the level of commitment that administrators and faculty are willing to bring to the task. This stresses the significance of the time and effort that faculty and administrators must spend to build trust and create a sense of community among our students, and between our students and faculty. If the teacher-student relationship is a mentoring one, then we should be modeling the rewarding life of nursing as part of our efforts to engage students into the nursing profession. Most second-degree students are enthusiastic learners, and we know that nursing is a rich and exciting profession. If faculty remain engaged and current in their field, engaging students in learning that field of study is easy. It has been said that accountability serves improvement. If so, we should expect improved learning by remaining engaged with our students as well as with our field of practice, and by maintaining the high expectations and standards deemed necessary by that practice.

## Innovative Teaching Methods

As previously stated, accelerated nursing programs need to customize as many experiences as possible to the needs of the second-degree student. This is an ongoing process of evaluation and modification. Although second-degree students have impressive backgrounds and excel in the classroom (AACN, 2005), they are novices in nursing, and have distorted views that lack an understanding of the complexities of the role of nurses in healthcare settings. But these students are eager to gain the clinical experience they lack. Attaining a balance between teaching students who are, on the one hand, experienced adult professionals, yet on the other hand, novice nursing students is certainly challenging. However, this balance is necessary to reduce the stress and allow learning to occur. Faculty must utilize the rich backgrounds of second-degree students, and build on their prior learning experiences while addressing their misperceptions. As these students acquire a more accurate picture of nursing they discover the more they learn, the more they need to learn. The following teaching-learning methods have been found to be particularly valuable in our accelerated programs.

## A Hybrid Inquiry-Based Learning (IBL) Clinical Instruction Model

Nurse educators are well aware of the challenges brought about by the increasing amount and complexity of content that students need to learn, faculty shortages, and larger class sizes (NLN, 2005). These challenges are confounded by the significantly shortened timeframes that are sharply contrasted with the compressed and taxing curriculum of accelerated programs. In response to these many challenges, our programs have implemented an innovative clinical instruction model using a hybrid inquiry-based learning (IBL) framework that combines inquiry with problem-based learning (Holaday & Buckley, in press). This has been a particularly useful teaching method, especially for the more mature, experienced students in the accelerated programs. It has been a very successful approach to teaching the accelerated students an enormous amount of information while quickly engaging them in the clinical setting and the profession of nursing. Working together as a team, the process draws upon the skills and resources of both students and faculty. This is particularly effective with the varied skills and resources the second-degree students bring with them to the teaching-learning environment. Students are challenged to assume responsibility for their own learning needs, which is something that most second-degree students do very well.

Holaday and Buckley (in press) describe the hybrid IBL clinical instruction model which involves actual clinical experiences and seminar tutorials. Each student presents a case study about one of their clinical patients to their seminar group members. Together, the seminar group explores the patient case data using a step-by-step process within the hybrid IBL guidelines. Hypotheses are reviewed, and students work toward solving problems presented in their cases. As ideas are generated and explored, critical issues are identified for further study. Faculty provide the structure for learning to occur by guiding their seminar group of students through difficult problem-solving issues when needed, while allowing the students to confront and wrestle with different perspectives. The faculty role is to assist students to identify what learning needs exist, and when appropriate, refer students to experts outside the classroom for problem-solving and inquiry. Students begin to understand the real meaning of teamwork and leadership during this process.

Faculty evaluations strongly indicate the hybrid IBL teaching method has helped to quickly identify gaps in the curriculum as well as gaps in student knowledge. Student course evaluations and anecdotal data also strongly indicate that faculty and students from both the authors' nursing schools regard the clinical instruction model as a valuable teaching-learning approach that strengthens the relationship between theory and practice, prepares students to think critically and act effectively, and grooms students and faculty for lifelong learning.

## Streaming Videos on Demand

A wonderful supplement to classroom teaching is the use of streaming media. This technology enables real-time, or on-demand, distribution of audio, video, and multimedia over a local network or the Internet. It is an ideal way to distribute, preserve, and manage teaching-learning information. A bank of lectures or other desired content can be created and received by students online as a continuous real-time stream. Videos can be indexed and accessed on demand, providing students the option of viewing the entire program or watching a shorter clip. The digital content data can be shared using a network streaming server and displayed by applications such as the Microsoft Windows® Media Player or the QuickTime® Player. Incorporating streaming video into the curriculum provides lectures, study tools, and educational programming to students anytime, anywhere. It provides a welcomed flexibility to second-degree students in emergency situations if a class can not be attended, and reinforcement when needed throughout the program as a study tool.

## Web-Based Instruction

Online courses offer accelerated students a much welcomed convenience. Kearns, Shoaf and Summey (2004) compared students' performance and satisfaction with the use of web-based versus traditional classroom instruction in a second-degree nursing program. These authors found the students in the Web-based course scored significantly higher on performance measures, but were less satisfied with this type of instruction. Although students reported strong dissatisfaction with the timeliness of instructor feedback and a strong sense of uncertainty about progressing with remaining coursework due to feedback delays, 87% of the students in the Web-based course stated they would take another online course because of the convenience and flexibility.

Faculty must approach Web-based instructional with accelerated students with great care. One of the challenges of the accelerated program is to engage students into the nursing profession. Physical presence, visual cues, and the non-verbal aspects of communication are lost with online courses, making it difficult to know the students and connect (Diekelmann & Schulte, 2000). Course evaluation data from our online nursing research course revealed the second-degree students were able to grasp such information as research terminology, research designs, the steps involved when conducting a research study, and criteria for critiquing an article. However, they had difficulty when reading, analyzing, and critiquing critical dimensions and issues specific to nursing. Qualitative response data from course reports also indicated these students needed a considerable amount of assistance interpreting and clarifying research articles in the practice of nursing.

Nursing students are faced with a daunting amount of new information. While looking at ways of streamlining an accelerated program and minimizing stress, we must also remember that very little "face-to-face" time is spent with these students. It is crucial to carefully select, design, and monitor the online courses we offer. Furthermore, when developing the courses, we must focus on incorporating availability and timeliness of instructor feedback to engage students who lack nursing knowledge, yet possess a high level of inquiry.

## Online Testing

Online testing can be used with Web-based instruction and with face-to-face courses. The design and administration of computerized examinations, using National Council Licensure Examination (NCLEX®) style questions has been found to be a successful approach in evaluating the knowledge of students in our accelerated programs. In several courses we used computerized exams that were programmed according to the same time limitations of the NCLEX, and were constructed so students cannot revisit previously answered questions. For the convenience of the student and faculty, these exams can be taken outside of class time in a proctored, computerized classroom if available. Blocks of time can be made available for students to take their exam, allowing them flexibility in scheduling. Exam scores are automatically computed, recorded, and sent directly to students electronically. Although computerized testing may require more time to develop, once established this approach has the advantage of allowing more time for classroom teaching.

## Assigned Demonstrations and Dialogues

Teaching in an accelerated nursing program requires faculty to streamline assignments to yield accurate assessment data for evaluation of students' knowledge and skills. Second-degree students are impressively intolerant of busy work (Anderson, 2002), so each assignment needs to have meaning. Assignments need to be streamlined and clinical situations need to be a partnership of direct intense study. We have found that clinical assignments that involve actual demonstrations and dialogue with faculty in the clinical setting are most effective. This allows faculty to assess students' knowledge and critical thinking skills directly, eliminating hours of writing for students and hours of grading for faculty. However, as with any assignment, it is important to provide students with clear guidelines and grading criteria for all demonstrations and dialogues, along with an explanation of the expected format.

An example of an effective clinical assignment is to require each student to conduct an in-depth patient assessment while the faculty assesses what the student does, says, and documents. During and following the assessment, the faculty engages the student in dialogue, asking questions and discussing findings, interventions, rationales, and expected outcomes. This enables the faculty to directly assess the students' knowledge, clinical skills, time management, communication, critical thinking and judgment, and provides the student the opportunity for immediate feedback.

Another effective clinical assignment that allows for direct student assessment and immediate feedback is to ask each student to present during clinical postconference, assessment data relating to an assigned patient. Following the presentation of data, the student uses a chalkboard or flip chart as they lead the conference group in constructing a concept map or care plan of the patient. During this exercise, the faculty participates by introducing important points, and questioning and clarifying information, while everyone in the group shares information and resources. This type of assignment provides clinical faculty the opportunity to assess group interaction, leadership skills, collaboration, communication, critical thinking, judgment, and decision-making skills. It also allows faculty to provide students with immediate feedback during the process about accuracies and inaccuracies as they arise.

In our experience, these assignments have accomplished much more than originally expected. Students and faculty became engaged in the learning process through a partnership. Together they explored possibilities for patient outcomes and determined how to implement various plans of care. Students "walked with faculty" in their educational journey, as clinical situations evolved. Students benefited from intensive learning situations, allowing faculty many opportunities to assess students' ability to think, make decisions, and perform in real-life clinical situations.

## Collaborative Relationships

It has been said that practice drives education. Throughout the years many creative approaches have been used to solve problems by establishing cooperative relationships in nursing and health care. The AACN (2007) urges hospitals, healthcare systems, and other practice settings "to form partnerships with schools offering accelerated programs to ease the financial burden of nursing students in exchange for a steady stream of new nurse recruits" (para. 13). Nurse educators and nurse employers have a responsibility to the public to join together in response to the AACN's call for solutions to the nursing shortage. Furthermore, the process of collaborative professional relationships is a major component of the nursing role and is, therefore, a valuable teaching-learning tool to incorporate into the nursing program to strengthen student engagement into the nursing profession.

## An Example of Collaborative Relationship

With the support and involvement of several agency contacts and childbirth educators throughout the community, our students were assigned to complete a series of childbirth classes as part of their maternity clinical. A brief written report of the experience was due following the experience. As with many nursing courses, there is not time to teach what is taught to the layperson, yet in maternity, the lay content is vital to understanding the complexities of the clinical expectations during childbirth. This collaborative assignment helped to close this teaching gap, enriched the maternity experience, and actively engaged students in clinical nursing practice.

Initially many students were unhappy about this assignment. One student stated, "I have had babies; I know what it's like". Another student asked, "Why do we have to go to the whole series of classes, can't you just put that information in a nutshell?" However, by completion of the childbirth classes, students reported only positive information. Many students encountered couples from their childbirth class again as they cared for them during their labor and delivery experience. They expressed how they felt closely connected while caring for patients and their families, reporting they felt more involved as part of the healthcare team caring for their patients. This was an important factor on such an intimate unit as labor and delivery, where many students find it difficult to become involved with direct patient care.

Written reports from the students revealed such thoughts as:
- "I never realized how different the whole perspective is when you are not the patient."
- "I don't know why I fought this."
- "I wouldn't trade this experience for anything".

Other comments expressed were, "These classes pulled together the entire childbirth experience among the patient, the family, and the provider", and "Whatever you do, don't drop the childbirth class assignment from the program, it was incredibly insightful".

## Preceptorships

Many nursing programs provide experiences and opportunities for their students to work directly with an expert RN preceptor from local agencies for a set period of time. This traditional preceptorship experience was expanded by several of our local hospitals to bring education and practice together through a collaborative mentoring program. Selected students received a full-tuition scholarship in exchange for completing all clinical experiences at the collaborative agency, and a two-year employment commitment following graduation. Students were paired with a nurse preceptor from the collaborative agency for each clinical course. A preceptor-student dyad could be extended for more than one clinical course if desired and appropriate for the course, or the student could be paired with a different preceptor at the collaborative agency for each clinical course. Upon entry into practice, the student may continue with a previous preceptor if desired and appropriate for their orientation period.

This type of collaborative relationship offers a number of benefits. In addition to the costs saved by the hospital on recruitment, the relationship-based preceptorship provides students with a personal and intense learning experience. Students develop an understanding of the assigned agency, resulting in a smoother, less stressful transition to the labor force. The orientation period is shorter than the typical orientation, offering a savings to the agency or extra time to spend on further strengthening the new graduates' skills and understanding of the care they provide.

It must be said, however, that there are no perfect partnerships, and like all collaborations, evaluation and modification must be ongoing, For example, one difficulty was encountered when students were asked to commit to a unit placement for the two-year work obligation upon receipt of the scholarship award. A commitment too early is unfair to the student and places them at a disadvantage, resulting in resentment and breach of contracts.

Most beginning nursing students, and especially second-degree students, do not have an idea of what the various unit environments and responsibilities entail, and they feel pressured when asked to commit to an area of nursing before having experienced that area. Not all new graduates are ready to be placed on specialty units such as critical care, labor and delivery, or the emergency department. Some need more time on a medical-surgical unit to assimilate and build upon the material they have learned. It is important for the student and the collaborative agency to wait until the latter part of the education program before a unit placement commitment is made.

Another obstacle occurs when communication, assessment, and evaluation are not a two-way process. Gaps and inconsistencies occur and the student falls behind. Regular face-to-face meetings with the faculty member, the student, and the preceptor, as well as an ongoing reporting system, are recommended. In addition to the face-to-face meetings, a written student report on academic performance should be sent on a regular basis from the academic institution to the collaborative agency, and a written student report on clinical performance from the collaborative agency to the academic institution. This assists faculty to guide the student experience and evaluate the student performance more objectively, using the written information documented by others involved. It also assists the agency in making decisions such as unit placements upon entry into practice.

Finally, when unforeseeable life events happen, the student or the preceptor must break the two-year commitment. Ongoing and open communication, flexibility, and a willingness to compromise when and if possible are suggestions for maintaining a smooth running collaboration during bumps in the road. A positive attitude and a sense of humor assist with mending disappointments. However, in the end, it is important not to lose sight of, or neglect the goals of, the student, the agency, and the collaborative relationship.

## Program, Course, and Student Evaluation

Evaluation at all levels requires a united front, accountability, and responsibility from all involved. A current challenge is to have courage, in the face of the need to produce more graduates in response to the nursing shortage. We caution faculty and administrators to deal responsibly, and not to neglect what really matters when being flexible or innovative in designing accelerated nursing programs or teaching, assessing, and evaluating students in those programs. We must not compromise quality for quantity.

Accelerated nursing students must be held to the same professional standards and outcome expectations as those required in traditional prelicensure nursing programs. Therefore, the only requirements, experiences and courses that should be eliminated when shortening timeframes in accelerated programs are those that are clearly comparable with, or match the requirements, experiences, or courses already obtained by the student upon entry into the accelerated program. If this can not be accomplished with certainty, then the requirement, experience, or course should not be eliminated, regardless of the time added to the program. This underscores the issue that if the requirements for a baccalaureate degree in an accelerated nursing program are lower then the requirements for a baccalaureate degree in a traditional nursing program, then the meaning of the accelerated nursing program degree is diminished.

Kravitz and Fathe (2006) discuss the importance of appropriately relating outcomes to inputs. Specifically, the time and effort required to complete assignments should be commensurate with the number of course credits. There should also be a relationship between the weight of an assignment toward a course grade and the effort required to complete the assignment. Also, the point value of exam questions should be commensurate with question difficulty, and the point value of tested material should be commensurate with the importance of the material. Because different students excel at different types of activities, Kravitz and Fathe recommend using a variety of assignments in an effort to account for individual needs, abilities and characteristics.

## Assessment and Evaluation

Assessment and evaluation is a process that requires ongoing attention. Nurse educators are responsible for helping students focus their attention on the critical information to be learned, the critical behaviors to be performed, and the expectations for assessing what is learned and performed. When students have a clear understanding of expectations and are evaluated by clear guidelines for levels of expected performance, there should be a resulting decrease in misinterpretation and misunderstandings, and an improvement in the quality of student learning and student performance. Moreover when expectations and levels of performance are defined according to a set of standards, faculty are able to assess and evaluate the student more objectively, accurately, and fairly.

To evaluate the written material generated by students at a fast pace, and their performance in the clinical settings, we have developed comprehensive guidelines and grading criteria or rubrics to measure the quality of the product or performance for all class and clinical assignments. These are included in all syllabi at the beginning of the course for students to use as a guide throughout the semester. We advise course coordinators to hold regular monthly meetings to establish consistency in expectations and the use of such grading rubrics.

Assessment and evaluation is about honesty, integrity, and fundamental fairness. We must strive to provide clear, honest, and ongoing feedback about student progress for students to grow and improve. Not all students perform exceptionally well, nor should they be convinced they have. This approach harms the student in the long-run, degrades the credibility of the faculty and the institution, and distorts the very essence of the evaluative process.

Faculty cannot afford to be silent about deficiencies in academic or behavioral performance, when those who fall behind in an accelerated program have a difficult time completing the work. Rather, faculty need to be candid with students and attend to their problem areas immediately and with integrity. This involves the sometimes difficult but necessary process of conversations to clearly describe any problems or concerns and to explain how the student can improve. Strengths as well as problem areas should be discussed with an opportunity for questions and clarification. If students express that faculty demands are unfairly high, it does not imply the faculty should automatically lower expectations, but it does stress the importance of clarifying and justifying faculty expectations (Kravitz & Fathe, 2006).

## Evaluation in the Clinical Setting

One of the most challenging questions regarding assessment and evaluation in the clinical setting is the appropriate evaluation tool to use in an accelerated program, and where to find it. Holaday and Buckley (2008) provide a detailed description of an innovative clinical performance evaluation tool-kit (Holaday, 2004) that serves as an organizing blueprint for nursing schools to develop clinical performance evaluation tools based on essential educational competencies for use as clinical outcome indicators. The tool-kit is designed to be used by any nursing school and all nursing programs, regardless of the degree offered. It is used by an increasing number of nursing schools to develop a clinical evaluation tool that is based on agreed-upon performance standards and customized to the individual mission and needs of their institution. The tool-kit also includes measurement scales that have been tested for validity and reliability to assess, evaluate, and measure student performance, growth, and competence across all clinical settings and at all levels of educational preparation in a nursing program. Benchmarks are also provided, for assessing course and program outcomes, which is important for accreditation.

Regardless of the instrument used, it is important for it to be valid and reliable, and tested in the clinical setting with second-degree students in an accelerated program. To conduct a meaningful and fair evaluation, students and faculty should be thoroughly oriented to the instrument and its use at the beginning of each clinical course. It is very important to allow ample time for discussion and questions to decrease user error and clarify expectations.

## Grading and Grade Inflation

The teaching, assessing, and feedback cycle must be completed with an evaluation for assigning a grade or symbol that reflects the student's achievement in a course. Nurse educators are obligated to graduate students who have demonstrated an accomplished level of competency aligned with the professional standards for entry into nursing practice. As previously stated, accelerated nursing students must be held to the same standards as students in traditionally-paced programs. This means that all students in course sections must be graded by the same expectations, principles, and standards for delivery of nursing care.

Most second-degree students communicate very well and appear very knowledgeable, and they are, in many areas. It is easy to grade these knowledgeable students based on this impression and the notation that accelerated students are stressed enough without the additional stress created by strict adherence to grading standards. However, it is vital not to forget the knowledgeable second-degree students are learning the profession of nursing, and students learn at different rates and levels. Deficiencies should not be ignored based on the thinking that second-degree students are a higher caliber nursing student than traditional students. Faculty should avoid developing a pattern of excusing or compromising when assigning grades.

When working with a talented and motivated group of students such as second-degree students, we must take care not to lose sight of what is considered average, above average, and below average as we are sprinting, and sometimes panting to keep up with the pace of grading assignments and clinical accomplishments. When the "A" no longer distinguishes the outstanding student from the good student, we weaken our standards, spiraling into the concealment of excellence and failure.

Rojstaczer (2003) reported significant grade inflation over the last thirty-five years, which has continued unabated at virtually every school for which data has been available. Grade inflation is contrary to the ideals and ethics of the nursing profession. It results in a serious quality issue, diminishing the meaning of the very pledge we are to uphold, ultimately causing harm to the public to whom we have pledged to provide care and to protect.

Nursing schools must take responsibility for the integrity of the degrees they award, and that includes the baccalaureate degree in nursing in an accelerated pathway. The authors encourage nursing schools to evaluate the grade distributions in all nursing programs that are offered, and engage in serious discussions about the nature of grades and grading. In addition to discussions and the provision of guidelines for grading, some suggestions provided by Manhire (2004) for addressing grade inflation problems include sharing grade distribution data within courses and programs, and posting all individual grades awarded in each course along with the mean or median grade and the number of students in the course.

## Summary

A quote by Albert Einstein sums up thoughts in reference to teaching second-degree students in an accelerated nursing program: "Everything should be made as simple as possible, but not one bit simpler". Accelerated programs provide an innovative approach for nursing education at a time when there is a significant nursing shortage. Although these programs appear to be successful in offering a fast track to nursing practice, they have their own set of challenges, as do the second-degree students who are enrolled in them. However, these challenges can be overcome with a careful screening of applicants, an ongoing supportive advisement system, and a core group of experienced faculty. Clear channels of communication, such as the use of electronic tools and open student forums help to alleviate student anxiety and strengthen the overall quality of the program. Innovative teaching methods that draw upon the varied skills and resources of the mature second-degree students, challenging them to actively assume responsibility for their own learning are a successful way of teaching an enormous amount of content, while engaging the fast-track students into nursing practice. These methods include inquiry-based learning, streaming media technology, web-based instruction, and assignments that involve collaborative relationships with professional nurses and organizations.

Nurse educators and administrators must form a united front and deal responsibly when teaching in and designing accelerated nursing programs. Students in these programs must be held to the same professional standards and outcome expectations as those required in traditional nursing programs. It is vital not to cut or neglect what really matters in nursing education when being flexible or using innovation. The time and effort required to complete assignments should be commensurate with the number of course credits, and there should be an appropriate relationship between the weight of an assignment toward a course grade and the effort required to complete the assignment.

Faculty must be clear and thorough about what is expected, and provide students with honest and ongoing feedback about their progress, assessing and evaluating all students in course sections using the same guidelines and principles. It is important to use evaluation tools that are based on professional standards and agreed upon competencies, and which are tested for reliability and validity when assessing and evaluating students. A thorough orientation for faculty and students to the evaluation instrument and process is essential to decrease user error and clarify expectations.

Finally, when working with a talented, motivated, and knowledgeable group of students such as second-degree students, we must not lose sight of what is considered average, above average, and below average in nursing education. It is vital to the integrity of the nursing program and to the competency of students in that program, that all students are graded fairly, accurately, and responsibly, according to guidelines and standards.

A personal message the authors would like to share is: if we as faculty strive to be that special person who taught a course that made a lasting difference in the lives of our students, or the person who inspired our students to learn – not only for that course or in that semester, but for a lifetime, at the very least we can expect to be greatly respected, and perhaps remembered for years to come. But most importantly, we can then believe we made a valuable contribution to the profession of nursing and to our society. As we strive for improvement in teaching, assessment, evaluation, and grading in our nursing programs, we recommend taking a deep breath every now and then, and reflect on our final quote, in the words of Albert Einstein: "not everything that can be counted counts, and not everything that counts can be counted".

## Learning Activities

1. Interview faculty of two different schools who teach in an accelerated nursing program. Develop three questions of interest that you developed after reading this chapter. Ask the faculty these questions. Compare and contrast their answers

2. Interview two students from two different schools who are enrolled in an accelerated nursing program. Develop three questions of interest that you developed after reading this chapter. Ask the students these questions. Compare and contrast their answers.

3. What do you perceive as the pros and cons of teaching in an accelerated nursing program?

## Educational Philosophy

"Education is not the filling of a pail," wrote W. B. Yeats, "but the lighting of a fire." As a nurse educator, I find it vital to prepare our nursing students to think critically and act effectively, and groom them for a lifetime of learning. A curriculum structured simply to convey knowledge is not enough. I believe that learning is most effective when students are actively involved and learn in the context in which the knowledge is to be used. Grounded in constructivism, my orientation toward teaching-learning is flexible and open, integrating education and experience while drawing on the varied skills and diverse talents of my students whenever possible. I encourage students to be active creators rather than passive receptors of knowledge, with the assumption that everyone holds the responsibility for his or her own learning. — Stephanie D. Holaday

Through a learner-centered approach, the teaching process must begin with an analysis of the learner's needs. Learning materials, resources, and environment are developed based upon explicit demonstrable objectives. The implementation and evaluation process includes feedback to ensure that the learning needs are being met as effectively as possible. — Kathleen M. Buckley

I believe that we are teachers and learners of each other. Each student brings gifts of curiosity and a yearning to be the best person and nurse she/he can be. Our role as educators is to enable the student to tap into the potential and power within, so as to flourish. I believe in order for students to learn that we must: (a) form "student-centered learning communities" in each class room; (b) create environments free of anxiety and fear which promote maximum discovery that can be made manifest in the student's nursing practice; (c) allow students to "make mistakes" in both clinical lab and clinical settings that will enhance their learning experience in foundational nursing practice; and (d) foster genuine excellence in the classroom and clinical settings through role-modeling for/to the students. — Margaret A. Miklancie

## References

Agho, A. O., Mosley, B. W., & Smith-Paul, B. (1998).Use of interview in selecting students for occupational therapy programs. *American Journal of Occupational Therapy, 52*(7), 592–594.

American Association of Colleges of Nursing (AACN). (2005). *Accelerated programs: The fast-track to careers in nursing.* Retrieved May 4, 2007, from www.aacn.nche.edu/Publications/issues/Aug02.htm

American Association of Colleges of Nursing (AACN). (2007). *Accelerated baccalaureate and master's degrees in nursing.* Retrieved May 4, 2007 from www.aacn.nche.edu/Media/FactSheets/AcceleratedProg.htm

Anderson, C. A. (2002). A reservoir of talent waiting to be tapped. [Editorial]. *Nursing Outlook, 50*(1), 1-2.

Byrd, G., Garza, C., & Nieswiadomy, R. (1999). Predictors of successful completion of a baccalaureate nursing program. *Nurse Educator, 24*(6), 33-37.

Diekelmann, N., & Schulte, H. D. (2000). Technology-based distance education and the absence of physical presence. *Journal of Nursing Education, 39*(2), 51-52.

Ferguson, E., James, D., & Madeley, L. (2002). Factors associated with success in medical school: Systematic review of the literature. *British Medical Journal, 324*(7343), 952–957.

Haring-Smith, T. (2004, April). Shifting paradigms require shifting policies: Creating a campus climate for engagement. Paper presented at the meeting of the Association of American Colleges and Universities, Chicago, IL.

Holaday, S. (2004). *Clinical performance evaluation tool-kit.* Copyrighted material: US Government Copyright Office. Reproduced by permission of Holaday, S.

Holaday, S. D., & Buckley, K. M. (2008). A standardized clinical evaluation tool-kit: Improving nursing education and practice. *Annual Review of Nursing Education, 6*(1), 123-149.

Holaday, S. D., & Buckley, K. M. (in press). Addressing the challenges of nursing education through an inquiry based learning (IBL) clinical instruction model. *Nursing Education Perspectives.*

Institute of Medicine (IOM) (2003). *Health professions education: A bridge to quality.* Washington, DC: The National Academies Press.

Institute of Medicine (IOM). (2004). *Keeping patients safe: Transforming the work environment of nurses.* Washington, DC: The National Academies Press.

Kearns, L. E., Shoaf, J. R., & Summey, M. B. (2004). Performance and satisfaction of second-degree BSN students in web-based and traditional course delivery enhancements. *Journal of Nursing Education, 43*(6), 280-284.

Kravitz, D., & Fathe, L. (2006, January). Who's the fairest of them all: Perceptions of fairness in the college classroom. Paper presented at the meeting of The Association of American Colleges and Universities, Washington, DC.

Kuh, G. D. (2003). What we're learning about student engagement from NSSE. *Change, 35*(2), 35-44.

Lewis, C., & Lewis, J. H. (2000). Predicting academic success of transfer nursing students. *Journal of Nursing Education, 39*(5), 234-236.

Manhire, B. (2004). Grade Inflation, ethics and engineering education. Proceedings of the 2004 American Society for Engineering Education Annual Conference & Exposition. Session 2560. June 20-23, 2004. Salt Lake City, Utah.

National League for Nursing (NLN), Board of Governors. (2005). Position statement: Transforming nursing education. *Nursing Education Perspectives, 26*(3), 196-197.

National League for Nursing (NLN). (2007). *Pre-Admission Examination (PAX)-RN*. Retrieved April 20, 2007, from www.nln.org/testproducts/preadmin/GeneralInfo/paxrngeneralinfo.htm

National Survey of Student Engagement (NSSE). (2004). *Student engagement: Pathways to collegiate success*. Retrieved May 10, 2007, from http://nsse.iub.edu/2004_annual_report/pdf/annual_report.pdf

Rojstaczer, S. (2003). Grade Inflation at American Colleges and Universities. Retrieved March 20, 2008 from www.gradeinflation.com.

Salvatori, P. (2001, 2006 revised). Reliability and validity of admissions tools used to select students for the health professions. *Advances in Health Sciences Education, 6*(2), 159-175.

Scott, A. H., Chase L. M., Lefkowitz, R., Morton-Rias, D., Chambers, C., Joe, J., Holmes, G., & Bloomberg, S. (1995). A national survey of admissions criteria and processes in selected allied health professions. *Journal of Allied Health, 24*(2), 95–107.

Seldomridge, L. A., & DiBartolo, M. C. (2005). A profile of accelerated second bachelor's degree nursing students. *Nurse Educator, 30*(2), 65-68.

Singham, M. (2007). Death to the syllabus! *Liberal Education, 93*(4), 52-56.

Speck, M. (1996). Best practice in professional development for sustained educational change. *ERS Spectrum, 14*(2), 33-41.

Spiezio, K. E. (2002). Pedagogy and political engagement. *Liberal Education, 88*(4), 14.

Tinto, V. (1993). *Leaving college: Rethinking the causes and cures of student attrition* (2nd ed.). Chicago, IL: University of Chicago Press.

## Acknowledgements

We are very grateful to Dr. Holaday's father-in-law Dr. Paul Smalley, cardiologist, medical school professor, pioneer of open heart surgery, and friend to nursing, for his generous sharing of expertise in teaching students to become healthcare professionals. His considerable insight and challenging questions deepened our understanding of theories and brought clarity to our ideas. His unconditional support, enthusiasm, humor, and kindness contributed greatly to the joy of writing this chapter. He is gone from us now, but he was here when it counted.

Special appreciation goes to Dr. Holaday's daughter-in-law, Amy Holaday, for her contribution as a second-degree nursing student. Her personal experiences provided a valuable perspective that otherwise would have been missing.

# CHAPTER 26

# GRADUATE EDUCATION IN NURSING

Marilyn Frank-Stromborg, MS, EdD, JD, RN, ANP, FAAN
Kenneth Burns, MS, PhD, RN

The content of this chapter relates to the following major content area and subconcepts on the Certified Nurse Educator Examination Detailed Test Blueprint:

**Participate in Curriculum Design and Evaluation of Program Outcomes**
- Demonstrate knowledge of curriculum development
- Design courses to reflect the philosophical and theoretical framework of the curriculum
- Maintain community and clinical partnerships that support the educational goals
- Create community and clinical partnerships that support the educational goals
- Analyze results of program evaluation and initiate curricular change

## Introduction

There are significant differences between undergraduate and graduate nursing programs relative to:
- Educational setting
- Faculty expectations
- Student expectations
- Curricular focus

This chapter details the differences typically found between graduate and undergraduate education and the trends that are emerging in graduate education.

## Educational Settings

Graduate nursing programs include master's, post-master's, and doctoral programs that take place in colleges or universities. There is tremendous variation within master's programs in terms of the students who are initially admitted. These include licensed practical/vocational nurses (LP/LVNs) to master's programs, registered nurses (RNs) to master's programs, and accelerated baccalaureate nurses to master's programs (Fang, Htut, & Bednash, 2008). The traditional student admitted to a master's in nursing program has a bachelor degree in nursing and typically has been clinically active for several years. There is also an increasing trend for schools to offer dual-degree master's programs with students obtaining a master's degree in nursing coupled with a master's in business administration, master's in public health, master's in public administration, or juris doctor.

Another trend is to admit RNs with baccalaureate degrees in other disciplines and award a master's degree in nursing. Master's programs in nursing also differ in terms of the final degree that is awarded and can range from a Master of Nursing (MN), Master of Science (MS) with a major in nursing, Master of Arts (MA) in nursing, and Master of Science in Nursing (MSN) (Fang et al., 2008). In 2007, there were 458 institutions offering master's programs. Of those 458 institutions, 344 offered master's and/or post master's nurse practitioner programs and 244 offered master's and/or post master's Clinical Nurse Specialist (CNS) programs. At the same time, there were 62,451 students enrolled in master's programs (Fang et al., 2008).

Post-master's certificate programs offer an educational approach to address the desire for nurses with master's degrees in areas that may no longer be marketable to retool. These programs are defined as formal postgraduate programs for the preparation of nurse practitioners that admit RNs with master's degrees in nursing and, at completion, award either a certificate or other evidence of completion, such as a letter from the program director. Completers are eligible to sit for a national nurse practitioner certification examination. (Berlin Stennett, & Bednash, 2003, p. xii)

There is also wide variation in doctoral education, which ranges from baccalaureate- to-doctoral programs, clinically focused doctoral programs awarding a Doctor of Nursing Practice (DNP), Doctor of Nursing (ND) degree, and research-focused programs that award a PhD, DNS, or DNSc. Historically, nurses obtained doctoral degrees in education (EdD) because there were no doctoral programs in nursing. Currently, with the plethora of nursing doctoral programs, many nurses have the option of pursuing a PhD, DNS, DNSc, as well as an EdD. Over the past 10 years, the proportion of DNSC (or doctor of nursing science or doctor of science in nursing), relative to PhD programs in nursing have declined. Initially, the number of nursing programs offering PhD and DNSc or DNS was about equal. In 2003, 86% of all doctoral nursing programs offered the PhD (Keithley et al., 2003); in 2007, 89% offer the PhD (Fang et al., 2008). The reasons for this dramatic change are that many programs that originally offered the DNSc changed to the PhD degree, programs that offered both degrees dropped the DNSc, and all but 3 of the 25 doctoral programs that have started since 1990 grant the PhD degree (Keithley et al., 2003).

Doctoral programs in nursing prepare graduates for one of two roles. These two roles are:

- Academic roles, which include expectations of research, education, and practice
- Careers as advanced clinicians, administrators, and researchers, and in public policy (Norbeck et al., 2002).

In 2007, 132 doctoral programs offered an emphasis on nursing: 97 PhD; 1 EdD; 10 DNS, DNSc, DSN; 1 ND, and 72 DNP. In 2007, 3,843 students were enrolled in research intensive doctoral programs (Fang et al., 2008). Since 1970, most new programs have been developed to offer a PhD degree in nursing.

Another trend is the growth in postdoctoral nursing programs and the desire for newly graduated doctoral students to continue their education. This trend replicates a practice that has been historically widespread in other disciplines such as liberal arts and sciences. The concept of postdoctoral education is to assist the postdoctoral fellow in the development of high-level research skills and the development of a program of research that becomes the cornerstone of their research career.

## Expectations of Graduate Faculty

One strong expectation of graduate faculty is that either they have a doctorate degree or they are close to obtaining this degree. Typically, graduate faculty are on tenure track with a ticking tenure clock. Tenure track faculty have a predetermined number of years to obtain tenure. Tenure is most typically obtained by evidence of significant scholarly contributions, strong teaching credentials, and demonstrated professional service. A major expectation of graduate faculty is involvement in scholarly activities that includes writing data-based articles in peer reviewed journals; contributing to books by writing book chapters; giving presentations at state, national, and international meetings; and obtaining external funds to assist in financing their program of research. With the advent of curricula to produce advanced practice nurses (APNs), the scholarship of practice has emerged as a critical component in the maintenance of clinical competency of faculty in university settings and the advancement of clinical knowledge in the discipline (AACN, 1999a). Practice roles for faculty in healthcare delivery systems may include direct caregiver, educator, consultant, and administrator.

How stringent requirements are for tenure varies among universities based on the research-intensive status of the institution (Feldman & Acord, 2002). "Integrating teaching, practice, and research within the faculty role promotes knowledge development, dissemination, and application. Immersion in each area, however, often is difficult logistically" (Fawcett, Aber, & Weiss, 2003, p. 20). To maintain national certification, doctorally prepared APNs must provide evidence of continued clinical practice. It is not uncommon for graduate faculty to experience role conflict and fragmentation as they try to balance all the components of scholarship, including maintaining clinical practice (Tolve, 1999).

Another graduate faculty expectation is the need for faculty to retool and acquire advanced practice skills so they can teach in a revised master's curriculum that has shifted from traditional nursing roles to APN roles. For example, at the University of Alabama School of Nursing at Birmingham, when the curriculum was first restructured to accommodate an advanced practitioner of nursing track, there were five nurse practitioners. After the advanced practice curriculum was implemented, 12 faculty members had completed the postmaster's nurse practitioner option and achieved national certification (Miers, 1998).

The National Organization of Nurse Practitioner Faculties (NONPF, 2000) has criteria for evaluating advanced practice curriculum. One requirement for graduate programs that offer advanced practice options is that faculty teaching courses directly related to the advanced practice role or clinical management courses:

- Have authorization by the state licensing entity to practice as nurse practitioners and are currently nationally certified as nurse practitioners
- Have demonstrated history and current practice to ensure clinical competence in the area of teaching responsibility (NONPF, 2008).

Although it is recognized that the need for experienced faculty to retool to become APNs has significantly expanded their faculty role, it has been stressful for many faculty as they transition from expert to novice (Margolius & Sneed, 1999).

A significant difference between undergraduate and graduate education is the role of national organizations in setting the agenda and expectations for APN graduate curriculum. The recommendations for what should be in a graduate curriculum preparing APNs are significantly more prescriptive than that found in undergraduate curriculum. All national guidelines reflect the involvement of a multitude of national specialty and accreditation organizations. A sample of those organizations includes the American Nurses Association, American Academy of Nurse Practitioners, National League for Nursing, and National Certification Board for Pediatric Nurse Practitioners and Nurses (this is only a sample list). The national guidelines for what should be in a graduate curriculum are the result of multiple organizations coming together and deciding what must be in these guidelines to graduate programs. The Essentials of Master's Education for Advanced Practice Nursing (AACN, 1996); Nurse Practitioner Primary Care Competencies in Specialty

Areas: Adult, Family, Gerontological, Pediatric, and Women's Health (NONPF & AACN, 2002); and Criteria for Evaluation of Nurse Practitioner Programs (NONPF, 2008) outline with a high degree of specificity the expectations for:

- Organization and administration
- Curriculum
- Resources
- Facilities and services
- Faculty and faculty organization
- Evaluation of the graduate program

Figure 1 shows the AACN recommended Model of Master's Nursing Curriculum.

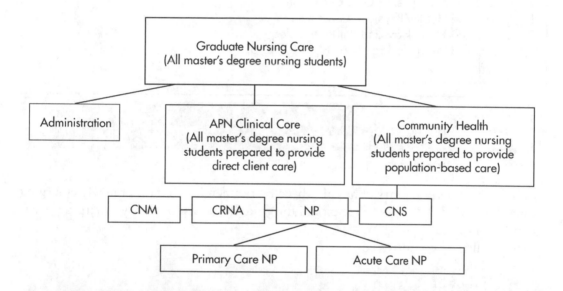

**Figure 1.** AACN Recommended Model of Master's Nursing Curriculum

The essential curriculum elements are outlined in Figure 2.

Graduate Core Curriculum Content

I.  Research
II. Policy, Organization, and Financing of Health Care
    A.  Health Care Policy
    B.  Organization of the Health Care Delivery System
    C.  Health Care Financing
III. Ethics
IV. Professional Role Development
V.  Theoretical Foundations of Nursing Practice
VI. Human Diversity and Social Issues
VII. Health Promotion and Disease Prevention

Advanced Practice Nursing Core Curriculum
I.  Advanced Health/Physical Assessment
II. Advanced Physiology and Pathophysiology
III. Advanced Pharmacology (AACN, 1997, p. 5)

Reprinted with permission.

**Figure 2.** Essential Curriculum Elements

In the last several years, it has also been recommended that other newly emerging topics be added to NONPF's curriculum guidelines. These newly emerging areas include:
- Cultural competence
- Genetics
- End-of-life care
- Community-based care
- Global health
- Business aspects of practice
- Evidence-based practice
- Distance education (Crabtree, 2002)

Other emerging topics which have been recommended for inclusion in graduate nursing curriculum include:

- Increasing competency in information literacy so that master's prepared nurses have the skills to be literate consumers of information in an electronic environment (Jacobs, Rosenfeld, & Haber, 2003)
- Increasing content on complementary and alternative therapies (Gaydos, 2001)
- Establishing standards of ethics education in MSN program (Burkempher et al., 2007).

Because of the profound demographic changes occurring in the American population there are increasing calls to have the diversity trend reflected in the graduate nursing curriculum. For instance, the US Census Bureau has projected that by 2020 the percentage of Americans of European descent will dramatically decrease which the number of Asian Americans and Hispanic Americans will triple and African Americans double (Speziale & Jacobson, 2005).

Due to the increasing competition for APN positions, it is essential that the business aspects of practice and securing employment be included within the graduate education experience.

## Expectations of Graduate Students

Graduate programs tend to be smaller than undergraduate programs. Over the past several years, some nursing programs have elected to downsize their bachelor's program and increase their master's and doctoral programs. Because students admitted to graduate programs demonstrate above-average academic performance, the level of expectations for student performance is higher than that of the student enrolled in an undergraduate program. Another change from the undergraduate experience is that graduate students are expected to be independent, goal-directed, and self-directed. It is not unusual for class assignments to be due at the end of a course to demonstrate a synthesis of knowledge.

Thus, students must adjust to not having assignments due throughout the term. They must pace themselves to successfully complete course requirements due at the end of the term.

Another expectation of graduate students in many advanced practice curricula is that students locate their own preceptors for their clinical experiences. In 2000, the majority of advanced practice programs reported their programs required a mean for supervised clinical practice clock hours of 651 clinical hours (AACN & NONPF, 2002). NONPF criteria for advanced practice curriculum mandate a minimum of 500 supervised clinical hours. Practice areas that provide care to multiple groups (e.g., family nurse practitioners) or prepare practitioners to function in multiple-care settings (e.g., primary and tertiary care) may require more than 500 clinical hours (NONPF, 2008).

Preceptors must be nationally certified in their specialty as well as possess clinical experience and expertise in their area of specialty. While many master's advanced practice programs allow students to have some of their experiences with physicians or physician's assistants, there is generally the firm requirement that the majority of the students' clinical experience be with nurses functioning in the role for which they are preparing. Locating a preceptor who is willing to provide a student with a semester or more of clinical experience and supervision can be a daunting assignment. In many areas, there is tremendous competition among graduate programs for preceptors because students in APN programs may be competing with students from physician's assistants programs also seeking preceptors. Graduate faculty are challenged by the limited supply of preceptors willing or able to provide graduate students with clinical experience. Faculty are also challenged by the lack of variety in traditional clinical resources necessary to expose the student to a holistic clinical experience: patients of various ages, diagnoses, cultural or racial groups, and socioeconomic status (Crabtree, 2002).

Because of the essential role of preceptors in the educational preparation of graduate students, NONPF developed a preceptor manual, Partners in NP Education (Dumas, 2000). This manual includes a sample clinical evaluation guide for faculty and preceptors to use when evaluating students' development as APNs and ability to meet the new competencies. Preceptors evaluate nurse practitioner students by direct observation of the students' skills in clinical training settings and by patient encounter information from various clinical log data collection strategies (Carney, Eliassen, & Harwood, 2002). Clinical log data are important to ensure the variety of patients and clinical conditions, but these are not easily amenable to review and reflection. However, if used effectively, clinical logs can guide subsequent student learning experiences or clinical placements (Jones & Clark, 1999). Many graduate students collect clinical log data using hand-held computers, PDAs, personal digital assistants. PDAs are increasingly required in graduate programs since they provide the nurse with access to a wide range of information at the point of care (Smith & Pattillo, 2006). Additionally, it is essential that graduate faculty assure the clinical competence of all graduate student preceptors as well as maintain a close working relationship with those preceptors.

Admission criteria for graduate school may include the following:
- Grade point average (GPA) of 3.0 or higher
- High Graduate Record Exam (GRE) score
- Letters of recommendation

- Interviews
- Evidence of writing skills
- Evidence of clinical accomplishments
- A stated research focus

Generally, graduate-level nursing students attend school part-time, are in their late 20s and early 30s, and struggle to balance full-time jobs and family responsibilities with increased academic demands. In 2002, 63% of master's students were enrolled part-time (AACN, 2003). Because students are required to balance multiple demands on their time, including rigorous academic course assignments, there is a high level of stress associated with the graduate student role. Faculty who advise graduate students need to assist them with the following:
- Developing time management skills
- Setting realistic academic goals
- Recognizing when work or family responsibilities require taking fewer courses per semester and altering their planned graduation date

## National Certification

Most state boards of nursing use professional nursing certification as a requirement for granting authority for advanced practice registered nurses (Hodnicki, 2002). National certification is also a requirement for reimbursement in many clinical settings. Therefore, upon graduation from a graduate program, students typically apply for and take a national certification examination. Graduate programs must demonstrate effective outcomes, and pass rates on national certification examinations have become an important benchmark in demonstrating those outcomes have been achieved. This is similar to the NCLEX® being an important outcome measure for undergraduate programs. Graduate programs are now routinely required to report to their university annual pass rates on national certification tests. Many commercial review courses are available to take by graduate students who do not pass national certification tests on the first try. Two organizations that offer certification examinations for nurse practitioners are the American Academy of Nursing and the American Nurses Credentialing Center (ANCC). The ANCC also offers certification examinations for a multitude of clinical nurse specialist's roles. Students can also obtain national certification from specialty organizations such as the American Association of Nurse Anesthetists, Oncology Nursing Society, American Association of Occupational Health Nurses, and National Association of School Nurses. State nurse practice acts for APNs typically list the national organizations that offer certification that the state recognizes. Certification by one of these recognized organizations is essential to obtain a license as an APN.

Hodnicki (2002) pointed out that as new and blended APN roles evolve, it is imperative that the educational program faculty consider how the graduates can meet national certification requirements and state credentialing criteria. She cautioned that graduate faculty must be cognizant of the certification requirements for all the applicable certifying entities. Students may desire to simultaneously take certification examinations in family, pediatrics, and adult advanced practice nursing. "There can be major legal problems if a graduate is declared ineligible to sit for a national certification examination because of a curricular deficiency. This situation can be avoided with comprehensive curricula planning and oversight" (Hodnicki, 2002, p. 101). The credentialing organizations require program directors to supply information on their programs to assure that all the essential components of an advanced practice curricula are offered and students complete sufficient clinical hours and didactic courses. There are states that license advanced practice nurses upon proof of passing a national advanced practice certification examination. Rhode Island, Illinois and California, for instance, provide both licensure for registered nurses and advanced practice nurses.

Perhaps one of the major differences between undergraduate and graduate education is the absence of guaranteed employment in the student's selected advanced practice role following graduation. Undergraduate students typically have multiple positions from which to select, often before they graduate. Students graduating from an advanced practice curriculum frequently work diligently to secure the exact type of position they desire. In some areas of the country, where there is an over-supply of nurse practitioners, graduates enter nonnurse practitioner positions. Because of the competition for securing advance practice positions, students need to spend considerable time during their graduate education establishing a network of contacts, learning how to market themselves and the role, and developing sophisticated entrepreneurial skills. Faculty have important roles in assuring that students have these skills as well as the requisite clinical skills before they graduate.

## Graduate Curriculum Focus

In the last decade, there has been a national move to restructure graduate curriculum to prepare nurses for APN roles. In fact, in 2007 as in 2002, the majority of enrollees and graduates from graduate programs were in nurse practitioner (NP), clinical nurse specialist (CNS), or combined NP/CNS programs. Nationwide, 458 institutions offered master's programs, with 344 (75%) offering master's-level NP and/or post-master's NP programs. NP or combined NP/CNS majors accounted for 45.4% of master's enrollees and 48.5% of master's graduates. In contrast, CNS, administration, nurse anesthesia, and education majors comprised 6.0 %, 10.5 %, 6.5%, and 16.8 % of master's enrollees, respectively (Fang, et al., 2008). Due to the increasing shortage of nursing faculty, many nursing programs are responding by:

- Developing educational tracks designed to prepare nursing faculty
- Developing postmaster's programs for master's prepared clinicians who want to transition into teaching roles

In the fall of 2004 the American Association of Colleges of Nursing (AACN) voted to move all advanced practice education to the practice doctorate model (Chase & Pruitt, 2006). The result of this vote was the AACN Position Statement on the Practice Doctorate in Nursing (2004). Terminal professional doctoral degrees are not academic research doctorates. The minimum term for a terminal professional degree is 3 years post baccalaureate, and the degree entitles the holder to pursue academic careers on par with holders of academic research doctoral degrees (Hathaway et al., 2006). The concept of the practice doctorate is designed for nurses seeking a terminal degree in nursing practice and offers an alternative to research-focused doctoral programs (AACN, 2009). The new role is not administratively focused but rather one that prepares the nurse to function within a microsystem and assume accountability for healthcare outcomes for a specific group of patients (population-focused) within a unit or setting (Radyminski, 2005). The AACN's goal is to transition advanced practice nursing preparation to the doctoral level by 2015 (Hathaway et al., 2006). Controversy surrounds this new role and has generated much debate in the nursing literature.

One notable change with curricular switch to prepare advanced practice nurses is the significant decrease in graduate students electing to write a thesis because of the focus on the development of sophisticated advanced practice clinical skills. This has implications for the nursing profession in terms of producing the next generation of nurse researchers. National discussion has been held on the need to increase writing and research activities in both master's and doctoral education (Diekelmann, Magnussen, & Ionside, 1998; Mill & Morris, 2000). Graduate faculty need to develop creative ways to provide graduate students with opportunities to participate in, design, or implement research projects so they develop research-related skills and an enthusiasm for incorporating research into their clinical roles.

Faculty have also been required to expand their teaching skills to include developing courses for on-line and distance technology (distance learning). There has been an explosion in graduate education in using nontraditional methods to deliver course content (AACN, 1999b; Larsen, Logan, & Pryor, 2003; Wambach et al., 1999).

For nurses in rural or remote areas, access to health care and health professional education is often limited. Therefore, distance learning and on-line courses may be the only viable means of providing nurses with the requisite knowledge and skills to become APNs. Further, community-based delivery of education where nurses live increases the likelihood that rural nurses or nurses in medically underserved areas will remain in their community after graduation, thus ensuring that providers will share the cultural values of the populations they serve (Robinson, 2002).

The use of technology is a significant means to increase access to education for adult, working students who represent a growing proportion of the graduate nursing student population. The use of technology in graduate education may provide an opportunity to increase the number of faculty-qualified nurses to support education, research, and practice (AACN, 1999).

Because of these reasons, many graduate programs have implemented multisite approaches to increase access to educational opportunities in advanced practice nursing for location-bound professional nurses. These multisite approaches include crossing state lines as well as international borders, which poses legal, professional, and cultural issues for faculty to solve prior to implementing these programs (Kim & Berry, 1998). Although these new approaches have opened up educational opportunities for nurses in remote areas, they have also presented new challenges to graduate faculty. One particular challenge is how to socialize students to new roles when there is no face-to-face contact. Safety and quality of education for advanced practice roles remain priority concerns with teaching adaptations that promote access and cost-effectiveness such as distance learning and online programs (Crabtree, 2002). The same benefits and concerns of distance education for all nursing students apply to graduate students as well.

Other issues facing graduate education include the aging of nursing faculty, lack of diversity, and need for more doctorally prepared faculty. In 2002, the average age of doctorally prepared faculty by rank was 56.2 years for professors, 53.8 years for associate professors, and 50.4 years for assistant professors (AACN, 2002b). During this same time, only 9.2% of nursing faculty identified themselves as a member of a racial/ethnic minority group, only 3.7% were male, and less than 50.0% were prepared at the doctoral level. One of the national implications of these statistics is that within the next decade, it is anticipated that there will be an unprecedented number of nursing faculty retiring. The National League for Nursing in 2002 predicted a shortfall of 20,000 faculty members needed nationwide to substantially increase undergraduate enrollment to stave off the nursing shortage (Tanner, 2006).

According to the report Oregon's Nursing Shortage: A Public Health Crisis in the Making (AACN, 2002b), 41% of the faculty in baccalaureate and higher degree programs in Oregon were projected to retire by 2005, with an additional 46% projected to retire by 2010. In associate degree programs, 24% were expected to retire by 2005, with an additional 33% retiring by 2010. This retirement pattern is likely to be experienced in other parts of the country as well (AACN, 2002b). The projected faculty retirements equal or exceed the rate at which we can prepare faulty at the doctoral level or in master's degree programs that provide preparation in nursing education (Tanner, 2006).

A significant problem contributing to the loss of graduate faculty are the higher salaries in clinical and private-sector settings that lure current and potential nurse educators away from the education setting. At the same time, graduates from master's and doctoral programs in nursing are decreasing. One of the most challenging factors contributing to the nursing shortage is the increasing shortage of master's-prepared and doctorally prepared nursing faculty. The faculty shortage, in turn, constricts the current pipeline for education of professional RNs (Livsey, Campbell & Green, 2007). This all translates to a smaller pool of potential nurse educators. Graduate faculty need to identify creative solutions to the emerging faculty shortage. The federal legislation, the Nurse Reinvestment Act, may assist in the crucial need to prepare more nursing faculty. The Nurse Reinvestment Act has multiple components, including a Faculty Loan Cancellation Program, Career Ladder Grant Program, and Nurse Scholarships (AACN, 2003).

Some initiatives that graduate programs have instituted to address diminishing faculty resources are limited-cohort distance-education programs and development of academic consortium. For example, four universities in Louisiana have formed a consortium for delivering graduate education in nursing. This group is called Intercollegiate Consortium for a Master of Science in Nursing (Lund, Tate, & Hyde-Robertson, 1998). The University of Minnesota developed a limited-cohort distance education graduate program to overcome geographic barriers and address the shortage of master's-prepared specialty nurses in rural areas of the upper Midwest. This program is to be offered for a limited period of time to meet the regional needs to prepare more APNs (Block et al., 1999).

Multiple challenges to graduate education are anticipated over the next few years. Some of these include the following:

- The need to provide specialization for graduate nursing students who choose to become indirect care providers, leaders in systems of care, or future nursing educators.
- The need for practice to become as integral to the faculty role as teaching, research, and service. Faculty need to have schedules that facilitate practice time.

- The need to increase the diversity of graduate faculty. The number of racial and ethnic minorities enrolled in master's degree programs that prepare nurses for advanced practice is only 12%. This representation remains a continuing challenge (AACN, 1999b).
- The need to continue blending roles and primary care content.
- This blending must continue in graduate programs so graduates can more flexibly serve populations across the care continuum.
- The need to address certification and credentialing issues. As new roles emerge and curricula are combined in innovative ways, there will continue to be issues related to certification and credentialing for both master's and postmaster's programs.
- The need to continue to emphasize the preparation of culturally competent faculty and students.
- The need to address technology issues. The widespread use of new technology to deliver education programs to distant, remote, or rural settings will create new issues of quality and clinical competence of students.

## Summary

Graduate education has changed dramatically in the past decade as graduate nursing programs have responded to the national need to prepare APNs. It can be anticipated there will be similar changes required of graduate nursing education in the coming years as the healthcare system changes and new nursing roles/expectations emerge. At the same time, it is essential that graduate nursing education responds to the changes that have occurred in the country, e.g., increasing diversity of the population, decreasing healthcare resources, aging of the baby boomers, and shortages of nursing faculty. Graduate educators will have to be flexible and creative to meet all the demands for curricular changes they will encounter in the coming years.

## Learning Activities

1. You have been asked to design and implement several new graduate courses for acute-care practitioners. Identify the national organizations and guidelines you would consult to ensure that the content will enable graduates to take national certification examinations.

2. Of all the identified challenges to graduate education, propose some effective strategies for two challenges that could be implemented with minimal resources.
3. You have taught in an undergraduate nursing program for several years and have recently accepted a position to teach in a master's degree nursing program. Discuss how your role as graduate faculty will be the same as and different from your role as faculty in the undergraduate program.
4. Compare and contrast the expectations of graduate faculty with those of faculty in undergraduate-only programs, and identify those aspects of the role that have the potential for conflicting with the teaching role. For example, how do faculty balance scholarship and teaching?
5. Visit the AACN website. Read the information on the CNL and the DNP. What do you perceive as the strengths of these degrees? What do you perceive as the limitations of these degrees?

## Educational Philosophy

Effective teaching is based on the personal interaction and caring between teacher and student. This interaction can occur anywhere, anytime, can last a lifetime, and has the potential to change the student's life significantly for better or worse. The role of teacher thus is a serious responsibility that should not be entered into lightly. — Marilyn Frank-Stromborg

An educator is a mentor and role model, whether in the classroom, practice, or research setting, who serves as a guide in the development of a student's knowledge about the profession and discipline. — Kenneth Burns

## References

American Association of Colleges of Nursing [AACN]. (1996). *The essentials of master's education for advanced practice nursing*. Washington, DC: Author.

American Association of Colleges of Nursing. (1999a). *Nursing education's agenda for the 21st century*. Retrieved April 11, 2003 from http://www.aacn.nche.edu/Publications/positions/nusgedag.htm

American Association of Colleges of Nursing [AACN]. (1999b). *Distance technology in nursing education* (AACN white paper). Washington, DC: Author.

American Association of Colleges of Nursing [AACN]. (2001). *AACN position statements: Indicators of quality in research-focused doctoral programs in nursing*. Washington, DC: Author.

American Association of Colleges of Nursing [AACN]. (2002a). *Assessing the annual state of the schools*. Washington, DC: Author.

American Association of Colleges of Nursing [AACN]. (2002b). *Backgrounder: AACN'S nursing faculty shortage fact sheet*. Washington, DC: Author.

American Association of Colleges of Nursing. (2004). *AACN position statement on the practice doctorate in nursing*. Retrieved May 16, 2006, from http://www.aacn.nche.edu/DNP/pdf/DNP

American Association of Colleges of Nursing. (2009). *AACN position statement on the practice doctorate in nursing*. Retrieved April 13, 2009 from http://www.aacn.nche.edu/Media/FactSheets/dnp.htm

American Association of Colleges of Nursing [AACN] and National Organization of Nurse Practitioner Faculties [NONPF]. (2002). *Master's-level nurse practitioner educational programs: Findings from the 2000-2001 Collaborative Curriculum Survey*. Washington, DC: Author.

American Association of Colleges of Nursing [AACN]. *Government Affairs. Nurse reinvestment act at a glance*. Retrieved April 11, 2003 from http://www.aacn.nche.edu/edia/nraataglance.htm

Berlin, L. E., Stennett, J., & Bednash, G. D. (2003). *2002-2003 enrollment and graduations in baccalaureate and graduate programs in nursing*. Washington, DC: AACN.

Block, D. E., Josten, L. E., Lia-Hoagberg, B., Bearinger, L. H., Kerr, M. J., Smith, M. J., Lewis, M.L., & Hutton, S.J. (1999). Fulfilling regional needs for specialty nurses through limited-cohort graduate education. *Nursing Outlook, 47*(1), 23-29.

Chase, S.K., & Pruitt, R.H. (2006). The practice doctorate: Innovation or disruption? *Journal of Nursing Education, 45*(5), 155-161.

Carney, P. A., Eliassen, M. S., & Harwood, B. G. (2002). Evaluating nurse practitioner students: State of the art approaches throughout the learning continuum. In M. K. Crabtree & R. Pruitt (Eds.), *Advanced nursing practice: Building curriculum for quality nurse practitioner education* (pp. 215-222). Washington, DC: NONPF.

Crabtree, M. K. (2002). Introduction. In M. K. Crabtree & R. Pruitt (Eds.), *Advanced nursing practice: Building curriculum for quality nurse practitioner education* (pp. 1- 6). Washington, DC: NONPF.

Diekelmann, N., & Magnussen Ironside, P. (1998). Preserving writing in doctoral education: Exploring the concernful practices of schooling learning teaching. *Journal of Advanced Nursing, 28*(6), 13471356.

Dumas, M. A. (Ed.). (2000). *Partners in NP education: A preceptor manual for NP programs, faculty preceptors, and students.* Washington, DC: NONPF.

Fang, D., Htut, A., & Bednash, G.D. (2008). *2007-2008 enrollment and graduations in baccalaureate and graduate programs in nursing.* Washington, DC: American Association of Colleges of Nursing.

Fawcett, J., Aber, C., & Weiss, M. (2003). Teaching, practice, and research: An integrative approach benefiting students and faculty. *Journal of Professional Nursing 19*(1), 17-21.

Feldman, H. R., & Acord, L. (2002). Strategies for building faculty research programs in institutions that are not research intensive. *Journal of Professional Nursing, 18*(3), 140-146.

Gaydos, B. (2001). Complementary and alternative therapies in nursing education: Trends and issues. *Online Journal Issues Nursing, 6*(2), 5.

Hathaway, D., Jacob, S., Stegbauer, C., Thompson, C., & Graff, C. (2006). The practice doctorate: Perspectives of early adopters. *Journal of Nursing Education, 45*(12), 487-495.

Hodnicki, D. R. (2002). National certification and credentialing. In M. K. Crabtree & R. Pruitt (Eds.), *Advanced nursing practice: Building curriculum for quality nurse practitioner education* (pp. 99-105). Washington, DC: NONPF.

Jacobs, S.K., Rosenfeld, P., & Haber, J. (2003). Information literacy as the foundation for evidence-based practice in graduate nursing education: A curriculum-integrated approach. *Journal of Professional Nursing, 19*(5), 320-328.

Jones, M. E., & Clark, D. W. (1999). Measuring nurse practitioner student clinical outcomes using a scannable log. *Journal of the American Academy of Nurse Practitioners, 11*(5), 200-205.

Keithley, J. K., Gross, D., Johnson, M. E., McCann, J., Faux, S., Shekleton, M., Horton, B., & Trufant, J. E. (2003). Why Rush will keep the DNSc. *Journal of Professional Nursing, 19*(3), 223-229.

Kim, S., & Berry, D. (1998). Models and strategies of collaboration across countries in doctoral education. *Nursing Leadership Forum, 3*(4), 130-135.

Larsen, L. S., Logan, C. A., & Pryor, S. K. (2003). Redesign of clinical nurse specialist role course for distance education: Development, implementation, and outcomes. *Clinical Nurse Specialist (CNS), 17*(1), 25-33.

Livsey, K. R., Campbell, D., & Green, A. (2007). Yesterday, today, and tomorrow: Challenges in securing federal support for graduate nursing education. *Journal of Nursing Education, 46*(4), 176-184.

Long, K. A. (2004). Preparing nurses for the 21st century: Reenvisioning nursing education and practice. *Journal of Professional Nursing, 20*(2), 82-88.

Lund, C. H., Tate, E. T., & Hyde-Robertson, B. (1998). Benefits and challenges of a graduate nursing consortium. *Nurse Educator, 23*(6), 13-16.

Margolius, F. R., & Sneed, N. V. (1999). From expert to novice: Doctorally prepared nursing faculty retooling for the future. *Nurse Educator, 24*(1), 9-11.

Miers, L. J. (1998). *Restructuring master's education: A contemporary and unique model. Innovations in master's nursing education. New ways of learning for the marketplace.* Proceedings of the American Association of Colleges of Nursing's Master's Education Conference, San Antonio, TX.

Mill, J. E., & Morris, H. M. (2000). The ambivalence of ownership: Nursing graduate students as collaborators in action research. *Educational Action Research, 8*(1), 137-149.

National Organization of Nurse Practitioner Faculties [NONPF]. (2008). *Criteria for evaluation of nurse practitioner programs: A report of the National Task Force on Quality Nurse Practitioner Education.* Retrieved June 6, 2008, from http://www.nonpf.org/NONPF2005/NTFCriteriaWebVersion0208.pdf.

National Organization of Nurse Practitioner Faculties [NONPF]. (2000). *Domains and competencies of nurse practitioner practice, newly revised.* Washington, DC: Author.

National Organization of Nurse Practitioner Faculties [NONPF] and American Association of Colleges of Nursing [AACN]. (2002). Nurse practitioner primary care competencies in specialty areas: Adult, family, gerontological, pediatric, and women's health. Washington, DC: Department of Health and Human Services, Health Resources and Services Administration Bureau of Health Professions, Division of Nursing (HRSA 00-0532 (P).

Norbeck, J. S., Krauss, J. B., Levin, R. F., Martin, E. J., Munro, B. H., & Starks, D. (2002). *A vision of baccalaureate and graduate nursing education: The next decade.* Washington, DC: AACN.

Radzyminski, S. (2005). Advances in graduate nursing education: Beyond the advanced practice nurse. *Journal of Professional Nursing, 21*(2), 119-125.

Robinson, K. (2002). Instructional technology and distance learning modalities for advanced practice nursing education. In M. K. Crabtree & R. Pruitt (Eds.), *Advanced nursing practice: Building curriculum for quality nurse practitioner education* (pp. 195-203). Washington, DC: NONPF.

Smith, C. M., & Pattillo, R. E. (2006). PDAs in the nursing curriculum. Providing data for internal funding. *Nurse Educator, 31*(5), 101-102.

Speziale, H. J. S., & Jacobson, L. (2005). Trends in registered nurse education programs 1998-2008. *Nursing Education Perspectives, 26*(4), 230-236.

Tanner, C. A. (2006). Changing times, evolving issues: The faculty shortage, accelerated programs, and simulation. *Journal of Nursing Education, 45*(3), 99-100.

Tolve, C. J. (1999). Nursing scholarship: Role of faculty practice. Clinical Excellence for Nurse Practitioners: *The International Journal of NPACE, 3*(1), 28-33.

Wambach, K., Boyle, D., Hagemaster, J., Teel, C., Langner, B., Fazzone, P., Connors, H., Smith, C., & Forbes, S. (1999). Beyond correspondence, video conferencing, and voice mail: Internet-based master's degree courses in nursing. *Journal of Nursing Education, 38*(6), 267-271.

# CHAPTER 27

## CULTURAL DIVERSITY: TEACHING STUDENTS TO PROVIDE CULTURALLY-COMPETENT NURSING CARE

### Linda Wilson, MSN, PhD, RN

---

The content of this chapter relates to the following major content areas and subconcepts on the Certified Nurse Educator Examination Detailed Test Blueprint:

**Participate in Curriculum Design and Evaluation of Program Outcomes**
- Actively participate in the design of the curriculum to reflect current nursing and healthcare trends

**Engage in Scholarship of Teaching**
- Use evidence-based resources to improve and support teaching

**Function Effectively within the Institutional Environment and the Academic Community**
- Identify how social, economic, political and institutional forces influence nursing and higher education
- Integrate the values of respect, collegiality, professionalism, and caring to build an organizational climate that fosters the development of learners and colleagues

---

## Introduction

Significant changes in demographics, ever increasing complexity of health care, coupled with a worsening nursing shortage have prompted concerns about increasing health disparities in nursing education and clinical practice. Subsequently, there has been a paradigm shift in nursing to provide culturally competent education, thus culturally competent care.

Health disparities are based on patient characteristics such as racial and ethnic minorities, mistrust of the care system, and interaction between patient and provider (Pacquiao, 2007). Therefore, to reduce health disparities, cultural competence education should be a vital element in nursing schools and all health care professional education.

The American Academy of Nursing Expert Panel on Cultural Competency, American Nurses Association (ANA) position statement, NLN competency statements regarding cultural competence, and the Council on Graduate Medical Education have all identified a link between cultural competence education and reducing health care disparities, suggesting cultural competence improves health outcomes. Meanwhile, The U. S. Office of Minority Health Development of the National Standards for Culturally and Linguistically Appropriate Services in Health Care and Healthy People 2010 initiatives have emphasized the significance of culturally competent care in reducing health disparities.

Nursing's primary goal is to provide holistic care. This is a multidimensional focus, which includes aspects of how patients relate to the environment and previous health/illness experiences. "Unfortunately, biases, stereotypes, systemic factors such as lack of language support services and policies, have contributed to fragmented care, especially for racially, ethnically, and linguistically diverse groups" (Pacquiao, 2007 p. 28S).

## Demographical Breakdown

At a time when demographics are drastically changing, it is estimated there will be a shortage of more than 480,000 nurses by the year 2020. Unfortunately, this shortage will be even greater for ethnic minorities. In a 2004 survey of nurses who identified their racial/ethnic background 88.4 % indicated White, non-Hispanic, while 11.6% identified with an ethnic minority group. Table 1 provides the breakdown.

| Group | Percent |
|---|---|
| Black/African-American | 4.6 |
| Asian or Pacific Islander, non-Hispanic | 3.3 |
| Hispanic | 1.8 |
| American Indian/Alaskan Native | 0.4 |
| Two or more racial | 1.5 |

**Table 1.** Breakdown of Nurses' Racial/Ethnic Background, 2004

Meanwhile, in 2000, 12.4% of the RN population was estimated to be members of minority groups. The declining trend of ethnic minority nurses is evident in nursing schools with only 10% of nursing faculty in baccalaureate programs projected to be from an ethnic minority group.

Minority distributions in the RN population contrast with the minority distribution of the general United States (US) population. Table 2 presents the distribution of minority groups in the U. S. population in 2004.

| Group | Percent |
|---|---|
| Black/African-American | 12.2 |
| Asian or Pacific Islander, non-Hispanic | 4.1 |
| Hispanic | 13.7 |
| American Indian/Alaskan Native | 0.7 |
| Two or more racial | 1.3 |

**Table 2.** Minority Groups in the United States, 2004

According to the Sullivan Report, the disparity between the population and healthcare workforce will continue to broaden. Consequently, the focus should be for all nurses to be prepared as a culturally competent nurse.

With the increasing minority population and decreasing minority representation in nursing, the American Academy of Nursing Expert Panel on Culturally Competent Nursing Care identified the significance of culturally sensitive care:
- Increased awareness and acceptance of diversity and willingness to maintain ethnic heritage
- Increased minority unemployment, which increases the number of uninsured, limits access to health care, and increases the homeless population
- Nurses, as the largest workforce in the healthcare system, have the greatest potential to impact changes related to inequities in accessibility to health care
- Increased number of consumers knowledgeable about what is competent and sensitive health care

Despite the desire for culturally appropriate care for members of diverse groups, nursing has not responded adequately to the demand. Consequently, as the minority population increases and nursing workforce decreases, disparities in healthcare outcomes continue to broaden (U.S. Department of Health and Human Services, 2005).

Health disparities in ethnic-minority groups in America has been compared to those of third world countries (Woods, 2000). According to Leininger (2002) everyone has the right to have their cultural values known, respected, and appropriately addressed in the healthcare environment. Although increasing the number of nurses from ethnic minority cultures will assist in achieving this goal, it is imperative that all nurses, regardless of cultural background, be competent to provide holistic care. Culturally competent care is holistic care, predicated on knowledge, respect, and understanding of the impact of culture on health behaviors, without stereotyping or being judgmental. Cultural competence is essential to meet the unique needs of individuals, thus reducing health disparities.

## Culture

Culture provides a framework for behaving and develops over time. Domains such as family roles, healthcare practices, death rituals, spirituality, childbearing practices, communication, and localities are essential attributes that define an individual's culture. According to Burchum (2002), culture is inseparable from the person. Culture guides thinking, doing, and being (Giger & Davidhizar, 2004). Leininger and McFarland (2002) defined culture as learned and shared values, beliefs, norms, and practices of a particular group which guides a pattern of thinking and actions. Culture influences perceptions, interpretations, decisions, actions, and healthcare practices. Ways of behaving are based on group identity, their nature, doctrines, and opinions. Culture is the totality of socially transmitted behavior patterns, art, beliefs, values, customs, life ways, products, and characteristics of a population that guide decision making (Purnell, 2004). Culture includes experiences, which shape values, knowledge, customs, emotions, rituals, traditions, and norms that exist to satisfy a need and allow survival in a specific environment. According to the Department of Health and Human Services, **culture** refers to integrated patterns of human behavior that include the language, thoughts, communications, actions, customs, beliefs, values, and institutions of racial, ethnic, religious, or social groups.

**Competence** refers to "capable, adequate ability and qualities to meet one's need" (Webster's Dictionary, p. 143). The concept of **cultural competence** is based on assumptions that we all represent a culture and have the capacity to work toward responding effectively to meet the needs of others. According to the Department of Health and Human Services **competence** implies having the capacity to function effectively as an individual and an organization within the context of the cultural beliefs, behaviors, and needs presented by consumers and their communities. Therefore, competence is a set of congruent behaviors, attitudes, and policies that come together in a system, agency, or among professionals that enables effective work in cross-cultural situations.

## Cultural Competence

Cultural competency is further identified as one of the main ingredients in closing the gap in healthcare disparities, the way patients and doctors can come together and talk about health concerns without cultural differences hindering the conversation, but enhancing it. Cultural competency is a means of providing respectful healthcare services that are responsive to the health beliefs, practices, and cultural and linguistic needs of diverse patients which can help bring about positive health outcomes. This requires a willingness to develop interventions that are based on knowledge of the culture. Outcomes are predicated on the provider and patient culture and experiences in the health care system which must be transcended to achieve equal access and quality health care. (U.S. Department of Health & Human Services, www.hrsa.gov/culturalcompetence).

To provide appropriate care for diverse groups, nurses must be culturally competent. Burchum (2002) identified attributes of cultural competence as cultural awareness, cultural knowledge, cultural understanding, cultural sensitivity, and cultural skills. It was further noted that cultural competence is a nonlinear, never-ending, and ever-expanding process. Morgan (2002) believes cultural competence is a conscious process, not an endpoint in which nurses continuously strive to work efficiently within the cultural context of an individual/community from a background that is different from their own. Knowledge, skills, and cultural appreciation are used to assist others in achieving contextually congruent goals. According to Campinha-Bacote (2002, 2007) cultural competence is a process in which healthcare professionals try to effectively work within the context of a individual, family, or community.

According to the American Nurses Association (1996), cultural competence is "having the ability to provide effective health care to any population and knowledge of the effects of culture on health beliefs, behaviors, and attitudes, while being aware of one's own culture and biases and understanding the impact on others" (p. 2). Culturally competent care requires the health professional to be sensitive to the differences between the outward behaviors, attitudes, and meanings attached to emotional events for groups (Seibert, Stridh-Igo, & Zimmerman 2002).

Although there are some differences in definitions, it is evident that cultural competence is a process that is nonlinear and encompasses knowledge and skills to provide holistic care. Therefore, cultural competence has significant implications for nursing education, practice, and research.

Cultural competence improves knowledge and skills of healthcare providers. Recent studies support the need for cultural competence education and the positive consequences that result from this knowledge. Pacquiao (2007) argues that culturally competent education improves knowledge, attitudes, and skills of healthcare providers, which allows for holistic care for persons from diverse populations.

Cultural learning does not occur in and of itself. It is a process which includes cultural encounters. A willingness to learn about, respect, and work with persons from different backgrounds to provide care that is compatible with their values and traditions must be a high priority. Superficial cultural knowledge can be perilous. Treating individuals in accordance to their unique needs reinforces the notion that nurses are not only expected to provide health care but also mandated to act as a liaison between the healthcare system and the patient. This can only be achieved through extensive awareness, knowledge, and respect for individuals from different cultures.

Thus, cultural competence decreases the potential for assumed similarity, which implies all people share the same beliefs. Self-awareness facilitates insightful interpretation of others' behaviors and attitudes. Without self-awareness, nurses from the majority culture have a false sense of security about diverse individuals (Digh, 2001). Understanding of one's own worldviews and those of the patient allows for culturally competent care, while avoiding stereotyping and misapplication of scientific knowledge.

## Cultural Research

Research supports culture as a factor in determining healthcare outcomes. Three dimensions of professional support that include information, comfort, and assurance were identified as essential for family members of patients in Intensive Care Units. Cultural group affiliation determined the degree to which each factor was most significant (Waters, 1999).

Pacquiao (2007) argues that culturally competent nursing education, which allows for holistic care for persons from diverse populations, improves patient outcomes. Other studies support a positive correlation between cultural knowledge, attitudes, and skills of healthcare providers. In a study by Lieu (2004), higher cultural competence scores correlated with practitioners who worked in areas with diverse populations. According to Green (2005), cultural and linguistically congruent services improve healthcare delivery for Asian-Americans. There was a positive correlation between trained interpreters and the satisfaction of Latino parents and their children with experiences in ambulatory care (Morales et al. 2002).

## Current Approaches to Integrating Cultural Competence Education in Nursing Programs

Boyle (2007) best said it when she stated "integrating cultural competence into nursing education is in a rather precarious state" (p. 21S). Several different methods are used to incorporate cultural competence knowledge and skills into the curricula. Lipson and Desantis (2007) described a variety of teaching and learning methods used in nursing education. Required and elective courses, immersion experiences, distance learning, and simulations are used in associate, baccalaureate, and master's nursing programs.

At the University of Washington, students complete five quarters of internship with clinical placements in cross-cultural settings. In the master's program at University of California, San Francisco, four cross-cultural courses – cultural concepts, theory, cross-cultural nursing research, and global health issues – are required. Students in the graduate program at the University of Miami School Of Nursing are required to take a two-credit, non-clinical courses related to cultural competence. Several undergraduate schools require courses such as transcultural nursing, cultural concepts in nursing, and health disparities. Meanwhile, in California, all Community Colleges and Board of Registered Nurses require cultural content to be threaded throughout the nursing program (Lipson and Desantis, 2007).

Leininger's Sunrise Model guides an elective course at Middle Tennessee State University. The Sunrise model facilitates understanding of health, illness, and dying when caring for patients from different cultures. In a graduate class, one student described use of Leininger's Transcultural theory in the following way:

Over the years, I have found many opportunities to "tailor make" care of patients to accommodate their cultural beliefs or needs. It was common practice in my last position to give patients the first dose of a medication in which they were being prescribed to take at home. One night, as I approached a particular patient with the tablet and a glass of water, he glanced at his wife and shifted uncomfortably after taking them from my hand. My first thought was that he had concerns about the medication, so I began to explain why the doctor has ordered it. He still hesitated. I offered to get him something else to drink. Still no go. Finally, I told him that if he would just prefer not to take it, that was fine. He smiled a big sigh of relief and explained that since it was Ramadan and not yet sundown, he was not supposed to eat or drink, but had not wanted to appear rude. I had made assumptions about the reasons for his hesitation rather than clarifying with him. In addition, we were trying to impose our schedules and routines without realizing that they were causing the patient a conflict of conscience.

Another example occurred one night when I approached a patient who was completely unresponsive to me, although obviously alert, breathing, and in sinus rhythm on the cardiac monitor. I repeatedly called his name and was reaching out to touch him when his daughter, who was at the bedside, explained that he was praying. In a few moments, he was done and I was able to complete my care. At that time, I confirmed the prayer times with him. We communicated this to the other staff members and developed a routine which accommodated his needs without interruption. This was an instance when an actual wrong clinical assumption could have been made because of the patient's clinical appearance and behavior.

Another aspect of cultural adaptation includes not assuming abuse or neglect because another culture's practice is unfamiliar to us. When examining the back of an elderly Asian man with bronchitis, I found many round, erythematous, almost ecchymotic areas, which could have appeared as light burns or areas where he had been hit. This was in actuality from the practice of cupping, which his wife believed helped to draw out the illness from his lungs. Should an elder abuse case have been initiated because of this, it would have been a grievous mistake.

Opportunities for common ground despite cultural differences abound in our ever-smaller world. Excellent care will enable our patients to partake in the practices that are comforting and helpful for them, as we are able to offer our own treatments and therapies, resulting in holistically beneficial outcomes.

## Models for Providing Culturally Competent Care Education

Several cultural theories and assessment guides on cultural diversity have been developed and revised over the past three decades, including Campinha-Bacote's Culturally Competent Model of Care/Cultural Competence in the Delivery of Healthcare Services, Giger and Davidhizar's Transcultural Assessment Model, Leininger's Transcultural and Sunrise Models, and Purnell's Model for Cultural competence.

**Campinha-Bacote's Model of care:** Process of Cultural Competence in the Delivery of Healthcare Services (Campinha-Bacote, 2007) is based on an evolving process in healthcare, which includes five constructs: cultural awareness, cultural knowledge, cultural skills, cultural encounter, and cultural desire. According to Campinha-Bacote's Model, **self-awareness** is a deliberate and cognitive means of becoming conscious about one's own beliefs and sensitive to the worldview of others. Self-awareness allows for an understanding of one's own culture and its impact on others. A culturally responsive approach to health care can result from examining one's own biases with an understanding of how they influence perceptions and interactions with culturally diverse patients. Thus, cultural awareness includes awareness of racism in healthcare delivery systems.

**Cultural knowledge** is the process that allows the nurse to obtain information about diverse worldviews, health, and illness belief systems. Intra-ethnic variations are examined to prevent the assumption that all members of a group respond in the same way. **Cultural skills** include the process of learning how to provide culture-specific care by including appropriate cultural assessment. Cultural knowledge, alone, does not ensure the required skills to provide culturally competent care. This phase includes learning how to perform a cultural based physical assessment. It allows for understanding of other's beliefs and values about health practices, perceptions, and management of illness. Awareness and knowledge guides the assessment to elicit culture-specific information. **Cultural encounter** promotes effective engagement in cross-cultural interactions. It allows for validating, refining, and modifying existing cultural knowledge, thus reducing the potential to stereotype. **Cultural desire** is the motivation to achieve cultural competence.

**Giger and Davidhizar Transcultural Assessment Model (2004).** This model evaluates cultural variables and their effect on health and illness behaviors: communication, space, social organization, time, environmental control, and biological variations.

### 1. Communication

Communication is a critical factor in achieving culturally competent care. Information is processed and perceived by groups based on experiences. Oral and written languages, gestures, and body movements all transmit culture. There are obvious differences in communications such as dialect, grammatical structure, and pronunciations. Conflicts in verbal communication intensify when interactions include those who speak different languages. This discord hinders the nurse-patient/ family relationship.

Not only does language or dialect interfere in the nurse-patient relationship but patterns of communication can also create problems. Nurses usually interact with patients using a linear, sequential, and compartmentalized thought process. Questions such as "What happened first, then next" are asked, and the answers usually require personal information. Physical assessment is typically performed quickly, in a sequential and unidirectional manner. This pattern conflicts with many ethnic cultures. In African-American, Hispanic, and Asian cultures, it is considered rude to initiate a business or personal discussion before establishing social courtesies. These actions are viewed as sequential data gathering, uncaring, and offensive.

Nonverbal communication such as eye movement, facial gestures, hand gestures, and body language are used extensively by some cultures. Nonverbal communication can be over-powering or misunderstood. For example, silence is valued as a sign of respect in some cultures, whereas, it is viewed as agreement, in others. Appropriateness of touch is influenced by culture. In Africa-American and Hispanic cultures, touch is extremely important; it conveys approval, caring, trust, and respect. In the Asian culture, touching the head is disrespectful because it is viewed as the seat of the soul. In some Hispanic cultures, admiring without touching a newborn is considered rude. The nurse should first assess the appropriateness of touch then observe the response of individuals to determine the outcome.

Facial expressions vary greatly among cultures. African-Americans, Italians, and those of Jewish culture tend to use a smile or other facial gestures to convey feelings. People from northern European countries are less likely to respond to strangers with facial gestures. Chinese use facial expressions to convey happiness or anger with friends and family, but show very limited expressions in formal settings. Voice intonation may be offensive. Speaking loudly to an Asian can imply anger or confrontation.

Eye contact is perceived as appropriate in Western cultures. It implies respect, self-confidence, and listening. On the contrary, lack of eye contact suggests lack of assertiveness and confidence, shyness, and insecurity. American Indians view direct eye contact as a lack or respect, rudeness, and an invasion of privacy. Direct eye contact is considered confrontational and adversarial in Japanese culture and as evil in some Hispanic cultures.

Gestures and body movements tend to be culturally specific. Bowing of the head in the presence of an elder, conveys respect in Asian cultures, while in western culture, it suggests suspicion. Use of hands and body movements are common with African-Americans and Hispanics. Hands are oftentimes used to demonstrate and/or amplify a topic of discussion. This amplification should not be perceived as aggression or anger.

## 2. Space

The concept of **space** is influenced by culture. Space is a concept that encompasses the individual, body, and surroundings. Ethnic groups differ in their need for space. For example, Hispanics and African-Americans are relational and tactile oriented. Touch and sitting or standing in close proximity to the patient is acceptable, especially in the African-American culture. In contrast, Asians perceive close contact as impolite and invasion of space. In Western cultures, the space around an individual is divided into zones: intimate, personal, social, and public. For people of some cultures, entering intimate or personal space results in an uncomfortable environment. Since many healthcare procedures require nurses to move through all zones, they must be aware of spatial behaviors during interactions. Explaining the need to enter a patient's space can decrease uncomfortable feelings.

## 3. Social Orientation

Cultural behaviors are patterns learned through socialization. Characteristics such as self-motivation, individualism, achievement, self-confidence, and youth are identified as Eurocentric. Meanwhile, cooperation, tolerance, accommodation, belonging, and respect for age (elderly) are attributes associated with many ethnic minority cultures. Family is the primary unit of society and extended families are important.

Patients from groups or interrelated-oriented cultures tend to be reluctant to ask questions, for fear of bringing attention to self, since group supercedes the individual. In Asian and Hispanic cultures, authority is rarely questioned; to do so is regarded as disrespectful. Nurses are considered authority in many minority cultures.

Behaviors associated with many ethnically diverse cultures, such as close proximity, touching, group orientation, and interdependence are also related to locus of control. In many of these cultures, families make health-related decisions, not individuals. Such action can present a problem for the nurse who expects the patient to be the decision-maker about health-related issues. In African-American culture, extended family and sometimes clergy are involved in decisions. Elders are consulted for decisions in Asian culture. Family is priority in Hispanic families, collective or group supercedes individual needs. Nurses must acknowledge elders and the extended family in the plan of care with ethnic minorities. The typical dominance pattern in Hispanic families is patriarchal. Men are viewed as having the strength. Understanding the patriarchal structure of the Hispanic family can reduce the chance of stereotyping women as passive.

## 4. Time

There are distinctive cultural differences in the way time is perceived. It is usually sequenced as past, present, and future. Time can also relate to patterns. Nurses tend to function in a monochromic pattern in which the focus is linear, task oriented, and sequential; prioritizing one task at a time. Whereas, many ethnic cultures tend to follow a polychromic pattern of time, in which the focus is on relationships and connections, rather than tasks.

Middle-class Western cultures value time specific activities, such as promptness and punctuality. In present-oriented cultures, time is viewed as relative. Hispanics focus on connecting rather than meeting deadlines. Arriving late for an appointment is viewed as acceptable in some Hispanic cultures. African-Americans tend to be more present than past or future oriented. Time is less defining. It is more important to arrive at an appointment than to be there at a given time. However, some African-Americans subcultures are past-oriented because it focuses on transmitting culture through history. Others are future-oriented with a greater emphasis on education and professions. For American Indians, especially in the Navajo culture, life relates to the environment without time boundaries. The sequence of importance for time is present, past, and future. Minimal planning is done since the future is considered to be outside of the person's control.

Nursing's conceptualization of time as sequential and monochromic may be incompatible with cultural patterns that view time as relative or without boundaries. Persons from cultures where being connected is valued more than deadlines, may consider efficient and time conscious nurses as task driven, rude, impatient, and impersonal. Discharge planning usually includes scheduled, timed interventions. Without considering cultural practices and beliefs, there is an increased potential that expected health outcomes would not be obtained.

## 5. Environmental Control

Environmental control refers to the ability of a group to plan and control nature. Traditional western cultures believe in self-determination and control over the environment. Illness has a scientific cause that can be diagnosed and treated or cured. The focus is on risk reduction and prevention. Meanwhile, in many ethnic minority cultures, disease and illness are viewed more fatalistically. Illness is viewed as disharmony and conflict. Illness is based on two theories: personalistic or naturalistic. Personalistic theory defines illness as a consequence of a sensate agent, such as an evil spirit or ancestor; resulting in punishment. Naturalistic theory characterizes illness in terms of equilibrium or harmony between body elements -- such as hot and cold -- and the individual's environment. Consequently, illness results from disequilibrium between body and environment.

## 6. Biological Variations

Biological Variations relate to differences that exist among individuals in various racial groups. This knowledge is particularly important to complete understanding of a group of people. There is a direct correlation between race, body structures, enzymatic and genetic variations, susceptibility to disease and nutritional alterations. "The strongest argument for including concepts on biological variations in nursing education and practice is the scientific fact that biological variations can assist nurses in providing culturally appropriate care" (Giger & Davidhizer, 2004, p.136)

## Leininger's Transcultural Theory

The goal of **Leininger's Transcultural Theory** is to provide culture-specific and universal nursing care practices when delivering health care to patients to help them face unfavorable human conditions, illness, or death in culturally meaningful ways. Leininger identified three concepts in her transcultural theory:

1. Cultural care preservation and maintenance for preserving and retaining a cultures'care values for health and well-being
2. Cultural care accommodation and negotiation, which pertains to a cultures ability to agree or adapt with medical providers to obtain a beneficial health outcome
3. Cultural care repatterning or restructuring: actions taken by the professional that are in agreement with the patient, showing respect for their cultural beliefs, while providing healthier lifestyles for them

The three concepts reflect respect, advocacy and partnership, which are core values of nursing.

## Purnell's Model for Cultural Competence (Purnell & Paulanka, 2003)

This model has an organizing framework that consists of 12 domains of culture the nurse assesses:

1. Healthcare-care practices
2. Healthcare-care practitioners
3. Overview/heritage
4. Communication
5. Family roles/organization
6. Workforce
7. Biocultural/bilological variations
8. High-risk behaviors
9. Nutrition
10. Pregnancy/fertility practices
11. Death rituals
12. Spirituality

Using the model, healthcare providers are identified as unconsciously incompetent, consciously incompetent, consciously competent, or unconsciously competent.

The degree to which the 12 domains are included in assessing patients determines cultural competence. According to Purnell, **unconsciously incompetent** indicates one is lacking knowledge about another culture and not aware of it. Being aware that one is lacking knowledge about another culture is described as **consciously incompetent**. When one learns about the patient's culture, verifies generalizations, and provides culturally specific interventions, this individual is deemed **consciously competent**. Automatically providing culturally congruent care to patients of diverse cultures is labeled as **unconsciously competent**.

## Strategies to Enhance Cultural Competence with Students and Faculty

The following lists provide strategies that faculty can use to enhance cultural competency in both self and students.

- Provide simulation experiences using problem-based learning with scenarios such as cultural practices related to death and dying.
- Offer preceptorship experiences with culturally diverse preceptors.
- Demonstrate application of the concepts of vulnerability, health disparities, and diversity of patients and preceptors.
- Provide reading assignments that focus on cultural competence.
- Require students to complete the standardized preparation for the Cultural Sensitivity and Alternative Medicine exam. Faculty should have a required set passing score (Boyle, 2007).
- Use cultural case scenarios without including a medical diagnosis so students will focus on culture (Purnell, 2007).
- Include group exercises such as bicultural observations that attempt to minimize superiority (negative stereotyping), fear and mistrust, in order to identify factors that interfere in teacher-student relationships.
- Provide or encourage educational sessions/sensitivity workshops to explore patterns of behavior and expectations of teachers. The workshop should identify hidden constraints in policies, procedures, and structures in nursing education that place minorities at risk for academic failure.

## Strategies to Enhance Cultural Competence in the Clinical Setting

- Identify own beliefs and values and determine the impact on provision of care.
- Open dialogue regarding the lack of knowledge of another's culture. Learn about beliefs, values, and meanings of health, illness, and death for cultures that are prevalent in your community.
- Introduce social conversation to gain trust before beginning the assessment of a patient from an ethnically diverse culture.
- Convey respect for patient's support system and locus of control for decision-making. It is the patient and/or family's right to make choices about health care.
- Be amenable to change and willing to incorporate indigenous or folk practices such as the medicine man/woman and folk healer into traditional nursing care.
- Be willing to adapt nursing interventions to meet the needs of the patient. For example, a culturally sensitive nurse would know that when a Pacific Islander dies, a window should be open if possible. This allows the soul to leave. Or, when a pregnant American Indian patient refuses to buy baby clothes before the birth of the baby, this is not because she does not want the baby, but because it is forbidden or taboo to purchase baby clothing before birth.
- Allow for flexibility in schedules. Focus more on the task being performed instead of the time it is done. For example, instead of telling a Hispanic patient to take a hypoglycemic agent at 7 AM each morning, focus more on encouraging the action, rather than the time of the act. Instructions to take the medicine each morning facilitates a better outcome than demanding the medicine be taken at exactly 7 AM.

## Communication Patterns and Cultural Beliefs about Health, Illness, and Death

In view of the fact that culture influences health practices and outcomes, it is imperative for students to learn to implement self-assessment and evaluate the potential impact of their beliefs on others prior to entering a nurse-patient relationship. Without a self-assessment, culturally competent care can not be attained. Beliefs and practices vary within subcultures of every culture. Several cultural groups are discussed in this chapter to assist students in understanding the significance of culture as it relates to providing culturally competent care.

## Providing Culturally Competent Care

Being an effective nurse cannot be achieved separately from a cultural context. Expectations and beliefs about health care enter into each nurse-patient interaction and impact health outcomes. The role that cultural competence plays in promoting optimal care cannot be over emphasized. It is imperative that clinical experiences be restructured to incorporate cultural diversity into all aspects of the nursing role. Cultural assessment should be as routine as physical, psychosocial, spiritual, and developmental assessments. This change in philosophy must be an integral part of nursing education.

Students should be required to purchase a reference book that describes various cultures and their cultural beliefs and practices. Students can then use this information to compare and contrast their patient's behavior with the norm of that group. A tool, such as that found in Appendix 1 of this chapter, can be completed by students in the clinical setting to assist them to provide patient-centered care. This tool can be accessed on the CD accompanying this book.

## Summary

Inadequate knowledge of the impact of culture on health can lead to false assumptions, which interfere with the nurse's ability to provide optimal care. Data support the lack of cultural knowledge increases health disparities for those from ethnic minority cultures. For this reason, students must broaden their skills to include an understanding of values, beliefs, and the impact of culture on health practices in all phases of the nursing process. Cultural knowledge and skills can assist students in identifying appropriate diagnoses and treatment plans. Identifying community resources is important to this process.

Effective communication is essential to the nurse-patient relationship. Treatment plans must be culturally sensitive and inclusive of the patient's concept of health and illness. Understanding cultural differences in treatment expectations, pharmacological interventions, and biological responses to medication is vital to a mutually acceptable plan of care. There must be an understanding that the patient and/or family have the right to make decisions about their own health care.

Cultural information should be critically examined and appropriately used in the context of individual relationships. The increased ethnic minority population in the healthcare system mandates that differences be recognized, valued, and appropriately addressed by healthcare providers. The linear and technological environment of the healthcare system increases the potential for cultural dissonance and disempowerment of ethnic minorities. Nurses must strive to be creative and willing to adapt nursing care to meet the needs of all. Self-awareness, knowledge of limitations, and understanding the influence of culture on health beliefs and practices are essential to becoming an effective nurse.

Commitment by nursing programs and the healthcare system to cultural competence is essential to reduce disparities in health outcomes. Because the nursing profession and nursing schools remain dominated by individuals from traditional western cultures; many students have little experience with persons of diverse ethnicity. Increasing the numbers of minority nurses and interpreters is only a start to providing culturally competent care. By the shear numbers of minority nurses, the likelihood of meeting the needs of all culturally diverse patients is limited if minority nurses are expected to be solely responsible for providing care to the minority population. Consequently, all nurses will need to become more knowledgeable and competent in providing culturally congruent care. Patient outcomes will improve and nurses will be enriched from an understanding and achievement of cultural competency.

Federal law requires all health care facilities to provide access to interpreters/translators if at least 5% of their patient population does not have English as a primary language. This access might be on site or through a telephone service language line. Any health care facility who receives reimbursement from a federal program is required to comply with this law.

## Learning Activities

1. Refer to the Appendix of this chapter. Assign students to use this tool during a clinical day. Discuss their entries during postconference.
2. Discuss possible areas where cultural dissonance may interfere with care for clients in your specialty area of nursing practice.
3. Interview two clients from the same culture and complete the tool in the Appendix. State how the entries are the same and how they are different.

## Educational Philosophy

As an educator, my role is to facilitate learning in a safe and caring environment that is conducive to creativity and critical thinking. I want to encourage a desire to seek answers and inspire a thirst for lifelong learning. — Linda Wilson

# References

American Academy of Nursing Expert Panel on Culturally Competent Nursing Care. (1992). Culturally competent healthcare. *Nursing Outlook, 40* (6), 277-283.

Boyle, J. (2007). Commentary on current approaches to integrating elements of cultural competence in nursing education. *Journal of Transcultural Nursing, 18*(1), 21S-22S

Campinha-Bacote, J. (2002). The process of cultural competence in the delivery of healthcare services: A model of care. *Journal of Transcultural Nursing, 13*(3), 181-184.

Campinha-Bacote, J. (2003). Many faces: Addressing diversity in health care. *Journal of Online Issues in Nursing, 8*(1). Online at : http://nursingworld.org/ojin/topic20/tpc20_2.htm

Campinha-Bacote, J. (2005). *A Biblically based model of cultural competence in the delivery of healthcare services.* Transcultural C.A.R.E. Associates Press. Order form online at: http://www.transculturalcare.net/Resources.htm

Campinha-Bacote, J. (2007). *The process of cultural competence in the delivery of healthcare services: The journey continues.* (5th ed.)Transcultural C.A.R.E. Associates Press Order form online at: http://www.transculturalcare.net/Resources.htm

Covington, L. (2001). Cultural competence for critical care nursing practice. *Critical Care Nursing Clinics of North America, 13*(4), 521-529.

Davidhizer, R., Dowd, S., & Giger, J. (1998). Educating the culturally diverse healthcare students. *Nurse Educator, 23*(2), 38-42.

Digh, P. (2001). Culture? What culture? *Association Management 2,* 43-48.

Giger, J., & Davidhizer, R. (2004). *Transcultural nursing: Assessment and interventions* (4th ed.) St. Louis: Mosby.

Leininger, M., & McFarland, M. (2002). *Transcultural nursing: Concepts, theories, research & practice* (3rd ed.). NY: McGraw-Hill Medical Publishing Division.

Leininger, M., & McFarland, M. R. (2006). *Culture care diversity & universality: A worldwide nursing theory* (2nd ed.). Boston, MA: Jones and Bartlett.

Pacquid, D. (2007). The relationship between cultural competence education and increasing diversity in nursing schools and practice settings. *Journal of Transcultural Nursing, 18*(1), 28S-37S.

Seibert, P. S., Stridh-Igo, P., & Zimmerman, C. G. (2002). A checklist to facilitate cultural awareness and sensitivity, *Journal of Medical Ethics, 28,* 143-146.

US Bureau of the Census statistics. Population estimates. URL: www.census.gov/population/fact finders, 2006.

U.S. Department of Health and Human Service, Office of Minority Health, www. hhs.gov, (2006)U.S. Department of Health & Human Services, HRSA) Cultural Competence Resources for Health Care Providers Office of Minority Heath, www.hrsa.gov/culturalcompetence.

U.S. Department of Health and Human Services, Bureau of Health Professionals, Division of Nursing, National Sample Survey of Registered Nurses, 2004.

U.S. Department of Health and Human Services, Office of Disease Prevention and Health Promotion (2000). Tracking Healthy People 2010 (2nd ed.) Pittsburgh: U.S. Government Printing Office.

Waters, C. M. (1999). Professional support questionnaire for critical-care nurses working with family members. *Research in Nursing & Health,* 22(2), 107-17.

Webster's II: New Riverside Dictionary, (1998). Office Edition. Houghton Mifflin: Boston, p 142.

Woods, D. (2001). Learning about difference. *Minority Nurse,* Spring: 46-50.

Wilson (Covington), L. (1996). Correlation between cultural inclusion, self-esteem and academic Success in African Americans attending predominantly White Universities. *Dissertation Abstracts.*

# Appendix 1
## Diversity Tool

| | Column 1 List behaviors typically associated with this culture, religion, and developmental level. | Column 2 List HEALTH behaviors typically associated with this culture, religion, and developmental level. | What behaviors does your patient display that are the same as those listed in columns 1 and 2? | What behaviors does your patient display that are not consistent with those listed in columns 1 and 2? | Considerations for nursing interventions. |
|---|---|---|---|---|---|
| Date: What is your patient's: | | | | | |
| Culture: | | | | | |
| Religion: | | | | | |
| Developmental Level: | | | | | |

As a result of this activity, I have learned how to:

This activity gave me insights into how diversity impacts nursing care by:

This activity shows that I have more to learn about:

This activity shows my growth because:

Reflections on the "Diversity Tool"

# Rubric for Grading the Diversity Tool

| | 3 | 2 | 1 | 0 |
|---|---|---|---|---|
| List behaviors typically associated with this culture, religion, and developmental level. | Lists at least 5 behaviors typically associated with the patient's culture, religion, and developmental level and documents source of information. | Lists only 3 behaviors typically associated with the patient's culture, religion, and developmental level and documents source of information. | Lists less than 3 behaviors typically associated with the patient's culture, religion, and developmental level but unable to document source of information. | Unable to list behaviors typically associated with this culture, religion, and developmental level. |
| List HEALTH behaviors typically associated with this culture, religion, and developmental level. | Lists at least 5 health behaviors typically associated with the patient's culture, religion, and developmental level and documents source of information. | Lists only 3 health behaviors typically associated with the patient's culture, religion, and developmental level and documents source of information. | Lists less than 3 health behaviors typically associated with the patient's culture, religion, and developmental level but unable to document source of information. | Unable to list any health behaviors typically associated with this culture, religion, and developmental level. |
| What behaviors does your patient display that are the same as those listed in columns 1 and 2? What behaviors does your patient display that are not consistent with those listed in columns 1 and 2? | Assesses patient and able to identify at least 5 behaviors the patient displays that are either the same or different than the behaviors typically associated with the patient's culture, religion, and developmental level. | Assesses patient and able to identify only 3 behaviors the patient displays that are either the same or different than the behaviors typically associated with the patient's culture, religion, and developmental level. | Assesses patient and able to identify less than 3 behaviors the patient displays that are either the same or different than the behaviors typically associated with the patient's culture, religion, and developmental level. | Unable to identify behaviors the patient displays that are either the same or different than the behaviors typically associated with the patient's culture, religion, and developmental level. |

| Considerations for nursing interventions. | Able to identify at least 5 factors to consider when planning patient care based on the patient's culture, religion, and developmental level and alterations in nursing interventions associated with those factors. | Able to identify at least 3 factors to consider when planning patient care based on the patient's culture, religion, and developmental level and alterations in nursing interventions associated with those factors. | Identifies less than 3 factors to consider when planning patient care based on the patient's culture, religion, and developmental level and alterations in nursing interventions associated with those factors. | Unable to identify factors to consider when planning patient care based on the patient's culture, religion, and developmental level and alterations in nursing interventions associated with those factors. |
|---|---|---|---|---|

# CHAPTER 28

## PORTFOLIO ASSESSMENT:
### ONE SCHOOL OF NURSING'S EXPERIENCE

Julie Fisher Robertson, EdD, RN
Jeanette Rossetti, EdD, RN
Bradley Peters, MS, EdD, PhD
Sharon Coyer, PhD, RN, CPNP, APRN
Mary Elaine Koren, PhD, RN
Judith Hertz, PhD, RN
Stacie Elder, PhD, RN

---

The content of this chapter relates to the following major content area and subconcepts on the Certified Nurse Educator Examination Detailed Test Blueprint:

**Participate in Curriculum Design and Evaluation of Program Outcomes**
- Demonstrate knowledge of curriculum developing including identifying program outcomes and selecting appropriate evaluation strategies
- Revise the curriculum based on evaluation of program outcomes
- Implement program assessment models
- Analyze results of program evaluation and initiate curricular change
- Critique the program evaluation methods and plan

---

## Introduction

The purpose of this chapter is to describe the evolution of Northern Illinois University (NIU) School of Nursing's portfolio program, which is one of several methods used to assess the effectiveness of the undergraduate nursing curriculum. This chapter includes:

- A brief review of the literature on the use of portfolios to assess student learning
- An overview of the School of Nursing's (SON) original portfolio program and the reasons for revising it
- Key features of the revised program
- Strategies used to promote the program's success
- Accomplishments of the revised program

The chapter concludes with important considerations to keep in mind when developing portfolio programs for large-scale, program-level assessment and learning activities that can be used to develop successful portfolio programs.

## Review of the Literature

### Portfolios Used for Authentic Assessment of Student Learning

Using portfolios to measure student learning has increased in popularity among educators in the last several decades. A major reason for this increased interest is the growing recognition that traditional assessment methods, such as standardized and teacher-developed tests, do not adequately measure skills such as critical thinking, communication, and problem solving (Banta, 2007; Braskamp & Schomberg, 2006; Chabeli, 2002). Using standardized tests also has been shown to produce a "teaching to the test" phenomenon (Johnson, McDaniel, & Willeke, 2000). As a result, a paradigm shift has occurred in educational assessment. More and more, the focus is on the use of authentic methods of assessment, such as student portfolios, for documenting learning. In contrast to traditional methods, which are based on recall and recognition, authentic assessment requires students to demonstrate their knowledge or skills through performance on scholarly tasks or by providing observable samples of their work. Authentic assessment provides concrete evidence that students can apply knowledge in real-life situations (Mueller, 2006; Wiggons, 1990).

The heightened interest in authentic assessment is intensified by the growing national concern that colleges and universities are not providing policymakers and the public with clear evidence of student outcomes (Association of American Colleges and Universities [AACU], 2002; U.S. Department of Education [USDE], 2006). The push for more direct proof of student learning is reflected in the recent report of the Commission on the Future of Higher Education, which was appointed by U.S. Secretary of Education, Margaret Spellings (USDE, 2006). The Spellings' Report emphasized the critical need for colleges and universities to use evidence-based assessment methods that clearly document students' abilities in critical thinking, writing, and problem solving. Authentic assessment methods, such as portfolios, can provide this kind of observable evidence of learning (AACU, 2002; Mueller, 2006; Wiggons, 1990).

The increased use of portfolios for assessing student learning also is consistent with the paradigm shift in educational methodology from reductionistic, teacher-centered approaches to constructivistic, student-centered learning environments

(Abate, Stamatakis, & Haggett, 2003; Chabeli, 2002). The constructivistic emphasis is on students taking responsibility for their learning and for documenting what they actually can do as a result of the educational experience. Developing a portfolio is student-driven. Students are responsible for choosing examples of their work that document sophisticated outcomes. Examples of these outcomes include changes in their ways of thinking, the ability to write effectively, growth in specific knowledge areas, evidence of required competencies, and the ability to engage in self-reflection and problem solving. Because students focus on their accomplishments, portfolios also can enhance students' self-image. Since portfolios can provide documentation of complex skills, portfolio assessment is one way nursing programs can evaluate students' abilities in key areas such as critical thinking, communication, and nursing interventions (Karlowicz, 2000; Kear & Bear, 2007).

## Portfolio Assessment in Undergraduate Nursing Programs

The use of portfolios for assessing student learning is not new to nursing education. Interest in this type of assessment began in the early 1980's (Alexander, Craft, Baldwin, Beers & McDaniel, 2002). Since that time, most of the published articles have focused on using portfolios as an assessment method for students to demonstrate course-embedded outcomes and nursing competencies (Chabeli, 2002; Dolan, Fairbairn & Harris, 2004; Emden, Hutt, & Bruce, 2004; McCready, 2006; McEwan & Taylor, 2007; McMullan et al., 2003; Schaffer, Nelson, & Litt, 2005; Spence & El-Ansari, 2004; Tiwari & Tang, 2003; Tracy, Marino, Richo, & Daly, 2000). Much of this work has been done internationally, with the United Kingdom taking the lead (Chabeli, 2002; Dolan et al., 2004; Emden et al., 2004; McCready, 2006; McEwan & Taylor, 2007; McMullan et al., 2003; Spence & El-Ansari, 2004; Tiwari & Tang, 2003). However, there is a paucity of literature on using student portfolios to assess large-scale, program-level curricular effectiveness in schools of nursing (Alexander et al., 2002; Karlowicz, 2000; Kear & Bear, 2005).

## NIU School of Nursing's Portfolio Program

This section includes details about the key features of the NIU School of Nursing (SON) portfolio program. We included the "early years" of our involvement in portfolio assessment because the history and the lessons learned from the original program helped to make the current program successful.

## The Early Years

Our SON began using student portfolios in 1994 in response to the National League for Nursing's (NLN) requirement for nursing programs to develop outcome assessment programs that document students' abilities in critical thinking, communication, and therapeutic nursing interventions. Because we had no experience in portfolio assessment, we decided to begin on a small scale and initially measured only one NLN criterion, critical thinking. The original portfolio program was designed to measure changes in critical thinking from the beginning to the end of the nursing program. The assignments chosen to evaluate changes in critical thinking were the Personal Professional Beliefs Papers (PPBP) that students wrote in the first-semester professional nursing course and again in the last-semester capstone seminar course. Standardized guidelines for writing the PPBP were developed for students in both courses to increase accuracy of assessment results. Portfolio assessment of a random sample of student portfolios was conducted once each academic year by the Curriculum and Evaluation Committee's Portfolio Subcommittee. A well-known critical thinking rubric (Facione & Facione, 1994) was the instrument used to score the PPBP.

Our portfolio program looked great on paper, but in reality, there were many problems. One problem was inconsistent follow-through with portfolio guidelines by faculty and students and an overall lack of buy-in from both stakeholder groups. Another problem was lack of a clear fit between the rubric criteria and the PPBP requirements. As a result, we had difficulty using the rubric to score our PPBP assignments. We also had concerns that the PPBP was not the best assignment to measure changes in critical thinking. We found that conducting portfolio assessment one time a year was not frequent enough to maintain satisfactory inter-rater reliability, and assessing only a sample of portfolios negatively impacted student buy-in and did not provide an adequate picture of the critical thinking skills of each student cohort. By 2001, it was clear the original portfolio program had run its course. It was time to explore another model of portfolio assessment.

## The New Definition of Portfolio Assessment

The revised portfolio program constituted a major shift in the definition of portfolio assessment in the SON. Our definition changed from an end-of-the program measurement of changes over time to a mid-program appraisal. The program is modeled after the nationally recognized Washington State University Portfolio Program (Condon, 2001), which is a one-point-in-time assessment of all student portfolios at the end of the junior year and is conducted by faculty teams. The revised portfolio program is designed to assess the effectiveness of the nursing foundational courses (curricular levels 1 and 2) in preparing students for their important senior year (level 3). The goal of the revised program is to provide authentic data about student competencies in all three undergraduate nursing program outcomes (critical thinking, therapeutic interventions, and communication) as indicators of curricular effectiveness. By assessing portfolios from every student rather than a random sample of portfolios, the new program provides a more complete profile of the collective strengths and weaknesses of each student cohort in relation to the undergraduate curriculum.

## Key Features of the SON Portfolio Assessment Program

**Student involvement and responsibilities.** When students enter the nursing program, they receive information about the portfolio program which provides a beginning understanding of the program and their responsibilities. Students then receive a more complete description of the program in one of the first semester nursing courses. At that time, they also receive a copy of the "Top Ten Questions" document (see Appendix A). This document was developed to provide students with important information about what the portfolio is, the purpose of the portfolio, documents to include in their portfolios, and students' responsibilities related to submitting portfolios. In addition, the syllabi of all level 1 and 2 nursing courses are standardized to include a description of the portfolio assessment program and student responsibilities.

Early in the second semester of the junior year, several members of the Portfolio Subcommittee (typically a faculty member and one or two student representatives) visit the classroom of the course designated for portfolio submission. Students are reminded they are required to submit the portfolio to pass the course. Students also receive specific directions for submitting their portfolios, a copy of the assessment rubric, and a folder to use for their portfolio documents. Students are instructed to write a cover letter "introducing" their portfolio to the faculty reviewers (see Appendix B). The cover letter offers students an opportunity to reflect on how the chosen assignments demonstrate their abilities in relation to the three outcome criteria. They also are asked to reflect on which of their abilities are strong and which ones need improvement.

In addition to the cover letter, students choose three completed written assignments they consider to be the best examples of their critical thinking, writing, and therapeutic interventions. They are encouraged to submit their best work and to make the changes recommended by the instructor who graded the assignment. They also attach the assignment guidelines to each submitted document. Examples of appropriate assignments for the portfolio include a concept map with related care plan, a review of the literature paper, and a process recording. To ensure anonymity, students are instructed to include their university identification number on the front of the portfolio folder, and to remove all identifying information from the documents they are including in their portfolios.

Originally portfolios were submitted during finals week of the last semester of the junior year. However, students indicated that finals week was too stressful and asked if they could submit their portfolios at the beginning of the following semester. We are now in the process of changing the portfolio submission time and designating a first-semester senior-level course as the class in which students would be required to submit their portfolios in the first two weeks of the semester.

**Faculty responsibilities.** An important characteristic of our portfolio program is that all faculty members are expected to be involved in the reading and scoring of portfolios. Nursing faculty meet twice a semester to conduct portfolio assessment which involves less than three hours of faculty time each semester. This three-hour time period includes the Portfolio Preparatory Session and the Portfolio Assessment Session, which are described below. Both sessions are held during regularly scheduled faculty meetings that all faculty members are expected to attend. Portfolio assessment is considered an integral part of curriculum development and improvement, and thus is viewed as an important faculty responsibility. In addition, the syllabi of all level 1 and level 2 courses are required to include statements from faculty indicating which course assignments would be appropriate for students to include in their portfolios.

## Portfolio Preparatory and Assessment Sessions

**The Portfolio Preparatory Session.** As preparation for grading current students' portfolios, the faculty conduct the Portfolio Preparatory Session. During this session faculty assess the two "practice" portfolios using a scoring rubric. (Practice portfolios are copies of previously assessed portfolios. After a cohort of portfolios are reviewed and scored, several portfolios are chosen to be practice portfolios for subsequent preparatory sessions.) After the review of each practice portfolio, faculty participants share their scores with each other and the range of scores is determined. This is an important exercise for promoting inter-rater reliability. Having portfolio reviewers periodically score the same pieces of student work using the same rubric is essential in maintaining reliable scoring (Perlman, 2002). Faculty reviewers also discuss the strengths and weaknesses of the practice portfolios in relation to the undergraduate curriculum. One of the Portfolio Subcommittee members records details of this discussion, which are later transcribed and retained as qualitative evidence. All portfolio reviewers are requested to complete an evaluation of the preparatory session experience.

**The Portfolio Assessment Session.** One or two weeks after the Portfolio Preparatory Session, the formal assessment of student portfolios takes place. The session begins with a review and scoring of a practice portfolio by all faculty reviewers and a comparison of faculty ratings. This review of a practice portfolio is done for inter-rater reliability purposes prior to the formal assessment of portfolios.

The formal assessment of student portfolios is then conducted by approximately six faculty teams, consisting of three to four faculty reviewers per team. The portfolios to be assessed are equally divided among the faculty teams. In each team, each portfolio is independently read and rated by two faculty reviewers according to the criteria on the rubric. Each reviewer reads the portfolio as a body of work. The reading is done quickly (about 10 minutes per portfolio) using the rubric as a framework. The reviewer then assigns a whole number rating to each rubric criterion and calculates an average rating for the portfolio, rounded to one decimal point. If the two average ratings for the portfolio differ by more than one whole point, the portfolio is read and rated by a third faculty reviewer. The final portfolio score is the average of all the reviewers' ratings.

Each team has a Table Leader who supervises the team's progress, checks the accuracy of the rating calculations from each reviewer, calculates the average rating for each portfolio, and determines if a third reader is needed. The Table Leader also enters the average rating for each reviewed portfolio on a tally sheet, which is then given to a trained graduate assistant who records the portfolio ratings on an Excel spreadsheet during the portfolio assessment session.

Immediately following the reading and scoring of the portfolios, faculty discuss strengths and weaknesses of the portfolios that were reviewed. This is when the assessment session gets exciting. It is during these faculty discussions that curricular issues are identified and solutions are considered. Issues also are identified for follow-up by the SON Curriculum and Evaluation Committee. The faculty discussion time is a great opportunity for sharing experiences, concerns, teaching strategies, and assignment ideas. It is also a time for faculty to individually reflect on what they are doing in their classes that might need improvement.

Details of the faculty discussion are recorded by one of the Portfolio Subcommittee members and then transcribed and retained as qualitative evidence. At the end of the Portfolio Assessment Session, faculty reviewers complete an evaluation of the session.

**Feedback to students and faculty.** After the assessment session is completed, portfolios are returned to the students. General feedback is given to students about the strengths and weaknesses of the entire cohort of portfolios. Students also receive individual feedback about their portfolios including feedback about which criteria indicate their strengths and those indicating further work is needed. Students are encouraged to focus on improving weaker areas during their last academic year. Faculty who teach the senior level courses are available to work with students who want to improve in the deficient areas identified in the portfolio review. Upon return of their portfolios, students are asked to complete an evaluation of the portfolio assessment process.

All the evaluation and outcome data generated by the portfolio review process are collated and analyzed by the Portfolio Subcommittee, and a report is sent to the Curriculum and Evaluation Committee for review and follow-up. The semester reports are also placed in a binder in the Faculty Lounge for general faculty access. In addition, the Chair of the Portfolio Subcommittee gives a portfolio report via a PowerPoint® presentation during the annual nursing faculty curriculum review day.

**The portfolio subcommittee responsibilities and membership.** The Portfolio Subcommittee is responsible for organizing and presiding over the Portfolio Preparatory Sessions and Portfolio Assessment Sessions. The Subcommittee develops and updates all the portfolio program protocols and collects, analyzes, and disseminates portfolio evaluation and outcome data. This Subcommittee works closely with nursing administration and the Curriculum and Evaluation Committee on curricular issues stemming from portfolio findings. In addition, the Subcommittee develops a mission statement to guide its activities (see Appendix C).

Membership on the Subcommittee is voluntary and consists of three full-time faculty members, one full-time faculty member who functions as a liaison to the Curriculum and Evaluation Committee, at least two undergraduate student representatives from levels 2 (junior year) and 3 (senior year) of the nursing curriculum, an administrative representative, a consultant with expertise in portfolio assessment, and a nursing faculty consultant with experience in the SON portfolio program. The nursing faculty consultant position was created for the purpose of continuity and ensuring the portfolio program vision and goals would be ongoing.

**Portfolio assessment participation as important faculty service.** The portfolio program also includes provisions for recognizing faculty participation in portfolio assessment as important faculty service. Faculty who participate receive annual recognition letters from the Chair of the nursing program thanking them for their participation and encouraging them to document their participation in their Tenure and Promotion Curriculum Vitae and annual Faculty Service Reports.

## Strategies Used to Develop a Successful Program

We learned many lessons from the problems experienced with our original program (Robertson, Elster, & Kruse, 2004). As a result, we made several strategic decisions which greatly contributed to the success of the revised program. Those decisions included the following actions.

### Using a Consultant

By 2001, it was clear we needed help redefining portfolio assessment in the nursing program. We were fortunate to have a Writing Across the Curriculum (WAC) Coordinator at NIU who also is an expert in portfolio assessment. In the spring of 2001, the WAC Coordinator became a consultant to the Portfolio Subcommittee and has provided invaluable counsel on all aspects of developing and implementing our new program. This was one of the best strategic decisions that we made because we discovered that consultants can be powerful catalysts for change. Consultants have a unique status. They can ask, do, and say things that no one else can! And they see things with a visitor's eyes. The WAC consultant helped us broaden our perspective and gave us the courage and support to venture into a new way of approaching assessment of the portfolios

### Developing Our Own Rubric

Because of the previous problems using a standardized rubric, we decided to develop our own rubric for assessing student portfolios. The Portfolio Subcommittee reviewed the literature on rubric design and followed the steps of rubric development recommended by experts in the field. The Student Portfolio Rubric underwent two years of pilot testing, which is discussed later in this section. Our rubric is based on the nursing process and measures all three outcome criteria. It is a 6-item instrument (see Appendix D). The first three criteria address the steps of the nursing process. Criterion 4 measures students' ability to present or develop logical arguments. Criterion 5 measures students' ability to write. Criterion 6 measures students' ability to engage in self-reflection.

The rubric is scored on a 3-point Likert scale for each criterion, where "1" indicates the portfolio was below expectations, "2" indicates the portfolio met expectations, and "3" indicates the portfolio exceeded expectations. We decided to use a 3-point scale because minimum scoring improves inter-rater reliability and is easier and more efficient for reviewers to use (Brualdi, 2002; Elbow, 1996). The 3-point scale also provided us what we needed. It is a rough estimate of how students are doing at the end of their junior year related to the three outcome measures, and it forms the framework within which to assess strengths and weaknesses of the nursing curriculum.

Due to faculty's request for a more detailed description of each rubric criterion, an expanded rubric was developed (see Appendix E). The expanded rubric is utilized as a supplement to the Student Portfolio Rubric to assist faculty in scoring portfolios.

## Involving Key Stakeholders

Another major lesson we learned from the original program was the importance of involving key stakeholders in the development and implementation of a portfolio program. These stakeholder groups included students, administration, and faculty.

**Students.** A most important decision was to invite students to join the Portfolio Subcommittee. We were surprised at how receptive students were to this request and often had a large number of volunteers. Student members represent both the second and third levels of the program (junior year and senior year, respectively). They are recruited on a semester-by-semester basis so that there is consistent student representation from those levels. Typically there are three to four student members serving on the Subcommittee at any one point in time. Students have an important voice in subcommittee discussions, and their contributions have been immeasurable.

**Administration.** Another important stakeholder group we involved was administration. An administrative representative serves as an ex-officio member of the Portfolio Subcommittee. The administrator has brought an important perspective to the table and has had a great impact on faculty buy-in. We learned that assessment programs will not survive without administrative support. Involving administration is vital for developing and maintaining a successful assessment program.

**Faculty.** The third important stakeholder group was faculty. From the very beginning, faculty members were involved in the development and implementation of the new portfolio program. In 2001, the WAC consultant met with nursing faculty to discuss the problems with the original program and the direction faculty wanted to take with portfolio assessment. As a result of that meeting, faculty gave the Portfolio Subcommittee approval to explore the Washington State University model. After the details of the revised program were determined, the Subcommittee developed a formal proposal that was presented to faculty for their consideration and vote. In 2003, faculty unanimously approved the key features of our new program.

We also increased the number of faculty serving on the Portfolio Subcommittee and increased membership terms from 2 to 3 years. We learned that rotating faculty through the subcommittee was important to increase faculty understanding and appreciation of the portfolio assessment process and their commitment to the program.

## Obtaining Grant Funding for Training Faculty and Building the Infrastructure

For the new program to work, faculty as a whole needed to be involved in the assessment of portfolios. However, they first needed to be trained to work in faculty teams and to assess portfolios as a composite of student work using a rubric. Also, the protocols and orientation materials for the new program needed to be developed. It was evident that funding was required if the revision effort was to be successful. Fortunately, the Portfolio Subcommittee obtained two $3000 university WAC Grants to develop the new program.

A major goal of the first grant year (Phase I) was to increase faculty involvement in the portfolio program and train them to do large-scale portfolio assessment in faculty teams. Faculty participated in several training sessions that introduced them to the process of evaluating a portfolio as a composite of several assignments using our newly developed rubric. Several students provided practice portfolios for faculty to assess that included writing assignments they had done in previous courses. This experience presented faculty the opportunity not only to pilot the new rubric, but also to evaluate which assignments seemed more appropriate for the portfolio. All faculty participants had the same portfolios to review and score. Faculty then shared their ratings and discussed the strengths and weaknesses of the portfolios they had reviewed in relation to the nursing curriculum. Faculty evaluations of the training sessions were very positive. Faculty indicated that practicing the new portfolio process was the most beneficial aspect of the session and that the rubric format was appropriate and easy to use.

In the second semester of Phase I, faculty participated in a Portfolio Assessment Workshop. The workshop experience was a simulation of how portfolio assessment would be done in the new program. The workshop involved faculty learning to work in teams to review and score model portfolios. The model portfolios were developed by all nursing students in the 2nd semester of the junior year. Each portfolio contained clean copies of three already-graded assignments that students believed best indicated their abilities in critical thinking, therapeutic interventions, and writing. Faculty participants were enthusiastic about the workshop experience and learning to work in teams. They also indicated they were becoming more comfortable using the rubric and assessing portfolios as a body of work.

The second WAC grant funded Phase II of the revision effort. Phase II focused on developing the infrastructure for the new portfolio program. This included developing protocols for the assessment sessions, orientation materials for faculty and students, portfolio program information for the Undergraduate Student Handbook, and protocols for data collection and evaluation. Faculty also participated in additional training sessions to further hone their skills in assessing portfolios.

Built into both WAC grants were provisions for monetary compensation to faculty members who attended the workshop and at least one of the training sessions. The Subcommittee strongly believed it was essential to recognize faculty participation in the assessment process and establish a precedent for rewarding faculty who participated.

## Working Collaboratively as a Faculty to Determine Appropriate Course Assignments

Toward the end of the original portfolio program, a growing awareness emerged that the two assignments chosen for portfolio assessment were not the best to showcase students' abilities. Therefore, one of our objectives for the new program was to determine appropriate assignments for the portfolio. From lessons learned in the past, we knew this needed to be a collaborative effort with the whole faculty.

One of the activities funded by the second WAC grant was a Writing Assignment Workshop for faculty that was presented by our consultant. Faculty participants brought assignments from courses they taught and were divided into workgroups. Each workgroup analyzed assignments from faculty members in their group and determined how the evaluation criteria of each assignment related to the criteria on the Student Portfolio Rubric. Findings showed that many of the course assignments addressed aspects the rubric criteria. Faculty feedback indicated they found it helpful to review what others were doing with assignments and which assignments were most congruent with the rubric.

While participating in the portfolio preparatory and assessment sessions, faculty members continue to have the opportunity to review assignments their colleagues are using. During the discussion portion of these sessions, faculty often share their approach to making their assignments appropriate for inclusion in the portfolio. Some participants have verbalized how they changed their course assignments to reflect the rubric criteria. Others have indicated that certain parts of the rubric were not reflected in their assignments, and they plan to add those criteria to their guidelines. This kind of sharing encourages other faculty to make similar changes in assignments; it also helps faculty make collective decisions about appropriate portfolio evidence.

We found that determining the best assignments is an evolutionary process, not only because we have become more knowledgeable about what assignments best reflect our rubric, but also because courses change, faculty change, and class sizes change. For example, we recently experienced increased class sizes, which resulted in the elimination of some writing assignments. To help with this problem, our consultant presented a workshop for faculty on how to develop writing assignments for large classes. Faculty found this workshop very helpful. To date, the quality of writing assignments has not decreased, even though class sizes continue to increase. We are ever vigilant about changes that are occurring around us that might affect course assignments, since not having adequate writing samples can have a detrimental effect on the quality of portfolio evidence.

## Accomplishments of the Nursing Portfolio Program

### Time-Efficient Assessment

After two years of training and five years of participation in our revised program, nursing faculty have developed expertise in large-scale portfolio assessment. The result has been a continuing decrease in the amount of time needed to assess an entire cohort of portfolios despite increased class sizes and the resulting increase in the number of portfolios. This is an extremely important development due to the escalating demands placed on faculty's time. We found that twenty faculty reviewers divided into six teams can assess 60 portfolios in less than two hours. The two-hour time period also includes the curricular discussion that occurs after the reading and scoring of portfolios. According to our consultant, we have successfully developed an "economy of assessment" program.

### Increased Student Buy-In

Student buy-in has greatly improved and is demonstrated by the active participation and support from the student representatives serving on the Subcommittee. When student and faculty Subcommittee members meet with 2nd semester junior nursing students to discuss student responsibilities in submitting their portfolios, the student representative is often the person who makes the presentation and answers students' questions. The student member also accompanies faculty into the classroom when portfolios are returned and assessment findings are reported to students. Student members help their classmates understand the importance of portfolio assessment, and consequently have had a huge impact on student follow-through with portfolio requirements.

Improved student buy-in also is demonstrated by students increasingly submitting their best work for the portfolio review. We have noticed that students are making better choices in selecting portfolio documents that demonstrate their abilities in critical thinking, therapeutic interventions, and writing. In addition, students' self-reflection cover letters have improved in quality since the revised portfolio program was implemented.

## Strong Faculty Involvement and Support

The portfolio assessment program has garnered strong support from nursing faculty. From the beginning, faculty members were an integral part of the development and implementation of the revised program. As a result, the vast majority of nursing faculty has consistently participated in the assessment sessions, and faculty evaluations of both the Preparatory and Portfolio Assessment Sessions have been very positive. Of course not all faculty attend these sessions. However, on average, 20 of the 26 full-time faculty are consistent participants.

## User-Friendly Rubric with Strong Inter-rater Reliability and Validity

As indicated earlier, the Student Portfolio Rubric was painstakingly developed and pilot tested for two years under the expert guidance of our consultant. We conducted extensive faculty training in how to use the rubric and developed the expanded rubric to facilitate greater understanding of the Student Portfolio Rubric by faculty scorers. Faculty evaluations consistently indicate they find the rubric easy to use. The rubric has undergone only one minor change in over seven years of use. We removed the APA format requirement from criterion 5 (the writing skills criterion) because faculty expectations for APA format were too varied, and some faculty reviewers placed too much emphasis on APA format in relation to other aspects of criterion 5 when assessing portfolios.

Because we conduct portfolio assessment both semesters of the academic year and include preparatory sessions with faculty scoring the same practice portfolios (Perlman, 2002), we have been able to sustain high inter-rater reliability (92.5% - 100%). Inter-rater reliability is determined by dividing the number of scorer agreements by the number of agreements plus disagreements (i.e. the number of required third readings of the portfolio). Using a shorter scale contributes to better inter-rater reliability, since scorers have fewer rating decisions to consider (Elbow, 1996; Perlman, 2002). Experts also indicate that reliability of rubrics may be increased when faculty work collaboratively to develop and implement portfolio programs because more involvement in the process may improve faculty understanding of what is being measured. Our faculty assessors are familiar with the writing assignments students include in their portfolios, which is another factor that can improve inter-rater reliability (Johnson et al., 2000).

The Student Portfolio Rubric also has strong validity. Experts indicate that the validity of a rubric needs a clear connection to the purpose of the assessment, and there needs to be clear linkages between the purpose and the rubric criteria (Moskal & Leydens, 2002). The purpose of our portfolio assessment was to measure students' abilities in critical thinking, therapeutic interventions, and writing. When developing the rubric, we were careful to make clearly identifiable linkages between the rubric criteria and our three outcome measures (see Appendix F). The rubric also is based on the nursing process, a process that is very familiar to the rubric developers. Validity is enhanced when rubrics are designed by experts in the field (Gadbury-Amyot et al., 2003).

## Portfolio Program Recognition on Local, National, and International Levels

An unanticipated, but exciting, accomplishment that occurred is the recognition our portfolio program has received on local, national and international levels. For instance, the SON Chair cited our portfolio program as the primary example of best practice in a recent departmental program review. The NIU Institutional Assessment Coordinator sponsored an article on student involvement in our portfolio program that appeared in the spring 2008 issue of the university's assessment newsletter. In fall 2007, an article on our portfolio program was published in the NIU faculty and staff newsletter, *Northern Today*. In addition, an article was published in the premier journal of English composition that focused on the interdisciplinary collaboration between the university WAC program and the nursing portfolio program (Peters & Robertson, 2007). Paper presentations about our portfolio program were given by Portfolio Subcommittee members at the 2007 Sigma Theta Tau International Biennial Convention (Robertson et al., 2007) and the 2008 Wisconsin League for Nursing Fall Conference that focused on evidence-based nursing education (Rossetti et al., 2008).

The recognition has been very exciting, but more importantly it has validated the importance of assessment as scholarship. Unfortunately, nursing programs historically have not valued the scholarship of assessment as much as the scholarship of research, and assessment is oftentimes unappreciated and misunderstood. However, those who are leaders in assessment can change that mindset. One way to do that is to disseminate the results of our assessment projects through publications and presentations. When we presented our program at national and international nursing conferences, the response from participants was overwhelmingly positive, with many participant questions. It was obvious the conference attendees were interested in developing good assessment programs, and they were eager to learn from our experiences. Disseminating findings from successful assessment programs can make significant contributions to the improvement of nursing education world wide.

## Closing the Assessment Feedback Loop in Record Time

The most significant accomplishment of our portfolio program is the ability to close the assessment feedback loop in just 3 ½ years, compared to the 5 to 7 years that is typical for new assessment programs (Nagin, 2003). Closing the assessment feedback loop means we have used portfolio evidence to improve our curriculum (American Public University System, 2005). For example, the portfolio assessment trend data and faculty discussions of portfolio findings indicated that students were doing well in the assessment aspects of the nursing process at the end of the junior year, but were weaker in the areas of interventions and evaluation. Self-reflection also was an area that needed improvement. As a result, some faculty changed assignments to include interventions and evaluation. Faculty also reported incorporating more self-reflection in assignment guidelines. In subsequent assessments, we observed students were including assignments in their portfolios that addressed more of the full range of rubric criteria, which included interventions, evaluation, and self-reflection. Also, more students were earning greater numbers of the "exceeding expectations" score in a greater number of criteria. Because faculty were willing to make changes in how they were teaching based on portfolio findings, nursing students in those classes obtained richer educational experiences.

Being able to close the assessment feedback loop is especially noteworthy in light of increased national emphasis on accountability in higher education and recent research findings that indicate few institutions of higher learning have been successful in using assessment results to improve their curricula (AACU, 2002; Wegner, 2002). Researchers indicate that establishing a "culture of evidence" is essential in creating quality educational programs and these programs are characterized by pedagogical environments in which faculty are willing to use assessment data to change their practices in the classroom (Braskamp & Schomberg, 2006; USDE, 2002; Wegner, 2002). Our nursing program has been successful in developing such a culture of evidence.

## Important Considerations in Developing a Portfolio Assessment Program

Developing a portfolio program for program-level assessment requires time, commitment, dedication, expertise, and fortitude. It is not an undertaking for the faint of heart! Portfolio assessment, when correctly implemented, requires faculty and administrators to work together and actively engage in self-reflection on both program and individual levels. This, of course, can be difficult and most likely will have political implications. Therefore, before embarking on the development of a portfolio program for large-scale program assessment, it is important to keep in mind several considerations:

- Portfolio assessment programs require strong buy-in from faculty, administrators, and students (Abate et al., 2003; Weaver-Kaulis & Crutsinger, 2006). These stakeholders need to be included in the development, implementation, and maintenance phases of the program; and good communication is essential among all parties.
- Administration is the key stakeholder in determining the success of a portfolio program. If administration is not supportive, developing and maintaining a portfolio program will be an up-hill battle (Abate et al., 2003).
- Assessment needs to become part of the culture of the institution (AACU, 2002; Abate et al., 2003; Braskamp & Schomberg, 2006); otherwise, a good program today may be gone tomorrow because of changes in the players (Abate et al., 2003).
- Outside consultation is a valuable resource and should always be considered (Abate et al., 2003).
- Developing a successful portfolio program for program-level assessment requires extensive pilot testing of instruments and protocols and adequate faculty training (McCready, 2007; Perlman, 2002).
- Obtaining grant funding not only provides important resources, but also increases the status of the portfolio program in the eyes of faculty and administrators.
- Reliable scoring is promoted when scorers are well trained and participate in periodic practice sessions to score the same student documents (Perlman, 2002).

- Regular discussion of assessment findings among faculty reviewers is essential for increasing reliability of portfolio scoring and developing solutions to improve curricula and classroom teaching. Faculty commitment to portfolio assessment and involvement in the scoring process leads to curricular enhancement (Abate et al., 2003; Braskamp & Schomberg, 2006; McCready, 2007; Wiggins, 1990).

- It is preferable to develop authentic assessment instruments and rubrics that are individualized and reflect the program's expected outcomes, rather than using standardized instruments, which may not be logically connected to program goals (AACU, 2002).

- Portfolio assessment programs should be directed by faculty who are knowledgeable and committed to the assessment process, but all faculty need to be involved if the portfolio program is to be successful (Abate et al., 2003).

- Faculty participation in portfolio assessment needs to be viewed as important faculty service, and faculty members who participate need recognition and reward.

- Faculty who spearhead the development and implementation of any assessment program should be recognized for their efforts and supported by their administrators and colleagues.

## Summary

We learned that assessing student portfolios is an excellent way to evaluate the effectiveness of an undergraduate nursing program (Alexander, et al., 2006; Karlowicz, 2000; Kear & Bear, 2007). We also found that assessing portfolios at the end of the junior year was ideal for determining assets and deficits of our foundational nursing courses and providing important feedback to students on their strengths and weaknesses. In this way, our assessment program is a type of formative evaluation, which helps both students and faculty bring about needed changes on both individual and program levels.

Our nursing school's Portfolio Assessment Program has experienced a significant transformation since 1994! It has been a fascinating journey, and we have discovered the powerful impact faculty can have on improving the integrity of a curriculum when they unite as a group to assess curricular effectiveness through assessment of student portfolios (Peters & Robertson, 2007).

We hope that after reading this chapter you will consider beginning a portfolio assessment program at your school of nursing. The Learning Activities provided at the end of this chapter were prepared to help guide you in the process of developing a program. One final consideration to keep in mind when developing successful portfolio programs is remembering that challenges which arise need to be embraced and viewed as opportunities for program improvement and growth. In the words of our esteemed consultant, "never forget that assessment is always in a state of evolution."

## Relevant Website

Washington State University Writing Portfolio: http://www.writingprogram.wsu.edu/units/writingassessment/midcollege/writingportfolio/

## Learning Activities

1. Identify important stakeholders to include in the planning and development of a Portfolio Assessment Program.
2. Recruit interested faculty members and students to serve on the initial Portfolio Committee. Consider the role of a consultant and who that consultant might be.
3. Develop a plan/proposal for a Portfolio Assessment Program. Include the following key areas:
   • Vision Statement
   • Goal
   • Rationale and Background
   • Benefits of the Proposed Portfolio Program
   • Details of the Proposed Program
   • Projected Development Stages
   • Future Plans
4. Identify grant funding sources for initial start-up monies.
5. Identify the program outcome criteria to be evaluated.
6. Develop a rubric that connects with the program outcomes. Develop a linkages document to show the connections
7. Determine which pieces of student writing will be included in the portfolio.
8. Develop the infrastructure of the program including:
   • Student cover letter with directions for students to follow
   • Protocols for the portfolio assessment sessions
   • Evaluation forms:

- o Faculty evaluation of Preparatory Session
- o Faculty evaluation of Assessment Session
- o Student Evaluation
- Orientation materials for students and new faculty
- Additional portfolio informational materials for master syllabi and student handbooks
9. Write a mission statement for a new portfolio assessment program.
10. Determine appropriate writing assignments to be included in your own portfolio program.
11. Identify several different uses for student portfolios (e.g. course embedded assessment, program-level assessment, job procurement). Describe how the methods of compiling and assessing the types of portfolios would vary.
12. Identify how an RN-to-BSN or graduate program's writing assignments might differ from an undergraduate program. List appropriate writing assignments for each.

## Educational Philosophy

I believe that teaching should include a passion for the subject matter, respect for students, high standards, humor, experiential application, continuous quality improvement, and a caring approach. I believe that teachers need to create classroom environments in which students can succeed in meeting course objectives, increase their confidence in themselves, become self-reflective learners, develop new ways of thinking, broaden their perspective of their professional role, and discover exciting possibilities for the future. — Julie Fisher Robertson

I believe in the importance of being able to motivate, enlighten, and inspire my students, thus creating a passion for learning. It is important to recognize that nursing students are adult, self-directed learners who excel in a nurturing, challenging, and supportive environment. Building rapport with my students is important to me and leads to increased communication during discussions in the classroom and on a one-to-one basis. This communication is vital in the teaching/learning process and in building relationships with my students. — Jeanette Rossetti

Writing serves as a cornerstone of critical thinking and should play an important role in shaping all student learning outcomes. — Bradley Peters

As a faculty member in the School of Nursing and Health Studies, I am deeply interested in contributing my experience and knowledge about nursing to student nurses. I want to share my love of the profession of nursing and the knowledge I have gained in my years of practice in the care of children and their families. In addition, I hope to foster critical thinking skills and lifelong learning skills. In the rapidly changing healthcare industry, I hope to prepare students to use information effectively and develop problem solving skills. There are multiple ways of learning and I try to offer alternative teaching methods to practice student-centered learning. Preparing students for a future role in nursing is achieved by modeling both very good nursing care, and very good teaching methods. Each semester is an opportunity to demonstrate both the role of the nurse and the role of the teacher to students who will lead our profession in the future. — Sharon Coyer

I can best describe my teaching philosophy through the words of the great philosopher, Kahil Gibran (1951) who said, "If he is indeed wise, he does not bid you enter the house of his wisdom, but rather leads you to the threshold of your mind." My intent is to help students achieve their full potential, open their minds to new ideas and ways of thinking, and further develop their critical thinking skills. — Mary Elaine Koren

Dr. Hertz believes that the role of educators is to promote student learning and that each learner has different life experiences and perspectives as well as preferences for learning. Therefore, she deliberately tries to incorporate a variety of teaching methods and learning activities in each course she teaches. In addition, she tries to build options into the learning activities to accommodate the unique experiences and interests of students; e.g., by allowing students to choose a topic of interest related to the focus of the course when writing papers, making presentations, etc. — Judith Hertz

Dr. Elder's philosophy of nursing education focuses on developing critical thinking through the synergism of knowledge from various courses in nursing, as well as in courses from various disciplines. She feels that the importance is focusing not only on nursing content, but also on how philosophy, religion, psychology, sociology, and various other courses enhance the impact of nursing in healthcare facilities and the community. — Stacie Elder

# References

Abate, M. A., Stamatakis, M. K., & Haggett, R .R. (2003). Excellence in curriculum development and assessment. *American Journal of Pharmaceutical Education, 67*(14), 478-501.

Alexander, J. G., Craft, S. W., Baldwin, S., Beers, G. W., & McDaniel, G. S. (2006). The nursing portfolio: A reflection of a professional. *The Journal of Continuing Education in Nursing, 33*(2), 55-59.

American Public University System. (2005). Writing student learning assessment reports. Retrieved June 24, 2008 from http://www.apus.edu/Learning-Outcomes-Assessment/Resources/Degree-Program-Assessment_Reports/Program-Assessment-Reports_Overview.htm

Association of American Colleges and Universities. (2002). *National Panel Report-Greater Expectations: A new vision for learning as a nation goes to college.* Washington, DC: Author.

Banta, T. W. (2007, January). A warning on measuring learning outcomes. *Inside Higher Ed, 27.* Retrieved June 24, 2008 from http://www.insidehighered.com/views/2007/01/26/banta

Braskamp, L., & Schomberg, S. (2006, July 26). Caring or uncaring assessment. *Inside Higher Ed.* Retrieved May 23, 2008, from http://www.insidehighered.com/layout/set/print/views/2006/07/26/braskamp

Brualdi, A. (2002). Implementing performance assessment in the classroom. In C. Boston (Ed.), *Understanding scoring rubrics: A guide for teachers* (pp. 1-4). College Park, MD: Clearinghouse on Assessment and Evaluation.

Chabeli, M. M. (2002). Portfolio assessment and evaluation: Implications and guidelines for clinical nursing education. *Curationis, 25*(3), 4-9.

Condon, W. (2001). Introduction: Why WSU? In K.B. Yancey & B. Huot (Series Eds.) & R.H. Haswell (Vol. Ed.). *Perspectives on writing: Theory, research, and practice: Vol. 5. Beyond outcomes: Assessment and instruction within a university writing program* (pp. xiii-xvii). Westport, CN: Ablex Publishing.

Dolan, G., Fairbairn, G., & Harris, S. (2004). Is our student portfolio valued? *Nurse Education Today, 24,* 4-13.

Elbow, P. (1996), Writing assessment in the 21st Century: A utopian view. In L. Bloom, D. Daiker, & E. White (Eds.). *Composition in the Twenty-First Century: Crisis and change.* (pp. 83-100). Carbondale, IL: Southern Illinois University Press.

Emden, C., Hutt, D., & Bruce, M. (2004, February). Portfolio learning. *Contemporary Nurse,* Article 2047. Retrieved April 29, 2008 from http://www.contemporarynurse.com/archives/vol/16/1-2/article/2047/portfolio-learning

Facione, P. A., & Facione, N. C. (1994). *Holistic Critical Thinking Scoring Rubric.* Millbrae, CA: California Academic Press.

Gadbury-Amyot, C. C., Kim, J., Palm, R. L., Mills, G. E., Noble, E., & Overman, P. R. (2003). Validity and reliability of portfolio assessment of competency in a baccalaureate dental hygiene program. *Journal of Dental Education, 67*(9), 991-1002.

Johnson, R. L., McDaniel, F., & Willeke, M. J. (2000). Using portfolios in program evaluation: An investigation of interrater reliability. *American Journal of Evaluation, 21*(1), 65-80.

Karlowicz, K. A. (2000). The value of student portfolios to evaluate undergraduate program. *Nurse Educator, 25*(2), 82-87.

Kear, M. E., & Bear, M. (2007). Using portfolio evaluation for program outcome assessment. *Journal of Nursing Education, 46*(3), 109-114.

McCready, T. (2007). Portfolios and the assessment of competence in nursing: A literature review. *International Journal of Nursing Studies, 44*, 143-151.

McEwan, A., & Taylor, D. (2007). Assessing practice through portfolio learning. *Journal of Community Nursing, 21*(8), 4-6.

McMullan, M., Endacott, R., Gray, M. A., Jasper, M., Miller, C. M. L., Scholes, J., & Webb, C. (2003). Portfolios and assessment of competence: A review of the literature. *Journal of Advanced Nursing, 41*(3), 283-294.

Moskal, B. M., & J. A. Leydens, (2002). Scoring rubric development: Validity and reliability. In C. Boston (Ed.), *Understanding scoring rubrics: A guide for teachers* (pp. 25-33). College Park, MD: Clearinghouse on Assessment and Evaluation.

Mueller, J. (2006). *Authentic assessment toolbox.* Retrieved June 24, 2008 from http://jonathan.mueller.faculty.noctrl.edu/toolbox/index.htm.

Nagin, C. (2003). *Because writing matters: Improving student writing in our schools.* The National Writing Project. San Francisco, CA: Jossey-Bass.

Perlman, C. (2002). An introduction to performance assessment scoring rubrics. In C. Boston (Ed.), *Understanding scoring rubrics: A guide for teachers* (pp. 5-13). College Park, MD: Clearinghouse on Assessment and Evaluation.

Peters, B., & Robertson, J. F. (2007). Portfolio partnerships betweenfaculty and WAC: Lessons from disciplinary practice, reflection and transformation. *College Composition and Communication, 59*(2), 206-236.

Robertson, J. F., Elster, S., & Kruse, G. (2004). Portfolio outcome assessment: Lessons learned. *Nurse Educator, 29*(2), 52-53.

Robertson, J. F., Hertz, J., Elder, S., Rossetti, J., Koren, M. E., Coyer, S., & Peters, B. (2007, November 4) *Changing definitions of portfolio assessment: One school of nursing's experience.* Sigma Theta Tau International 39th Biennial Convention, Baltimore, MD.

Rossetti, J., Robertson, J. F., Hertz, J., Elder, S., Koren, M. E., Coyer, S., & Peters, B. (2008, October 3). *Using portfolio assessment evidence to improve undergraduate curricula: An innovative approach.* Wisconsin League for Nursing Fall Conference, Pewaukee, WI.

Schaffer, M. A., Nelson, P., & Litt, E. (2005). Using portfolios to evaluate achievement of population-based public health nursing competencies in baccalaureate nursing students. *Nursing Education Perspectives, 26*(2), 104-112.

Spence, W., & El-Ansari, W. (2004). Portfolio assessment: Practice teachers' early experience. *Nurse Education Today, 24,* 388-401.

Tiwari, A., & Tang, C. (2003). From process to outcome: The effect of portfolio assessment on student learning. *Nurse Education Today, 23,* 269-277.

Tracy, S. M., Marino, G. J., Richo, K. M., & Daly, E. M. (2000). The clinical achievement portfolio: An outcomes-based assessment project in nursing education. *Nurse Educator, 25*(5), 241-246.

U.S. Department of Education. (2006). *A test of leadership: Charting the future of U.S. higher education.* A report of the Commission Appointed by Secretary of Education Margaret Spelling. Washington, DC: Author.

Weaver-Kaulis, A., & Crutsinger, C. (2006). Assessment of student learning outcomes in FCS programs. *Journal of Family & Consumer Sciences, 98*(1), 74-80.

Wegner, G. R. (2002) *Beyond dead reckoning: Research priorities for redirecting American higher education.* National Center for Postsecondary Improvement, Stanford University, Retrieved 5-24-08 from http://www.stanford.edu/group/ncpi/documents/pdfs/beyond_dead_reckoning.pdf

Wiggins, G. (1990). The case for authentic assessment. *Practical Assessment, Research & Evaluation, 2*(2). Retrieved March 20, 2008 from http://PAREonline.net/getvn.asp?v=2&n=2

**Appendix A**
Northern Illinois University
School of Nursing
**TOP TEN QUESTIONS**
**About Your Portfolio Program**

1. What is a portfolio?

   A portfolio is:
   - Something you create from work already done.
   - A place to keep representative samples of your work from courses successfully completed.
   - A portable showcase for your skills in writing, critical thinking, and therapeutic decision-making.
   - A reflection of your educational accomplishments.
   - An opportunity to participate in self-evaluation of your professional growth.

2. What is the purpose of the portfolio program?

   The purpose is two-fold:
   - To evaluate the nursing program.
   - To provide you with input to see how you can improve your writing skills, critical thinking, and other nursing skills.

3. What should I put into my portfolio?

   - Choose three (3) different written assignments that reflect your best work. They can be from any nursing classes. For example:
     i. Concept map with its related care plan
     ii. Care plan
     iii. Research literature review
     iv. Case study analysis
     v. Process recording
   - Provide a copy that does not include your name, written comments, or grades.
   - Attach the course assignment to each document you chose.
   - Include a cover letter explaining why you selected these three documents.

4. Does this mean I have to do extra work?

- No. You will already have completed the projects that you select.
- However, because you should submit your "best" work, you are encouraged to revise a previously completed assignment.

5. When do I submit my portfolio?

- You will be expected to submit your portfolio at the beginning of your fourth semester in one of your assigned courses.

6. Will I be graded on my portfolio?

- No. Your work will be assessed using the attached Student Portfolio Rubric.

7. Who evaluates my portfolio?

- Two or three faculty members will read and evaluate each portfolio.
- Place only your Z-ID number on your paper, not your name.

8. What happens to my portfolio after it is evaluated?

- It will be returned to you.

9. Why is a portfolio important for me to do?

- You will receive feedback that indicates your strengths and weaknesses related to the 6 criteria on the Student Portfolio Rubric. You can use this valuable information in your self-assessment of your growth in the nursing program. Your portfolio feedback highlights areas that would be important to focus on in your senior year.
- You will be making an important contribution to the assessment of the NIU School of Nursing program.
- Share your portfolio with potential employers when requested as part of the interview process or to provide examples of writing.

10. Is my participation in this program required or optional.

- Your participation is required.

Date

Dear Undergraduate Student,

As you know, students who are in the third semester of the nursing program are required to submit a portfolio at the end of the semester as a requirement for passing NURS 317. Following the review of your portfolio, which will be conducted in the beginning of the next semester, you will receive results of the assessment process. This assessment does not affect your grade point average, but it does provide important information to you about areas for you to address in your senior year. This assessment also provides the School of Nursing with critical information about how well the nursing program is preparing students.

This is what you need to do:

- Using the folder provided for you, develop a portfolio that contains <u>three</u> documents <u>that you feel best demonstrate your abilities in critical thinking, written communication, and therapeutic nursing interventions</u>. These documents are assignments that you have already completed. We would like you to choose assignments from your 3rd semester nursing courses. However, if you have completed assignments from previous courses that you feel demonstrate your abilities in critical thinking, therapeutic interventions, and communication, you can include those. The following is a list of possible documents to include:
  1. Concept map or care plan
  2. Case study
  3. Paper of your choice
  4. Process recording

- Remove (blacken) any patient identifying information from the documents that you submit.
- For each document, <u>attach the assignment guidelines</u> you received from your professor.
- A cover letter should be included that addresses the following information:

Keep in mind the cover letter speaks your portfolio's first words, portrays your commitment to nursing, and engages your reader. Please indicate in the cover letter some reflections about how the documents you have selected demonstrate what you have learned during your education in the School of Nursing and where you still need to grow in your professional development. The following questions can assist you in this self reflection. You do not have to answer all the questions.

1. How do the documents selected demonstrate your abilities in critical thinking, writing, and therapeutic interventions?
2. What are the strengths or weaknesses of each selection?
3. What are the areas in which you personally changed including: biases, cultural sensitivity, caring or other values?
4. What are the areas in which you professionally changed including: collaboration organization, prioritization, time management, leadership, or professional role behaviors?
5. Describe the major strengths you have developed during your School of Nursing experience.
6. What are the areas you need to grow in over the next year?

- **To preserve anonymity, we are asking you to:**
  1. <u>Remove your name</u> from all submitted documents
  2. Submit <u>un-graded copies</u> of assignments

- **Place your Z-ID number on the portfolio folder label.**
- **Submit your portfolio folder with the above documents to your N317 professor by the deadline date determined by your professor.**

Following the faculty portfolio review, your folders will be returned to you. We hope the portfolio assessment provides useful information to you for your senior year studies. School of Nursing faculty are always available to assist you in any way they can.

Thank you for your participation,

School of Nursing Portfolio Subcommittee

## Appendix C
### Northern Illinois University
### School of Nursing
**Mission of the Portfolio Subcommittee**

The mission of the Portfolio Subcommittee is to develop and maintain a state-of-the-art portfolio assessment program that is progressive, responsive to students' and faculty's needs, and congruent with successful national portfolio assessment models. The Subcommittee is dedicated to providing a portfolio program that promotes the School of Nursing's commitment to excellence and serves as a model for other departments in the university. The Subcommittee coordinates the portfolio assessment process; collects and analyzes portfolio data to show trends in students' abilities in critical thinking, therapeutic interventions, and communication; and facilitates faculty review and discussion of portfolio assessment outcomes to address curricular deficiencies and build on curricular strengths.

## Appendix D
### Northern Illinois University
### School of Nursing
### **Student Portfolio Rubric**

1. The student's portfolio demonstrates an ability to **gather appropriate data**, **analyze situations**, and **formulate appropriate diagnoses/conclusions**.

   Exceeds Expectations         Meets Expectations         Is Below Expectations
            3                            2                           1

2. The student's portfolio demonstrates an ability to **transfer information** or **apply principles** from one context to another **in establishing therapeutic nursing interventions** or in **developing implications** for professional nursing.

   Exceeds Expectations         Meets Expectations         Is Below Expectations
            3                            2                           1

3. The student's portfolio demonstrates an ability to **evaluate the effectiveness of therapeutic nursing interventions**, **conclusions drawn from professional resources**, or **other kinds of decision making**.

   Exceeds Expectations         Meets Expectations         Is Below Expectations
            3                            2                           1

4. The student's portfolio demonstrates an ability to **present or develop logical arguments or cases**.

   Exceeds Expectations         Meets Expectations         Is Below Expectations
            3                            2                           1

5. The student's portfolio meets professional expectations of readers in the field of nursing in terms of **adequate referencing**, **grammar and spelling**, **format**, and **professional language**.

   Exceeds Expectations         Meets Expectations         Is Below Expectations
            3                            2                           1

6. The student's portfolio demonstrates an ability to **reflect upon what the student has learned and still needs to learn**.

   Exceeds Expectations         Meets Expectations         Is Below Expectations
            3                            2                           1


Raw Score:_____
Average Score:_____
Initials _____

## Appendix E
### Northern Illinois University
### School of Nursing
### Expanded Explanation of Criteria in SON Portfolio Rubric:

| Criterion | Exceeds expectations=3 | Meets expectations=2 | Doesn't meet expectations=1 |
|---|---|---|---|
| 1 | Data are unusually thorough and appropriate; analysis is superior and meticulously detailed; diagnoses and conclusions show high degree of professional rigor. | The student's portfolio demonstrates an ability to gather appropriate data, analyze situations, and formulate appropriate diagnoses/conclusions. | Data are inappropriate or insufficient; analysis is poor or incomplete; diagnoses or conclusions are wrong or aren't adequately supported. |
| 2 | Therapeutic nursing interventions/ implications for professional nursing are extremely well formed based on research and current practice; principles are applied with exceptional accuracy and judgment. | The student's portfolio demonstrates an ability to transfer information or apply principles from one context to another in establishing therapeutic nursing interventions or in developing implications for professional nursing. | Therapeutic nursing interventions are inappropriate, absent, or not based on sufficient information; principles are misapplied; implications for professional nursing are underdeveloped or missing. |
| 3 | Criteria for evaluating effectiveness of therapeutic nursing interventions are especially clear and exact; conclusions or decisions reflect a masterful understanding of professional resources. | The student's portfolio demonstrates an ability to evaluate the effectiveness of therapeutic nursing interventions, conclusions drawn from professional resources, or other kinds of decision making. | Inadequate or insufficient criteria established for evaluating the effectiveness of therapeutic nursing interventions; conclusions or decisions do not utilize professional resources accurately or well. |
| 4 | Arguments or cases are logical and compellingly thought through. | The student's portfolio demonstrates an ability to develop logical arguments or cases. | Arguments or cases demonstrate significant gaps in development and logic. |

| 5 | The student's portfolio is consistent and polished in every area of professional conventions. | The student's portfolio meets professional expectations of readers in the field of nursing in terms of adequate referencing, grammar and spelling, format, and professional language. | The student's portfolio does not meet professional expectations of readers in the field of nursing due to inadequate referencing, errors, lack of editing, inattention to format, and/ or inaccurate use of professional language. |
| --- | --- | --- | --- |
| 6 | Reflection is detailed and pertinent, demonstrating an outstanding self-awareness of progress and future learning goals in the nursing program; reflection may even revise or pose alternatives to points raised in contents of portfolio— or explain improvements made to individual papers. | The student's portfolio demonstrates an ability to reflect upon what the student has learned and still needs to learn. | Reflection merely summarizes the material of the portfolio and inadequately addresses self-awareness of progress or future learning goals. |

## Appendix F
Northern Illinois University
School of Nursing
**Linkages Among Rubric Criteria and School of Nursing Outcomes**

| Outcome | #1 Criterion: Data Collection/ Analysis | #2 Criterion: Knowledge Application | #3 Criterion: Evaluation | #4 Criterion: Logic | #5 Criterion: Language Conventions | #6 Criterion: Self-Reflection |
|---|---|---|---|---|---|---|
| Critical Thinking | X | X | X | X | | X |
| Therapeutic Nursing Interventions | X | X | X | | | |
| Communication | | | X | X | X | |

# CHAPTER 29

# ENGAGING STUDENTS FOR AFFECTIVE LEARNING THROUGHOUT THE CURRICULUM

Lynn Norman, MSN, EdD, RN
Arlene Morris, MSN, EdD, RN

---

The content of this chapter relates to the following major content areas and subconcepts on the Certified Nurse Educator Examination Detailed Test Blueprint:

**Facilitate Learning**
- Implement a variety of teaching strategies appropriate to desired learner outcomes
- Use teaching strategies based on educational theory; evidence-based practices related to education

**Facilitate Learner Development and Socialization**
- Foster the development of learners in the affective domain
- Adapt teaching styles and interpersonal interactions to facilitate learner behaviors

**Participate in Curriculum Design and Evaluation of Program Outcomes**
- Demonstrate knowledge of curriculum development including identifying program outcomes; selecting appropriate learning activities; selecting appropriate evaluation strategies

---

## Introduction

Due to the rapidly expanding body of nursing knowledge, nursing faculty are challenged with the demand to determine appropriate theory content and learning strategies to be included in nursing curricula. Selecting the specific content for courses and placing these concepts within the curriculum triggers discussions for novice and experienced faculty members. Krathwohl, Bloom, and Masia (1964) developed a comprehensive list of instructional objectives, divided into the following three major domains: cognitive, psychomotor, and affective. Nursing curriculum design must account for student achievement in the cognitive domain of learning, such as that tested in traditional examinations, and in the psychomotor domain, such as performance of nursing skills in clinical settings. In developing curriculum concepts, the tendency may be to overlook the affective domain of learning (Martin and Briggs, 1986). Keeping pace with affective learning outcomes may be even more evident in the current era of ever-changing evidence-based nursing practice.

## Affective Learning

The beginning point of teaching in the affective domain is gaining the attention of the individual nursing student to some concept. As the nursing student pays attention to that concept, an awareness of it begins. The socialization of nursing students progresses along levels of attaining professional nursing values and attitudes and putting these into practice. Shephard (2008) points out that the actual outcomes at the top of the affective learning hierarchy include self-reliance, cooperation, leadership, and confidence in making choices. Each of these outcomes is essential to the practice of nursing.

### Krathwohl's Levels of Affective Learning

Krathwohl et al (1964) differentiate levels of affective learning that progress from receiving, responding, and valuing, to the organization of values into a system with the ultimate development of a characteristic lifestyle. Included in their definition of affective learning is the principle of internalization, " . . . the process by which the phenomenon or value successfully and pervasively becomes a part of the individual." (Krathwohl, et al. 1964, p. 28). The lowest level is **receiving** in which a gradual emotional connection is formed with the concept. The next level is **responding,** in which the nursing student's reaction becomes more consistent in reacting to similar stimuli.

Professional nursing **valuing** continues to form in an internalization process as the student develops a preference or commitment to the concept. The next step involves the nursing values being organized into a personal value system. Successful **internalization** of the values taught in the beginning nursing courses enables the student to use these values in situations throughout the curriculum to continue the valuing process to the point that his/her individual value system for the nursing profession becomes organized. Finally, the values are interrelated, or **organized,** in a structure or worldview that the student brings as a set to new problems and the student responds consistently to value laden situations as a professional nurse.

Faculty may encounter difficulty in planning for inclusion of affective teaching strategies and methods to evaluate the learning attained from those strategies. Measurable student learning outcomes should be specified for each affective level of attainment. The **receiving** level involves the student attending to a stimulus and can be evaluated by observation of student engagement in the content. The **responding** level entails the student showing a behavior such as answering questions. The **valuing** level includes the student showing involvement or commitment, and may be evaluated by the student beginning to use the newly learned concept. The **organization** level occurs as the student incorporates the behavior into nursing practice, and may be evaluated by observation in classroom or clinical settings. The characteristic lifestyle level of affective learning has associated behavior changes in which the concept is more consistently demonstrated (Krathwohl, et al. 1964). Emphasis on evaluation of the **responding** and **valuing** levels allows more immediate evaluation; whereas, the **organization** and development of a characteristic lifestyle level may occur post-graduation or later in the graduate's nursing practice. The goal is to recognize the need for affective learning in nursing curriculum design, identify strategies to engage students in affective learning, and offer methods for effective evaluation.

## Schulman's Table of Learning

Shulman (2002) suggests that taxonomies not be considered theories of learning, and that learning may occur other than in the sequential order of the hierarchy in Bloom's cognitive and Krathwohl's affective domains. Shulman proposes a heuristic, or model of learning, involving six interacting elements which can all be considered to have a cyclical quality

1. engagement and action
2. knowledge and understanding
3. performance and action
4. reflection and critique
5. judgment and design
6. commitment and identity

Teaching strategies, according to Shulman (2002), can be designed to promote involvement of each of the elements in the learning model to attain specific learning objectives. For example, one learning objective is for students to be able to assess a patient with a particular illness. During the lecture/discussion of content regarding the illness, students could become **engaged and motivated** by facts regarding patient outcomes presented as stories, or case studies, or by the educator asking if students wanted to share personal examples. **Knowledge and understanding** of the illness could be promoted by discussion of the process in class and observation of patients in clinical settings. The **performance and action** element in this model of learning would involve students motivated to use the knowledge to actually assess the patient for behaviors in a clinical setting. **Reflection** following the clinical would allow self-critique of both knowledge and performance, and identification of any additional learning desired. The student can use **judgment and design** by working within time and budget constraints, comparing multiple factors of the patient's values and the student's values, standards of nursing, etc to intervene with the patient in the most appropriate manner for the situation and desired outcomes of the interaction. The student may then internalize the value of interacting with patients to assess the illness and promote compliance to the point that a **commitment** to integrating this in the student's personal practice of nursing exists without external prodding, with the desire (**engagement**) to continually re-examine actions for improvement. The process would then recycle.

## Fink's Taxonomy of Significant Learning

Fink (2003) presents the need for college level learning to be significant to result in a lasting change that is important to the learner. This significant learning involves internal and external changes, similar to Krathwohl's valuing of content and behavior change. The six categories in Fink's taxonomy can be used for nursing course or curricular design:

1. **Foundational knowledge** (specific facts and ideas necessary as a basis for other kinds of learning)
2. **Application** (engaging in useful intellectual, physical or social action)
3. **Integration** (the power to make connections such as between ideas or areas of life)
4. **Human dimension** (learning about themselves or others that increases effective functioning)
5. **Caring** (new feelings, interests, or values, that provide energy for making a change)
6. **Learning how to learn** (determining how to continue learning with greater effectiveness)

Each of these categories of learning is extremely pertinent in the discipline of nursing, and specific learning objectives for each could be developed. For example, fundamental nursing concepts, pathophysiology, assessment, and pharmacology provide **foundational information** for the practice of nursing. Both **application and integration** of these facts occur in reflection, discussions, and clinical experiences. The **human dimension** of determining more about self and others includes finding ways to more effectively interact with patients, families, interprofessional staff, and building teams in clinical or classroom settings. The category of **caring** can be the source for energy to provide safe, quality nursing care in a life-long career throughout practice settings. The category of **learning how to learn** can foster application of various forms of information used by nurses for evidence-based practice, such as from research studies, systematic reviews, and practice guidelines.

## Reasons to Incorporate Affective Learning

The inclusion of the affective domain of learning throughout the nursing curriculum is imperative to the practice of nursing. Affective learning assists in the formation of the character of the professional nurse. The American Association of Colleges of Nursing (AACN) (2008) includes development of professional as one of their 9 *Essentials of Baccalaureate Education.* The central concept is caring, consisting of the following suggested sample professional values for nursing education:

- altruism
- respect for patient autonomy
- respect for human dignity
- integrity
- respect for social justice.

Certain disciplines, such as nursing, involve interpersonal interactions that must be based on a set of values that are vital to the caring perspective (Zimmerman & Phillips, 2000).

Martin (1989) adds that affective learning may also be overlooked because of the ethical question "Should teachers teach values?... Should indoctrination be part of the instructor's role?" (p16). Davis (2003) cautions that simple character education may emphasize behaviors, rather than actual moral reasoning that includes deliberation of intentions or motives for the chosen behavior(s). This author's discussion of "a generalized tendency to deliberate in a certain way (at length when there is time, quickly when there is not) – with deliberation ending in action" (Davis, 2003, p. 42) is most certainly pertinent to nursing education. In fact, in a study of perioperative nurses, Killen (2002) found that moral motivation and moral character are related to moral action, and that an education background in ethics that stimulated moral imagination was related to moral actions essential for nursing. Students must be prepared prior to patient interactions in varying situations to critically think about their own values and develop the ability to make ethical judgments and take action based on those judgments.

## Enhancing Cognitive Retention through Affective Learning

Martin and Briggs (1989) researched the integration of the affective and cognitive domains. They claim that for a change in behavior to occur, an attitude of valuing the behavior must be developed. It is important that the instructional design be planned to enable the student to develop the desired value. Valuing increases motivation to change behavior.

Goleman (1995) also suggests that emotions and cognition are not separate processes. Belanger and Jordan (2000) state that using the affective domain enhances cognitive retention. In their work on evaluation and implementation of distance learning, they assert that affective strategies raise the level of interest and engagement of the student in the instructional content. They further maintain that affective learning engages the learner through multiple senses integrated into the instructional material. Learners feel, see, and touch along with the cognitive learning, enabling the learner to use more senses than learners sitting passively in lecture-based course environments. Therefore, engaging the learner through multiple senses raises the level of interest and engagement with the instructional content. Brookfield (2006) proposes that "developing understanding, assimilating knowledge, acquiring skills, exploring new perspectives, and thinking critically are activities that prompt strong feelings" (p. 75).

Goulet & Owen-Smith (2005) suggest the cognitive and psychomotor domains are involved in the **explicit** curriculum, while the affective abilities such as self-reflection, cultural or social awareness, and advocacy are **implicit** in curricula. Furthermore, the affective domain may not be specified in course or program outcomes, except perhaps in psychosocial components. Because learning may endure more over time when emotions are involved, these authors propose a commitment to explicit program goals in the affective domain, consideration of methods to evaluate affective goal attainment, and increased focus on cognitive-affective interaction.

Oermann and Gaberson (2006) assert that learning in nursing involves lower level cognitive behaviors such as recall and comprehension, progressing to higher level cognitive skills (application, analysis, synthesis, and evaluation) in which "students apply concepts, theories, and other forms of knowledge to new situations, use that knowledge to solve patient and other types of problems, and arrive at rational and well-thought-out decisions about actions to take" (p. 111). Decisions involved in clinical judgment involve evaluation of multiple courses of action. The evaluation level of the cognitive domain necessitates determining importance (valuing), and thus integrates the affective domain.

# The Climate for Affective Learning

Consideration of the teaching/learning climate for affective learning is essential. Nursing faculty must take into account the learners' prior attitudes, values, and experiences. Instruction in the affective domain may be disorienting if the student's prior attitudes, values, or experiences conflict with those of the nursing profession, or if the student has not reflected on personal values prior to the content presented (Mezirow, 2000). The following suggestions are offered for consideration:

- Provide a climate of acceptance of student differences in attitudes and values.
- Allow time for student reflection, discussion, or pondering of issues (Brookfield, 2006). Classroom or hall discussion, peer group discussion, clinical conferences, or appointment with faculty may be helpful, especially if strong feelings have been aroused.
- Curriculum planning must include opportunities to be quiet and engage in self-reflection prior to journaling or recording reactions to clinical, simulation, or classroom experiences.

> Giving permission and opportunities to students to self-reflect and work out personal meanings of course materials or of learning opportunities conveys to them the significance and legitimacy of their previous life experiences and of their personal interpretation to their learning (Goulet & Owen-Smith, 2005, p. 69).

- Identify the value to be gained prior to structuring the assignment, then structure the assignment to achieve the goal of value development. Design lessons to simultaneously influence achievement of both affective and cognitive behaviors (Martin, 1989).
- Present persuasive messages in a credible manner, through a respected role model (Miller, 2005).
- Consider what is happening during the learning activity. Is there so much activity that the situation will be distracting and cloud the value being taught? Simple to complex educational strategies are more effective when teaching in the affective domain.
- A segment of lecture may introduce the content, followed by relevant and vivid examples such as video clips with the opportunity for discussion and critiquing.
- The learners may be involved in the planning, production, or content delivery (Miller, 2005).

- Although more time may be involved, writing tasks such as reflection papers, summary paragraphs, or online discussions may promote student articulation of understanding and valuing (Russo & Ford, 2006).
- Learning activities that allow opportunities for students to evaluate thinking and valuing should be included in each course. Mezirow (2000) used the term cognitive dissonance for the emotional disturbances that occur in education when a person is exposed to a different possibility than had been previously considered. However, the learner then experiences emancipatory learning by choosing to (or not to) integrate new learning into personal valuing or behaving. Time for reflection and consideration of options may occur over multiple exposures to the content.

Timing in the curriculum is also highly important for students to relate the intended value to actual life experiences. First semester nursing students need stories, role play, or interactive activities because a background of experiences with patients may not yet be formed. Students in successive semesters may recall experiences with patients from previous semesters, and be able to associate new learning with the prior experience. For example, the value of human dignity may be introduced as a role play in which there is an obvious lack of respect for an individual in a healthcare setting. Students may then brainstorm methods to improve the interaction to include respect for human dignity. Thus, an early example can provide a basis for interaction with patients in successive semesters or settings.

The importance of planning activities to engage students throughout the curriculum enables an opportunity to encourage development of the values in proximity to the time the student will be experiencing similar situations in clinical settings, and to allow reflection on how the values can be applied in various situations. The dignity of patients and empathy are recurring themes in all nursing content. Reinforcement of affective content in courses throughout the curriculum promotes revisiting "valued" concepts in successive semesters. Also, revisiting issues assists in determining if behavioral changes have occurred.

Structured learning activities allow students to experience the dilemmas of potential value conflict in the environment of the traditional classroom, nursing laboratory, or web-based distance learning environment. Exploration of alternative feelings is encouraged, with peer and faculty feedback (Mezirow, 2000). The internalization of the value to the point that it becomes a characteristic of the student's lifestyle, or part of nursing practice, may actually occur later in the curriculum following several experiences, much like building blocks (Martin and Briggs, 1986).

## Evaluation Strategies to Determine Outcomes

Evaluation is actually two-fold. Outcomes are characteristics students should display at a designated time (Billings & Halstead, 2008). Did the learner achieve the outcome? Evaluation also needs to determine the effectiveness of the teaching strategy. To assess affective learning, affective outcomes are written. Goulet and Owen-Smith (2005) suggest that affective outcomes and evaluation tools should be developed to measure student progress throughout the curriculum, although time and effort are required to develop affective teaching strategies.

The short-term outcome is: Did the students affectively experience, or feel, the content? Miller (2005) suggested that students' interest is necessary for them to be engaged or value the content. Goulet and Owen-Smith (2005) state:

> Cognitive-affective learning should be fostered through student motivation, engagement, active experimentation, and critical self-reflection, …[including] more active learning time to create disorienting moments and disorienting disturbances. Some classroom time needs to be devoted to preparation to and debriefing of the learning experience to increase self-efficacy and allow students to feel their emotions, to reflect on their understanding, and to figure things out. (p. 71)

However, the long-term outcome is: Do the students use the outcome in actual nursing practice? The actual use of the outcome requires the valuing of the content enough to change behaviors consistently when engaged in the practice of nursing.

To assess the effectiveness of affective learning, several methods could be used (Martin and Briggs, 1986):
- questionnaires
- self-reporting strategies such as interviews
- behavioral observations

Additionally, attitudinal-oriented written test items can be included in the classroom examinations or case studies.

Oftentimes, the development of a value takes longer than the time the students spend in the classroom. That is why assessment of attainment of the objectives may occur several months or years after the value has been introduced. Behavioral changes are the best indicators that a change in affective learning has taken place. For nursing, the student outcome is heightened awareness of potential patient needs and the development of attitudes for providing higher quality nursing care – the change in behavior. A post graduation survey may be needed to evaluate long-term changes in behavior.

## Suggested Affective Learning Strategies Throughout the Curriculum

A variety of affective teaching strategies can be incorporated throughout the curriculum.

### Nursing Concepts Course

The nursing concepts course in the beginning semester includes a values clarification exercise by the individual student. Students identify values that are deemed most important to them and incorporate these values into a personal nursing philosophy. Students review their personal nursing philosophy throughout the curriculum and make revisions based on newly learned material or new experiences. Senior students in the capstone course complete a final review of their nursing philosophy. Students reflect on the comparison of the beginning personal nursing philosophy and senior nursing philosophy.

Caring is another concept introduced in the beginning nursing course. Students can be exposed to the broad concept of caring with many teaching strategies. Probably the most important teaching method is student modeling of the caring attitudes and behaviors of teachers, peers, and staff nurses. Early clinical experiences provide opportunities for students to record observations of caring activities by interprofessional team members when interacting with patients and families. Other learning activities can be included in the presentation of course content. Small groups of students brainstorm synonyms for caring and write brief narratives of a time when caring was personally experienced. The narratives are then reviewed to determine what aspect of caring was effectively demonstrated. Students can be assigned to write a response to an article such as Benner's "The Wisdom of Our Practice" (2000), which provides exposure to caring concepts discussed by a professional nurse leader. Photos and brief summaries of nurses' experiences such as those included in Smeltzer and Vlasses' (2003) *Ordinary People, Extraordinary Lives: The Stories of Nurses* can be used as introductions to various topics.

During the first semester nursing concepts course, a role-play is used in which the students act as a patient in the admission process for a routine surgery and the healthcare providers who are encountered (Alderman & Brien, 1987). In the script, calling the patient by terms referring to the service to be provided – the broccoli dietary tray, the gall bladder x-ray, the broken call bell, the red pill, etc. – provides opportunity for students to identify a need for dignity, respect, and courteous interaction with all patients. The scripted interaction of interprofessional healthcare providers rapidly entering the patient's hospital room to focus on tasks instead of patient needs provides an opportunity for beginning nursing students to respond to the need to address the patient as a holistic person. The placement of this activity is prior to the initial clinical experience. The intended learning outcome is the valuing of human dignity by creating an awareness of healthcare team members' verbal and non-verbal communication and transmission of attitudes to a patient in the vulnerable situation of hospital admission.

Cultural awareness is promoted by many teaching strategies. Online discussion postings provide valuable insight toward student perceptions and learning. International nursing classes can link via the Internet to discuss cultural and healthcare issues. Interviews with persons on campus from a cultural background different than that of the nursing student can be scheduled. The interviews include topics on local health care and how it affects the cultural customs of that person. Students present their findings during class or small group settings. Following presentation of content that may be culturally sensitive, students may desire to express feelings, especially if a disorienting dilemma has occurred (Mezirow, 2000). Planned opportunities for continued discussion may be needed. Bafabafa (Shirts, 1977) is an interactive game developed to promote sensitivity to various cultural customs and offers insight into cultural differences. Although this game offers simulated diversity, students reflect on their feelings during the game.

## Fundamental Nursing Skills

Technical nursing skills easily cover the cognitive and psychomotor domains. Affective components of technical skills should be explicitly included in the curriculum. The basic skill of handwashing is taught with an emphasis on the affective domain. The affective learning objectives for handwashing are to impact the student's attitude regarding the importance and relevance of proper handwashing technique. A teaching strategy utilized to demonstrate the importance of the thoroughness of handwashing involves the use of Glo Germ™ (1968) and fluorescent lighting. Students are instructed in handwashing, rinsing, and drying techniques. Glo Germ™, an oil based liquid that glows under ultraviolet light, is then placed on their hands. Students wash hands, then view the hands under the fluorescent lighting. The remaining orange glow simulates the bacteria that would have remained on the hands. Initially, students are startled as to how thoroughly hands were washed only to see the "bacteria" remaining. At the end of the semester, a follow-up questionnaire assesses any change in behavior regarding handwashing in all areas of their student and personal lives. Students state increased awareness of the importance of thorough handwashing, and report changes in behaviors such as washing hands more diligently and more often.

Changing soiled gloves is another skill important to aseptic technique in a nursing skills course. Teaching a student to remove gloves requires little innovation unless affective learning is a goal. Using chocolate pudding to demonstrate soiled gloves is an effective strategy (G. Langham, personal communication, September 12, 2003). Students don clean gloves then are asked to close their eyes and place both hands opened out in front of them. The instructor places a dollop of chocolate pudding in the palm of each student's hands and tells the student to gently rub hands together. With the student's eyes still shut, the instructor describes a scenario of emptying a bed pan or attempting to dislodge a fecal impaction. The students are instructed to look at the gloves, and then to remove gloves using proper technique. Students comment on the impact of the chocolate pudding and the need to be cognizant of the correct way for removing gloves. Evaluation is evidenced by student comments and behavior in the clinical setting.

Beginning nursing students typically have had limited contact with touching and caring for strangers. Morning care, which includes bathing, oral care, and hair care is a common routine that students perform on themselves every day. To incorporate affective learning, students are required to brush each other's teeth in the nursing laboratory prior to attending clinical. Students choose a partner and each brings a toothbrush and toothpaste. Each student performs oral care on the partner. Students comment that it is easier to perform the skill on themselves than on each other. Performing the skill on each other enhances awareness of how it feels to have someone provide supportive care for them, prior to facing an actual situation in which supportive care is provided to a patient. Learning outcomes of empathy can be evaluated by student comments and actual behaviors in the clinical setting.

Catheterization is a technical skill taught in the skills course using cognitive and psychomotor domains of learning. Emphasis on the affective learning component for this skill is enhanced with the use of the Cath Triad (R. Coker, personal communication, February 18, 2008). After the initial demonstration, practice, and return demonstration for the skill, students are divided into groups of three. Each student participates in role-play as the patient, nurse, and evaluator. The patient lies fully clothed in the nursing laboratory bed in the correct position for catheterization. Using the removable male or female genitalia from the practice manikins, the patient positions the genitalia in the correct anatomical position on the body and holds the part in place. The nurse performs the procedure using the practice catheterization tray and proper technique. The evaluator assesses for correct procedure and for the amount of time it took to perform the procedure. After each student has played each role, the students reflect on how it felt to be in each of the roles. Some of their comments included:

- The patient did not like the positioning they were in or the amount of time they were "exposed".
- The nurse liked the extra practice without an instructor watching and was able to experience the actual time it takes to set up the sterile field.
- The evaluator did not like playing the role of the instructor.

A post conference activity during initial clinical courses could involve discussion of what moral or ethical foundation nurses use in making clinical decisions. Students could reflect on the experiences during the clinical day, and discuss or journal regarding situations that elicited consideration of moral or ethical concerns. For example, exposure to patients with physical disabilities, limited resources, or difficult life situations may prompt students to express their thoughts, as could situations regarding interprofessional or patient-caregiver conflict.

## Maternal/Newborn Nursing Course

An apron made with canvas material, a partially inflated beach ball, and scuba diving weights are props used for an affective learning strategy used in the maternal/newborn course to simulate the changes of late pregnancy. The inexpensive apron and 8 pounds of scuba weights together represent the last few weeks of pregnancy. The weights are placed in pockets so when the student wears the apron, pressure from the weights lies on the student's bladder. The ball is inflated to the extent needed to represent the effect of a term or near term uterus pushing up on the diaphragm. The students wear the apron for 1 to 2 hours during class. They experience the challenge of getting in and out of the small desks and retrieving a pencil from the floor.

At the end of the course, students are surveyed for their reaction to this experience, and to ascertain if their behavior changed when caring for maternal patients at the end of a pregnancy. The responses were positive. Several students, including the male students, stated this strategy gave them a better appreciation of pregnant patients and influenced their provision of care. The students stated they allowed more time for maternal patients to change positions, ambulate, and perform simple activities.

## Pediatric Nursing Course

Assisting grieving parents is often difficult for students. In the pediatric course, parents speak to students about the intense feelings they experienced when their child required care for serious health problems or when their child died. Inviting those who have first hand experience with the feelings can effectively engage students to become more aware of family needs. The affective learning outcome at the receiving level is achieved as students engage in listening then questioning the parents regarding experiences with nursing care of an infant with major anomalies and subsequent death. Evaluation of the affective learning level of responding is also evident by the students' emotional reactions, including attempts to comfort the parent as students and speaker share tears. The level of valuing may be evaluated in clinical settings as needs of family members are addressed.

Providing nursing care for children with a disability in long term care is an opportunity in pediatric course to meet affective learning goals. Students assess the developmental level of the child and learn the various medications and dosages prescribed for the children. Following the clinical experience an extensive post conference provides time for the students to reflect on their feelings. Discussions by the students include their personal feelings for the children's level of functioning and feelings felt for the parents who had the difficult decision of placing the child in the long term care setting. Students often describe this experience as being outside their comfort zone. After this experience, students are better equipped to care for these children should they require hospitalization in the acute care setting.

## Care of Older Adults/Chronicity Nursing Course

Several teaching strategies can promote the nursing value of human dignity when providing nursing care to older adults. The teaching/learning strategy of role taking where students take on the role of the patient is very effective. These activities provide students the opportunity to experience how older patients perceive the environment and/or deal with physical changes (Tsushima & Gegas, 2001). Sensory alterations of aging can be simulated with:

- Construction paper glasses with "lenses" to create the effect of multiple eye disorders
- Cotton in the ears
- Audio tapes in which consonants are less audible than vowels
- Masking tape around fingers to limit flexibility

With these alterations, each student is asked to retrieve a dime, not a penny, from a small plastic bag. Students realize the intended affective learning goal of valuing the challenges of functionality when dealing with effects of aging or chronic illness.

Another role-taking strategy for the older adult is having students sit through a class in a wheelchair with vest and wrist restraints. The students comment at the end of an hour that position changes "are really needed!" Students also comment about the feelings experienced while watching other students leave the room for a break.

Video viewing is another teaching strategy helpful in conveying respect for the dignity of older adults. Short clips may provide a model of caring behaviors of caregivers toward older adults. For example, the portion of the motion picture *Driving Miss Daisy* (Zanuck, Zanuck, & Beresford, 1989) in which the gentleman feeds pie to an older resident in a nursing home can promote discussion regarding meaningful interaction with older adults and methods of providing feeding. The videotape *Tucked in Tight* (Caputi & Gauldin, 2001), uses music and images to depict caring interactions of nurses with an older adult. For a preview of this video, see the CD accompanying this book.

## Mental Health Nursing Course

Reflective journaling can be utilized throughout the nursing curriculum, and is especially useful in mental health nursing. Personal stories about coping with stressful events by students and patients encourage contemplation, and promote student attainment of the affective level of valuing of effective interventions. Reflective journaling can also be used throughout the curriculum for students to identify areas in which they have demonstrated professional growth, thereby providing a method to evaluate the organization level of attainment of professional nursing behaviors and values.

The online environment can be used to provide more time to reflect on, and respond to, value-laden assessments. The on-line environment also affords privacy with responses that is not possible in the classroom.

## Community Health Nursing Course

Student involvement in community assessments promotes awareness of the needs of individuals and groups in various communities. Communication with individuals and community leaders fosters interaction and development of students caring for populations possibly different from the students' background. The empathy developed can enhance the socialization of nursing students to be more aware of the professional nursing value of social justice. Planning effective community interventions enables students to achieve the affective learning level of valuing the residents' needs as well as efforts to achieve change.

Curriculum requirements of completing community service hours best illustrates the affective domain goals. Students become engaged and committed by self-selecting, with faculty approval, a particular community service project or organization (Shulman, 2007). Each semester, students organize or participate in community blood drives, or blood pressure, scoliosis, or other wellness screenings. Other community service projects chosen include escorting adults and children with disabilities to the zoo or museum, participating in the senior center dances, or holding reading classes for elementary school children. An appreciation of the chosen community organization is evident as the students share their experiences.

Another community course affective learning strategy centers around art. Individuals or small groups of students identify an art medium that portrays the word community. Examples of art media used by students include quilts, paintings, music, poems, disasters, or videos. This strategy is fun and enables students to fully conceptualize the essence of community (R. Coker, personal communication, February 15, 2008).

## End of Life Issues Course

A faculty-created role-play may be used during the semester in which acute care or end-of-life issues are taught. Several members of the nursing faculty play the role of a patient who is near death, while inter-generational family members are in conflict regarding end-of-life decisions. Exaggerated costumes and dramatic acting quickly engage the students' attention in the learning activity. End-of-life issues can be emotionally charged for students as well as faculty, and a role-play learning activity promotes a safe environment in which to explore personal feelings prior to encountering the situation in an actual clinical setting. Portrayal of diverse family members' conflicting desires related to end-of-life issues presents the value of respect for the patient's autonomy and informed consent. This role-play is performed once with faculty making blatant errors in dealing with the patient, family, healthcare team members, and the actual nursing care and environment. Students individually list identified errors, compare the list with a peer, and then engage in a class discussion to problem-solve more effective methods of dealing with the difficult and emotionally-charged situation of end-of-life. The role-play and discussion promote recall of personal experiences, and exploration of effective methods of interacting with patients and family members. Immediately following the class discussion, a second role-play is performed with several student volunteers who play the role of the healthcare providers – with the same faculty playing the patient and family members. Prompts from students who are not participating in the role play are welcomed. End-of-life issues students once regarded as depressing become real in the situation, and an opportunity to provide the ideal nursing care for patient and family is realized. The classroom provides a safer environment for reflection on the emotionally charged concepts than occurs with an unexpected clinical situation with an actual patient. The outcomes of valuing patient autonomy can be evaluated immediately by student discussion comments, and then later evaluated in the clinical setting when similar situations occur.

## Summary

Goleman (1995) states that increased empathy can be linked to increased motivation to intervene. Those engaged in nursing as a discipline must develop motivation to intervene and provide quality care for their patients. Planning educational strategies to promote affective learning is a necessary component in nursing education. Planning strategies to incorporate the affective domain can be integrated with teaching content for the cognitive or psychomotor domain.

Effectiveness of affective teaching and learning must be evaluated using different criteria than is used in either the cognitive or psychomotor domains. The teaching strategy must be evaluated for its effectiveness. Learner participation, enjoyment, or motivation encouraged by the activity are outcomes for measuring the receiving and responding levels of affective learning, the engagement element of Schulman's (2002) heuristic, and the caring category of Fink's (2003) significant learning.

- Did the student reflect on or critique the learning experience?
- Did the teaching strategy achieve the intended outcome of student valuing and internalizing the concept?
- Was the student involved in making judgments or designing actions?
- Are professional nursing behavioral patterns being formed that can be observed in student interactions with patients?
- Is the student demonstrating commitment to the actions that have been prompted by the understanding gained?
- Is the behavior and commitment becoming part of the student's identity, yet the student exhibits an openness and motivation to continually seek additional learning?

The educational strategies presented in this chapter are intended to provide suggestions for incorporating the affective domain in nursing education, with the hope that ideas for many more "effective affective" strategies will be sparked in creative nursing educators. These strategies can be used as a springboard for developing your own "effective affective" educational strategies.

## Learning Activities

1. Write two to three student learning objectives in the affective domain.
2. Associate the learning objectives in #1 to Krathwohl's levels of attainment in the affective domain (receiving, responding, valuing, organization, or characterization).
3. Plan teaching strategies to promote attainment of the student learning objective in #1.
4. Observe a group of junior and senior nursing students in the skills lab. Identify which element of Schulman's model each student is experiencing.
5. In a clinical setting, assess students for behaviors that reflect each of Fink's categories of Significant Learning.
6. Develop a survey tool that can be used to evaluate learning in the affective domain, focusing on both immediate and long-term behavior changes. The following chart may be helpful in completing these learning activities:

| Student Learning Objective | Level of Affective Attainment | Teaching Strategy | Method of Evaluation |
|---|---|---|---|
|  |  |  |  |
|  |  |  |  |
|  |  |  |  |

7. Identify teaching strategies for the affective domain that can be used for distance learning.
8. Develop affective learning goals for a clinical nursing elective course.

## Educational Philosophy

Nursing students enter the classroom and clinical setting with a variety of backgrounds and personal experiences that make each individual unique. The nursing instructor uses this uniqueness as a building block to help the learners achieve their learning goals. The instructor employs cognitive, psychomotor, and affective teaching strategies in a climate conducive to making learning safe, practical, and fun. — Lynn Norman

My teaching philosophy includes two core values that are also inherent in my nursing philosophy: the dignity of each individual and an emphasis on quality. Each student brings valuable attributes and experiences to the learning environment, and educators build on these to assist the student to develop a commitment to learning and a self-expectation of providing quality nursing care. Transformation occurs through collaboration and active engagement as both learner and faculty seek knowledge, understanding, and quality nursing. — Arlene Morris

## References

Alderman, S., & Brien, A. (1987). *I am the broccoli.* Customer Communication Systems, Inc.

American Association of Colleges of Nursing. (2008). *Essentials of baccalaureate nursing education.* Washington, DC: Author.

Belanger, F., & Jordan, D. (2000). *Evaluation and implementation of distance learning: Technologies, tools, and techniques.* Hershey, PA: Idea Group.

Benner, P. (2000). The wisdom of our practice. *American Journal of Nursing, 100*(10), 99-105.

Billings, D. M., & Halstead, J. A. (Eds.). (2009). *Teaching in Nursing: A guide for faculty* (3rd ed.). St. Louis: Mosby.

Brookfield, S. D. (2006). *The skillful teacher: On technique, trust, and responsiveness in the classroom* (2nd ed). San Francisco: Jossey-Bass.

Caputi, L., & Gauldin, D. (2001), *Tucked in Tight.* [DVD]. Glen Ellyn, IL: College of DuPage.

Davis, M. (2003). What's wrong with character education? *American Journal of Education, 110*(1), 32-58.

Fink, D. L. (2003). *Creating significant learning experiences: An integrated approach to designing college courses.* San Francisco: Jossey-Bass.

Goleman, D. (1995). *Emotional intelligence.* New York: Bantam.

Goulet, C., & Owen-Smith, P. (2005). Cognitive-affective learning in physical therapy education: from implicit to explicit. *Journal of Physical Therapy Education, 9*(3), 47-72.

Glo GermTM (1968), Moab, UT  84532 (telephone 435-259-5931; 1-800-842-6622). www.glogerm.com

Killen, A. R. (2002). Morality in perioperative nurses. *Association of Operating Room Nurses AORN Journal, 75*(3), 532-549. Retrieved June 20, 2008, from ProQuest Nursing & Allied Health Source database

Krathwohl, D. R., Bloom, B. S., & Masia, B. B. (1964). *Taxonomy of educational objectives: The classification of educational goals. Handbook II: Affective Domain.* New York: David McKay Co.

Martin, B. L. (1989). A checklist for designing instruction in the affective domain. *Educational Technology, 29,* 7-15.

Martin, B. L., & Briggs, L. J. (1986). *The affective and cognitive domains: Integration for instruction and research.* Englewood Cliffs, NJ:  Educational Technology Publications.

McCausland, L. L. (2002). A precepted perioperative elective for baccalaureate nursing students. *Association of Operating Room Nurses.* Retrieved January 31, 2008, from http://findarticles.com/p/articles/mi_m0FSL/is_6_76/ai_95681589

Mezirow, J. & Associates (2000). *Learning as transformation: Critical perspectives on a theory in progress.* San Francisco: Jossey-Bass.

Miller, M. (2005). Teaching and learning in affective domain. In M. Orey (Ed.) *Emerging perspectives on learning, teaching, and technology.* Retrieved June 15, 2008, from http://projects.coe.uga.edu/epltt/

Oermann, M. H., & Gaberson, K. B. (2006). *Evaluation and testing in nursing education* (2nd ed.). New York: Springer Publishing.

Russo, T. C., & Ford, D. J. (2006). Teachers' reflection on reflection practice. *Journal of Cognitive Affective Learning, 2*(2), 1-12.

Shephard, K. (2008). Higher education for sustainability: Seeking affective learning outcomes. *International Journal of Sustainability in Higher Education, 9*(1), 87-98.

Shirts, R. G. (1977). *BaFaBaFa: A cross culture simulation.* Del Mar, CA: Simulation Training System.

Shulman, L. S. (2002). Making a difference: A table of learning. *Change, 34,* 36-44.

Shulman, L. S. (2007). Making differences: A table of learning. *The Carnegie Foundation for the Advancement of Teaching and Learning.* Retrieved February 15, 2008 from www.carnegiefoundation.org/publications/sub.asp?key=452&subkey=612

Smeltzer, C. H., & Vlasses, F. R. (2003). *Ordinary people, extraordinary lives: The stories of nurses*. Indianapolis, IN: Sigma Theta Tau International.

Tsushima, T., & Gegas, T. (2001). Role taking and socialization in single-parent families. *Journal of Family Issues, 22,* 267-288.

Zanuck, R. D., & Zanuck, L. F. (Producers), & Beresford, B. (Director). (1989). *Driving Miss Daisy.* [Motion picture]. (Available from Warner Home Video, 4000 Warner Blvd., Burbank, CA 91522)

Zimmerman, B. J., & Phillips, C. Y. (2000). Affective learning: Stimulus to critical thinking and caring practice. *Journal of Nursing Education, 39,* 422-428.

# UNIT 4: TEACHING SPECIAL TOPICS IN THE NURSING CURRICULUM

# CHAPTER 30

# TEACHING CARING

## JoAnne Duffy, PhD, RN

---

The content of this chapter relates to the following major content areas and subconcepts on the Certified Nurse Educator Examination Detailed Test Blueprint:

**Participate in Curriculum Design and Evaluation of Program Outcomes**
- Actively participate in the design of the curriculum to reflect current nursing and healthcare trends

**Engage in Scholarship of Teaching**
- Use evidence-based resources to improve and support teaching

**Function Effectively within the Institutional Environment and the Academic Community**
- Identify how social, economic, political and institutional forces influence nursing and higher education
- Integrate the values of respect, collegiality, professionalism, and caring to build an organizational climate that fosters the development of learners and colleagues

---

## Introduction

Caring is an elusive concept. On the one hand, it is a common word used in all cultures and among human beings as they live and work in society. In this larger context, caring is associated with positive feelings or empathetic concern, but it also has meanings associated with protective actions, providing for or assisting others, and often involves responsibility such as the case with parents and children. On the other hand, the word, caring, is specific to nursing as both a moral ideal (Watson, 1988) and a way of being (Swanson, 1991) with patients and families. Used in this context, its meaning connotes a human way of relating that includes specific knowledge, actions, and demeanors or attitudes. The profession of nursing has considered the concept of caring to be fundamental to good practice. It is often cited as one of the central concepts in nursing curricula and is frequently "taught" through faculty role-modeling or embedded in classes on therapeutic communication. It is assumed that nursing faculty value caring and students grasp its importance to patients and the profession of nursing. Yet, the literature is replete with accounts of faculty and student incivility (Clark, 2007; 2008; Ehrmann, 2005) and non-caring nursing practices (Duffy, 2009).

Caring relationships with patients and families have preliminarily been linked to improved patient outcomes (Burt, 2007; Duffy, 1992; Latham, 1996; Swan, 1998; Wolf, Colahan, & Costello, 1998; Yeakel, Maljanian, Bohannon, & Coulombe, 2003) and recently have been highlighted as critical to meaningful work for nurses (Duffy, 2009). It is through relationships that information is exchanged, feelings and concerns are shared, interventions are provided, and outcomes are attained. Likewise, relationships among healthcare professionals caring for specific patients have been demonstrated to be associated with improved health outcomes (Brewer, 2006). For nursing, caring has been called the essence or central tenet (Watson, 1979; 1985) and has been cited as a moral imperative (Hartman, 1998). One would expect that a concept considered so crucial to a profession would be extensively taught by highly competent experts, in a rigorous manner, with multiple ways of assessing its achievement.

The teaching of caring, however, has been debated since the late 1980s, when the curriculum revolution first established the need for a more flexible, reflective, and empowering way of educating nurses (Bevis & Watson, 1989; National League for Nursing [NLN], 1989; Tanner, 1990b). The importance of grounding nursing education in caring was seen as a way to meet the challenges of an ever-changing, disease-oriented, technologically-driven healthcare system. The available literature has provided nursing faculty with some preliminary evidence about teaching and learning caring. For example, in Beck's (2001) metasynthesis of caring within schools of nursing, 14 qualitative studies in schools of nursing were analyzed. Using a meta-ethnographic method, four major themes emerged:

- caring among faculty
- faculty–nursing student caring
- caring among nursing students
- caring between nursing students and patients

The central component of these themes was "reciprocal connecting," which consisted of presencing, supporting, sharing, competence, and uplifting effects. This inductive approach implied that experiencing caring in the educational environment is contagious and even has a "trickle down effect" that can be translated into the practice environment (Beck, 2001 p. 108). Faculty caring through role modeling has been studied and seems to enhance students' caring behaviors (Gramling & Nugent, 1998; Grams, Kosowski, & Wilson, 1997; Schaffer and Juarez,1996), while students' knowledge of caring practices has been shown to increase through innovative teaching methods (Hoover, 2002; Pullen, Murray, & McGee, 2001).

However, due to limitations in terms of sample size, methodology, and analytical approaches, gaps and inconsistencies in how best to teach caring remain.

Recent ideas such as integrative learning, liberating pedagogies, and problem-based and experiential learning have added to the repertoire of nursing faculty as they go about teaching this construct so central to nursing. And, the complex, more interdependent and global practice environment has heightened the need for a more relationship-centered professional nurse with knowledge, skills, and values that embrace interaction and connection, systems thinking, collaboration, teamwork, and reflective awareness (Duffy, 2009). The purpose of this chapter then is to highlight the most current thinking about teaching caring within the unpredictable, nonlinear nature of today's health systems.

## Complex Health Systems

A more realistic view of health system systems is emerging today, based on complexity science (Cohen & Stewart, 1994). In this way of thinking, health systems are living systems that contain patterns of relating, the ability to self-organize, and eventually the capability to self-sustain (Zimmerman, Plsek, & Lindberg, 2002). The word, **complex**, suggests multifaceted, complicated connections among a wide variety of parts. **Adaptive** suggests change or modification or the ability to adjust. And lastly, **system** represents a collection of many interdependent factors, which in the case of health care can connote persons, diseases, organisms, and the many relationships among them. In a complex system, there is no central controller; rather, individuals with their own multifaceted characteristics, contribute to the system through their many complex connections or relationships. Thus, it is not the individual that is most critical but the relationships between individuals.

However, most well-meaning members of the health system interact in a variety of ways that oftentimes end up fragmented, specialized, and isolated. Relationships, especially the nature of the relationships among the members is invisible to most and not considered noteworthy. Yet, those who can "see the whole," who view the patient as a living system, and understand that both patients and healthcare providers are multidimensional humans living in diverse communities are able to comprehend the significance of the many daily relational processes that can eventually have sizeable results. And the quality of these relationships adds value to complex systems. As masters of caring relationships, nurses have a unique opportunity to contribute to health systems.

With such a view, educators, particularly nursing educators, have the challenge of helping students notice the relevance of caring relationships versus more mechanistic procedures as the central subject matter of nursing. Curricula need to focus more attention to knowledge, skills, and attitudes in relationship-building, interactions among members, teamwork, and interdependency. As this content becomes the dominating theme, students become better able to interact, engage, and participate in decision-making.

## The Relationship Nature of Teaching and Nursing

Understanding nursing as a practice is fundamental to teaching caring. In the clinical setting, where practice is showcased, nursing knowledge, professional skills, and values converge to create situations or encounters that contribute to the health of individuals and groups. After prolonged learning, repetitive practice, and interaction with experts (faculty and other nurses), nurses perform what they know and value "in relationship."

Likewise, the transmission of knowledge and resulting growth (learning) in students occurs "in relationship." This is accomplished between student and teacher, student and the self, or between student and others, most often peers or clinical role models and preceptors. And it is often the quality of the relationship/s that determines the success of the teaching (learning). As such, relationships hold a central place in learning nursing and may be a critical factor in the ongoing development of caring capacity. The dependency of learning on relationship/s is important to consider, especially in nursing, where competencies such as caring relationships, collaboration, and engagement are so vital for expert professional practice. The subject matter of nursing and the way it is taught, however, is often fragmented as well-meaning faculty see the curriculum as separate from the practice.

Blending the subject matter of nursing, caring, with the relationships inherent in learning can help students to cultivate caring approaches and develop caring dispositions. "Teaching is more than imparting knowledge; it also is about openness, connection, and creativity" (Duffy, 2009, p. 135). The nature of relationships is at least two-way; thus simply imparting information to students does not take advantage of the built-in nature of teaching-learning situations. Attending to what students bring to the classroom or clinical setting, the content and conduct of their interactions, the sociocultural context, and the unique characteristics of patients, families, and clinical settings that occur in nursing educational programs are vital responsibilities of effective teachers. But relationships tend to be messy and complex, and nursing educators often overlook the power of this aspect of teaching and learning. Yet, using relationship as a context for learning caring helps students and faculty develop shared meanings, elicit relevant data, listen, notice cues, establish rapport, and develop mutually trusting interactions. To use the student-teacher relationship effectively in nursing education, a comprehensive understanding of the content area of nursing is required.

## Requirements for Caring Professional Practice: Content

The view of this author includes nursing as a relationship-oriented profession that best advances health when those relationships are caring in nature (Duffy & Hoskins, 2003; Duffy, 2009). "In healthcare situations, persons with health needs meet in relationship with healthcare providers who function independently and collaboratively with them. Independent relationships are those between patients and families and a healthcare provider, in this case, the professional nurse. Furthermore, collaborative relationships among the healthcare team are necessary to cohesively provide services that are holistic and complementary" (Duffy, 2009, p. 195). Depicted as the Quality-Caring Model© (Duffy & Hoskins, 2003; Duffy, 2009), a significant proposition of the model, "feeling cared-for influences the attainment of intermediate and terminal health outcomes" (p. 199) best sums up the relationship nature of nursing (See Figure 1). Nursing's role in this model is to engage in caring relationships with self and others to engender feeling "cared for." Feeling "cared for" helps patients and families feel secure, take risks, self-disclose and assume self-healing or self-caring ways. In this model, professional nurses focus on the person rather than the disease and have an appreciation for the larger system in which they work.

To practice in a manner that results in recipients feeling "cared for" requires specialized knowledge, behaviors, values, and attitudes (See Table 1). First learning how to care requires an understanding of human beings as they interact with self and communities. This includes the human nature of the student. As multidimensional beings, humans live, work, and grow "in relationship." An understanding of the many different relationships (biologic, emotional, sociocultural, and spiritual) humans form during their lives, the integration of them into unique whole persons, and the possibilities inherent in human persons is paramount. Helping students learn to appreciate the relationship nature of humans including their evolution over the lifespan is a prerequisite to caring for others. Grasping how humans relate in families and communities is part of this content area as well.

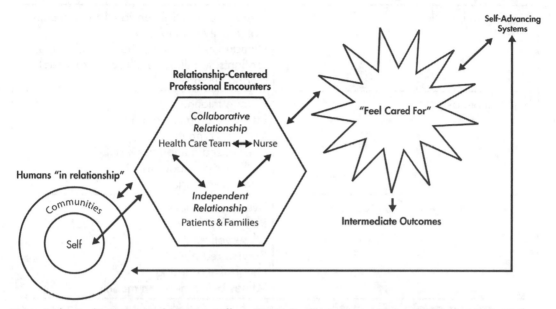

Figure 1. The Quality-Caring Model.© From Duffy, J. (2009). Quality Caring in Nursing: Applying a Middle Range Theory to Clinical Practice, Education and Leadership. New York: Springer Publishing. Published with permission.

**Figure 1.** The Quality-Caring Model

Second, comprehending the human person's experience of health and illness including the adjustment to an illness, changes in social roles and responsibilities, family relationships, and the many personal losses associated with illness is necessary to adequately respond to health needs. Learning how to experience another's world is important to effectively help them feel "cared for," an antecedent to healthy outcomes (Duffy, 2009).

Third, understanding the factors inherent in caring relationships must be mastered. These factors have been identified by nursing theorists (Watson, 1979; 1985) and more recently by empirical research (Duffy, Hoskins, & Seifert, 2007).

**Mutual problem solving** connotes behaviors that help patients and families understand how to think about their health and illness. Nurses and patients decide, after weighing options, how to approach and solve health problems. Behaviors such as providing information, reframing, helping patients learn, exploring alternative ways of dealing with health problems, and validating what patients know about

| Nursing Knowledge | Interacting, Multidimensional Human Beings<br>Community Relationships<br>Human's experience of health and illness<br>(patients, families, health care providers)<br>Caring Factors |
|---|---|
| Nursing Behaviors | Human relating<br>Effective communication<br>Cultural competence<br>Specialized human need skills<br>Authentic collaboration<br>Community engagement |
| Nursing Values/Attitudes/Meanings | Lived experiences<br>Reflective Analysis<br>Observation<br>Service Learning<br>Integrative Learning<br>Values-based decision models |

**Table 1.** Requirements for Caring Professional Practice

their illnesses are important. Accepting feedback from patients and families, and experimenting with different ways of doing things, are also activities that communicate this factor. Listening to how patients care for themselves at home or how they approach life challenges implies that nurses are continuously learning and engaging patients and families in mutual discussions of their health problems.

The second factor, **attentive reassurance**, refers to nurse availability and hopeful outlook (Duffy et al., 2007), even in the face of poor prognoses. Evidence of nurses' continued availability affects expectations of future availability; it assures patients and families that they can rely on the nurse, resulting in a sense of security about the healthcare situation. Nurses who are confident and encourage possibilities convey this factor. Helping students to understand the significance of authentic noticing, active listening, and focusing on the person of the patient is the content important to this factor. Providing reassurance to a patient also includes the choice to "be with" and "do for" together. This is especially difficult for newer nurses who are concerned about mastering specific procedures.

**Human respect**, another caring factor, refers to honoring the worth of humans, including the unique person experiencing an illness or health-related concern. It includes honoring the rights and responsibilities all human persons as significant members of society. Using an **encouraging manner** refers to the demeanor or attitude of the nurse. It assumes that human persons are intrinsically motivated and have abilities to grow and change. Nurses who allow patients to express their feelings, whether good or bad, while remaining open to multiple points of view convey this factor. Providing a supportive stance, offering non-judgmental encouragement, and using congruent verbal and non-verbal behaviors are important to this factor. **Appreciation of unique meanings** is concerned with a patient's understanding of the world. Knowing what is important to patients including their sociocultural context avoids making assumptions about patients and families. Rather, as nurses use those features that are important to patients and families in the provision of care, it helps them feel capable and confident in self-caring. Facilitating a **healing environment** refers to the setting where caring is taking place and the structures for maintaining privacy, safety, and comfort. Maintaining safety in the health setting is a major role of professional nurses and this factor is tied to content that ensures healing and protective situations. **Basic human needs** include the well-known physical needs (air, food and fluids, elimination, sleep, and rest), safety and security needs, social and relational needs, self-esteem needs, and self actualization needs (Maslow, 1954, 1971). Understanding, recognizing, and attending to the primacy of these needs during acute illness along with **affiliation needs**, persons' needs for belonging and membership in families or other social contexts, helps students to comprehend their responsibility for meeting them. These eight caring factors form the basis for competent expert professional nursing and under gird all nursing interventions. Viewed in this manner, they form the in-depth content pertinent to the practice of nursing. Helping students explicitly comprehend their meanings is the work of nursing educators.

## Using the Caring Behaviors

The behaviors essential for caring professional practice must be repetitively rehearsed in multiple settings. These include human relating skills, particularly effective communication, ways of being with others in differing contexts, congruence between verbal and non-verbal behaviors, cultural competence, specialized skills related to human needs, authentic collaboration, and community engagement. Typically, nursing skills laboratories are used to teach specialized nursing skills. Yet, if caring as the central concept pertinent to professional nursing is to be learned, behaviors associated with it must be rehearsed. Thus, nursing skills laboratories are essential places to help students develop the caring skills required for good practice. Role playing, simulation, and case study approaches followed by videotaped actions are useful in helping students to process their actions and learn how to improve. Intentionally integrating caring professional practice within common psychomotor skills requires revising common competencies to integrate caring with other specific psychomotor skills.

Such an approach to learning caring behaviors was reported by the Minnesota Baccalaureate Psychomotor Skills Faculty Group (2008). In this multisite study, investigators used the well-known blood pressure measurement as a way to integrate caring behaviors into a professional psychomotor skill. First, they revised the behaviors usually assessed during blood pressure skill evaluation to incorporate caring behaviors such as "faces patient throughout procedure, maintains eye contact, voice is congruent with patient's emotions, physical contact is performed with a gentle touch" into the procedure (p. 102). Then they provided an assigned reading, a class on caring, and evaluated the students as they demonstrated blood pressure measurement. Using a pre – post test design, they found significantly higher caring behaviors in those students who used the revised procedure. These faculty members were innovative and created a skills lab experience very similar to the practice situation where nurses continuously blend psychomotor skills with cognitive and affective dimensions of practice (**being** and **doing** together). In this way, the process of human caring was operationalized in an integrated fashion where human caring and a specialized technique worked together to provide expert caring professional practice. Similarly, the vital behavior of collaboration between health care personnel can be developed using an intentionally-designed simulation.

Finally, developing caring attitudes and meanings occurs through one's lived experiences of caring as well as through learning human caring acts by studying, self-reflecting, and observing members of one's profession. Helping students think about and interpret their relationships with patients through engaged discussions or reflective analysis assists students to attach significance to relationships. In summary, **caring content** includes specific knowledge of the self, the holistic nature of human beings as they relate to others over a lifetime, the experience of illness, the caring factors, specialized behaviors such as active communication and collaboration, and the development of a caring value system. This content is mastered over time through lived experiences of caring as well as through learning human caring by studying, self-reflecting, and observing members of one's profession. Personal caring experiences and external sources of caring knowledge combined with the more internal understanding of the self enhance caring capacity or competence.

## Caring Pedagogies

Pedagogy refers to specific methods or strategies of teaching. "A caring pedagogy utilizes the caring factors to create an environment of engagement that is genuine and student centered. **Caring,** as one of the core values of professional nursing, is honored, given high regard, and lived through the behaviors of faculty and staff. Faculty members who continuously reflect on the nature of nursing, themselves as teachers, and integrate the caring value of nursing with their words and actions set the tone of a school and become powerful role models for students" (Duffy, 2009, p. 138). In other words, teaching caring begins with the faculty member. In the role of teacher, the nursing educator who values caring will help students learn by example, looking for and pointing out "caring moments," and facilitating shared application of caring. Cultivating student-teacher caring relationships, including the use of the caring factors in classroom and clinical settings may enhance both students' and teachers' personal and professional growth. Using caring student–faculty relationships as the core of learning may decrease student anxiety and create more cohesive learning (Pullen, Murray, & McGee, 2001; Schaffer & Juarez, 1996). Such learning experiences demonstrate the essential nature of caring and offers students the chance to witness caring in action. The ultimate goal of the nursing educator is to help students become independent learners who continuously search for ways to increase their caring knowledge.

Caring pedagogy emphasizes relationships and implies that both subjective and objective components of learning are valued and used to adequately develop the knowledge-base. Simply put, caring knowledge is partially learned in the classroom or online through innovative teaching strategies followed by additional learning in the simulation laboratory. For example, a difficult scenario could be presented involving deep conflict among a nurse, physician, and respiratory therapist concerning the course of treatment for a patient who is dependent on a ventilator. The student is directed to work with the team and patient in making a safe and quality health decision. Behaviors such as: focusing, questioning techniques, active listening, clarification, assertiveness, gathering facts, readiness to engage, deep breathing, the congruence between verbal and non-verbal messages, use of humor, and demonstration of the caring factors can be observed by peers and faculty members to assess the student's skill in relating to others in challenging situations. Such a scenario would then be followed by a group reflection. Both the classroom or online and laboratory learning experiences are then perfected in clinical courses where students are confronted with real patient situations.

Subjective or internally focused knowledge helps one to see clearly how life experiences shape thoughts and behaviors. Helping students develop and understand themselves – in other words – to be self aware, lifelong learners is a pertinent strategy for both classroom and laboratory learning. Approaches such as subjective reflection, reflective analysis, mindfulness practices, and supervision can be helpful. Connecting to the self through special sensory learning activities – witnessing art, listening to music, writing poetry – accesses the often untapped wisdom within.

Learning how to effectively interact and build relationships, however, requires more objective, learner-centered activities including experiences designed to teach the patient's perspective. For example, having students get into a vacant intensive care unit (ICU) bed and remain there for 4 hours, tape recording the sounds and undergoing the many sights and smells of an ICU provides insight into a similar patient experience. Having students become "disabled" for a day by tying one arm behind the back or ambulating via wheelchair provides a more comprehensive understanding of patients' lived experiences. Sharing these experiences with the larger group of students allows many to learn the care needs of special groups of patients and families.

Merging information gained from external situations together with internal reflection is dependent on relationships – with each other, the larger system, and with the self. Schon's (1983) seminal work in learning a practice, helps to frame learning for the health professions. He advocated that professional practice required the ability to "think on your feet" and that learning together in relationship with a coach-like teacher maximized professional behaviors. In his view, reflection is considered a hallmark of understanding a professional practice. The faculty member's role is to design, facilitate, and evaluate the learning experiences in the context of relationship.

The modern term, integrative learning (Huber, Hutchings, Gale, Breen, & Miller, 2007), is a teaching approach receiving national attention as the Carnegie Foundation and the American Association of Colleges and Universities join in an innovative national project aimed at fostering students to integrate learning (The Carnegie Foundation, 2007). Integrative learning leads students to synthesize learning from a wide array of sources, learn from experience, and make significant and productive connections between theory and practice. Integrating knowledge from multiple sources is a skill necessary for quality care, so performing this activity early and repeatedly is wise. Examples of innovative educational strategies that provide opportunities for more integrative, intentional, connected learning include: first-year seminars, learning communities, cooperative group learning, inter-disciplinary studies, capstone experiences, portfolios, and student self-assessment.

Values-based experiential activities such as service learning or participating in caring groups help students accept and embrace the importance of caring as the cornerstone for professional nursing practice. Using a values-based decision model for case discussions addresses conflicts that frequently occur in practice settings and fosters values-based (caring) choices. Faculty members using such techniques help students see a course of action that best aligns with caring and produces the greatest benefit to patients and families.

Helping students learn the caring factors through focused study, simulations, and modeling creates situations where students can test their interactions in a safe place under the guidance of experts. Grounding nursing simulations in caring allows faculty to create lifelike environments where the uniqueness of the human person and the fullness of nursing practice can be understood. Likewise, in the online course environment, faculty must ensure the wholeness of patients and families is preserved.

At the graduate levels, students (who are often actively working in demanding positions) come to educational programs seeking alternatives. The faculty member who models caring and uses the power of relationship in the teaching-learning function allows graduate students to renew the meaning of nursing and perhaps "recharge" their careers. At this level of nursing education, spending time looking inward and sharing nursing experiences through reflection and interpretive activities among faculty, preceptors, and students is affirming and helps students frame new perspectives and approaches. At the same time, learning activities focused on appraising caring research adds to the knowledge of caring relationships while shaping appraisal skills. At the graduate levels, courses in health systems and reflective leadership together with clinical experiences advance caring knowledge and skills. Facilitating knowledge development of caring at the doctoral level requires faculty role models who are using the research process to answer clinical questions and advance caring theory.

Finally, acknowledging the importance of clinical teaching where caring relationships are showcased is essential. "It is in the practice setting where a sense of caring professionalism is internalized, teamwork is learned, safety and quality is ensured, accountability is developed, and an appreciation for the larger system is formed." (Duffy, 2009, p. 137). The richness of the clinical experience for nursing students cannot be overemphasized for it is in this environment that students learn what is important to pay attention to, how to react safely, and internalize caring values (See Figure 2). Caring experiences with patients and families during praxis help students appreciate its value to healthcare outcomes and their own growth as a caring person. Designing such experiences is a role of the faculty. Clinical education offers faculty members the opportunity to role model, invite thinking, create safe space for exploration, and evaluate the effectiveness of their teaching. Stimulating questions during practicums, such as what is happening in this relationship? or what seems to be important to this patient?, provide opportunities for students to reflect on their growing caring capacity.

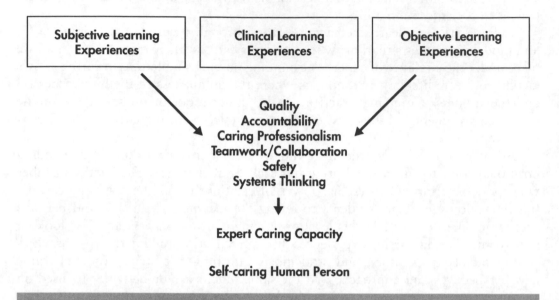

**Figure 2.** Valuable Clinical Learning Experiences

Caring pedagogy realizes that not all healthcare content can be taught in a particular nursing program. Rather, concepts considered central to practice (in this case, caring) are taught in depth and learned over time (See Table 2 for an example baccalaureate curriculum). Increasing expectations of performance are emphasized and evaluation becomes more advanced including deep understanding, connections, and context. Eventually, capacity or competency is developed that can be assessed and applied.

| Year | Fall Semester | Spring Semester |
|---|---|---|
| 1 | Knowing the Self as Caring Person<br>The Human Experience of Health and Illness | Humans in Relationship<br>Specialized Caring Behaviors I<br>Relationship-centered Caring |
| 2 | Specialized Caring Behaviors II<br>Clinical Caring I | Clinical Caring II<br>Caring Research |
| 3 | Clinical Caring III | Clinical Caring IV |
| 4 | Clinical Caring V | Caring Leadership |

**Table 2.** Example Caring Courses Threaded throughout a Baccalaureate Program of Study

## Assessing Caring Knowledge

Ensuring caring capacity or competency through formative and summative evaluation helps prepare professional nurses "to be" as well as "to do" nursing. Formatively, ensuring that all domains of learning (Bloom, 1956) are evaluated is essential. An increase in knowledge of caring, for example, does not ensure adequate performance of caring behaviors or internalization of caring values. Therefore, formative assessment of caring must include comprehensive evaluation of all domains. Using specific caring objectives that increase in complexity over a curriculum, faculty can design evaluation mechanisms that are inclusive. For example, whereas a sophomore student may "interact with patients and families," a senior student may "independently monitor and modify their interactions with patients and families." Multiple evaluation techniques, such as written essays, critical analyses, concept mapping, role modeling, peer review, asynchronously delivered simulation followed by reflective analysis, taped observation/s of behaviors, and special applications versus the rote multiple choice testing format allow for a more comprehensive evaluation of caring. In addition, self and peer reviews offer a differing perspective that enhances the faculty-only assessment.

In summary, nursing faculty have an obligation to ensure caring competency in their graduates. Formal evaluation of this learning outcome can be accomplished through a 360 degree assessment in the final semester. Student self evaluation, peer and faculty reviews, and patients' perceptions of students' caring abilities form a broad and in-depth overview of a potential graduate's caring capacity. For a review of the latter component – the patient's view – see *Want to Graduate Students Who Care?* (Duffy, 2005). These four levels of data provide the evidence from which to revise curricula. Finally, understanding students' perceptions of faculty caring provides important data for individual faculty members and the structural and process components of an educational program.

## Summary

Caring, as the most often described value associated with nursing, must remain the major thrust of nursing education in order to meet the needs of patients and families in complex health systems. A strong liberal arts foundation combined with increasingly difficult caring courses spread throughout a nursing curriculum will strengthen caring knowledge, behaviors, and attitudes. Frequent opportunities for critical reflection (both individual and group) integrated with rich caring experiences provide curricular balance and enhance caring capacity.

Educational program evaluation including assessment of student caring competencies will better inform faculty how to revise curricula to meet the caring learning needs of students. Ultimately, teaching, learning and validating caring knowledge, behaviors, and attitudes at all levels of nursing education will build a more confident workforce that can positively contribute to the evolution of complex health systems. Finally, educational research aimed at better understanding the nature and consequences of caring pedagogies is paramount.

## Learning Activities

1. Review three syllabi from a nursing program. In these syllabi, find examples of how caring is taught in the curriculum.
2. Using the same three syllabi, compare what is taught based on those syllabi to what you are teaching regarding caring. How is it the same? How is it different?
3. Ask three students to define caring in nursing practice. Ask three faculty to define caring in nursing practice. How are the definitions of the groups the same? How are they different?

## Educational Philosophy

I believe that teaching and learning are processes that are essential for growth and benefit both the teacher and the learner. Furthermore, I believe that learning occurs best in the context of a caring relationship fostered by the teacher. I believe learners are psycho-socio-cultural-spiritual individuals who have unique needs, beliefs, and experiences that influence their learning styles. Teachers have similar characteristics; they have the social responsibility to respond to learners' unique needs by maintaining expertise, providing a variety of learning experiences, and offering ongoing guidance and support in the context of a caring relationship. I believe the teaching role is to create a caring environment for learning to occur. In this environment, a spirit of cooperation, sharing, active participation, creativity, and honoring the strengths of all participants should prevail. In this way, learners become active participants who respond to each others' unique perspective/s. Through this caring relationship, both the teacher and the learner establish mutual goals, acquire new knowledge, attain skills and independence, and develop values and attitudes that contribute to improved patient outcomes and advance the profession of nursing. Teaching and learning within a caring milieu advances an appreciation for lifelong learning and the growth of both participants. — JoAnne Duffy

## References

Beck, C. T. (2001). Caring within nursing education: A metasynthesis. *Journal of Nursing Education, 40,* 101–109.

Bevis, E. O., & Watson, J. (1989). *Toward a caring curriculum: A new pedagogy for nursing.* New York: National League for Nursing.

Bloom, B. S. (1956). *Taxonomy of educational objectives, Handbook I: The cognitive domain.* New York: David McKay Co Inc.

Brewer, B. (2006). Relationships among teams, culture, safety, and cost outcomes. *Western Journal of Nursing Research, 28*(6), 641–653.

Burt, K. (2007). The relationship between nurse caring and selected outcomes of care in hospitalized older adults. *Dissertation Abstracts International* (UMI No. 3257620).

Clark, C. M. (2007). Student voices on incivility in nursing education: A conceptual model. *Nursing Education Perspectives, 29*(5), 284-289.

Clark, C. M. (2008). Student perspectives of faculty incivility in nursing education. *Nursing Outlook, 6*(1): 4-8.

Cohen, J., & Stewart, I. (1994). *The collapse of chaos: Discovering simplicity in a complete world*. New York: Viking Publishers.

Duffy, J. (1992). The impact of nurse caring on patient outcomes. In D. Gaut (Ed.). *The presence of caring in nursing* (pp. 113–136). New York: National League for Nursing.

Duffy, J., & Hoskins, L. (2003). The Quality-Caring Model©: Blending dual paradigms. *Advances in Nursing Science, 26*(1), 77–88.

Duffy, J., Hoskins, L. M., & Seifert, R. F. (2007). Dimensions of caring: Evaluation of the caring assessment tool. *Advances in Nursing Science, 30*(3), 235-245.

Duffy, J. (2009). *Quality caring in nursing: Applying a middle range theory to clinical practice, education, and leadership*. New York: Springer Publishing.

Duffy, J. (2005). Want to graduate nurses who care? Assessing nursing students' caring competencies in *Annual Review of Nursing Education, 3,* 73-97.

Ehrman, G. 2005). Managing the aggressive student. *Nurse Educator, 30*(3), 98-100.

Gramling, L., & Nugent, K. (1998). Teaching caring within the context of health. *Nurse Educator, 23*(2), 47–51.

Grams, K., Kosowski, M., & Wilson, C. (1997). Creating a caring community in nursing education. *Nurse Educator, 22*(3), 10–16.

Hartman R. L. (1998) Revisiting the call to care: An ethical perspective. *Advanced Practice Nursing Quarterly, 4*(2), 14–18.

Hoover, J. (2002). The personal and professional impact of undertaking an educational module on human caring. *Journal of Advanced Nursing, 37*(1), 70–86.

Huber, M. T., Hutchings, P., Gale, R., Breen, M., & Miller, R. (2007). Leading initiatives for integrative learning. *Liberal Education, 93*(2), 57–60.

Inui, T. (2003). *A flag in the wind: Educating for professionalism in medicine*. Washington, DC: Association of American Medical Colleges.

Latham, C. P. (1996). Predictors of patient outcomes following interactions with nurses. *Western Journal of Nursing Research, 18,* 548–564.

Maslow, A. (1954). *Motivation and personality*. New York: Harper.

Maslow, A. (1971). *The farther reaches of human nature*. New York: The Viking Press.

Minnesota Baccalaureate Psychomotor Skills Faculty Group. (2008). Nursing student caring behaviors during blood pressure measurement. *Journal of Nursing Education, 47*(3), 98 –104.

National League for Nursing. (1989). *Curriculum revolution: reconceptualizing nursing education*. New York: Author.

National League for Nursing. (1989). *Curriculum revolution: Redefining the student-teacher relationship*. New York: Author.

Pullen, R., Murray, P., & McGee, K. (2001). Care groups: A model to mentor novice nursing students. *Nurse Educator, 26,* 283–288.

Schaffer, M., & Juarez, M. (1996). A strategy to enhance caring and community in the learning environment. *Nurse Educator, 21*(5), 43–37.

Schön, D. (1983) *The Reflective Practitioner. How professionals think in action,* London: Temple Smith.

Swan, B. (1998). Postoperative nursing care contributions to symptom distress and functional status after ambulatory surgery. *Medical Surgical Nursing, 7*(3), 148–158.

Swanson, K. M. (1991). Empirical development of a middle-range theory of caring. *Nursing Research, 40*(3), 161–166.

Tanner C. A. (1990b) Reflections on the curriculum revolution. *Nursing Outlook, 29*(7), 295-299.

The Carnegie Foundation. (2007). *Integrative Learning: Opportunities to Connect.* Retrieved October 2, 2008 from www.carnegiefoundation.org/files/elibrary/integrativelearning/index.htm on

Watson, J. (1979). *Nursing: The philosophy and science of caring.* Boston: Little, Brown and Company.

Watson, J. (1985). *Nursing: Human science and human care: A theory of nursing.* Norwalk, CT: Appleton-Century-Crofts.

Waston, J. (1988). New dimensions of human caring theory. *Nursing Science Quarterly, 1,* 175-181.

Wolf, Z. R., Colahan, M., & Costell, A. (1998). Relationship between nurse caring and patient satisfaction. *Medical Surgical Nursing, 7*(2), 99–105.

Yeakel, S., Maljanian, R., Bohannon, R., & Couloumbe, K. (2003). Nurse caring behaviors and patient satisfaction: Improvement after a multifaceted staff intervention. *Journal of Nursing Administration, 33*(9), 434–436.

Zimmerman, B., Plsek, P.,k & Lindberg, C. (2002). A Complexity Science Primer. Retrieved October 2, 2008 from www.plexusinstitute.org/ideas/show_elibrary.cfm?id=150

# CHAPTER 31

# INCORPORATING SPIRITUALITY INTO THE CURRICULUM

**Diann A. DeWitt, MS, DNS, RN, CNE**

---

The content of this chapter relates to the following major content areas and subconcepts on the Certified Nurse Educator Examination Detailed Test Blueprint:

**Participate in Curriculum Design and Evaluation of Program Outcomes**
- Actively participate in the design of the curriculum to reflect current nursing and healthcare trends

**Engage in Scholarship of Teaching**
- Use evidence-based resources to improve and support teaching

**Function Effectively within the Institutional Environment and the Academic Community**
- Identify how social, economic, political and institutional forces influence nursing and higher education

---

## Introduction

We had just talked about providing spiritual care in class on Monday and on Tuesday one of my senior students (Carole) was caring for a man (Mr. Jones) about to have a craniotomy. (Names were changed to maintain confidentiality.) During that morning, Mr. Jones was very restless. The usual interventions of answering questions related to the upcoming surgery did nothing to abate his anxiety. Even having his family present did not seem to help him. When Carole asked if she could accompany him to the pre-anesthesia area, Mr. Jones and I readily agreed. During post conference Carole reported the events occurring in the pre-anesthesia area. "When we got in there, Mr. Jones seemed even more upset and nothing I did seemed to make any difference. I remembered what you said in class about spiritual care and thought maybe that would help him, but I wasn't really sure what to do. Finally, Mr. Jones asked me to pray for him. I almost panicked. I thought, now what do I do? Just then I looked up on the wall and saw a plaque that had a prayer on it. I told Mr. Jones that I wasn't very good at praying but I would be glad to read him the prayer on the plaque if that was OK with him. He agreed. I'm not even sure what that prayer said but it had something to do with asking for God's protection and healing. After I read the prayer, Mr. Jones visibly relaxed. He was no longer restless or anxious and he said, 'I feel much better now. Thank you' and you could just tell that he was ready for surgery."

Preparing students to provide spiritual care is a challenge for nurse educators. Even when the curriculum includes information regarding spiritual care, many students such as Carole in the preceding story, are uncomfortable with this aspect of patient care. Nursing students are not alone in feeling unprepared to provide spiritual care. Practicing nurses report recognizing that spiritual care is a vital aspect of caring for the whole person, yet they indicate they are ill-prepared to deliver this care (Harrington, 1995; Narayanasamy, 1993; Piles, 1990; Schnorr, 1988). Some report a lack of inclusion of spiritual care in their nursing programs (Harrington, 1995; Pullen, Tuck & Mix, 1996; Sellers & Haag, 1998). Additionally, nurse educators agree, in theory, with the need to address spiritual issues; however, many are unsure about the content, unaware of effective instructional methods to use, and, to varying degrees, uncomfortable with the topic (Lemmer, 2002).

The aim of this chapter is to provide nurse educators with salient information regarding preparing student nurses to provide spiritual care. Initial information addresses what spiritual care is and why it needs to be included in the curriculum. Subsequently, evidence to support the preparation of nursing students is discussed. Finally, information concerning transitioning spiritual care from the classroom to practice is presented.

## What is Spirituality and Spiritual Care?

The story of Mr. Jones and Carole at the beginning of the chapter illustrates one way to provide spiritual care; however, praying with a patient, while very important to many people, is not the only way to provide spiritual care. To understand the many forms of spiritual care, an exploration of the concept of spirituality is essential. Prior to discussing spirituality and spiritual care definitions, a brief tour of worldviews, or philosophical perspectives, may be beneficial.

What is a worldview? Simply put, a worldview is how we see the world around us. The American Heritage Dictionary of the English Language (2000) defines worldview as "the overall perspective from which one sees and interprets the world." This complex way one interprets what is visible and not visible in this universe is formed by multiple factors. Those factors include, but are not limited to:

- Personality
- Other people
- Genetic make-up
- Environmental influences

- Community
- Culture

Often persons from similar backgrounds form views of the world that are congruent. When discussing spirituality and spiritual care, it is essential to be cognizant of a variety of philosophical perspectives or worldviews. Worldview is closely associated with the culture in which persons live. Therefore, it is beneficial to obtain common beliefs about life and the world from others to more fully understand the differences. It follows that persons with different worldviews will likely differ in their concepts of spirituality and spiritual care. An example of how worldviews may impact the meaning of spirituality is presented subsequently.

There is no universal definition of spirituality or spiritual care. Lemmer (2002), in a survey of baccalaureate-nursing programs, reports that: "Most (nursing) programs did not have an 'agreed on' definition of spirituality (87.4%) or spiritual care nursing (93.8%)" (p. 484). Persons over the centuries have attempted to define spirituality. In 1981, Colliton defined spirituality as "the life principle that pervades a person's entire being, including volitional, emotional, moral-ethical, intellectual, and physical dimensions, and generates a capacity for transcendent values" (p. 492). Stoll (1989) proposes that the spiritual involves "a vertical dimension (i.e. a person's relationship with God, the transcendent, supreme values) and a horizontal dimension (i.e. the living out of the vertical dimension through one's beliefs, values, life-style, quality of life and interactions with self, others and nature)" (p. 7). Reed (1992) states, "Spirituality refers to the propensity to make meaning through a sense of relatedness to dimensions that transcend the self in such a way that empowers and does not devalue the individual. This relatedness may be experienced:
- Intrapersonally (as a connectedness with oneself)
- Interpersonally (in the context of others and the natural environment)
- Transpersonally (referring to a sense of relatedness to the unseen, God, or power greater than the self and ordinary resources) (p. 350)

Similarly, Pesut (2003) includes worldviews with key features for the commonalities in spirituality definitions.

Considering the variety of definitions, it is no wonder that confusion abounds! There is hope, however, because there are common themes contained within the definitions of spirituality. These common themes are:
- Meaning and purpose
- Transcendence
- Connectedness or relatedness (Carson, 1993; Emblen, 1992; Reed, 1992; Stallwood & Stoll, 1975).

Meaning and purpose are viewed as the seeking of relevant experiences and direction in life and work, or as the reason for being and doing (Carson, 1993). Transcendence means going beyond the material world or the search for someone (e.g. God) or something (e.g. values) outside of and greater than ourselves (Carson, 1993). Connectedness refers to relationships with self, others, community, and the environment.

With those concepts in mind, the following could be a broad definition of spirituality. "Spirituality is the invisible, unseen core of individuals that contributes to their uniqueness and communes with a transcendent being (a higher power or God) or transcendent values that provide meaning, purpose, and connectedness" (DeWitt-Weaver, 2001, p. 8). Please note this definition is not confined to one worldview, rather it allows for differences in worldview. For example, persons who espouse a New Age philosophy may choose the transcendent value of self-actualization as the source of meaning, purpose, transcendence, and connectedness. On the other hand, persons with a Christian perspective would likely identify their source of transcendence as God through Jesus. In other words, persons embracing various philosophies or religions would likely find their source of transcendence, meaning, purpose, and connectedness in a higher power or values.

With the broad definition of spirituality in mind, providing spiritual care is focused on the uniqueness at the very core of each person. Spiritual care seeks to assist individuals to remain connected to their source of transcendence, discover or reaffirm their meaning and purpose in life, as well as impact connectedness (with God or a higher power, self, others, and the environment). What would this mean for a person suffering with a terminal illness? How would spiritual care be implemented for a grieving mother who has just lost her baby? What about spiritual care for the nursing student who is failing in clinical?

You may be saying to yourself, "Those situations would benefit from some good psychosocial care." You may be right. However, it is critical that we remember we are whole persons. While we arbitrarily divide human beings into parts for study, we sometimes fail to put the pieces back together to care for the person in a holistic manner. Realistically, we are complexly integrated persons and therefore, our mind, body, and spirit are interconnected in such a way that they are difficult to address separately. Frankl (1975) said that the spirit is the core of a person's being expressed through the mind, emotions, and body. Stallwood and Stoll (1975) echo this belief and indicate a person's spirit enables awareness of and establishment of a relationship with God (as defined by the person). They also provide a model that explicates the inter-relatedness of humans. In the model of concentric circles, spirit is in the center surrounded by the psychosocial first, then the biological. The view that the spirit is the core of the person and is expressed through the body, mind, and emotions sheds light on the seeming allusiveness of the spirit as a separate and distinct aspect of individuals.

Where does religion fit with spirituality? Some would equate the two terms; however, when Emblen (1992) examined the nursing literature for use of the terms, the two terms were delineated differently. She concluded that spirituality was the broader term and the words most frequently associated with it were personal, life, principle, animator, being, God (god), quality, relationship, and transcendent. The words most frequently used to define religion were system, beliefs, organized, person, worship, and practices. Based on Emblen's analysis of the literature, she concluded that "religion has to do with a person's belief system and worship practices. On the other hand, spirituality has to do with meaning and purpose in life, maintaining personal relationships and transcending a given moment" (Emblen, 1992, p. 47). While spirituality is not the same thing as religion, most persons express their spirituality through a specific religion. Catanzaro and McMullen's (2008) study supports that while there is often a close relationship between spirituality and religion, they are not synonymous terms.

Using the aforementioned definition of spirituality and spiritual care provides a focus for planning spiritual care. In addition, assessment of religious affiliation is also pertinent to providing spiritual care as many persons express aspects of their spirituality through a formalized religion. It is also important to be aware of cultural differences and their impact upon the worldview of persons.

### Spiritual Well-Being, Spiritual Needs, Spiritual Distress, and Spiritual Formation (Development)

In nursing literature, several terms are used to describe patients' spirituality. The most commonly used terms are spiritual well-being (including potential for enhanced spiritual well-being), spiritual needs, spiritual distress, and spiritual formation (development).

According to the National Interfaith Coalition on Aging (1975) spiritual well-being is "the affirmation of life in relationship with God, self, community and environment that nurtures and celebrates wholeness" (p. 12). Ellison (1983) conceptualized spirituality as multidimensional containing both horizontal and vertical components that interact dynamically within the person. To measure these dimensions, Ellison constructed a Spiritual Well-Being (SWB) scale that has two major components. They are existential well-being and religious well-being. The former focuses on psychosocial aspects of SWB while the latter describes a person's relationship with God or a higher being.

Spiritual needs are the second approach to spirituality in nursing. They include the need for:

- Meaning and purpose in life
- Love, including giving and receiving love, unconditional love, relatedness and trust
- Hope and faith
- Forgiveness from God, self, and others (Fish & Shelly, 1978; Highfield & Cason, 1983; Stallwood & Stoll, 1975).

The third approach to spirituality identified by Carson (1993) is spiritual distress and is defined as "disruption in the life principle which pervades a person's entire being and integrates and transcends one's biological and psychosocial nature" (Ackley & Ladwig, 2002, p. 711). Spiritual distress is an accepted nursing diagnosis and may be evident in a variety of situations. Defining characteristics of spiritual distress is examined later in this chapter.

The last approach to spirituality noted in the literature is spiritual formation or development. It is logical to conclude that individuals progress in the spiritual dimension much the same as through psychosocial and moral development. We often talk of each person being on a journey in this life. If we are truly multidimensional and yet holistic beings, how we progress on this journey is also multidimensional. While there is a paucity of research to support this approach, theologians have addressed spiritual development and compared it to Erickson's stages of psychosocial development (Carson, 1989). In addition, the idea of moral development, which has a strong research base, is closely aligned with spiritual development (Gilligan, 1982; Rest, 1986). Further exploration of spiritual formation or development may assist nurses in better understanding themselves as well as others.

## Why Spirituality and Spiritual Care in the Curriculum?

In this section the historical roots of spirituality in nursing, standards for inclusion of spiritual care in nursing practice, and research related to spiritual care are presented.

### Historical Roots of Spirituality in Nursing

Care of the whole person is at the heart of nursing and has its roots in nursing history. Carson (1989) states that many historians credit the earliest nurses with "...a holistic but intuitive response to health needs..." (p. 54). "Spiritual care was not seen as separate but as woven into total nursing interventions" (Carson, 1989, p. 55).

The practice of holistic care also was noted in ancient civilizations when religion and health care were combined and administered by priest-healers (Donahue, 1996). While many religions followed this pattern, the combination of religion and health care was clearly evident with the advent of Christianity as the care of the sick and suffering took on a spiritual meaning (Donahue, 1996). Barnum (2003) further credits Christianity as "the first religion to understand care of the ill as an important spiritual charge" (p. 30). Christian hospitals were founded in the fourth century as places for the poor, sick, strangers, and the aged. Florence Nightingale promoted holistic care as she advocated treating the person, not just the disease.

The focus on the whole person continued throughout nursing history until early in the twentieth century when significant scientific advances and the scientific view flourished. Implied in this worldview was the idea that whatever was real could be tested empirically (Barnum, 2003). The spiritual was not considered a matter for scientific inquiry and, therefore, was discounted. This worldview impacted nursing, as well as medicine, and the treatment of individuals became fragmented (Donahue, 1996). "Nurses no longer took care of the mind, body and spirit; instead, they cared for the biopsychosocial animal" (Barnum, 2003, p. 4). Consequently, any form of spirituality was included within psychology and sociology. Often spirituality became relegated to a person's specific religious affiliation or beliefs. Fortunately, the past twenty years has brought a changing world paradigm that has shaped nursing as well as society at large. This post-modernistic worldview refutes earlier modernistic (scientific) ideas about what is real. The impact of the changing world paradigm in nursing is evident in renewed interest in a holistic approach with patients, including the spiritual dimension.

## Standards for Inclusion in the Curriculum

Nurses are not only encouraged to provide spiritual care, there are codes and standards to guide nursing practice. The International Council of Nurses Code for Nurses (2000) states, "the nurse promotes an environment in which the human rights, values, customs, and spiritual beliefs of the individual, family, and community are respected." The American Nurses Association includes assessment of the spiritual dimension of persons in The Standards for Clinical Nursing Practice (1998). The Essentials of Baccalaureate Education for Professional Nursing Practice (American Association of Colleges of Nursing [AACN], 2008) maintains that graduates should provide multi-dimensional care, and that spirituality is one of those dimensions. In addition, the Joint Commission on Accreditation for Healthcare Organizations

(Joint Commission) mandates spiritual support, based on assessment, is provided to all patients. This emphasis on spirituality may be operationalized in a nursing curriculum by including it as a major concept.

## What the Research Says

According to Taylor (2005), nursing research regarding spiritual care reveals that:
1. Nurses believe patients have spiritual needs but they often go unmet
2. Patients desire nurses to provide spiritual care by being present, respectful, and caring
3. Nurses must be sensitive to their own spirituality to be effective
4. Ongoing research is needed

Additionally, Taylor suggests that integrating spiritual care with other nursing care could be more effective and would address the barrier of lack of time for providing spiritual care.

Pesut (2008) examined fundamentals textbooks to determine what was being taught to nursing students about spirituality and spiritual care. The findings indicate that comprehensive information is provided in these sources; however, Pesut asserts there are marginally examined and troubling conceptual issues that require exploration. Among the issues mentioned are the separation of spirituality and religion; definitions of spirituality that are exclusively positive while omitting the reality of suffering; and, definitions of spirituality that depend upon cognitive capacities thereby neglecting those with diminished capacities in this area. Recommendations from Pesut's study include educator recognition of the lack of clarity related to spirituality, religion and spiritual care necessitating students to critically reflect on these concepts, and use of case studies and journaling to aid student learning as opposed to exclusive use of the nursing process format.

A survey examining the inclusion of spiritual care in the curriculum was conducted using a stratified random sample of 250 baccalaureate-nursing programs in the United States (Lemmer, 2002). Of the 152 programs completing surveys, 47.7% were public (Public), 38.6% were private, religious sponsored (Religious), and 12.1% were private, nonsectarian institutions (Private). The majority of all programs surveyed (81.5%) integrated spiritual care throughout the curriculum, 3.8% required a spiritual care course, and 15.9% offered an elective spiritual care course. The most frequently included content reported was assessment of spiritual needs, the needs of dying persons, and spirituality as a component of holism or culture. Instructional methods used role modeling of spiritual care by faculty, although there were varying levels of faculty knowledge and comfort with the topic (Lemmer, 2002).

In a national survey of Registered Nurses (RNs) using a stratified random sample, Piles (1990) reported that 62% of the respondents indicated that spiritual care content was included in their nursing curricula. However, 66% of the same respondents reported feeling inadequately prepared to provide spiritual care (Piles, 1990). Additional studies report similar results (Lemmer, 2002). Denham (1990) surveyed nursing faculty in Ohio and reported a relationship between perceived abilities and teaching practices concerning spiritual care.

Several studies link the nurses' own spirituality with providing spiritual care. Taylor, Highfield, and Amenta (1994) surveyed oncology nurses to assess their attitudes and beliefs about spiritual care. Those who had the most positive attitudes toward spirituality reported including spiritual care in their practice more frequently. Similarly, Deane, Cross, and Barber (1990) found a positive relationship between the spiritual well-being of nursing students and their attitudes about providing spiritual care. Soeken and Carson (1986) reported a positive correlation between perceptions about the role of health professionals and providing spiritual care. Chung, Wong, and Chan (2006) examined the relationship of nurses' spirituality to their understanding and practice of spiritual care. Their study provides evidence to support the influence of nurses' own spirituality in providing spiritual care. Further, they assert the need for nurses to continuously care for their own spirituality.

## Preparation to Provide Spiritual Care

In a grounded theory study, DeWitt-Weaver (2001) reports that baccalaureate student nurses, in describing experiences of providing spiritual care, progressed through three stages in **becoming ready**. Initially, students in this study described their experience of **learning faith**. This stage occurred primarily in their developmental years prior to attending college and is marked by spiritual receptivity, role models, personal value development, and spiritual formation. The next phase, **thinking it through,** occurred as nursing students sought to integrate their faith with the nursing profession. In this stage, students reported the importance of sensing permission to integrate spirituality into the professional role. A supportive environment, role models, information, and group support strengthened professional and spiritual integration. The last phase of **becoming ready** is termed, **trying it out**. In this stage, nursing students described instances of providing spiritual care and reflected on the factors influencing comfort when providing spiritual care in the clinical setting. Levels of knowledge, skills, motivation, and confidence aided students in recognizing opportunities to provide spiritual care. Once opportunities were recognized, an environment supportive of providing spiritual care is essential. With increased provision of spiritual care, students described increased comfort and confidence in the professional role.

A quantitative study conducted by Meyer (2003) examined the effectiveness of nurse educators in preparing students to provide spiritual care. One finding is that little time (e.g. less than 6% of classroom and 10% of clinical) was spent in the curriculum addressing spiritual care issues. However, students' spirituality and religious commitment were the two strongest predictors of students' perceived ability to provide spiritual care. The most significant environmental influence reported by students and faculty was the emphasis in the nursing program about spiritual care.

In Schnorr's study (1988), nurses described several methods helpful in preparation to provide spiritual care. They were religious education, role modeling, personal experience, patient experiences, readings, and nursing classes.

VanLeeuwen and Cusvellar (2004) advised a framework for spirituality education in nursing that includes developing student self-awareness, therapeutic use of self, and integration of spirituality in the nursing process. Further, six key competencies were suggested:
1. Managing one's own beliefs
2. Addressing the subject of spirituality
3. Collecting data
4. Discussing and planning the impact of spirituality on the patient situation
5. Assimilating new information regarding spirituality into policy
6. Assessing outcomes of the expanded use of spirituality

Certain authors assert that spirituality and spiritual care should be taught in a holistic manner that incorporates a variety of teaching strategies (Callister, Bond, Matsumaru, & Magnum, 2004; Pesut, 2008). Examples of such teaching strategies include reflection, journaling, case studies, and conferences. Catanzaro and McMullen (2001) report using reflection and journaling to increase BSN students' spiritual sensitivity in a community health nursing course. Students reflected upon their relationship with God or any higher power and the need to be sensitive to patients' spirituality, they used journaling to assist in the process. Additionally, in conferences students dialogued with each other, faculty, parish nurses, parish social minister, and clergy. Upon completion of the course, students reported increased spiritual sensitivity and personal growth that often continued upon graduation.

Wallace, Campbell, Grossman, Shea, Lange, and Quell (2008) conducted a project integrating spirituality into the undergraduate nursing curricula, then measuring spiritual knowledge and attitudes as an outcome. Recommendations include providing definitions of and dialogue about spirituality. Further, incorporating spirituality in health assessment and throughout each clinical course in the program provides opportunities to use the nursing process in relationship to spiritual care (Wallace et al., 2008).

While additional research is needed in the area of student nurse preparation to provide spiritual care, there are some important guidelines to glean from the aforementioned studies.

- Support faculty development in the area of spirituality along with inclusion in nursing programs
- Provide students with basic information and dialogue about spiritual care that is developed further throughout the curriculum
- Encourage student self-assessment and spiritual development
- Facilitate student development of excellent therapeutic communication skills
- Assist students to integrate spirituality into nursing practice
- Provide a supportive environment both in the classroom and the clinical setting
- Encourage group support, role modeling spiritual care in the practice setting
- Use a variety of teaching strategies to facilitate the abilities of students to provide spiritual care

## Spiritual Care: From Classroom to Practice

It is essential to move from the theoretical to the practical. What do we, as nurse educators, include in the nursing curriculum? How do we become confident in our own spirituality so we are able to teach the provision of spiritual care? Beyond that, how do we best assist our students in becoming ready to provide spiritual care? In this section, spiritual self-assessment, essential information to include in the curriculum, the use of the nursing process in addressing the spiritual dimension, and support for personal spiritual development are presented.

### Spiritual Self-Assessment

For nurses to provide effective spiritual care, they must understand their own spirituality. This concept of self-awareness applies in many areas in nursing. For example, to effectively care for a person who is dying, nurses must examine their thoughts and feelings regarding their own mortality. Spiritual self-awareness may be determined through various methods. There are a variety of formal spiritual assessment instruments (e.g. Spiritual Well-Being Scale, JAREL Spiritual Well-Being Scale, and Spiritual Assessment Scale) as well as informal ways to assess one's own spirituality. Spiritual self-assessment can focus on the three main concepts of meaning and purpose in life, connectedness, and transcendence. Table 1 presents questions related to each of these broad areas and may stimulate nurses to more closely examine their own spirituality.

---

Meaning and purpose in life:

1. What gives most meaning to your life? What is the most important thing in your life?
2. What motivates you to deal with difficult life situations?
3. What has been the primary influence in shaping your life goals?

Connectedness (relatedness):

1. What relationships are most important in your life?
2. Who are you able to depend upon to help you when you need assistance?
3. What are some of the ways you perceive that someone loves and cares about you?
4. How do you handle feelings of guilt, anger, resentment, and bitterness? Do these feelings affect your relationships? Do these feelings affect your overall attitude toward life?
5. Do you believe in God or a higher power? If so, describe your beliefs. What is your God or higher power like?
6. Do you feel loved by others? Do you feel loved by God or a higher power?

Transcendence:

1. What hopes and dreams do you have (unrelated to material things)?
2. Who or what provides you with strength, hope, and faith?
3. Describe how you make it through difficult times in life.
4. What do you do to nurture your spirit?

---

**Table 1.** Questions Related to Spirituality

The questions in Table 1 are adapted to this framework from a variety of sources (Carson, 1989; Fish & Shelly, 1988; O'Brien, 1999; Taylor, 2002; Wilt & Smucker, 2001). Please note this is not a comprehensive list, but questions to stimulate self-reflection about spirituality. It may be helpful to discuss questions such as these with a trusted colleague or friend. Ongoing spiritual self-assessment is essential to personal and professional development.

## Theoretical Information Needed in the Curriculum

What should be included in the nursing curriculum related to spiritual care? A discussion of the concepts of spirituality, religion, and spiritual care is foundational. Further, when providing spiritual care, as with any nursing care, progressing through the nursing process is useful.

### Assessment

Spiritual assessment not only includes direct questions similar to the ones suggested under spiritual self-assessment, but observations as well. While establishing a rapport with patients, it is essential to listen closely to the content and context of what they say and do not say. For example, does the patient mention friends and loved ones? Does the patient talk about God, Allah, or a higher power? Does the patient express anxiety or fear about pain, suffering, or death? Is there any mention of a specific religion, belief system, or spiritual practices (e.g. prayer, communion)?

Clarifying feelings, thoughts, and information assists the nurse to better understand the patient's lived experience. It is also critical to monitor the patient's non-verbal communication and explore those observations as appropriate.

Assessment of behaviors may reveal spiritual needs or concerns. For instance, if a patient is reading an inspirational book or card, this is an opportunity to explore the meaning of this type of item to the person. A patient may be observed praying at specified times of the day or with visitors. Certain foods may be requested and others avoided depending on spiritual beliefs and practices. Similarly, there may be cues in the environment that suggest spirituality is important to the patient. For example, the presence of a rosary, Bible, Koran, inspirational literature, special clothing, paintings, and sculptures may indicate specific religious connections and offer opportunity for discussion with the patient.

Direct questions provide another means to collect assessment data from patients about spiritual concerns. In addition to the questions under the heading "Spiritual Self-Assessment," the nurse may ask how to assist the patient with spiritual concerns. Other questions may relate to specific religious practices (since most persons express their spirituality through religion) and to beliefs about the relationship of spirituality and health.

## Analysis

Analysis of assessment data may lead to a nursing diagnosis related to spirituality. Currently spiritual distress and potential for enhanced spiritual well-being are the most commonly used nursing diagnoses for the spiritual dimension. Defining characteristics for spiritual distress include, but are not limited to:

- Expresses concern with meaning of life/death and/or belief systems; questions moral/ethical implications of therapeutic regimen
- Verbalizes inner conflicts about beliefs
- Anger toward God
- Alteration in behavior/mood (Ackley & Ladwig, 2002, p. 712)

Related factors for spiritual distress could include a challenged belief or value system or separation from religious or cultural ties (Ackley & Ladwig, 2002, p. 712).

The defining characteristics for potential for enhanced spiritual well-being include, but are not limited to:

- Inner strengths…such as a sense of awareness
- Sacred source
- Harmony with self, others, higher power/God and the environment (Ackley & Ladwig, 2002, p. 718).

Related factors might include a challenging health problem or crisis.

## Goals and Outcomes

Identifying goals and outcomes related to the nursing diagnosis is the next step of the nursing process. Outcomes may include spiritual well-being and be stated as, "The patient will demonstrate spiritual well-being as demonstrated by expression of faith, hope, meaning, and purpose in life." The outcomes should relate to the specific defining characteristics that are identified. As Pesut (2008) asserts, it may be difficult to identify realistic and achievable outcomes related to the deep nature of the issues. Additionally, decreased acute and home care times for patients may negatively impact observation of goal achievement.

## Interventions

Spiritual care interventions are ways of connecting with patients and can be divided into two major categories. According to Carson (1995) spiritual care interventions can be indirect or direct. Indirect spiritual care includes listening attentively, demonstrating deep respect and value for others, responding in ways that affirm the person, and clarifying information and feelings which, in essence, compose the nurse's therapeutic use of self. Communicating in a therapeutic manner is an essential part of holistic nursing care. Providing spiritual care often depends on the value the nurse places on his/her own spirituality and perception of its importance to the patients for whom care is provided. In the study by DeWitt-Weaver (2001), several participants conveyed the importance of their own spirituality and its influence on their willingness to even try to provide spiritual care. One nursing student added, "I didn't know it (spirituality) was important to so many people" (DeWitt-Weaver, 2001, p. 57).

Referrals to a community of faith, clergy, inspirational readings, and prayer are examples of direct spiritual care. According to Carson, indirect spiritual care is always appropriate and does not require explicit patient consent. On the other hand, direct spiritual care requires the patient's permission. Nursing students report not wanting to "cross the line" into private and personal issues the patient does not wish to discuss (DeWitt-Weaver, 2001). As with any intervention, the nurse needs to carefully assess what the patient's needs are prior to providing care.

Cone (1994) reports provision of spiritual care by nursing students and nursing faculty as the basic social process of **connnecting**. The three stages of connecting are accepting, supporting, and caring. Within the deepest level of caring Cone describes a **spirit-to-spirit** connecting between the patient and the nurse. This process of connecting further explains the levels of spiritual care that may be given.

### Evaluation

The nursing process is incomplete without evaluation. Has the expected outcome been achieved? What nursing interventions were beneficial? Which ones were not? If the goal has not been achieved, does it need to be changed? Are there additional strategies that may assist the patient in making progress toward the goal? Is there new assessment information to include?

### Practice Providing Spiritual Care

A student once succinctly reported that she learned from her nursing faculty "... you do not force your beliefs on anyone else and ... you ask permission to pray (with the patient)" (DeWitt-Weaver, 2001, p. 50). This exemplifies some of the priorities for providing spiritual care. Further, it addresses the issue of whose needs are being met, the nurse's or the patient's.

The clinical setting is a fertile ground for learning to provide spiritual care. Students report that observing spiritual care modeled is helpful to them in learning to provide spiritual care (DeWitt-Weaver, 2001). They further report that faculty most often model spiritual care. As educators, we need to develop our spiritual care skills to be more effective in teaching students. Using post-conference time to discuss spiritual care needs and interventions based on actual patient situations may allow for students to debrief as well as gain support for their efforts.

## Support for Personal Spiritual Development

I am convinced that it is the character of the nurse that is evident in the care given to patients. As we progress on our individual life journeys, it is important that we take time to develop ourselves personally and professionally. In the area of spirituality, nurturing our spirits every day is as vital as caring for our physical bodies. How can this be accomplished? For some, it is by reading a holy book and praying to a personal and living God or gods. For others, it is taking a leisurely stroll in a park to enjoy nature. What lifts your spirits? What helps you maintain a positive outlook on life? What helps you deal with the difficulties that are inevitable? What helps you transcend the moment? Discover those activities that aid your spiritual development and commit to include them in your life on a routine basis. Encourage your students to do the same.

## Summary

While it is beyond the scope of this chapter to provide a comprehensive guide to teaching spiritual care in nursing education, the hope is that it has stimulated further exploration in this area. There are many excellent resources that provide more depth in the spiritual care arena. An asterisk (*) prefaces the sources in the reference list that are highly recommended. While specific religious beliefs and practices are not addressed in this chapter, some of the sources asterisked contain specific information about various religions and cultures that may assist you in teaching students to address those precise spiritual needs.

In the vignette at the beginning of the chapter, we hear Carole's description of providing spiritual care to Mr. Jones. This example gives us one story of delivering spiritual care. There are many more stories that also illustrate spiritual care in nursing. Hopefully, as you apply the information in this chapter, you will add your stories and those of your students to make the picture more complete. It is my hope this chapter provided you, as educators, with resources to assist students in becoming ready to provide spiritual care.

## Learning Activities

1. Have students compare and contrast various definitions of spirituality and journal about their reflections as well as their own spiritual self-assessment.
2. Ask students to focus on spirituality and spiritual care in patient care situations and use the SO, SO WHAT, and WHAT NOW format for journaling (Callister et al., 2004). Have them share their experiences in a clinical conference.
3. Using the guidelines provided, develop a care plan/concept map using a case study related to a patient experiencing spiritual distress.
4. Look at the nursing process forms used in a healthcare institution. Where does spirituality fit in? What interventions are used on the nursing care plan?

## Acknowledgements

During my many years of employment at St. John's College, I have explored and developed much of the material presented in this chapter. It is with deep gratitude that I thank my wonderful colleagues, administrators, and staff at St. John's College in Springfield, Illinois. Each, in their way, has provided me with timely assistance in my journey of exploring spiritual care in nursing. In addition, nurses associated with Nurses Christian Fellowship have provided tremendous inspiration and support as I progressed both personally and professionally through the journey of doctoral education. God has richly blessed my life through knowing and working with them. Last, but certainly not least, I am especially grateful for the nursing students who volunteered to participate in my dissertation as well as those who have helped me to learn more about spiritual development and spiritual care each and every year.

## Educational Philosophy

In order for teaching to be effective, it is essential that the learner be actively involved in the process and value what is taught. Students blossom in an environment where there is communication of expectations that are high, yet clear, respect for students and their diverse talents and ways of learning, timely feedback, encouragement of teacher/student contact, and development of cooperation among students so that knowledge can be shared (adapted from Chickering and Gamson, 1991). It is essential for teachers continually and accurately to assess student learning as well as the effectiveness of specific teaching strategies. — Diann A. DeWitt

## References

Ackley, B. J., & Ladwig, G.B. (2002). *Nursing diagnosis handbook: A guide to planning care*. St. Louis: Mosby.

American Association of Colleges of Nursing. (2008). The essentials of baccalaureate education for professional practice. Washington, DC: Author.

American Heritage Dictionary of the English Language (4th ed.). (2000). Retrieved April 15, 2003 from  www.bartleby.com/61/741/W0227400.html

Barnum, B. S. (2003). *Spirituality in nursing: From traditional to new age* (2nd ed.). New York: Springer.

Callister, L., Bond, A., Matsumuro, G., & Magnum, S. (2004). Threading spirituality throughout nursing education. *Holistic Nursing Practice, 18*(3), 160-166.

Carson, V. B. (1989). *Spiritual dimensions of nursing practice*. Philadelphia: Saunders.

Carson, V. B. (1993). Spirituality: Generic or Christian? *Journal of Christian Nursing, 10*(1), 24-27.

Carson, V. B. (1995, June) *Providing spiritual care*. Paper presented at Nurses Christian Fellowship Conference, Cedar Campus, MI.

Chung, Y. F., Wong, K. Y., & Chan, M. F. (2007). Relationship of nurses' spirituality to their understanding and practice of spiritual care. *Journal of Advanced Nursing, 58*, 158-170.

Cone, P. (1994). *A qualitative study of the experience of giving spiritual care*. Unpublished Master's Thesis. Azusa Pacific University, Azusa, CA.

Deane, D., Cross, J. R., & Barber, S. (November, 1990). *Spiritual well-being and role attitudes of nurses*. Paper presented at Third Biennial Neuman Systems Model International Symposium, Dayton, OH.

Denham, S. A. (1990). *Spiritual care: Ability, attitudes, and role in educating students as perceived by nursing faculty*. Unpublished Master's Thesis. Bellarmine College, Louisville, KY.

DeWitt-Weaver, D. (2001). *The experience of Christian student nurses becoming ready to provide spiritual care*. Unpublished doctoral dissertation. Indiana University. IN.

Donahue, M. P. (1996) *Nursing: The finest art: An illustrated history* (2nd ed.). St. Louis: Mosby.

Ellison, C. W. (1983). Spiritual well-being: Conceptualization and measurement. *Journal of Psychology and Theology, 11*(4), 330-340.

Emblen, J. (1992). Religion and spirituality defined according to current use in nursing literature. *Journal of Professional Nursing, 8*(1), 41-47.

Fish, S., & Shelly, J. (1988) *Spiritual care: The nurse's role.* Downer's Grove, IL: Intervarsity Press.

Fulton, R. A. (1992). *Spiritual well-being of baccalaureate nursing students and faculty and their responses about well-being of persons.* Unpublished doctoral dissertation. Widener University, Chester, PA.

Fulton, R. A. (1996). Spirituality and nursing education. As published in K. R. Stevens, (Ed.). *Review of Research in Nursing Education Volume VII,* New York: National League for Nursing.

Harrington, A. (1995). Spiritual care: What does it mean to RNs? *Australian Journal of Advanced Nursing, 12*(4), 5-14.

International Council of Nurses. (2000). *The ICN code of ethics for nurses.* Geneva, Switzerland: Author.

Joint Commission on Accreditation for Health Care Organizations. (2000). *Hospital accreditation standards.* Oakbrook, IL: Author.

Lemmer, C. (2002). Teaching the spiritual dimension of nursing care: A survey of U.S. baccalaureate nursing programs. *Journal of Nursing Education, 41*(11), 482-490.

Meyer, C. L. (2003). How effectively are nurse educators preparing students to provide spiritual care? *Nurse Educator, 28*(4), 185-190.

Narayanasamy, A. (1993). Nurses' awareness and educational preparation in meeting their patient's spiritual needs. *Nurse Education Today, 13,* 196-201.

O'Brien, M. E. (1999). *Spirituality in nursing: Standing on holy ground.* Boston: Jones & Bartlett.

Pesut, B. (2003). Developing spirituality in the curriculum: Worldviews, intrapersonal connectedness, interpersonal connectedness. *Nursing Education Perspectives, 24*(6), 290-294.

Pesut, B. (2008). Spirituality and spiritual care in nursing fundamentals textbooks. *Journal of Nursing Education, 4*(4), 167-173.

Piles, C. (1980). *Spiritual care as a part of the nursing curriculum: A descriptive study.* Unpublished master's thesis, St. Louis University, St. Louis, MO.

Piles, C. (1990). Providing spiritual care. *Nurse Educator, 15*(1), 36-41.

Pullen, L, Tuck, I., & Mix, K. (1996). Mental health nurses' spiritual perspectives. *Journal of Holistic Nursing, 14*(2), 85-97.

Reed, P. G. (1992). An emerging paradigm for the investigation of spirituality in nursing. *Research in Nursing and Health, 15*, 349-357.

Sellers, S. C., & Haag, B. A. (1998). Spiritual nursing interventions. *Journal of Holistic Nursing, 16*, 338-354.

Schnorr, M. A. (1985). *The spiritual dimension: The philosophies and curricula of professional nursing programs in Illinois*. Unpublished graduate research paper, Northern Illinois University, DeKalb, IL.

Schnorr, M. A. (1988). *Spiritual nursing care: Theory and curriculum development*. Unpublished doctoral dissertation, Northern Illinois University, DeKalb, IL.

Soeken, K. L., & Carson, V. J. (1986). Study measures nurses' attitudes about providing spiritual care. *Health Progress, 67*(3), 52-55.

Stallwood, J., & Stoll, R. (1975). Spiritual dimensions of nursing practice. In I. L. Beland and J.Y. Passes (Eds.), *Clinical nursing: Pathophysiological and psychosocial approaches* (pp. 1086-1098). New York: Macmillian.

Taylor, E. J., Highfield, M., & Amenta, M. (1994). Attitudes and beliefs regarding spiritual care: A survey of cancer nurses. *Cancer Nursing, 17*(6), 479-487.

Taylor, E. J. (2002). *Spiritual care: Nursing theory, research and practice*. Upper Saddle River, NJ: Prentice-Hall.

Taylor, E. J. (2005). What have we learned from spiritual care research? *Journal of Christian Nursing, 22*(1), 22-28.

Taylor, E. J. (2007). Patient perspectives about nurse requisites for spiritual caregiving. *Applied Nursing Research, 20*, 44-46.

Wallace, M., Campbell, S., Grossman, S. C., Shea, J. M., Lange, J. W., & Quell, T.T. (2008). Integrating spirituality into the undergraduate nursing curriculum. *International Journal of Nursing Education Scholarship, 5*(1), 1-13.

Wilt, D. L., & Smucker, C. J. (2001). *Nursing the spirit: The art and science of applying spiritual care*. Washington, D.C.: American Nurses Association.

# CHAPTER 32

# TEACHING NURSING ETHICS

Kathleen F. O'Connor, PhD, RN, CNE

---

The content of this chapter relates to the following major content areas and subconcepts on the Certified Nurse Educator Examination Detailed Test Blueprint:

**Participate in Curriculum Design and Evaluation of Program Outcomes**
- Actively participate in the design of the curriculum to reflect current nursing and healthcare trends

**Engage in Scholarship of Teaching**
- Use evidence-based resources to improve and support teaching

**Function Effectively within the Institutional Environment and the Academic Community**
- Identify how social, economic, political and institutional forces influence nursing and higher education

---

## Introduction

Nursing education involves three domains: psychomotor, cognitive, and affective. Often times the affective domain is the least emphasized. Teaching ethics is an important area that can be used as an area of content to emphasize the importance of attitude and fair thinking. Teaching ethics involves teaching about the subject matter of ethics, but it also encourages a way of thinking that is important when developing the professional role of the nurse. This chapter presents ways the educator can address the teaching of nursing with the secondary gain of helping the student nurse develop approaches to thinking and decision making that were perhaps not previously considered.

After reflecting on this chapter, it is the intent that the nurse educator will be able to:

1. Relate principles important to bioethics/nursing ethics (respect for autonomy, beneficence, nonmaleficence, and justice) to nursing practice
2. Apply ethical/moral theories commonly used in bioethics: utilitarianism, deontology, and care to case studies
3. Use discussion/narrative pedagogy to evaluate and resolve nursing ethics situations

4. Use reflective thinking in decision making about ethical situations

## Teaching Nursing Ethics

Current health care, including nursing, involves increasingly complex use of technology, major shifts in the composition of population groups, and restricted financial support. In the midst of these realities, the core of nursing is focused on care (American Association of Colleges of Nursing (AACN), 1996; 2008), and care is supported by ethical/moral behavior. Jameton (1984 classic) stated that nursing is called "the morally centered health care profession" (p. xvi), and care is the basis of that moral center.

Nurses begin their education in ethics and morals immersed in the thinking of their families, friends, faith communities, educational institutions, and society. Learning to acknowledge personal moral views, to analyze and evaluate moral opinions, to reflect on moral situations, to defend moral choices, and to work with other healthcare team members on resolutions of ethical/moral situations and dilemmas is critical to the development of the ethical nurse.

The purpose of including nursing ethics in the curricula of nursing schools, and in staff development, is to prepare nursing students, and nurses already in practice, to perform more competently and more comfortably in ethically charged environments. To function this way, nurses must be cognizant of the history, language, theories, and application of bioethics in a multitude of clinical settings. The basic information needed by nurses to strengthen their ethical performance includes: evolution of nursing ethics, language/theories of bioethics, recognizing ethical situations, and applying ethical information to practice. To be able to apply knowledge in this way, learners must be open to the many perspectives: of patients, families, other nurses, administrators, and the general public, in a context of care.

This ethics work serendipitously strengthens the students' ability to recognize personal values, to think critically, to collaborate with others, and to avoid any hint of breaks in academic integrity; such as plagiarism. With the assistance of faculty as facilitators, teaching/learning nursing ethics strengthens the student's socialization to the profession of nursing.

## Evolution of Nursing Ethics for Nursing Education

Nurse educators form the group of nurses who role model ethical practice to their students (Woods, 2005). These faculty must be prepared to facilitate thinking about ethics in their students; by acting as ethical persons of integrity, personally and professionally. Faculty also must be steeped in the nursing ethics literature, starting with the history of nursing ethics, and the documents from professional nursing organizations. The genesis of ethics, as the study of what is right action, can be traced back to the earliest philosophers, bioethics back to the Hippocratic Oath, and nursing back to the Nightingale Pledge by Gretter (www.countryjoe. com/nightingale/pledge.htm).

The following URLs provide historical information about these beginnings:
- www.lifestudies.org/bioethics.html
- www.lifeissues.net/writers/irv/irv_36whatisbioethics01.html
- http://science.jrank.org/pages/8456/Bioethics-History-Bioethics.html
- www.richard-t-hull.com/publications/defining_nursing_ethics.pdf

The roots of nursing are in the soil of the military and of religious communities. These dual roots focused on the ethical virtue of obedience, and the requirement for strict obedience fell upon nurses of the day. These nurses were judged by their commitment to long hours, to strict following of the physician's orders, and to their own social virtue.

Nightingale moved the notion of ethics related to the nurse forward (Dossey, 2000), with her focus on competence, devotion, and virtue. In addition, she engendered one part of the beginning idea of evidence-based practice with her use of graphical statistics, demonstrating the benefits of fresh air, handwashing, and nourishing food, when searching for funds to support nursing practice. Faculty can use this ethically sound tactic, using research statistics displayed as graphics, particularly when working with students preparing for nursing administration, and when trying to garner the allocation of scarce resources.

The explosion of technology primarily in the 1960s moved ethics and bioethics forward and nurses were an integral part of the resulting changes in health care. The interest in nursing ethics reached a peak in the 1980s. However, much of the literature for nurses during this time focused on discrete issues such as nursing representation on ethics committees, the lack of bioethics in the nursing curriculum, and staffing in healthcare organizations. Discussion about the existence of a specific nursing ethics continues to occupy theorists. In this chapter, the author considers that nursing ethics is a unique, sometimes overlapping, phenomenon; with relevance for the ethical behavior of nurses and for relationships with patients. Figure 1 shows a brief representation of the progression of ethics.

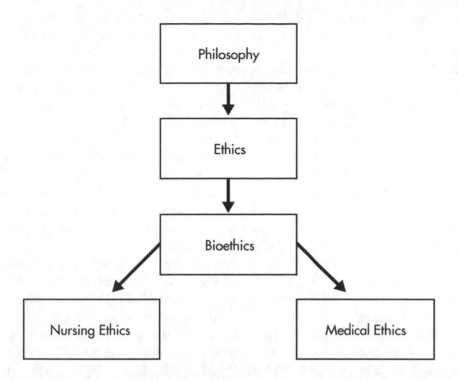

**Figure 1.** Genesis of Nursing Ethics

The American Nurses Association (ANA), in 2001, published the most current edition of *The Code for Nurses with Interpretive Statements* (http://nursingworld. org/ethics/code/protected-nwcde813.htm). This document forms the universal basis for American nurses to function ethically in practice. The code guides the members of the nursing profession in their interactions with patients, families, administration, and other healthcare providers, as the "non-negotiable professional standard". Nursing faculty will be able to gain expert help from the recently released ANA document: *Guide to the Code of Ethics for Nurses: Interpretation and Application* (ANA, 2008).

The American Association of Colleges of Nursing (AACN) spoke to the issue of ethics in the preparation of nurses in the 1996 document, *The Essentials of Master's Education for Advanced Practice Nursing*. This document was followed in 1998 by *The Essentials of Baccalaureate Nursing Education*, and the thinking about ethics, has been carried forward in the current, updated version (AACN, 2008). The inclusion of ethics in these documents supports the inclusion of ethics in the nursing curriculum.

The *Code of Ethics from the International Council of Nurses* (www.icn.ch/ icncode.pdf) was first released in 1973, and the latest revision was published in 2005. This code is designed to guide the practice of nurses throughout the world (Doborowoiska, Wronska, Fidecki, & Wysockinski, 2007).

Including selected professional documents in the early curricula of nursing programs helps to focus students on the importance of ethical competence in their practice, and on socialization to the profession. *The American Nurses Association Code for Nurses with Interpretive Statements* (ANA, 2001) is appropriate for concerted use at all nursing educational levels and in staff development. The Essentials documents and the ICN Code may be more appropriate for consideration at the baccalaureate, masters, and doctoral levels.

Nursing students will need further in depth study of the *ANA Code of Ethics with Interpretive Statements* (ANA, 2001), and the updated *Essentials of Baccalaureate Education for Professional Nursing Practice* (AACN, 2008). This study will enhance their comprehension of their role as an ethical professional nurse, the rationale behind the inclusion of ethics in their curriculum, the application of nursing ethics in their practice, and beginning consideration of the ethics of nursing research.

Students at the master's and doctoral levels will expand their in-depth consideration of the *ANA Code of Ethics with Interpretive Statements* (ANA, 2001), the *Essentials of Masters Education for Advanced Practice Nursing*, and the implications of the ICN Code, and other specialty documents. This study will enable them to present themselves as ethical nurses of integrity in their chosen special area of practice such as Nursing Education, Nursing Administration, Nurse Practitioner, Clinical Nurse Leader, Nurse Anesthetists, and in subspecialties. They will be able to apply what they have reflected on to their interactions with patients/families, staff, other healthcare workers, administration, and the public. These nurses with advanced preparation also will be prepared to influence social and healthcare policy in an ethical way.

Again the role of the nurse educator is to guide students in the understanding of the words contained in the documents, and how those words relate to a variety of nursing practice areas and situations. Confidence in their ethical role assists nurses to perform at all levels of the healthcare system.

# Nursing Ethics Course Development

As faculty work to incorporate an ethical perspective into the curricula for nurses at all levels, the reality of limited time to teach is always present. As a course progresses through the curricular approval process, buy in from all faculty is a most valuable element. The available options for including content about nursing ethics in nursing curricula include:

1. Stand alone nursing ethics courses, either classroom based or online: this may be limited to educational levels with longer programs depending upon the availability of units for the topic.
2. Integration of nursing ethics information into all other courses, following a stand alone ethics course.
3. Integration of nursing ethics information into all courses, following an introduction in an orientation to the program, or the fundamentals course.

The most difficult issue in incorporating ethics into the curriculum may well be that of "where will the teaching time come from"? Most faculty members believe strongly in the importance of the content they already teach, and do not want to give up the time allotted to it (Diekelmann, Ironside, & Gunn, 2005). Some discussions which may ease the way are:

1. Orientations: present academic integrity topics not just as university or program requirements, but also as professional ethical behavior. Include ethical work in important documents from professional nursing organizations, e.g. ANA Code, NLN statements about integrity, AACN material about ethics in academic curricula.
2. Work in faculty groups on case studies which incorporate the pathophysiological, psychological, spiritual, and ethical aspects of patient care.

For example, issues around ethical pain management can be included in case studies from all areas of practice: patients who seem to be seeking pain medications for some reason other than what might be considered "real" pain (justice); dealing with patients who do not want to ambulate, deep breathe, turn post operatively (beneficence/nonmaleficence); and patients who refuse pain medications when physiological parameters indicate that pain relief is needed (autonomy).

As any approach to the incorporation of ethical content progresses through the curricular approval process, real ethical situations from nursing practice should be used, rather than "made up"/hypothetical situations, e. g., the classical ethical case used by some philosophers, including Kohlberg (1969), of a porcupine seeking winter refuge in an underground warren with other species who would not benefit from or enjoy being "poked" by the porcupine; or a man who has to rob to try to save his wife from death despite all the ramifications of theft, e.g. separation from his wife.

## Academic Integrity

In their role modeling, faculty will want to treat students with respect, while molding ways of critical thinking about ethical situations. Some practical ethical activities will include, from the first day of the nursing program, a focus on what academic integrity means (Bellek, 2004). This focus forms the base for professional ethical behavior, and includes information related to such topics/issues as:

1. Lying: falsification of the student's own records, or those of patients; exaggerating information; making up content; patient health assessment, reporting completion of assignments
2. Cheating: quizzes, examinations, physical assessment
3. Stealing: medications from patients/nursing units; books/articles from library
4. Plagiarism: presenting the work of others as one's own
5. Respect for others: student colleagues, faculty, patients, families, and administrators; meeting academic obligations; avoiding unsafe actions, threats, avoiding gossip, revealing confidential information on a need to know only basis

O'Connor's (2007) *Academic Integrity* PowerPoint® (included on the CD accompanying this book) may be helpful to stimulate student and faculty thinking/ discussion about integrity as a nursing program/agency requirement, as part of the role of the nurse, and as doing what is right. The language/words included in academic integrity are powerful.

## Ethical Language

Nurses need to know the language of bioethics to collaborate with each other, and with healthcare personnel from other disciplines. The basic language links nursing ethics to bioethics and medical ethics, and bioethics to ethics. It seems best for students to read and compare the definitions of these terms, and then to spend significant time discussing what the words in the definitions mean in everyday language. This discussion will help the students to recognize ethical situations in real practice. Examples of such language include, but are not limited to, ethical theory, moral principles, and values.

Ethical/moral theory usually forms the basis of the thinking individuals in the healthcare professions use when working through ethical situations. The primary theories noted among these groups include: deontology, utilitarianism, virtue, and care ethics (Beauchamp & Childress, 2001). **Deontology** is rule based, focuses on doing what is right guided by rules and duty, and the outcome is incidental to the following of the "rule" (DeWolf Bosek & Savage, 2007).

**Utilitarianism** is outcome based, and focuses on the outcome(s) of the ethical decision. Utilitarianism is a consequentialist theory, and requires that healthcare professionals do whatever results in the good for the most people.

**Virtue** ethics focuses on the traits of good character that individuals develop over years, influenced by family, faith communities, education, and society. When faced with ethical situations virtuous individuals make decisions based on their character/virtues.

**Care ethics** focuses on the interaction of the individual nurse and the individual patient. The nurse is expected to consider the context of the situation, maintain relationships between individuals, and see that no one is left alone (Gilligan, 1987).

It is clear that resolving an ethical situation in the face of each healthcare worker adhering to a different ethical theory is challenging. Students, guided by faculty, can learn to navigate these difficult waters through discussion and appropriate compromise.

A simple example of a case study that could be used is that of a patient in a large ICU, who wishes to have her relatives with her. The patient has many relatives who are resistant to following any rules relating to visiting. The nurse following a **deontology** perspective would make a case for, "but the rule says", "patient needs rest", and "it is not fair to the other patients". Another nurse, following **utilitarian theory**, makes a case for the patient having many visitors because this will make the most people happy (patient and family members) stating the other patients are sedated and not having many visitors.

A third nurse, following **virtue theory**, makes a case for compassion and kindness for the patient, the family, and the other patients. This nurse attempts to think through what constitutes compassion and kindness for all involved, including: do not deliberately antagonize the visitors, work out a plan to space all the visitors over time, and spend special time with each one.

And finally, the nurse, following **care ethics** considers the relationship most valued, how often can the patient tolerate visitation without becoming exhausted, the geographical space available around the patient without impinging on other patients and visitors, and the maintenance of required health promoting nursing care. This nurse describes the most effective way of working with the visitors to follow a reasonable visiting plan.

Each of these plans has some pros and cons. Students and their faculty will discuss each pro and each con, identify commonalities, take an individual position on which approach is best, decide which compromise can be "lived with", and "where is the line in the sand". This discussion may well profit from inclusion of Butts and Rich's (2007) presentation of four topics with which to analyze situations: aspects of the patient's medical condition, what the patient prefers, quality of life, and context. The final resolution should be based on the analysis of the entire situation, and finding a resolution which will be accepted by all involved. If this is not possible, the case may have to be referred to the agency ethics committee for recommendations. While this case seems simple, it soon becomes clear how complex it can become.

Moral principles usually affect each available ethical theory. The four principles of respect for autonomy, beneficence, nonmaleficence, and justice are presented by Beauchamp and Childress (2001), the authors of the "gold standard" text on bioethics, as the four principles most important to nursing. Faculty and students can focus on recognizing these moral principles in reports of case studies. The words included in the case study will reveal the principles as listed in Table 1.

| Moral Principles | Language/Words |
|---|---|
| Respect for Autonomy | Control, respect, decide for self, confidentiality, privacy, preserve reputation, independence, self rule |
| Beneficence | Protect, comfort, relief, medicate, assuage, helped me, did not abandon me, paid attention, trust, availability, flexibility |
| Justice | Legal, fair, allocation of scarce resources, unfair, truth telling, giving information, not a clue, equal treatment, treatment according to need, staffing, not enough of_____. |
| Nonmaleficence | Pain, suffering, agony, therapy, hurt, harm, damage, injury |

**Table 1.** Examples of Bioethical/Ethical Language

Figure 2 places these moral principles in the schema of nursing ethics.

**Teaching Strategies for Nursing Ethics Education**
**Case Studies**

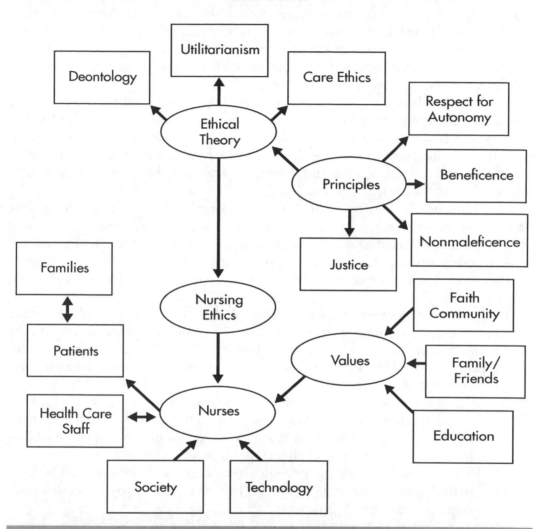

**Figure 2.** Overview of Nursing Ethics

## Signs and Symptoms of Ethical/Moral Situations/Issues/Dilemmas

Ethical situations that nurses experience are signaled by the experience of conflict and distress. This element of conflict can be experienced between the patient and health care provider(s) about care, between the family and the patient about care decisions, between the patient and family about information to be shared, and conflict between/among healthcare providers about care and/or information to be shared. Research implies these areas of conflict can be presented as themes of suffering, secrets, and struggles (O'Connor, 1991).

Case studies have long been used in teaching nursing and teaching nursing ethics. Researchers such as Kohlberg who have affected nursing ethics and moral development related to nursing ethics used case studies which were not real events, much less nursing events. There are so many real ethical/moral situations that occur in nursing, including clinical practice for nursing students, there does not seem to be any need to use "made up" case studies.

Initially students may want to focus on "large" ethical events that appear regularly in the news, e.g. war, stem cell transplant, or the death penalty. It is more advantageous for student growth in the profession of nursing for the faculty member to focus on equally important, nursing appropriate, ethical situations. Some of these situations can soon be revealed if students are asked questions (Brown & Keeley, 2001) such as,

1. If you were the nurse in a war situation, what ethical role would you have in deciding which patients need care first? Explore the ethical criteria/theory you would use to ground your thinking. Then discuss decisions about prioritizing patient care in times of need to allocate scarce resources, e.g. the ethics of staffing situations.
2. What would you do if you were the nurse when a patient asked about your opinion of stem cell transplantation? What effect would care theory have on your reflection? Then lead students in the discussion of to case studies related to the nurse's role in choosing patients for transplants.
3. What guidance for nurses related to the death penalty is available from nursing's professional organization? Then lead students to case studies built around issues of death and dying.

The complexity of the case studies is developed/chosen as the level of education increases, but the focus is always on issues important to nursing. Beginning generic students should be focused on commonly occurring nursing ethics problems such as:

1. **Honesty in recording assessment data.** Students may have a difficult time reporting what they actually observed in vital signs when the patient's record indicates that other, more experienced nurses have obtained different results; either higher or lower BP for example. In a parent/child clinical area, students may find it difficult to admit they are unfamiliar with monitoring equipment. In medical/surgical units students may have some difficulty acknowledging they are having trouble with any kind of new equipment, despite being oriented to that equipment.

2. **Honesty in performance on quizzes and exams.** Students may be tempted to cheat because they believe the faculty member has given them too much work, or that, as a student once said to the author, "I'm paying a lot of money to go to school here, and I deserve to be able to do whatever I can to get an A". Unfortunately, students may try to use cell phones to copy exams to share with others, and strict "ground rules" and "monitoring" need to be set and enforced. It may be helpful, as a faculty role model, for students to know that even their faculty were made to leave all books, cell phones, PDAs, etc. on a table in the front of the room when the faculty were taking the Certified Nurse Educator Examination for certification by the National League for Nursing. This is also a good time to begin letting students know the realities of the environment when taking licensing exams. It may be helpful to present information such as this from the aspect that, when stress is as high as it is in situations such as examinations at whatever level, all persons need external support to maintain their integrity.

Research implies these areas of conflict can be presented as themes of suffering, secrets, and struggles (O'Connor, 1991).

## Suffering, Secrets, and Struggles

The author's research (O'Connor, 1996; 1998) investigated the ethical/moral situations experienced by oncology nurses. While the participants were limited to one nursing practice group, the findings are informative. The 70 nurses involved in the first study (O'Connor, 1991), all female, randomly selected from all over the nation, described situations around the themes of suffering, secrets, and struggles. These same themes appeared in the second study with male oncology nurses (O'Connor, 1998).

**Suffering** primarily includes times/issues related to the end of life, especially enduring pain during the death and dying process; to other side effects of medical and nursing care and therapy; to futile care; and to the psychological trauma noted in behavioral health/psychiatric issues. The theme of suffering is supported by the moral principles of beneficence and nonmaleficence, and the moral virtues of gentleness, compassion, and kindness (Butts & Rich, 2005). The educator will undoubtedly encounter many situations of suffering on which to build case studies for student discussion, analysis, and planning. One example of such a case study is as follows:

"This particular night it was obvious that the end was near. By midnight we were expecting each breath to be the last. Her mother was with her and **all night** stood at the bedside holding her daughter's hand and speaking to her in a loving tone of voice, telling her daughter "It's all right to die honey. You won't need to suffer any more." It was extremely touching, and as the hours wore on, I was hoping the patient would die quickly to end her mother's labor of love. But she lingered on. About 7:00 her father arrived. He went in the room, saw his daughter, and immediately came out to the nurses' station demanding in a loud tone of voice, "You've got to give her something now—she can't go on like this—I can't stand to see her suffer...The patient had Ativan IV ordered for restlessness. I knew if I gave it to her it would push her on out. On the other hand, she could die any second anyway. After watching this daughter slowly die all night, I took the Ativan back to her room and slowly pushed it IV. I walked back to the nurses' station, and within seconds, her parents came out and said she was gone" (Anonymous personal communication, 1991).

The students and faculty could discuss this case in relation to the ANA Code for Nurses with Interpretive Statements, to the moral principle and virtues noted above, and to ethical theories.

The theme of **Secrets** primarily involves the patient and/or family being denied information to make clinical and personal decisions, and is supported by the moral principle of respect for autonomy and the moral virtue of truthfulness. Some patients are lied to, either by healthcare personnel or family. In some cases nurses found ways to deal with this problem of secrets in creative ways that could be used by nursing faculty and the nursing learner. One of the situations many student nurses are most anxious about is the episode of the patient asking for information the physician or family does not want the patient to have. The physician and/or the family may tell the nurse the patient is not to be informed of a serious diagnosis/prognosis. An effective way to deal with the situation when the patient asks about his/her diagnosis/prognosis, is to reflect back to the individual, "what concerns you most?". With this question, the nurse may acquire valuable information with which to approach the patient, family, and doctor. This intervention also offers the beginning nurse a way to deal with the situation that all parties will accept.

A student in the author's clinical group was providing care for a patient with extensive disease who was scheduled for radiation therapy 5 days a week. The student, faculty member, and staff all were sure the patient would be concerned she was going to die. When the student asked her "what concerns you most", the patient revealed that she was most concerned that her car would not be able to make the 30 mile curving, mountain drive 5 days a week for 6 weeks.

Another case study that may be helpful for discussion of the theme of secrets was shared by a nurse who had been caring for a woman in her mid-forties with urinary tract cancer. She said:

"The oncologist does not like to give chemotherapy in these situations because he believes uremia is a faster, easier death for the patient. The physician told the patient if she wanted further treatment her death would be 'horrible, painful, and prolonged', and there would be frequent hospitalizations, infections, etc. When I spoke to the patient about hospice, she told me she had not been told of any other palliative treatment such as chemotherapy. This patient was in good physical condition, had a son in college whom she wanted to see graduate, and she was not in any pain. I was torn between my desire to tell her about possible chemotherapy treatment and my desire to support her emotionally. I was also angry at the doctor for painting such a gruesome picture and for not giving her any hope. She was denied her choice in the matter by virtue of a very one-sided view of the physician's opinion about palliative chemotherapy. The physician and I had a heated discussion over this patient in his office later that day. The physician threatened me that he would prevent me from talking to terminally ill patients if I was going to confuse them by telling them of alternative therapies. I told him I had a moral, ethical, and professional responsibility to ensure patients are informed of their choices" (Anonymous personal communication, 1991).

The theme of **Struggle** involves conflict among healthcare providers about care to be delivered, and is affected by the moral principle of justice, and the moral virtue of courage (Butts & Rich, 2005). Conflict with administrators about such issues as staffing, (floating), and conflict with families/significant others can be involved. One of the most painful situations of struggle was reported in O'Connor's (1991) dissertation research, and narrative pedagogy is an appropriate teaching/learning strategy for faculty to have conversations (Diekelmann & Diekelmann, 2000) about interpreting the implications of the case. The attending physician for a seriously ill/dying patient was not available. There was no "Do Not Resuscitate" order. The resident spoke with the family, who did not want anything extraordinary done. The resident consulted with the medical doctor. The nurse wrote:

"The medical doctor wanted the patient transferred to the MICU and started on a dopamine drip. I made the appropriate phone calls to the nursing supervisor and bed utilization, and prepared myself for the response I would get from the MICU staff. When they called back the response was much as I expected. They said, 'You've got to be kidding, that is the most stupid thing we've ever heard of.' When they finally arrived with the stretcher to take the patient upstairs, one glared at me as soon as she entered the room. I told her it was not my idea, that if it had been up to me I would never have wanted this, and I would have kept her with us and let her go in peace. One of the nurses continued to express her displeasure by swearing and saying how ridiculous the whole thing was...a waste of bed space and what would happen if they needed a bed for someone who "really" needed it. ..By the time they transferred her, I was filled with outrage, anger, and frustration...I am still filled with outrage whenever I think about the whole episode, and especially about the cold, uncaring attitude of the ICU nurses" (Anonymous personal communication, 1991).

## Discussion groups

Using student discussion groups is one of the most effective experiences in nursing ethics education (Ellenchild-Pinch & Graves, 2000). While students may be uncomfortable with this teaching strategy when they begin the course, the facilitation of the faculty can help them to feel safe and open with each other (Brookfield & Preskill, 1999). The major purposes of these discussions are:

- Exposure to the ideas, beliefs, values, and thoughts of others
- Control of behavior in the face of conflict
- Reaching agreement on the resolution of ethical problems
- Respect for the autonomy of others, including patients
- Learning how to express personal thoughts/opinions in a professional and logical way
- How to grow as a scholar from interacting with peers

Assessment of group discussion learning performance is based on the following criteria which are made clear to students in the course syllabus, and are explained by the instructor at the first session of the course.

Acceptable participation is indicated by the following performance:

- Presents for session on time and for whole session
- Demonstrates critique of readings and completion of learning activities
- Demonstrates thought about topic in preparation for discussion
- Demonstrates interest in the discussion
- Engages in discussion in a thoughtful way

Faculty should provide participation grades and advice to students each week so they feel confident about their performance. Interestingly, it is easier for the faculty to calculate weekly discussion performance in online courses than classroom based courses. In online courses the faculty is able to read each posting to the discussion board that the students make. It is much more difficult for the faculty to keep track of student participation when there are multiple discussion groups working at the same time. One suggestion might be to have each group keep track of the essence of what each participant is presenting, and to summarize the results for submission at the end of the session. The online and suggested classroom-based strategies encourage students to actively participate in the discussion to achieve the major purposes of discussion. Other teaching strategies which can support discussion/narrative pedagogy/discussion include the use of concept mapping and the development of PowerPoint® presentations by the students.

Concept mapping is suggested for capturing thought processes in the discussion of ethical case studies. The following sites provide information for faculty and students to determine the uses of concept mapping and the potential presentation:

- http://users.edte.utwente.nl/lanzing/cm_home.htm
- www.socialresearchmethods.net/mapping/mapping.htm
- www.mindjet.com
- www.inspiration.com/vlearning/index.cfm?fuseaction=concept_maps
- http://learn.sdstate.edu/nursing
- http://classes.aces.uiuc.edu/ACES100/Mind/c-m2.html

This teaching strategy enables the faculty and students in their groups to capture the ideas of each student as they are shared. Since the concept mapping software often provides for variety, students can choose colors, shapes, and positions for their thoughts, which adds a fun or relaxed aspect to serious ethical work.

Students in discussion groups can summarize their class discussions, review their concept maps, then develop a PowerPoint® presentation to share with the class. After reflection on the content of the PowerPoint® work, students and the faculty can discuss the commonalities and differences noted, make a class decision on potential ethical actions for resolving the case studies, and move on to the particular ways to implement the plan. The combination of discussions/narrative pedagogy/conversations, concept mapping, and PowerPoint® presentations helps students to learn using their preferred learning style, e.g., auditory (discussion), visual (PowerPoint®), and kinesthetic (the mechanics of recording group work in a concept map/PowerPoint). The group work expands the students' thinking in preparation for knowledge application in clinical practice and postconferences, and to demonstrate their scholarly ability to express their thinking in writing.

## Scholarly Papers

Written paper-analyses of cases reveal where each student is in the ethical learning process, and how each student can express their thinking in writing. Papers should be developed around the discussion of the following issues:

- Perception of the ethical situation
- Perceived relationship to selected moral principles
- Ethical theory base(s) for considering the situation
- Potential barriers to a resolution
- Strategies to overcome the barriers
- Application of positive strategies to resolve ethical situations

A scoring rubric may be helpful to guide review of scholarly papers. (See Figure 3.) Grading these paper is different from grading papers reporting pathophysiological ideas, which are quantitatively measurable. Ethics papers report thoughts about difficult and complex human situations to which it is difficult to attach numbers. A rubric, transparently shared and discussed with students, may be helpful in determining a grade for the honest expression of ideas.

## Interviews

Students in nursing research courses could be assigned (with approval from the IRB as needed) to interview, in confidence, nurses with whom they work, or nurses who are in the functional areas to which they aspire. The development of a consent form (Christenbery & Miller, 2008) which meets or is based on federal guidelines (www.med.umich.edu/irbmed) can be developed with input from the class/groups.

It is helpful with this learning strategy to focus on qualitative methodology. A question/statement such as, "Tell me about an ethical/moral situation you have experienced in your practice. Tell me all you can remember about the situation until you have nothing left to say", can be asked and the answer audiotaped or written. The response is then analyzed to determine the essence of the situation, the theoretical basis reflected, the moral principles used, and the resolution to the situation.

|  | Excellent =4 | Satisfactory/ Adequate =3 | Fair =2 | Poor/ Unsatisfactory/ Inadequate = 0-1 |
|---|---|---|---|---|
| Presentation of ethical situation | • Is an ethical/ moral situation<br>• Is related to nursing<br>• Clear<br>• Concise | • Is mostly an ethical/moral situation<br>• Is primarily r/t nursing<br>• Majority clear<br>• Majority concise | • Limited r/t ethical/moral situation<br>• Some not r/t nursing<br>• Rarely clear<br>• Rarely concise | • Not r/t ethical/ moral situation<br>• Not r/t to nursing<br>• Unclear<br>• Scattered |
| Relationship to moral principles | • Related to at least one of four major moral principles<br>• Relationship is accurately presented | • Limited r/t any of the major moral principles<br>• Majority of the presented relationship is accurate | • Superficially r/t major moral principles<br>• Some of the relationships are not accurate | • Not related to major moral principles<br>• Presentation is not accurate |
| Ethical theory base | • Is accurately related to at least one ethical theory | • Limited r/t ethical theory<br>• Majority of r/t are accurate | • Superficial r/t any ethical theory<br>• Some of the r/t is not accurate | • Not r/t ethical theory<br>• Presentation is not accurate |
| Barriers to a resolution | • Barriers clearly identified<br>• Related to nursing | • Barriers clearly identified<br>• Related to nursing | • Superficial presentation of barriers<br>• Some not r/t nursing | • Barriers not appropriate/ accurate<br>• Not r/t nursing |

**Figure 3.** Nursing Ethics Scholarly Paper Scoring Rubric

| Strategies to overcome barriers | • Presentation of at least two strategies clearly presented<br>• Related to nursing | • At least one strategy clearly presented<br>• At least one r/t nursing | • Superficial presentation of strategies<br>• Questionable r/t nursing | • Strategies are not appropriate/accurate<br>• Not r/t nursing |
|---|---|---|---|---|
| Presentation of solution to ethical situation | • Solution is clearly related to situation<br>• Practical/reasonable | • Solution moderately r/t situation<br>• Practical/reasonable | • Superficial r/t situation<br>• Limited practicality/reasonability | • Solutions are not appropriate/accurate<br>• Not practical or reasonable |
| Scholarly writing | Follows APA for:<br>• Correct spelling/grammar Reference list Neat appearance<br>• Writing at appropriate level<br>• Reference List<br>• Neat Appearance | Follows most APA:<br>• Occasional spelling/grammar errors<br>• Occasional errors in reference list<br>• Occasional errors in neat appearance<br>• Most writing at appropriate level | Follows some APA:<br>• Many spelling/grammar errors<br>• Many reference list errors<br>• Many lack of attention to detail errors<br>• Writing not at student's educational level | • Does not follow APA |

**Figure 3 continued.** Nursing Ethics Scholarly Paper Scoring Rubric

## Summary

The rapidity of change in the healthcare system offers a multitude of ethical situations in which nurses will be involved. The information included in this chapter was offered to stimulate thinking, to provide resources for further study, and to encourage faculty who wish to teach nursing ethics to nurses who are beginning their practice. Professional documents, academic integrity, professional socialization, discussion of case studies, and the use of other teaching strategies are all part of the preparation of nurses to protect the humanity of patients.

## Learning Activities

1. Interview two nursing faculty asking about how they teach nursing ethics. Compare and contrast the two approaches.
2. Select one of the teaching strategies discussed in this chapter. Implement it in a course you are teaching. Develop an evaluation tool to solicit feedback from students about this method. Analyze the results. Describe the effectiveness of the teaching strategy.

## Educational Philosophy

I believe that teaching is the faculty/student partnership for facilitation of student learning. This partnership is based on adequate assessment, creation of a supportive environment, full disclosure of measurable objectives, transparent expectations, use of a variety of teaching/learning strategies, and fair evaluation of student and faculty achievement in the partnership for the ultimate benefit of patients. — Kathleen F. O'Connor

## References

American Association of Colleges of Nursing (AACN). (1996). *The essentials of master's education for advanced practice nursing.* Washington, DC: Author
American Association of Colleges of Nursing (AACN). (1998). *Essentials of baccalaureate nursing education.* Washington, DC: Author.

American Association of Colleges of Nursing (AACN). (2008). *The essentials of baccalaureate education for professional nursing practice*. Washington, DC: Author.

American Nurses Association (ANA). (2001). *Code of ethics for nurses with interpretive statements*. Silver Spring, MD: Author.

American Nurses Association (ANA). (2008). *Guide to the code of ethics for nurses: Interpretation and application*. Spring, MD: Author.

Beauchamp, T. L, & Childress, J. F. (2001). *Principles of biomedical ethics* (5th ed.). New York: Oxford

Belleck, J. P. (2004). Why plagiarism matters. *Journal of Nursing Education, 43*, 527-528.

Brookfield, S. D., & Preskill, S. (1999). *Discussion as a way of teaching*. San Francisco, CA: Jossey-Bass.

Browne, M. N., & Keeley, S. (2001). *Asking the right questions: A guide to critical thinking* (6th Ed.). Upper Saddle River, NJ: Prentice-Hall.

Butts, J., & Rich, K. (2005). *Nursing ethics: Across the curriculum and into practice*. Sudbury, MA: Jones and Bartlett.

Christenbery, T. L., & Miller, M. R. (2008). A strategy for learning principles and elements of informed consent. *Nurse Educator, 33*, 75-78.

DeWolf Bosek, M. S., & Savage, T. A. (2007). *The ethical component of nursing education: Integrating ethics into clinical practice*. Philadelphia: Lippincott Williams & Wilkins.

Diekelmann, N. L. (2003). *Teaching the practitioners of care*. Madison, WI: University of Wisconsin Press.

Diekelmann, N., & Diekelmann, J. (2000). Learning ethics in nursing and genetics: Narrative pedagogy and the grounding of values. *Journal of Pediatric Nursing, 15*, 226-231.

Diekelmann, N. L., Ironside, P. M., & Gunn, J. (2005). Recalling the curriculum revolution: Innovation with research. *Nursing Education Perspectives, 26*, 70-77.

Doborowoiska B., Wronska, I., Fidecki W., & Wysockinski, M. (2007). Moral obligations of nurses based on the ICN, UK, Irish and Polish codes of ethics for nurses. *Nursing Ethics, 14*, 171-180.

Dossey, B. M. (2000). *Florence Nightingale: Mystic, visionary, healer*. New York: Springhouse.

Ellenchild-Pinch, W. J., & Graves, J. K. (2000). Using web-based discussion as a teaching strategy: Bioethics as an exemplar. *Journal of Advanced Nursing, 32*, 704-712.

Gilligan, C. (1987). Moral orientation and moral development. In E. Kittay & D. Meyers, (Eds.) *Women and moral development*. Savage, MD: Rowan and Littlefield.

International Council of Nurses. (2006). *ICN code for nurses*. Geneva, Switzerland: Author.

Ironside, P. M. (2003). Trying something new: Implementing and evaluating narrative pedagogy using a multimethod approach. *Nursing Education Perspectives, 24*, 122–128.

Jameton, A. (1984). *Nursing practice: The ethical issues*. Englewood Cliffs, NJ: Prentice-Hall.

Kohlberg, L. (1969). Stage and sequence: The cognitive-developmental approach to Socialization. In D. A. Goslin (Ed.). *Handbook of socialization theory and research*. Chicago: Rand McNally.

National League for Nursing (n.d.). Core values. NY: Author www.nln.org/about-nln/corevalues.htm

O'Connor, K. F. (1991). *The ethical/moral language of cancer nurses (Dissertation)*. Claremont, CA:  Claremont Graduate School.

O'Connor, K. F. (1996). The ethical/moral experiences of oncology nurses. *Oncology Nursing Forum, 23*, 787-794.

O'Connor, K. F. (1998). *The ethical/moral experiences of male oncology nurses: A pilot study*. Carson, CA: CSUDH.

O'Connor, K. F. (2007). *Academic integrity PowerPoint*. Carson, CA: CSUDH

O'Connor, K. F. (2007). *Ethics as a discipline*. PowerPoint Presentation. Carson, CA.

University of Michigan. (2007). Consent to be part of a research study. Ann Arbor: MI: Author.  www.med.umich.edu/irbmed

# CHAPTER 33

# CHALLENGES AND OPPORTUNITIES FOR TEACHING RESEARCH

Sharon Cannon, MSN, EdD, RN, ANEF
Carol Boswell, MSN, EdD, RN, CNE, ANEF

---

The content of this chapter relates to the following major content areas and subconcepts on the Certified Nurse Educator Examination Detailed Test Blueprint:

**Facilitate Learning**
- Implement a variety of teaching strategies appropriate to content; learner needs; desired learner outcomes
- Use teaching strategies based on evidence-based practices related to education

**Participate in Curriculum Design and Evaluation of Program Outcomes**
- Actively participate in the design of the curriculum to reflect current nursing and healthcare trends

---

## Introduction

Throughout the years, research has been perceived as the something reserved for professors in colleges/universities or researchers associated with drug companies. In addition, trying to read and comprehend research was like trying to read and use a foreign language. As a result, even saying the word "research" is likely to elicit a "deer caught in the headlights" look. Consequently, teaching research successfully has been a daunting task. However, this chapter proposes several approaches to turn that perception around.

## Clarification of Terms

The first consideration for teaching research requires a clarification about research, evidence-based practice (EBP), research utilization (RU), practice-based evidence (PBE), and evidence-based nursing (EBN). These terms are often used interchangeably and yet, each term brings a different perspective for faculty to consider when teaching research.

According to Boswell and Cannon (2007), **research** is defined as "a methodic examination that uses regimented techniques to resolve questions and decipher dilemmas" (p. 346). True research is that process of carefully and methodically addressing each step in a carefully developed plan. **EBP** as defined by Boswell and Cannon (2007) is "a research-based, decision-making process used to guide the delivery of holistic patient care by nurses" (p. 340). EBP brings more to the table with decision making and patient preferences. **Research utilization** is considered to be a component in making clinical decisions that impact the outcomes of the care provided by nurses but is not the whole of EBP (Boswell & Cannon, 2007). Research utilization (RU) is simply using research outcomes while practicing clinically. RU is frequently a "catch all" term incorporated as the current direction for improving the quality of health care.

**Practice-based evidence** is another approach that looks at evidence (results found in practice) to guide clinical decisions. This concept was discussed at the Council of Advanced Nursing Sciences (CANS) conference, and again RU was a component. The latest trend is evidence-based nursing (EBN). Ireland (2008) defines EBN as "a client care approach that uses problem-solving methods to integrate the best research evidence with clients' preferences and values and clinician's expertise" (p. 90). EBN drives home the idea of nursing as the center within the provision of patient care based on the evidence located.

Although most of these concepts have emerged in the past 30 years, research in nursing can be traced back to Florence Nightingale. The evolution of nursing research has prompted multiple approaches to encourage nursing practice to critically examine factors influencing the nurse making clinical judgments at the point of care.

## Considerations When Teaching Nursing Research

Two aspects must be considered when teaching research. Vital to the successful teaching of research is that both faculty and students believe that research is valuable and relevant to nursing practice. How a faculty has been taught research often is the guiding force for teaching methodologies. Prior methodologies and approaches must be examined for relevance in the current healthcare arena. Finding unique strategies may be one of the biggest hurdles for faculty to overcome. Being complacent and believing, "it's the way I was taught" can be detrimental when teaching research. Students who believe that research is remote, ivory tower, and not applicable to the real world will have a difficult time understanding the language and process of research. The research course would be considered as just "something I have to get through to graduate."

The second aspect that is paramount to both faculty and students is relevance. Research has to be significant to nursing so it can be applied regardless of the setting. Understanding that faculty and students may already have knowledge about the value and relevance of research is critical to teaching research. Engagement of both faculty and students in the teaching/learning process, by capitalizing on what each brings to the table, allows for the exchange of information which is vital to the teaching/learning milieu.

Multiple challenges face the nurse educator who accepts the opportunity for teaching research. As faculty endeavor to provide exciting learning opportunities, a consensus about active learning needs to be formulated. According to Nielsen, Stragnell, and Jester (2007), "active learning is recognized as a strategy that promotes understanding of complex subject matter, as well as transfer of learning to new situations" (p. 514). The faculty must sift through the various concepts to determine the comfort level related to their own values and beliefs regarding research, as well as their students' values and beliefs. Selecting an EBP, RU, PBE, or EBN focus will determine the direction for the variety of teaching discussions required, i.e. textbook, course objectives, teaching strategies, and evaluation of student learning. This is true whether the research course is taught online/classroom, undergraduate, or graduate.

## Undergraduate (AD, Generic BSN, and RN-to-BSN)

Nursing research is frequently perceived as a boring, overwhelming, and complex process which requires the knowledge provided at upper levels of education. Too often, the message which seems to be transmitted by faculty is that research can only be done by highly-educated individuals in research institutions. With the incorporation of evidence-based practice into the health care arena, this message must be put to rest. Each and every nursing professional must embrace the idea that the process of research is within everyone's grasp. Every student nurse does not have to conduct research, but must engage with the process of research in some manner. Research is often extremely frightening to students; it is stunning and having a vastness of considerable intensity.

Faculty must carefully and frequently reassess the learners and their characteristics. At the current time, faculty engage an eclectic student population which includes individuals from the Baby Boom Generation (born 1943-1960), Generation X (born 1961-1981), and Millennial or Net, Generation (born 1982-2000). Each of these generations has unique characteristics that must be considered when planning a course. McNamara (2005) stated "the unique experience of these generations can create not only age discrepancies but value differences, gender issues, tension between cultures, and problems with team building and active participation in general" (p. 1149). Since the different generational characteristics are based upon life experiences, each generation holds specific values, beliefs, and expectations. These life experiences at times can result in the clashing of the generations. The Millennial generation is considered to be multitaskers, collaborators, and see the Internet as a tool not technology (Mangold, 2007; Skiba, 2005). As faculty work with the Millennial generation, awareness that this generation believes that to be "able to search and manipulate information to generate knowledge is more important than the attainment of knowledge" (Mangold, 2007, p. 22). Because the Millennial generation is very comfortable with the Internet and gaming, faculty understand these students have learned to solve problems by the "trial and error" format. The video games which are common place for this group are managed by trial and error, not by reviewing information and critical thinking about the material provided. According to Russell, Burchum, Likes, Jacob, Graff, Driscoll, Britt, Adymy, and Cowan (2008), the current students are "poor at distinguishing mass marketing from authoritative sources, identifying biased Web content, and discerning irrelevant results" (p. 79). Since contemporary undergraduate students are very comfortable with, and accustomed to, the Internet, they do not challenge or scrutinize for accuracy the information found on the web.

Faculty must change the way they teach research as these challenges arise. Ryan, Hodson-Carlton, and Ali (2005) state that "rethinking courses results in an increased awareness of course outcomes, design, and content" (p. 359). As the profession advances and evidence-based practice becomes increasingly important, the direction for the teaching and facilitating of research at the undergraduate level has to be revamped to move forward instead of staying stagnant. Our learners within each generation require innovative management of the instructional process. Faculty members tend to teach as they were taught. This process of relying on how we were taught must be changed. The idea that each student has to prepare an individual critique of a research article is no longer reflective of the practice arena. Within the practice arena, committee or group work is the norm. Evidence-based practice is crucial. Students' engagement with the process of research should address these aspects – committee/group activities within the realm of evidence-based practice. Faculty must accept the responsibility for engaging the current learners in the manner needed, not in the manner that was used for past generations.

Evidence-based practice, practice-based evidence, research, research utilization, and evidence-based nursing are each important aspects within the context of research at this time. Depending on the undergraduate level – AD, BSN, or RN-to-BSN – the level of instruction needs to be fluid and appropriate. Each level has expectations and responsibilities to advance the profession of nursing. The instruction process for research can not be left to only the integral parts of the research process. The concepts and ideas imperative to evidence-based practice, practice-based evidence, research utilization and evidence-based nursing have to be incorporated successfully into the nursing curriculum.

Within a study completed by Cannon, Boswell, and Robinson (2007), the primary yardstick to be addressed related to incorporation of research by bedside nurses was the need to make the research process important in the practical world. In translation of this important finding into the teaching of research at the undergraduate level, faculty must determine real world application of the process. The purpose for teaching research at any level has to be carefully considered and addressed. At the Associate degree nurse level, the expectation should reflect the reading and initial critique of research studies. The baccalaureate level student nurse is expected to utilize research findings within the day-to-day functioning in the practice arena. For either of these levels to exist, the faculty involved in the instructional process of research must reflect an excitement for the process while ensuring that it is functional. The requirements for stimulating an enjoyment for research include the need for the process to be engaging, match the learners' level of understanding, reflect a value within the profession, and be user friendly.

At the undergraduate level, functionality of the process is the driving force, instead of the complexity of the process. Each student must understand the utilization of the research within the work world. The process presented by the faculty has to demonstrate a practicality for it to be readily embraced and employed. One preliminary way to engage the learner within the research process is to excite the learner within the realm of research results. A demonstration of the responsiveness of the research endeavor, related to identified challenges within the workplace, is paramount to captivating the next generation of critical thinkers. When research is presented as a complex, convoluted process that takes time, energy, and resources with minimal short-term compensation, undergraduate learners turn their attention to other productive endeavors. If the research process is presented in this manner, nurses at the bedside tend to leave the entire process to other individuals who have more time, energy, and resources for research endeavors. Time is precious to the nurse at the bedside, so any process has to be serviceable and realistic. Faculty must carefully consider examples where the use of the research process was efficient and purposeful.

## Graduate

Teaching research to graduate students has many of the same requirements as are seen within the undergraduate level. As is common to all levels of learning, the student must be challenged to seek additional knowledge and understanding while excited at the potential to improve the practice arena. Graduate level work aspires to attract the student toward the active involvement within a research process. Faculty, at this level, must trigger the desire for knowledge investigation within the students. As students are stimulated to engage in the research process, innovative projects and studies will result. Making sure the students understand the value of mentoring with seasoned researchers is a win/win solution to the overwhelming nature of conducting research. The dialogue related to research must be engaging at all levels. The material provided needs to match the learner's level while addressing the expectation of being user friendly. Once again, if the topic is not seen as relevant to the learner, the material will not be retained nor utilized. Faculty members have to clarify for themselves the appropriate level of research involvement prior to initiating the course. After clarifying in their own minds the outcomes and expectations for the course, faculty members must effectively communicate information and rationales to the students. The students must understand why engaging in the research process is important to the profession of nursing. The master's-prepared nurse should be able to participate in research projects and direct initial pilot projects. Realizing the master's-prepared nurse does not have to conduct research alone, but can utilize a team/group approach, is one method that can make involvement with research more palatable.

## Delivery of a Research Course: Online, Enhanced, or Classroom

The decision regarding the mode of delivery of a course is frequently determined by the school. As a result, faculty could be assigned to teach an online, enhanced, or classroom venue. Each delivery methodology has differences, similarities, and challenges for the faculty. One obvious difference is that in teaching online, faculty cannot experience the students' nonverbal reaction to information. The frown, nod of understanding, or blank looks are missing from the communication process. Consequently, faculty must be ever diligent in assuring that students are synthesizing the concepts being explored. Asking for feedback is essential. Questions must be worded so the depth of the student responses reflects understanding.

Another difference in teaching research online is that the faculty member is no longer the "sage on the stage" but rather the "guide on the side". The teacher is not standing in front of the class giving a lecture. Imparting knowledge has to be approached differently and may require converting lecture notes to a link within the course that specifies tasks associated with the content.

Students may be more comfortable learning in a classroom. Online and web-enhanced courses require skills in maneuvering in a platform that may be unfamiliar. In an online course, faculty and students do not have the opportunity to develop close relationships as they would in the classroom setting. Students may be across state, national, or international geographic boundaries. In a study conducted by Sitzman and Woodard-Leners (2006), eight themes related to student satisfaction with online nursing courses were identified. The eight themes were frequent feedback, timeliness, reciprocal caring, personal connection and empathy, clarity, multiple contact opportunities, commitment to learning, and second-fiddle worries. Faculty members often reflect that "it is hard to get to know the students". Students often feel isolated. Developing meaningful student/teacher and student/student relationships requires online faculty to be creative in learning about the students and providing opportunities for students to interact with each other.

Online, web enhanced, or classroom delivery methodologies share common issues surrounding the teaching of research. Regardless of the method, the complexity of the material crosses all three. Designing activities, student feedback, and demonstration of comprehension require faculty and students to be engaged. Discussion can occur in the classroom or in a discussion forum. Questions can be asked in chats, emails, or the classroom. Debates can be lively and conducted in all settings. Posters can be presented online with discussions or delivered live in a classroom. Students can have discussions on a bulletin board or in the classroom. The point here is that many teaching techniques have application in all three areas.

## Teaching Tips for Practical Applications

Elder and Paul (2007) stated "no matter what your circumstance or goals, no matter where you are, or what problems you face, you are better off if your thinking is skilled" (p. 1). Clarity of thinking is a key factor within the conduction of, or reflection on, research undertakings. The process of engaging in research necessitates the orderly, balanced attention to details. Paul and Elder (1996) documented eight guidelines for developing reasoning abilities. These guidelines can be effectively applied to research as students seek to comprehend which research projects are advantageous and beneficial for evidence-based practice (see Table 1).

| Guidelines for Reasoning Abilities | Research Application |
|---|---|
| All reasoning has a purpose. | Research has to have a purpose stated via research statements, research questions, and/or hypotheses. |
| All reasoning is an attempt to figure something out, to settle some question, to solve some problem. | The significance to nursing is delineated clearly and effectively. |
| All reasoning is based on assumptions. | Assumptions and limitations to any study are clearly explained to document any biases which may be involved. |
| All reasoning is done from some point of view. | Researchers acknowledge any biases held by the researcher or research team. |
| All reasoning is based on data, information, and evidence. | The researcher must clearly and systematically document the statistical results and/or qualitative results when discussing validation of the results. |
| All reasoning is expressed through, and shaped by, concepts and ideas. | Within the documentation of the research process, the conceptual foundation for the study is explained. |
| All reasoning contains inferences or interpretations by which conclusions are drawn and meaning is given to data. | Within the establishment of the conclusions and meaning of the data, an understanding of the operational and conceptual definitions for each variable and concepts are effectively acknowledged to allow for generalizability. |
| All reasoning leads somewhere or has implications and consequences. | Effective dissemination of a research endeavor includes implications and recommendations for future directions. |
| (Paul & Elder, June 1996). *Foundation for Clinical Thinking*. Online at website: www.criticalthinking.org | |

**Table 1.** Applying Guidelines for Reasoning Abilities to Research

Faculty have the responsibility to translate the ideas of reasoning abilities as demonstrated by research dissemination. Since evidence-based practice is a key function of research, students need to associate the aspects of the research process and results to reasoning and critical thinking. When this connection can be firmly grounded, an excitement for the incorporation of research into the practice arena can be seen. The process of reviewing and analyzing research accomplishments becomes paramount to the inclusion of evidence into the workplace. Research becomes commonplace instead of some grand, complex process that is unattainable by the common healthcare provider. Practical application of research has to be a primary goal within the teaching of research to a student population. As students are challenged to question and seek the researched foundation for the healthcare practices used within the workplace, education must "foster a spirit of inquiry, an independence of thought, an ability to question prevailing assumptions, and a confidence with which to meet the complexities of a dynamic health care system" (Myrick & Tamlyn, 2007, p. 301).

The practical side of research for the undergraduate student is to ensure they emerge from the classroom experience with a willingness to question and scrutinize the data, outcomes, and findings available from the professional journals, websites, and other informational avenues. The entire process of exciting nurses to the possibilities of advancing the profession of nursing through critical thinking, research, and evidence-based practice is constructed on the understanding that cognitive skills are required to address the complexity of the healthcare needs encountered by today's engaged nurse (Riddell, 2007; Zygmont & Moore Schaefer, 2006). Each assignment and activity included within a course should easily be coupled to a reasoning skill. In addition, each assignment needs to build toward a final product. Although the grading of each assignment is unique for that assignment, the final outcome for the course needs to use each and every assignment. Assignments which have the appearance of being busy work, since they can not be connected to the final outcome, are frequently met with frustration and defensiveness by the students. The Millennial generation, as well as adult learners, expect and demand that each assignment interconnects to the final outcome. For faculty, a clear understanding of the final outcome provides single-mindedness for each and every assignment and activity within the course.

Another innovative approach to using research concepts is the process of nursing grand rounds. Furlong, D'Luna-O'Grady, Macari-Hinson, O'Connel, and Pierson (2007) champion the use of nursing grand rounds to "link the evidence-based practice literature to the clinical practice of nursing" (p. 288). Particularly at the undergraduate level, the use of an environment reflecting this forum allows the growth of each member of the group. The use of a process like nursing grand rounds permits the different members of the class to present evidence-based research articles related to a topic. For a research class, the focus would remain on the research aspects of the article while showcasing the clinical aspect. Since increased numbers of hospitals are implementing a process such as grand rounds, the use of the process in a class allows the students to become comfortable and confident within the environment.

An additional pointer for teaching research ideas recognizes the need to insure that students have academic writing skills. Academic writing skills can readily be assessed through the use of critical analysis of research related materials. According to Knowles and McGloin (2007), "critical analysis is the argument based on what theories were used, what is the evidence, how it is analyzed and evaluated to show how the students reached their conclusion" (p. 36). The expectation that students will effectively communicate rational and logical thinking concerning an interpretation of research-based literature reflects their critical thinking abilities. Within a critical analysis writing process, students are expected to pull from the different aspects within their knowledge and experiences to reflect and integrate information from a variety of perspectives.

When teaching research online, the use of chat time is an effective technique for initiating dialog (academic exchange). According to Reynaud (2007), "dialog requires the working of ideas towards a knowledge-based learning outcome" (para. 4). For focused instructional exchange to take place within a chat session, the faculty must spend time and planning in preparing the process. The chat session can not be left to chance. The crucial components to be covered within a session have to be carefully and thoroughly prepared concerning:

1. Questions to lead the discussion and understanding
2. What principal aspects are to be addressed

Faculty may find the incorporation of a whiteboard within the chat session a useful tool for insuring the presentation and/or brainstorming is effectively captured.

Boswell and Cannon (2007) stated that "to simply accept that a task has always been accomplished a specific way without understanding the evidence behind that task is no longer tolerated by the public, by health care entities, or by the health care system as a whole" (preface para 1). To engage students in the thought process, realistic conditions must be presented in a manner that will inspire the student to strive for new knowledge. Ideas such as "thinking outside of the box" and "red flags" are two mechanisms which can engage individuals to move to a different level of inquiry. By challenging students to move from the normal traditions of research thinking to innovative evidence-based activities allows a creativity to be realized. Students will rise to the level expected by the faculty. Faculty must ensure they are setting the level of expected behavior at an intensity that will challenge but still be reachable. The level should not be so high that it is not attainable by the majority of the students.

So often the idea of research is closely aligned with critical thinking. According to Twibell, Ryan, and Hermiz (2005), the cognitive skills needed for critical thinking include "information gathering, synthesis, reflection, assignment of meaning, problem solving, predicting, planning, and applying knowledge to new contexts" (p. 77). The process of understanding research articles and thus arriving at evidence-based nursing practice requires each of these skills. Within the content related to research and research utilization, each of these skills should be addressed and supported. The assignments and delivery method for teaching research at any level need to champion these cognitive skills. Within the study documented by Twibell, Ryan, and Hermiz (2005), several methods of imparting these skills were identified, such as questioning, conferencing, writing, and journaling. Each of these methods of cultivating cognitive skills can easily be integrated into the assignments used within the teaching of research.

As faculty contemplate the different aspects of any research course, the assignments need to incorporate these skills. Above and beyond just using these skills, the skills need to be coupled to the content and outcomes for the course. Care must be given to insure that each assignment is practical and beneficial to the student and not just an assignment because that was the way the faculty member learned to do it.

## Application

Consider the following situation. Using the following scenario as a springboard for discussion concerning teaching application of research and evidence-based practice, your workload assignment is to facilitate an undergraduate research course. The three semester credit hour course has 30 students enrolled. After approximately three weeks, a student raises the following situation for discussion.

During a clinical rotation, a student in your research class is assigned to care for an Hispanic patient who has just returned from the recovery room for placement of a stent during angioplasty. The policy/procedure calls for the use of manual compression after removal of the arterial sheath. The student hears the staff nurses discussing the use of Perclose® versus manual compression. The student asked you which approach would be appropriate.

When the scenario was presented, you recognized the value of using this practical example within the confines of the course. The potential teaching strategies for addressing this scenario in two different venues are offered.

## Face-to-Face Delivery

Directing students to examine how to apply research to this example can be achieved in either the classroom or a clinical pre/post conference. The faculty can direct students to use the PICOT (Population, Intervention, Comparison, Outcome, Time) format. Following the formulation of a question, the students decide who will investigate the literature to locate research on the topic. The students are then allowed to complete their portion and report the results in the next class/conference session. Faculty members are challenged to direct the students – not to provide the answers. Discussion allows for students to critically examine the evidence and what the implications are for practice.

Another teaching strategy is to assign students to debate whether manual compression produced better outcomes than Perclose®. Students are directed to choose which side to debate and are referred to the literature, policies, procedures, and interviews with nursing staff, the physician, and the Quality Assurance Department for data from the institution, as well as research conducted by vendors. Once the pros and cons have been discussed, the class will determine what the evidence shows. The faculty serves as a resource, guide, and moderator throughout the process.

The idea behind these approaches is involvement. The teaching strategies help students to establish themselves as a community of learners who are achieving an educational goal by working together where each member is valued, respected, and involved in a common task. Faculty must expect some resistance to this type of group work. Students frequently dislike having to be graded as a group. As a result, the faculty should devise a grading tool that reflects each individual student's work toward a grade. This process requires assigning individual grades rather than a group grade. Students will be more receptive to group work when the grade reflects their individual work.

Specific guidelines must be given to the students. They must choose a leader who may organize the work. This assigning of roles within the group provides an opportunity for the development of leadership. The members assume responsibility for the group work involved. As the project is conceptualized, a member is selected as a spokesperson to deliver the results. The spokesperson may or may not be the group leader. In fact, having someone other than the group leader is often the best approach to allow other members to develop leadership skills.

Another useful approach is to assign students to complete a reflective journal throughout the course of the class. Students are then asked to state what their original thoughts were when the course began and what their thoughts are at the end. This journaling provides opportunities to examine critical thinking, reasoning, and clinical decision making processes over a period of time.

Group results can be delivered by PowerPoint® or posters in face-to-face settings. One nice aspect of PowerPoint® or posters is that they can be used in other classes or even as a presentation to the hospital staff who originated the question about manual compression versus Perclose®. Disseminating the student work back to staff may result in changes in policies and procedures in the institution. Students and staff can experience how evidence-based decisions can impact nursing care.

## Online Delivery

Within an online course, the engagement of students in the research content is coupled to the connectedness between the faculty member and the students. With any teaching strategy used in an online course, it is imperative the faculty carefully and consistently cultivates higher order questions to challenge the students. Chat rooms and discussion/bulletin boards are common strategies used with the delivery of content within an online course. Conscientious attention to the wording within the entries posed in either setting compels students to strive for greater knowledge to confront and expand understanding. Although these two strategies are convenient and functional to use within online delivery, other tactics can be effectively utilized. Student led discussions are one mechanism for actively engaging students in the process. Because the student identified the concern and brought it to the attention of the faculty member, allowing the student to take the lead within a chat or discussion board provides an opportunity to encourage and support the student toward success. As the student is offered the lead within the discussion supported by the faculty, confidence is developed. The faculty provides guidance for the students as they network within either venue to identify ways of seeking the information. By having a topic identified by the students, the process of learning research technique develops from the seeking of answers instead of the lecturing of facts. The "need to know" drives the process through which the research techniques can be reflected through a practical application.

A debate is another way to support the material gained by the student-led discussion or chat session. In any setting, a debate has specific steps or levels. One side provides an argument which is countered by the opposing team. Each side responds to the position presented by the other team. This back and forth countering with opposing arguments within a chat or discussion provides a realistic platform for the documentation of the differing sides. Because students document the arguments in written format, careful attention to each supporting line of reasoning must be substantiated by evidence-based information. Within a chat session, the development of a responding argument is more akin to a face-to-face session. A debate conducted within a discussion platform allows additional time to organize and sustain the points of reasoning. When a debate forum is incorporated into an online course, the faculty member has to establish the guidelines for the documentation of the arguments and the counter-arguments. Each side may be given a specific time period to post arguments and counter-arguments. The number and depth of the postings related to a debate side are included within the guidelines. Clear instructions regarding the level of expertise included within the argument related to the research process must be delineated before the debate is conducted within the chat room or on the discussion board. Since a research course is endeavoring to provide a foundation of knowledge about research, the information used to support the arguments has to reflect attention to research concepts.

Within an online delivery venue, particular care to ensure that all guidelines are clear, concise, and understandable is imperative. Because students and faculty do not have the advantage of observing non-verbal communication, care concerning the clarity of any guideline is of utmost importance. Students must be able to read and assimilate the assignments through a written format. Group work and the learning community necessitates that faculty take extra care and time in the preparation of the instructions for each and every assignment. Another important consideration for faculty is to ensure the feedback provided to the students reflects the content focus.

## Summary

Teaching a research course offers multiple challenges and opportunities for faculty to stimulate students to participate in learning activities that have relevance and value to the practice of nursing. Regardless of the setting, teaching methodologies can bring excitement to students through a variety of approaches. Student-led discussions, debates, journals, nursing rounds, PowerPoint® presentations, and posters are offered as examples of activities for faculty to utilize when teaching research. Teaching research in ways different from the traditional approaches provides satisfaction for both faculty and students. Most importantly, evidence-based practice becomes a reality.

## Learning Activities

1. Examine each of your assignments within a research course for practicality. Determine which aspect of reasoning skills are developed through the completion of each assignment.
2. For each assignment in a research course, carefully review the description to determine the rationale for the assignment. Does the rationale for the assignment clearly state how this assignment builds toward a final product?
3. Consider your student population. Classify the members of your class into the generational levels that are based upon birth year as presented in this chapter. For each of the generations you identify, develop a list of four to five characteristics embraced by that group. Look at your assignments and course schedule to determine if you have included activities to challenge students in each of the generations. Carefully consider what aspects within the course could be changed to more effectively compel that group to excel.

## Educational Philosophy

Teaching is an interactive process that should be enjoyed by all. I believe that an emphasis on fun, or at least enjoyment, is essential to provide a positive environment for learning in nursing education. Interacting with students and observing their progress is a reward to be treasured. Helping students achieve their educational goals and apply new knowledge to enhance their practice is fundamental to my approach to teaching. — Sharon Cannon

Lifelong learning is the hallmark of the educational experience. To help individuals understand the necessity of continuing to grow and learn is the ultimate reward for an educator. Helping learners develop the skills and confidence to persevere in the learning environment should be the aspiration for every teacher and facilitator. The teacher's role has evolved into that of a facilitator for the student's learning experience. By fostering the concept of lifelong learning, teachers can help students become self-motivated, passionate, and dedicated to advancing the practice of holistic nursing care and evidence-based practice for the patients they encounter. — Carol Boswell

# References

Boswell, C., & Cannon, S. (2007). *Introduction to nursing research: Incorporating evidence-based practice*. Sudbury, MA: Jones and Bartlett.

Cannon, S., Boswell, C., & Robinson, M. (2007). Making research come alive at the bedside. *Nursing Management, 38*(10), 16-17.

Elder, L., & Paul, R. (2007). Becoming a critic of your thinking. Retrieved on December 21, 2007 from www.criticalthinking.org/articles/becoming-a-critic.cfm.

Furlong, K. M., D'Luna-O'Grady, L., Macari-Hinson, M., O'Connel, K. B., & Pierson, G. S. (2007). Implementing nursing grand rounds in a community hospital. *Clinical Nurse Specialist, 21*(6), 287-291.

Gruendemann, B. J. (2007). Distance learning and perioperative nursing. *AORN Journal, 85*(3), 574-586.

Ireland, M. (2008). Assisting students to use evidence as a part of reflection on practice. *Nursing Education Perspectives, 29*(2), 90-93.

Knowles, J., & McGloin, S. (2007). Developing critical analysis skills in academic writing. *Nursing Standard, 21*(52), 35-37.

Mangold, K. (2007). Educating a new generation: Teaching baby boomer faculty about Millennial students. *Nurse Educator, 32*(1), 21-23.

McNamara, S. A. (2005). Incorporating generational diversity. *AORN Journal, 81*(6), 1149-1152.

Myrick. F., & Tamlyn, D. (2007). Teaching can never be innocent: Fostering an enlightening educational experience. *Journal of Nursing Education, 46*(7), 299-303.

Nielsen, A., Stagnell, S., & Jester, P. (2007). Guide for reflection using the clinical judgment model. *Journal of Nursing Education, 46*(11), 513-516.

Paul, R., & Elder, L. (1996). *The analysis and assessment of thinking*. Online at www.criticalthinking.org.

Reynard, R. (2007). *Tips for using chat as an instructional tool*. Retrieved on November 2, 2007 from http://campustechnology.com/printarticle.aspx?id=52470.

Riddell, T. (2007). Critical assumptions: Thinking critically about critical thinking. *Journal of Nursing Education, 46*(3), 121-156.

Russell, C. K., Burchum, J. R., Likes, W. M., Jacob, S., Graff, J. C., Driscoll, C., Britt, T., Adymy, C., & Cowan, P. (2008). WebQuests: Creating engaging, student-centered, constructivist learning activities. *CIN: Computers, Informatics, Nursing, 26*(2), 78-87.

Ryan, M., Hodson-Carlton, K., & Ali, N. S. (2005). A model for faculty teaching online: Confirmation of a dimensional matrix. *Journal of Nursing Education, 44*(8), 357-365.

Sitzman, K., & Woodard-Lener, D. (2006). Student perceptions of caring in online baccalaureate education. *Nursing Education Perspectives, 27*(5), 254-259.

Skiba, D. J. (2005). The Millennials: Have they arrived at your school of nursing? *Nursing Education Perspectives, 25*(6), 370-371.

Twibell, R., Ryan, M., & Hermiz, M. (2005). Faculty perceptions of critical thinking in student clinical experiences. *Journal of Nursing Education, 44*(2), 71-79

Zygmont, D. M., & Moore Schaefer, K. (2006). Assessing the critical thinking skills of faculty: What do the findings mean for nursing education? *Nursing Education Perspectives, 27*(5), 260-268.

# CHAPTER 34

## TEACHING EVIDENCE-BASED PRACTICE

Diane Whitehead, EdD, RN, ANEF
Lynne E. Bryant, MSN, EdD, RN

---

The content of this chapter relates to the following major content areas and subconcepts on the Certified Nurse Educator Examination Detailed Test Blueprint:

**Facilitate Learning**
- Implement a variety of teaching strategies appropriate to content; learner needs; desired learner outcomes
- Use teaching strategies based on evidence-based practices related to education

**Participate in Curriculum Design and Evaluation of Program Outcomes**
- Actively participate in the design of the curriculum to reflect current nursing and healthcare trends

**Function Effectively within the Institutional Environment and the Academic Community**
- Identify how social, economic, political and institutional forces influence nursing and higher education

---

## Introduction

The preface of Goodman's text (2004) *Ethics and Evidence-Based Medicine* begins by asking the following question: Why do you believe what you do and not something else (p. ix)? Although this might seem like a simple question, Goodman challenges us to find easy answers when we are talking about life, health, and death. He goes a step further by stating that although the answers are not always easy, healthcare providers have a duty to respond to the question.

Whether you are reading this chapter as a novice or expert teacher, you have probably already heard the term evidence-based practice (EBP). The majority of textbooks in nursing and other healthcare disciplines incorporate this terminology into at least one chapter. We believe our responsibility as nurse educators is threefold:

1. To understand the concepts related to the development and implementation of evidence-based practices

2. To effectively communicate what we have learned to our students, peers, and other healthcare providers
3. To remain informed of the current research and literature related to evidence-based practice

At some point many of you will go a step further and actually participate in evidence-based practice research.

## History of EBP

As nurses, we would like to think that all clinicians make decisions based on high-quality scientific evidence. Do we not agree there is a moral imperative that all healthcare providers know what they are doing? Do we not all practice with evidence to support our decisions? On the other hand, might we also agree that scientific knowledge is expanding at a rate that makes it impossible to keep up with changing information, that humans are fallible, and that decisions we make can prolong life or even cause death. How do we go from the moral imperative to practice using evidence to evidence-based practice?

The concern about making decisions using evidence was revealed as early as the twelfth century when the physician, rabbi, and philosopher Moses Maimonides encouraged physicians to "always correct what we have acquired, always to extend its domain; for knowledge is immense" (Goodman, 2004, p. 2).

The eighteenth-century physician, Thomas Beddoes, is credited with the intellectual birth of evidence-based practice. Dr. Beddoes believed medicine had become stagnant and secretive, arguing for the systematic collection, indexing, and sharing of medical facts. Shortly thereafter, another physician, Pierre Charles Alexandre Louis, introduced the numerical method, a precursor to clinical evaluation and chart reviews. However, it was not until the 1970's that the true EBP movement began.

The British epidemiologist, Dr. Archie Cochrane challenged the public to pay only for care supported by evidence, especially evidence supported by randomized clinical trials. Although Dr. Cochrane died in 1988, his influence continues. In 1992 the Cochrane Center was formed followed by the Cochrane Collaboration in 1993 (www3.interscience.wiley.com/cgi-bin/mrwhome/106568753/HOME). The mission of the Cochrane Collaboration is "to improve healthcare decision-making globally, through systematic reviews of the effects of healthcare interventions, published in The Cochrane Library" (www3.interscience.wiley.com/cgi-bin/mrwhome/106568753/HOME).

Fueling the fire for EBP was the 1996 Institute of Medicine's (IOM) effort to improve the nation's quality of health care. The IOM defines quality as "the degree to which health services for individuals and populations increases the likelihood of desired health outcomes and are consistent with current professional knowledge" (www.iom.edu/?id=8089&redirect=0). A result of the IOM's efforts was a series of reports, known as the *Quality Chasm Series*. These reports support the importance of closing the gap between what is recognized as quality care and what is actually practiced. The IOM's 2003 publication, *Transforming Health Care Quality*, identified evidence-based practice as one of the core competencies. The IOM website maintains up-to-date information on the IOM's Health Care Quality Initiative at www.iom.edu.

Numerous position statements have been published linking EBP to the preparation of the 21st century workforce. Among them are the American Nurses Association's (ANA) (1994) position on education for participation in nursing research; the American Association of Colleges of Nursing's (AACN) Essentials of Baccalaureate/Graduate Education for Professional Nursing Practice (2008, 1998, 1996), and the report of the Pew Health Professional Commission (1998).

## Defining Evidence-Based Practice

There are numerous definitions of EBP in the literature. One of the most widely published (and shortest) definitions was written by Dr. David Sackett. Often referred to as the man behind the current buzz word - evidence based medicine, Sackett (2000) defines EBP as "the integration of best research evidence with clinical expertise and patient values" (p. 1).

Another widely used definition is presented by Stevens (2004). Evidence-based practice may be defined as "Finding, appraising and applying scientific evidence to the treatment and management of health care". EBP includes the discovery of underlying knowledge developed from the accumulation and refinement of a large body of science. The processes of EBP create new, state of the science knowledge, summarized and clarified for translation into best practice.

This seems simple enough. We look at the evidence and then we integrate it into our practice, incorporating our expertise and the values of the patient—right? In reality, the solution is not so simple. Think about each time you perform a literature review. You input only a few key words and you still may produce thousands of hits. Most of these references will only be nursing related and in English, but then compound these results with information in many languages and written by many disciplines. Besides the fact that the volume of information is unmanageable, much of it is in forms not applicable to direct practice. Who has time to weed through all this? How does one prioritize? Should you look at all disciplines and all languages? The solution is EBP. "Evidence summaries, including systematic reviews and other forms, reduce the complexity and volume of evidence by integrating all research on a given topic into a single, meaningful whole" (Stevens, 2004).

What constitutes the most relevant evidence? Evidence from systematic reviews of randomized clinical trials (RCTs) and evidence-based clinical practice guidelines are viewed as the strongest level of evidence. A systematic review is a summary of evidence, usually by an expert panel. The panel follows a very rigorous process for this review prior to publishing the information into a summary. The most comprehensive database of systematic reviews and clinical trials are found in the Cochrane Library (www3.interscience.wiley.com/cgi-bin/mrwhome/106568753/HOME). There is a fee for full text reports; however abstracts of reviews are free. Most healthcare facilities and universities have subscriptions to the Cochrane Library. The advantages of evidence summaries are described in Box 1.

- Takes volumes of information and puts it in a manageable format
- Identifies generalizability among participants, settings, treatments, designs
- Identifies consistencies and inconsistencies among studies
- Reduces bias from random and systematic error
- Increases efficacy in time between research and implementation
- Provides for continuous updates
- Much less time consuming to obtain information
- Integrates existing information in order to make clinical, economic, research and policy decisions

Mulrow, C. D. (1994). Systematic reviews: Rationale for systematic reviews. British Medical Journal, 309, 6954, pp. 597-599.

**Box 1.** Advantages of Using Evidence Summaries
Adapted from Stevens, 2005.

A meta-analysis is a statistical technique for combining numerous quantitative studies to yield overall summary statistics. Often used in EBP to combine the results of numerous RCTs, the summary study statistics are more precise than the statistics of each independent RCT. Again, the strength of the meta-analysis will depend on the strength of each RCT (Davie & Crombie, 2007) (www.evidence-base medicine.co.uk/ebmfiles/WhatisMetaAn.pdf).

Evidence from descriptive and qualitative studies, expert panels, evidence-based theories, and opinions of leaders in the field should also be recognized as evidence. Box 2 summarizes a widely accepted rating scale for the hierarchy of evidence. The Centre for Evidence-Based Medicine has a similar, more detailed rating scale at www.cebm.net/index.aspx?o=1025.

| Level | Evidence |
|-------|----------|
| I | Systematic review of all relevant RCTs<br>Meta-analysis of all relevant RCTs<br>Clinical practice guidelines based on systematic reviews of RCTs (clinical pathways, protocols, algorithms, standards of care) |
| II | At least one well-designed RCT |
| III | Well-designed controlled trials without randomization |
| IV | Well-designed case-control and cohort studies |
| V | Systematic reviews of descriptive and qualitative studies |
| IV | Single descriptive or qualitative study |
| VII | Expert opinions or reports of expert committees |

**Box 2.** Rating Scale for the Hierarchy of Evidence
Adapted from Guyatt & Rennie, 2002

Remember the old saying "garbage in, garbage out"? The Agency for Healthcare Research and Quality (www.ahrq.gov/clinic/epcsums/strengthsum.htm), through its Evidence-based Practice Center (EPC), works with a group of 12 EPCs throughout the United States to advance the understanding of how best to review clinical and related literature to ensure quality and rigor in each review.

One of the challenges as educators is to ensure that our students (and our peers) understand the difference between research utilization and EBP. Many of us can recall critiquing the qualitative and quantitative studies in our research classes and finding articles from CINAHL and other nursing references to support our clinical decisions. This process of using research finding as a basis for decision making (research utilization) is often used interchangeably with the term EBP. Besides using the terms interchangeably, we often assume that when we introduce students to research utilization they will automatically understand how to move into EBP. Consider this question: What is more powerful in clinical decision making, one study with a low sample size or a systematic review of multiple studies across disciplines? Unlike reviewing one article (research utilization), EBP involves not only the best evidence, but takes into consideration the context in which care is provided, resources, practitioner skills, and patient values.

## Teaching EBP

Before integrating concepts of EBP into your program's curriculum or into your individual course, you need to conduct an assessment of yourself, your program, and your institution. What are the strengths and weaknesses? How can you capitalize on the strengths and address the weaknesses?

### Institution

One of the first questions you must ask is "does my institution have the resources to support my teaching EBP successfully?" Box 3 lists questions for evaluating the institution's readiness. We encourage you to take time to evaluate your institution, your department, and yourself. Do not be discouraged if you do not have the human, fiscal, and technology resources to the level you feel you need. There are many resources available to assist you. Every year numerous conferences supporting evidence-based practice are available. Seek help and advice from programs that have been successful in implementing EBP into their programs.

1. Will the philosophy and mission support EBP?
2. Will the faculty and administration promote my commitment to teaching EBP?
3. Do any of my colleagues have the knowledge and skills to teach EBP?
4. Will the students and faculty have access to computers with Internet access?
5. Are the faculty and students computer literate?
6. Will the library support EBP resources?
7. Are the librarians knowledgeable in searching for EBP resources?
8. What is the status of EBP currently in our program?
9. What is our program's goal related to practicing and/or promoting EBP?
10. Are my colleagues supportive of this change?

**Box 3.** Evaluating the Institution's Readiness
Adapted from Melnyk, B. & Fineout-Overholt, E. 2005). Evidence-Based Practice in Nursing & Healthcare: A Guide to Best Practice. Philadelphia: LWW.

## Teaching Models

It is important that content related to EBP be included in the curriculum. "Foundations for practice improvement based on EBP should be initiated during undergraduate education, expanded in master's education, and advanced in doctoral education" (Stevens, 2005, p. 5). The following two models promote practice and are useful for teaching the EBP process.

## ACE Star Model of Knowledge Transformation

The Academic Center for Evidence-Based Practice (ACE) was established in 2000 at the University of Texas Health Science Center in San Antonio, Texas. The center focuses on workforce development for EBP and the study of the processes within EBP (Stevens, 2005). The ACE Star Model of Knowledge Transformation depicts the conversion of research findings from primary research results, through a series of stages and forms, to impact health outcomes by way of evidence-based care (www.acestar.uthscsa.edu/Learn_model.htm).

The ACE identifies the following premises related to knowledge transformation:

1.  Knowledge transformation is necessary before research results are useable in clinical decision making.
2.  Knowledge derives from a variety of sources. In health care, sources of knowledge include research evidence, experience, authority, trial and error, and theoretical principles.
3.  The most stable and generalizable knowledge is discovered through systematic processes that control bias, namely, the research process.
4.  Evidence can be classified into a hierarchy of strength of evidence. Relative strength of evidence is largely dependent on the rigor of the scientific design that produced the evidence. The value of rigor is that it strengthens cause-and-effect relationships.
5.  Knowledge exists in a variety of forms. As research evidence is converted through systematic steps, knowledge from other sources (expertise, patient preference) is added, creating yet another form of knowledge.
6.  The form (package) in which knowledge exists can be referenced to its use; in the case of EBP, the ultimate use is application in healthcare.
7.  The form of knowledge determines its usability in clinical decision making. For example, research results from a primary investigation are less useful to decision making than an evidence-based clinical practice guideline.
8.  Knowledge is transformed through the following processes:

- summarization into a single statement about the state of the science
- translation of the state of the science into clinical recommendations, with addition of clinical expertise, application of theoretical principles, and patient preferences
- Integration of recommendations through organizational and individual actions and evaluation of impact of actions on targeted outcomes (Stevens, 2004. Ace Star Model of EBP: Knowledge Transformation. Academic Center for Evidence-based Practice. The University of Texas Health Science Center at San Antonio www.acestar.uthscsa.edu/Learn_model.htm).

The ACE Star Model of Knowledge Transformation provides a framework useful in teaching the application of EBP (Figure 1). This model depicts the five stages of knowledge transformation. Focusing on the form of knowledge at each stage, the learner will have a context within which to understand EBP.

1. **Discovery.** Star Point 1 focuses on primary research. At this point new knowledge is discovered through a traditional research study using a variety of research designs.
2. **Evidence summary.** Star Point 2 introduces EBP. At this point evidence summaries are generated. The strength of the summary will dictate the credibility and reproducible results of the findings.
3. **Translation.** Star Point 3 transforms the evidence summaries into actual practice. This is done in two stages. First, translation of evidence into a clinical practice guideline (CPG). The CPG may be represented as a care standard, clinical pathway, protocol, or algorithm. The second stage is the actual integration of the CPG into practice.
4. **Integration.** Star Point 4 represents integration and sustainability of the change by the organization.
5. **Evaluation.** Star point 5, the final stage, is the evaluation of the EBP on health outcomes, provider and patient satisfaction, efficacy, efficiency, economic analysis, and health status input (Stevens, 2005).

The Academic Center for Evidence-Based Practice has published *Essential Competencies for Evidence-Based Practice in Nursing* (2005). These competencies were developed by a national panel of EBP experts. The competencies are described by educational level (undergraduate, masters, doctoral) and by each Star Point. These competencies are very useful as a starting point to begin integrating EBP into your program. This publication is available for purchase through the www.acestar.

# ACE Star Model of Knowledge Transformation

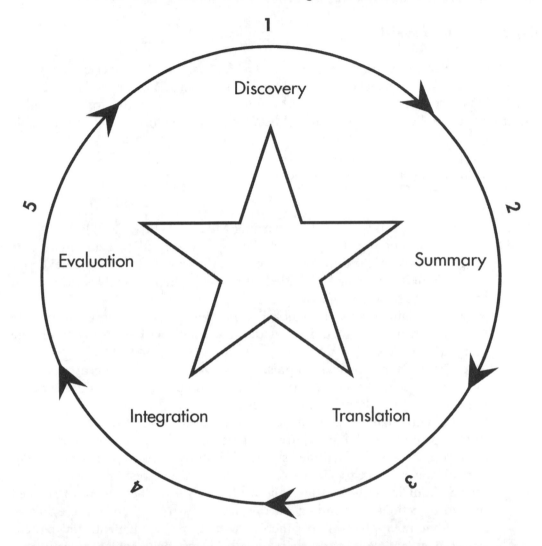

**Figure 1.** ACE Model
Stevens, K. R. (2004). Ace Star Model of EBP: Knowledge Transformation. Academic Center for Evidence-based Practice. The University of Texas Health Science Center at San Antonio. www.acestar.uthscsa.edu/Learn_model.htm

uthscsa.edu/Competencies.htm. We will be referring to these competencies as we discuss integrating EBP concepts into your curriculum.

## Cycle of Learning Model

The Cycle of Learning model is also used for teaching EBP. Developed at the University of Rochester School Of Nursing, this model is similar to the ACE Star model in addressing learners' needs through the cycle from the formulation of questions to application of evidence. The foundation of this model is a triangle depicting
1. Knowledge of research methods
2. Clinical experience and judgment
3. A context of caring

There are six steps to the Cycle of Learning Model (Melnyk, 2005):
1. **Step 1: Formulating the question.** Focuses on formulating an answerable and searchable clinical question. Step 1 is the foundation for the next four steps. The PICO format, explained later in this chapter, enables the student to formulate the question.
2. **Step 2: Applying search strategies.** Enables the student to apply appropriate search strategies. The focus is on evidence synthesis with the use of Cochrane systematic reviews.
3. **Step 3: Initiating critical appraisal.** Involves a critical appraisal of the evidence. Much more in depth than the traditional research critique, evidence is examined for validity and usefulness.
4. **Step 4: Synthesizing valid evidence.** Synthesizes research from step 3. This is not a repeat of step 3, but requires the student to identify commonalities and the uniqueness of the identified studies. It is during this step that the student puts all the evidence together to answer the clinical question.
5. **Step 5: Applying or generating valid evidence.** Allows the student to proceed in two directions. Depending on the outcomes from Step 4, the evidence will either be applied in conjunction with clinical judgment, and patient preferences and values, or there will be insufficient evidence to answer the clinical question. In the latter case, an outcomes management/quality improvement initiative might be instituted to generate internal evidence. Or, more rigorous research might be conducted to general external evidence.
6. **Step 6: Evaluating interventions or initiatives.** As with the ACE Star Model, this final step is one of evaluation. In either model the cycle begins again as the process surrounding quality outcomes continues.

## Key Elements for Including EBP in the Curriculum

Before you decide how to incorporate EBP in the curriculum faculty the following actions must be considered:

- Faculty write a definition of EBP
- Incorporate EBP in the philosophy
- Develop program student outcomes inclusive of EBP
- Assure the faculty has adequate EBP knowledge and skills
- Identify faculty who are fervent about EBP (Melnyk & Fineout-Overholt, 2005)

Once these tenets are established, approaches to including EBP in all courses can be identified. At present, no evidence exists as to what are the best approaches to use to include EBP in the curriculum (Ciliska, 2005). Faculty should select a model for teaching EBP that fits the needs of their curriculum, faculty, and students.

## Approaches to Integrating EBP in the Nursing Curriculum

Undergraduate students should be viewed as consumers of research and EBP. Their role is not to generate this evidence, but to know how to use it and apply it to their practice. Furthermore, all nurses, regardless of their educational background are expected to use the best available evidence as a basis for their nursing practice (Levin, 2006). Most baccalaureate nursing programs have a research course within the curriculum. In many cases, students perceive research as a course they must endure to get through their education to achieve their goal of graduation. Research concepts may or may not be threaded throughout the curriculum. In programs where research is threaded throughout the curriculum, a typical student assignment might be to locate and critique a research article that relates to course content. This technique does not promote student understanding or interest in research. With the paradigm shift to EBP, many faculty are at a loss about how to integrate this concept in courses. How can beginning students look at the Cochrane Collection and understand it? In our curriculum, the research course is in the second year. How will these beginning students learn to integrate EBP in the fundamentals course?

In the next section of this chapter, we include ideas about how to integrate teaching EBP into your curriculum and make EBP come alive for you and your students! Included are sample concepts, objectives, and activities for typical courses in a baccalaureate curriculum to help you get started integrating EBP. However, these ideas can be adapted for use in an associate degree program as well. Additional resources are included within the text as well as at the end of the chapter. We have divided this discussion by level of student: in to first, second and third year, but this approach can be adapted by semester or courses to fit your curriculum.

An important part of incorporating EBP in the curriculum is to develop teaching strategies, class activities, and assignments that build on those found in previous courses. The goal is to encourage the student to develop an attitude of inquiry. Additionally, students need to develop critical thinking skills. A carefully orchestrated curriculum can accomplish both.

Before we begin, we would like to address a common question that arises when considering how to integrate EBP in the curriculum: Where should the research course be placed in the curriculum? There is no right answer to this question. It should be placed wherever your faculty believes it should be placed! There are proponents of placing it at the beginning of the program, and others who believe it should be taught later in the curriculum. In the latter case, as in the sample that follows, concepts of EBP can be integrated in the curriculum even though students have not taken a research course. The important point is that faculty have rationale for their decision, then design the research portion of the curriculum around that rationale. As with any component of the curriculum, if outcome measures indicate the approach is not working, then faculty should reconsider. Change is based on data.

## First Year Students

Beginning students are introduced to EBP in their first course. At this level, the teacher is the expert and students are not asked to locate or critique any type of nursing evidence. Table 1 contains concepts, objectives, and course activities related to first year courses.

In a course focused on an introduction to nursing, faculty can introduce the concept of EBP and it relevance to nursing practice. The focus is to define EBP as well as the role of the nurse in seeking evidence. The types of evidence can be described in very basic terms. The faculty serves as a role model, and students are introduced to critical thinking and its relationship to EBP.

Using situations that students are familiar with can help students understand the concept. For instance, students can be placed in groups and assigned a consumer situation such as buying a car. The students then search for evidence in several consumer resources to help them make an informed decision. Some groups are assigned situations where there is a large amount of evidence, and others where there is minimal evidence. Students then present their evidence or lack of evidence to the class. The faculty relates this exercise to EBP. To further relate EBP to nursing,

| Course | Concepts | Objectives | Activities |
|---|---|---|---|
| Introduction to Nursing | 1. Nursing practice supported by evidence – what does that mean?<br>2. Role of the nurse in seeking evidence<br>3. Critical thinking –question what you are doing<br>4. Instructor as role model | 1. Define EBP<br>2. Discuss the relationship between critical thinking in nursing and EBP<br>3. Describe the role of the nurse as a participant in an evidence-based approach to nursing practice | 1. Consumer Group Activity<br>2. Storytelling related to the use of the CPG in their clinical experience |
| Fundamentals of Nursing Health Assessment | 1. Connecting evidence to skills<br>2. PICO introduced | 1. Utilize the PICO format to develop clinical questions<br>2. Describe the relationship between CPG and selected clinical skills | 1. Develop a clinical question using the PICO format<br>2. Paper on how a CPG influences the performance of the skill |
| Pharmacology | 1. Evidence related to drugs reaching and leaving the market<br>2. How drugs get on clinical practice guidelines | 1. Discuss how EBP influences the development of drugs and their inclusion/omission of drugs from the market and CPG | 1. Instructor examples<br>2. Class discussion |

**Table 1.** First Year Courses

the faculty uses storytelling and describes how EBP was used for decision making in his/her own practice.

Health assessment and nursing skills courses are usually placed in the first year of nursing curricula. In these courses, the focus is the introduction of evidence for some basic nursing practices. This evidence can be in the form of clinical practice guidelines (CPG). Several guidelines are explained to the students as examples. At this point in the curriculum the students have probably not taken a research course. Therefore, the faculty acts as the expert, and is the one to appraise the validity of the CPG.

To assist students to understand the use of these guidelines and to develop their critical thinking skills, students are assigned to compare a simple CPG with what they actually witness in practice. They examine why a CPG may or may not be followed in specific situations. This demonstrates that evidence is used in conjunction with the practitioner's expertise and also patient preferences and values (Levin, 2006). This can be a discussion, or a short one-page paper, or both. The faculty should demonstrate this activity before it is assigned as a paper. Many level appropriate Evidence-based Care Sheets can be located in CINHAL. Examples of these include Urinary Catheter Use and Prevention of Infection (Pinto, 2004), Fever Management (Rutledge, 2004), or Hand Hygiene, Standard Handwashing vs Alcohol Rubs (Buckley, 2004). The article Intramuscular Injection: An Integrative Research Review and Guideline for Evidence-Based Practice (Nicoll & Hesby, 2002) can be assigned as another source for a CPG. Another source that is appropriate for this level student is Best Practice Guideline for the Subcutaneous Administration of Insulin in Adults with Type 2 Diabetes (Registered Nurses Association of Ontario, 2004).

In these courses, students may be entering the clinical area for the first time. At this point, they are encouraged to ask questions about nursing practice. To assist the student to frame the question in a way in which evidence can be located, the PICO format is introduced.

- **P** refers to patient population
- **I** is intervention or area of interest
- **C** is comparison
- **O** is outcome (LoBiondo-Wood & Haber, 2006; Melnyk & Fineout-Over-holt, 2005).

This is completed at a very basic level and is demonstrated by the faculty. For example, a question might be: For healthcare workers, how effective is an alcohol-based rub versus soap and water in cleansing hands? A typical assignment might be to assign students to write a question using the PICO format for specific situations.

For these assigned situations, the faculty has already located related clinical practice guidelines. Although students may not be searching for the answer to the PICO question, they are learning how to ask the question in a focused format.

In a pharmacology course, students are introduced to the concept of clinical trials as they relate to the process of drug development. Another concept that can be included in this course is the presence of drugs in CPGs for disease treatment. The faculty can provide examples of CPGs related to specific drugs taught in the course and discuss how they are used in practice. An example is Adult Diabetes Clinical Practice Guidelines (Kaiser Permanente Care Management Institute, 2005).

## Second Year Students

The focus in the second year shifts from the faculty member as one who locates evidence to the student. In a research class at this level, students can begin to delve into the EBP process in more depth as a more complete base is formed in this course. See Table 2 for examples of the concepts, objective, and activities for courses in the second year.

In a research course, students are typically introduced to the basic concepts of research and research utilization. In addition to those basic concepts, research utilization and its relationship to EBP are examined. The different types of evidence and how to locate evidence should be included in this course. Students should be introduced to the concepts of meta-analysis and systematic review. Additionally, the process of learning how to evaluate evidence is begun as students explore the hierarchy of evidence. It is helpful to have the reference librarian come to class to explain which databases and other resources are available and how they can be accessed at your institution. It is important for students to discuss ethical principles as they relate to EBP. Additionally, a class discussion about reasons the availability of more medical guidelines than nursing based guidelines is appropriate for this course. This course should also include a discussion about what resources the student should use if no CPG can be located. It is important that students understand the difference between research utilization and evidence-based practice, and this can be emphasized by assigning students to compare the impact on practice using a systematic review and a research article. The systematic review and the article are selected by the faculty. By the end of the course students should be able to locate a CPG and evaluate the strength of evidence for the guideline. These abilities can be demonstrated in a written assignment. Burns and Foley (2005) describe such an assignment in which students are given an article on handwashing, and are given an instrument developed by faculty that will assist them to critically appraise the

| Course | Concepts | Objectives | Activities |
|---|---|---|---|
| Theories/Research | 1. Where to find types of evidence<br>2. How to evaluate evidence<br>3. Relationship between EBP and research utilization<br>4. Introduction to databases<br>5. Ethical principles<br>6. Explore reasons for more medical than nursing guidelines | 1. Locate systematic reviews and evidence summaries<br>2. Recognize the hierarchy and strength of levels of scientific evidence<br>3. Distinguish between EBP and research utilization<br>4. Discuss ethical issues related to differences in practice and EBP<br>5. Explore differences between medical and nursing guidelines | 1. Paper on strength of evidence to CP<br>2. Paper comparing the impact on practice using a systematic review and research article |
| Medical/Surgical Specialties | 1. Utilize agency adopted clinical practice guidelines, clinical pathways, or algorithms<br>2. Access databases | 1. Compare evidence with current care practices for assigned patients<br>2. Describe the use of an EBP approach in your clinical decision making | 1. Clinical experience<br>2. Compare and contrast a CPG with current care practices |

**Table 2.** Second Year Courses

article. Burns and Foley describe a second assignment that is designed to assist students to locate EBP literature for preselected (by faculty) topics.

Many agencies have adopted evidence-based guidelines for practice for use within that particular facility. In their clinical courses, students should be assigned to access these guidelines and compare the use of these guidelines in the practice they observe on that unit. Their findings can be discussed in post conference or in a written paper. This same activity can be assigned using either nursing or medically-based CPGs found in the literature for their assigned patients. This assignment helps students to think critically about why certain aspects of the guidelines were incorporated to the patient's care and conversely reasons why certain aspects of the guideline were not applied to that patient's care.

Other sources of evidence besides CPGs should be included in these courses. Students may use CINAHL, MEDLINE, or the Cochrane Collection to locate systematic reviews or meta-analyses. There are several assignments which can make use of these searches. Levin (2006) proposes that students be required to develop a clinical question for each clinical experience. These questions could be discussed in postconference and a plan developed to determine the answer. Students are assigned to locate the answer, which could be in the form of a systematic review, meta-analysis, or a CPG. This process helps students develop a questioning attitude. Levin also proposes conducting EBP rounds. In this assignment, rounds are made and students develop a clinical question for every patient. A few of the questions are selected, and evidence is located to answer the question. This information is presented during postconference, along with a discussion about how this might be implemented in practice.

In courses about nursing and medical practice, faculty should refer to the evidence used for common practices. For example, the technique for CPR was changed in 2006. The evidence supporting the change in practice should be discussed in class. Whenever possible, evidence for a particular practice should be discussed. An assignment whereby students are directed to locate the evidence for specific nursing practices is useful in helping students identify that many practices are based on tradition rather than evidence. Students may be frustrated by their inability to locate higher levels of evidence other than textbooks or one research article. However, the student is exposed to the need for nursing to build evidence for nursing practice (Rambur, 1999).

A classroom activity may include a case study about a course related topic and students locate, or are assigned, appropriate evidence for class discussion of the case study. Some examples of CPGs that are appropriate for this level student are:

- Diabetic foot disorders: a clinical practice guideline (2006 revision) (Frykberg, 2006)

- Clinical guideline for adults with diabetes (Joslin Diabetes Center, 2006)

For additional information about EBP activities refer to:
- Integrating quality and safety content into clinical teaching in the acute care setting by Day and Smith (2007) contains a discussion of additional ways to integrate EBP that are appropriate for second year students
- Weaving Undergraduate Research into Practice-based Experience (Kenty, 2002)

## Third Year Students

As students enter their final year of nursing education, their ability to apply principles of EBP should increase. Table 3 includes course related concepts, objectives, and activities.

In an advanced medical-surgical nursing course, the students begin to look for evidence-based approaches to care, and use these as the basis for the care they provide. Students in the critical care areas might locate and critique a systematic review or a CPG and present their findings to the clinical group. They can also present a summary of a CPG to the nursing staff. Examples of appropriate CPGs are:
- Guidelines for preventing healthcare-associated pneumonia, 2003: Recommendations of CDC and the Healthcare Infection Control Practices Advisory Committee (Tablan, Anderson, Besser, Bridges, & Hajjeh, 2003)
- Rotational bed therapy to prevent and treat respiratory complications: A review and meta-analysis (Goldhill, 2007)

Another activity in the advanced medical-surgical course focuses on the investigation of the need to develop CPGs that are appropriate for the students' assigned clinical units. This assists students to realize the need for continued research and to identify how they can be part of the solution. Students should continue to ask questions about nursing practice.

In the leadership or practicum course students begin to role model using EBP to clinical nursing staff. Students should begin to explore the culture of the organization for integrating EBP in practice, and examine the extent of its use on their unit. In a written paper, students describe their findings. If EBP is not used, or used minimally, on their unit they can develop a plan to introduce or enhance the use of EBP. If EBP is used extensively on the unit, they can discuss the factors that support its use. In their clinical journal, students should reflect upon the influence of role modeling EBP.

| Course | Concepts | Objectives | Activities |
|---|---|---|---|
| Advanced Medical/ Surgical Courses | 1. Choose EBP approaches over routine for own decision making<br>2. Investigate need for additional CPG in your clinical area | 1. Utilize EBP approach for own decision making<br>2. Investigate need for additional CPG in your clinical area<br>3. Present a brief summary of a systematic review or practice guideline to nursing staff | 1. Develop an in-depth critique of a systemic review or CPG (written paper)<br>2. Post conference report.<br>3. Present the summary to nursing staff |
| Leadership/ Practicum | 1. Student as role model | 1. Evaluate client outcome related to application or non-application of CPG or systematic review<br>2. Evaluate culture of the organization for integrating EBP<br>3. Identify area of nursing practice in need of a CPG<br>4. Develop recommendations for implementing change<br>5. Role model behaviors that contribute to inclusion of EBP in nursing care | 1. Clinical journal activity<br>2. Written paper to meet objectives 2, 3, 4 |

**Table 3.** Third Year Courses

These are just a few ideas to help you get started incorporating EBP in the curriculum. Consider the references used in this chapter for more ideas, such as the article by Schmidt and Brown (2007). Any of these assignments can be modified to fit your curriculum and course structure. We are sure you will add your own assignments and approaches as you build your knowledge base.

## Challenges

Incorporating EBP in the curriculum can be both rewarding and challenging. In this section, we focus on some of the challenges faced by educators as they seek to include these concepts in the curriculum.

Many educators are unfamiliar with the concept of EBP. It is uncomfortable to teach a topic with which the educator is unfamiliar. In addition, this lack of understanding hinders the incorporation of concepts within the curriculum. Faculty may understand the concept of EBP, but they lack the skills to locate or evaluate evidence. The lack of knowledge may cause resistance to including EBP in courses. Educational programs that are mentored by faculty experienced in EBP may decrease this challenge. A librarian can be a key resource to assist in this area (Klem & Weiss, 2005).

Faculty often thinks of EBP as time consuming. This challenge is not without merit. For those beginning to use EBP in their course, the educator must first locate and evaluate evidence relevant to that course and the level of the student. This is the same process used by the student (Erikson-Owen & Kennedy, 2001). The teacher must decide how to incorporate EBP in class materials and then design activities and assignments for the course. Fortunately, there are examples in the literature with suggestions about class activities and assignments, as well as those reported in this chapter.

Not only is a lack of knowledge about EBP a challenge, but a lack of excitement or passion for EBP present a challenge to this effort. Having a few champions of EBP who encourage and assist others in this effort may lessen this challenge (Chaboyer, Willman, Johnson, & Stockhausen, 2003).

Faculty may resist including EBP into the curriculum or their courses because they believe their course is so content saturated there is no room for one more thing. Government mandated policy related to use of evidence in care makes it necessary that students learn how to use EBP (Cilska, 2005). Reexamining how content is taught may help faculty incorporate EBP in their course.

Another challenge that Ciliska (2005) cites is that students do not see EBP used in the clinical area. However, that argument lacks merit as the clinical environment is changing. Additionally, nursing education needs to be a leader in this effort and educate nurses who will become change agents in the clinical area to promote the use of EBP.

The lack of nursing focused evidence is another challenge faced by nurse educators. When examining most nursing textbooks for evidence, one usually finds secondary sources or references to only one research article. When searching databases for evidence, the large majority are medically based, not nursing. All of this highlights the need for nurses to become active in the generation of evidence.

Finally, there is a lack of evidence regarding nursing education. Nurse educators use many creative teaching strategies for which there is no evidence (Ferguson & Day, 2005). This is definitely an area for further study. The National League for Nursing has a long-established focus on developing the science of nursing education. Refer to the chapter by Shultz in this book for information on evidenced based teaching in nursing education.

## Summary

The process by which nurse educators incorporate EBP in the curriculum is challenging, but imperative in today's educational and practice climate. Through careful planning, education of faculty, and development of resources, you can be successful!

## Learning Activities

1. Interview nursing faculty. Ask them what approach they take to teach EBP.
2. Develop a learning strategy for EBP for courses you teach. Develop a tool for evaluating this strategy. Implement the strategy. Evaluate the learning strategy. Was it successful? Why or why not?
3. Develop a plan for integrating EBP into the program where you teach or into a program that you are otherwise associated with. Present your plan to the other faculty in the program. What was their reaction?

## Educational Philosophy

I see my relationship with students as a partnership where teaching and learning are shared. Throughout this process, I believe in providing an atmosphere of caring, commitment, and enthusiasm for nursing. I want students to understand both the art and science of nursing, seeking evidence to support their practices. Above all, I hope to inspire them to understand what an honor it is to say "I am a nurse". — Diane Whitehead

I believe that students learn when they are challenged to think and are actively engaged in the learning process. As an educator, my role is to facilitate learning by providing innovative experiences that challenge students to think, be creative, and build their confidence level. These experiences should be built on sound educational practices and should not be boring and teacher-centered. I believe that as an educator, I need to continue to learn new ways to teach. — Lynne E. Bryant

## References

ACE: Learn About Evidence-Based Practice Academic Center for Evidence-Based Practice www.acestar.uthscsa.edu/Learn_model.htm

The Agency for Healthcare Research and Quality. (2002). *Systems to rate the strength of scientific evidence*. Retrieved February 4, 2008 from (www.ahrq. gov/clinic/epcsums/strengthsum.htm)

American Association of Colleges of Nursing. (2008). *The essentials of baccalaureate education for professional nursing practice*. Retrieved February 4, 2008 from www.aacn.nche.edu/Education/pdf/BaccEssentials98.pdf

American Association of Colleges of Nursing. (1996). *The essentials of master's education for advance practice nursing*. Retrieved February 4, 2008 from www. aacn.nche.edu/Education/pdf/MasEssentials96.pdf

American Nurses Association Position Statement. Retrieved February 4, 2008 from ainMenuCategories/HealthcareandPolicyIssues/ANAPositionStatements/research.aspx

Burns, H. K., & Foley, S. M. (2005). Building a foundation for an evidence-based approach to practice: Teaching basic concepts to undergraduate freshman students. *Journal of Professional Nursing, 21*(6), 351-357.

Buckley, L. (2004). Hand hygiene, standard handwashing vs alcohol hand rubs. CINAHL information systems. Retrieved February 24, 2008 from web.ebsco-host.com.ezproxy.barry.edu/ehost/pdf?vid=6&hid=15&sid=73aa5849-6690-4765-bf1f-e38a77a60558%40sessionmgr8

Centre for Evidence Based Medicine (1998). *Levels of evidence*. Retrieved February 4, 2008 from www.cebm.net/index.aspx?o=1025

Chaboyer, W., Willman, A., Johnson, P., & Stockhausen, L. (2004). Embedding evidence-based practice in a nursing curriculum: A benchmarking project. *Nurse Education in Practice, 4*, 216-223.

Ciliska, D. (2005). Educating for evidence-based practice. *Journal of Professional Nursing, 21*(6), 345-350.

Cochrane Library. Retrieved February 4, 2008 from www3.interscience.wiley.com/cgi-bin/mrwhome/106568753/HOME

Crossing the Quality Chasm: The IOM Health Care Quality Initiative www.iom.edu/?id=8089&redirect=0

Davie, H., & Crombie, I. (2007). *What is meta-analysis? What Is Series*, 1(8) p. 1 Retrieved February 4, 2008 from www.evidence-based-medicine.co.uk/ebm-files/WhatisMetaAn.pdf

Day, L., & Smith, E.L. (2007). Integrating quality and safety content into clinical teaching in the acute care setting. *Nursing Outlook, 55*(3), 138-143.

Erikson-Owens, D.A., & Kennedy, H.P. (2001). Fostering evidence-based care in clinical teaching. *Journal of Midwifery & Women's Health, 46*(3), 137-145.

Ferguson, L., & Day, R.A. (2005). Evidence-based nursing education: Myth or reality? *Journal of Nursing Education, 44*(4), 107-115.

Frykberg, R. G. (2006). Diabetic foot disorders: A clinical practice guideline (2006 revision), *Journal of Foot & Ankle Surgery, 45*(5): Supplement: S-2-66 (journal article) CINAHL AN: 2009311690.

Funk, S. G., Tounrquist, E. M., & Champagne, M. T. (1989). A model for improving the dissemination of nursing research. *Western Journal of Nursing Research, 11*(3), 362-367.

Goodman, K. (2004). *Ethics and evidence-based medicine*. United Kingdom: Cambridge University Press.

Goldhill, D. R. (2007). Rotational bed therapy to prevent and treat respiratory complications: A review and meta-analysis. *American Journal of Critical Care 16*(1), 50-62.

Guyatt, G., & Rennie, D. (2002). *Users' guides to the medical literature*. Washington, DC: American Medical Association Press.

Institute of Medicine. Retrieved February 4, 2008 from www.iom.edu/?id=8089&redirect=0

Institute of Medicine. Retrieved February 4, 2008 from www.iom.edu

Kenty, J. R. (2001). Weaving undergraduate research into practice-based experiences. *Nurse Educator, 26*(4), 182-186.

Klem, M. L., & Weiss, P. M. (2005). Evidence-based resources and the role of librarians in developing evidence-based curricula. *Journal of Professional Nursing 21*(6), 380-387.

Levin, R. F. (2006) Teaching evidence-based practice throughout an undergraduate curriculum: Here, there, and everywhere. In R. F. Levine & H. R. Feldman (Eds.), *Teaching evidence-based practice in nursing* (pp. 221-227). New York: Springer.

LoBiondo, G., & Haber, J. (2006). *Nursing research: Methods and critical appraisal for evidence-based practice.* St. Louis: Mosby.

Melnyk, B., & Fineout-Overholt, E. (2005). *Evidence-based practice in nursing & healthcare: A guide to best practice.* Philadelphia: LWW.

Mulrow, C. D. (1994). Systematic reviews: Rationale for systematic reviews. *British Medical Journal, 309,* pp. 597-599.

Nicoll, L. H., & Hesby, A. (2002). Intramuscular injection: An integrative research review and guideline foe evidence-based practice. *Applied Nursing Research, 16*(2), 149-162.

Pew Health Professions Commission (1998). Recreating Health Professional Practice for a New Century. Retrieved February 4, 2008 from www.futurehealth.ucsf.edu/pdf_files/recreate.pdf

Pinto, S. (2004). Urinary catheter use & prevention of infection. CINAHL Information Systems. Retrieved February 24, 2008 from http://web.ebscohost.com.ezproxy.barry.edu/ehost/pdf?vid=13&hid=15&sid=73aa5849-6690-4765-bf1f-e38a77a60558%40sessionmgr8

Rambur, B. (1999). Fostering evidence-based practice in nursing education. *Journal of Professional Nursing, 15*(5), 270-274.

Rutledge, D. (2004). Fever Management. CINAHL Information Systems. Retrieved February 24, 2008 from http://web.ebscohost.com.ezproxy.barry.edu/ehost/pdf?vid=7&hid=15&sid=73aa5849-6690-4765-bf1f-e38a77a60558%40sessionmgr8

Sackett, D. L., Straus, S. E., Richardson, W.S., Rosenberg, W., & Hayes, R. B. (2000). *Evidence-based medicine: How to practice and teach EBM.* London: Churchill Livingstone.

Schmidt, N. A., & Brown, J. M. (2007). Use of innovative-decision making process teaching strategy to promote evidence-based practice. *Journal of Professional Nursing, 23*(3), 150-156.

Stevens, K. R. (2004). *Ace star model of EBP: Knowledge transformation.* Academic Center for Evidence-based Practice. The University of Texas Health Science Center at San Antonio. www.acestar.uthscsa.edu/Learn_model.htm

Tablan, O. C., Anderson, L. J., Besser, R., Bridges, C., & Hajjeh, R. (2003). Guidelines for preventing health-care-associates pneumonia, 2003: recommendations of CDC and the Healthcare Infection Control Practices Advisory Committee. MMWR Recommn Rep 1997 Jan3:22(RR-!: 1-79. Retrieved

February 24, 2008 from www.guideline.gov/summary/summary.aspx?doc_id=4872&nbr=003506&string=health-care+AND+associated+AND+pneumonia

# UNIT 5: TEACHING AND LEARNING IN THE CLASSROOM

# CHAPTER 35

# TEACHING IN THE CLASSROOM

## Linda Caputi, MSN, EdD, RN, CNE

The content of this chapter relates to the following major content areas and subconcepts on the Certified Nurse Educator Examination Detailed Test Blueprint:

**Facilitate Learning**
- Implement a variety of teaching strategies appropriate to content; learner needs; desired learner outcomes
- Use teaching strategies based on evidence-based practices related to education
- Modify teaching strategies and learning experiences based on consideration of learners' past educational and life experiences
- Create opportunities for learners to develop their own critical thinking skills
- Create a positive learning environment that fosters a free exchange of ideas

**Facilitate Learner Development and Socialization**
- Foster the development of learners in the cognitive and affective domains
- Adapt teaching styles and interpersonal interactions to facilitate learner behaviors

## Introduction

A walk through the hallways of any college or university reveals that present-day education largely consists of using the lecture method to deliver instruction. In other words, the lecture format remains the most used teaching methodology. A single teacher stands in front of a fairly large number of students to deliver information. Teachers may relate to this method and be comfortable with this method because this is the way they were taught. Just as people often parent as they were parented, teachers teach as they were taught.

When I give presentations at nurse educator and staff development conferences, I often ask how many teachers use lecture. Approximately 90% of any given audience indicates that lecture is their primary method for delivery of educational content. Their reasons for using this method vary, and most say they would rather not lecture but believe they have no other choice. Closer examination of this method reveals lecture may not be all that bad.

Even if teachers would like to use other methods, they are frequently prohibited by institutional policy. For example, many colleges require a minimum number of students to be enrolled in a class. This number can range from a few to hundreds. Depending on the content, it becomes difficult for teachers to use methods other than lecture as the number of students in the classroom increases.

Lecturing will remain a prevalent teaching method in colleges and universities. It is not a bad method, just an oftentimes misused one. It is my hope that after reading this chapter, teachers will look at lecturing in a new light, realizing once again it is not the method that is good or bad, but how it is used.

This chapter discusses classroom instructional events, including lecture. It then describes additional enhancements for making the classroom an enriched environment for both teacher and students. Although many of these strategies have been used primarily in undergraduate courses, they can be adapted for use in graduate level courses.

## Advantages and Disadvantages of the Lecture Method

### Advantages of the Lecture Method

Teachers still use the lecture method because there are advantages. A lecture does not have to be boring. An enthusiastic teacher can motivate students and enliven information that may seem technical and tedious in a book. Some of the advantages of the lecture method include the following:

- Provides the teacher with maximum control
- Keeps all students focused on the same point
- Ensures efficient use of time and enables a teacher to cover a large amount of material in a short amount of time
- Is a familiar methodology for both teachers and students
- Is cost effective; student-to-teacher ratio can be very high
- Presents a common base of knowledge to all students

### Disadvantages of the Lecture Method

The disadvantages of the lecture method can provide a very convincing case for not using lecture. Some of the disadvantages include:

- A poor method for promoting retention; 80% of information is forgotten within the first 24 hours
- Learners become passive

- Student attention wanes quickly; makes it difficult for students to be attentive for longer than 25 to 30 minutes at a time
- Inhibits creative thinking
- Creates boredom and disinterest in the learner, if poorly delivered
- If done effectively, lecturing is a difficult skill to master
- Lack of learner participation may make the lecture session dull and boring

Most teachers who lecture are able to identify with each of the items in these lists. Enhancements can be included in a lecture presentation to help eliminate the disadvantages. This chapter presents many such enhancements. However, before incorporating enhancements into a lecture, it is imperative to master effective presentation skills. The following section briefly covers these skills.

## Effective Presentation Skills

Effective presentation skills are a must for a successful lecture. A list of guidelines related to basic presentation skills follows:
- Know the material
- Present the information in an organized manner; provide an overview or outline of the lecture
- Be comfortable with being the center of attention
- Know the audience; accommodate the message to students' unique characteristics, such as age, knowledge base, diversity of gender, race, and background
- Be aware of the rate, volume, and pitch of your speech
- Maintain eye contact with all students in the room
- Monitor students' nonverbal feedback regarding their perception and understanding of the material
- Use purposeful movement; avoid shifting and pacing
- Use gestures to create an open environment and release tension
- Eliminate non-words such as "um," "uh," and "oh" and verbal garbage such as "y'know", "like", and "okay"
- Use vocal variety, such as pausing and intonation, that raise and lower vocal pitch and place emphasis on individual words
- Articulate words clearly
- Show enthusiasm
- Monitor your physical appearance to be sure it is not distracting to the students and projects a professional image

For more presentation skills refer to Ryan (2010) listed on the reference page of this chapter.

## Two Major Challenges When Using the Lecture Format

Using effective presentation skills is the first step toward improving lecture skills. With these skills mastered, the obstacles listed as disadvantages of the lecture method can be addressed. These disadvantages result in two major challenges:
- Keeping students attentive
- Promoting recall of information

### Keeping Students Attentive

One major challenge for the lecturer is keeping students attentive. Learners easily become bored. Attention is greatest in the first 10 minutes of the lecture; therefore, this time is used to capture the students' interest. After the first 25 minutes, attention wanes then rekindles for a final spurt at the end (Fuszard, 1995).

Varying the stimuli presented during class is necessary to increase the attention span and receptivity of students. This chapter builds on a fundamental fact of human behavior – attention is drawn to what is novel, to whatever stands in contrast to immediate past experience or to lifelong experience. To sustain learners' attention, teachers must use a variety of instructional strategies that are qualitatively different. These can include cartoons, humorous stories, games, animation, videos, music, and role playing.

It is important to note the intent of the strategies discussed in this chapter is to arouse student attention and assist with the learning process; the strategies are not a substitute for a well-organized, logical, carefully planned presentation of material. This is the work of a master teacher; this is the teaching aspect of the educational process. The strategies in this chapter enhance the learning aspect of the educational process. Integrating active (sometimes referred to as interactive) teaching/learning strategies provide powerful teaching strategies that not only keep students attentive but encourage higher level thinking. These student-centered activities promote an active, rather than a passive, role for students in the classroom with faculty facilitating learning, rather than controlling it. This requires a flexible and accepting environment with a supportive, non-threatening faculty (Ridley, 2007).

## Promoting Recall of Information

A second challenge for the lecturer is to promote student retention for later recall. Retention of information presented in a strictly lecture format is limited. Students cannot recall 80% of the lecture information one day after the lecture (Fuszard, 1995). Strategies must be incorporated into the lecture to enhance retention.

A simple but important lesson to keep in mind is this: good teaching is but many small littles (Stalheim-Smith, 1998). Lecture enhancements do not have to be huge, expensive, earth-shaking adventures. Even small changes, systematically implemented over time, can have a significant impact.

Types of enhancements include:
- Active learning strategies
- Humor
- Visuals

## Active Learning Strategies

An active learning strategy refers to anything that involves students in doing things and thinking about the things they are doing (Bonwell & Eison, 1991). Active learning incorporates concepts from arousal theory. Arousal has both physiological and psychological components. It is basically excitement. Students are excited about learning and excited about the classroom environment. Students are alert and vigilant to the stimuli presented in the classroom. When the stimuli are meaningful and novel, the students are more attentive. The **amount** of stimulation is less critical than the **nature** of stimulation. The teacher should make a conscious effort to incorporate changes in stimulation throughout a lecture to engage the minds of the learners (Bonwell & Sutherland, 1996).

Classroom learning is not a spectator sport. Students should be active in their learning by constructing learning that is meaningful to them. Students should do more than look and listen; they need to participate. When they participate, they become more interested in the message (Hanks & Pulsipher, 1991). Active participation results in deep cognitive processing of the information being taught. By allowing some degree of participation, students are better able to respond, organize, and process the material.

Several disadvantages of the lecture method create the need for students to actively participate. First, during a lecture, it is assumed that all students are learning at the same pace; in fact, there is only one pace offered, that of the lecturer. Second, the lecture format provides little feedback to students regarding how well they are comprehending the lesson (Fuszard, 1995). Encouraging student participation helps to overcome both these disadvantages. The problem with student participation is that it potentially negates one of the major advantages of the lecture, that of economy of time.

Research evidence supports incorporating active learning approaches as an effective way to facilitate student learning (Bonwell & Sutherland, 1996). Some of these strategies do not involve a lot of time, but students are more likely to internalize, understand, and remember material learned through active engagement in the teaching/learning process (Bonwell, 1996).

Another approach to active learning is to have students form cooperative learning groups and work on teams to solve problems and complete projects. Cooperative learning in the classroom enhances learning but also facilitates development of other skills, such as communication, decision making, and conflict management (Stalheim-Smith, 1998).

### Reasons to Implement Active Learning Strategies

Research has shown the following about active learning strategies (Bonwell & Eison, 1991; Bonwell & Sutherland, 1996; Sutherland, 1996):

- Students show a great deal of enthusiasm in a class with active learning strategies.
- Students report having fun.
- Active learning is preferable to traditional lecture in developing higher-order thinking. Active learning strategies are as effective as lectures with respect to mastery of content but superior to lectures in developing students' thinking and writing skills.
- Students learn best when their intellectual engagement is high.
- Active learning strategies help to create inclusive learning environments.
- Active learning approaches may create more productive learning environments for the increasingly diverse student populations found in nursing education. Supportive social climates fostered by active learning strategies can be beneficial for students of diverse backgrounds. All students are engaged and participate when active learning strategies are used.

### Planning and Incorporating Active Learning Strategies

When a variety of active learning strategies are used, all of Bloom's (Anderson & Krathwohl, 2001) levels of cognitive skills are addressed. Some strategies promote mastery of functional, knowledge-based content. Others apply this content to new problems and situations. The following steps have been suggested by Bonwell and Sutherland (1996) for incorporating active learning strategies into a lecture:

1. Consider the course objectives
2. Consider your teaching style
3. Determine what active learning strategies best meet your needs
4. Work these into whatever format you choose to use in the classroom – lecture, small group work, etc.

### Sample Active Learning Strategies

Active learning strategies come in many forms. Some require very little preparation by the teacher; others require substantial advanced planning. Following is a list of examples of active learning strategies that can be used in the nursing classroom.

**The pause procedure.** Every 15 to 20 minutes, pause for a two-minute break to allow students to compare and rework their notes. A variation is to ask students to discuss with a partner what was just presented. Having students compare notes works best because two people working together are likely to take better notes and remember content than one student working alone.

**Think-pair-share.** In this activity, the teacher proposes a question to the class. The students think quietly about the answer for a minute and then form pairs and spend two to three minutes discussing the answer. The students then share their answers with the rest of the class.

**Formative quizzes.** The teacher projects questions similar to those used on exams, giving students time to respond. For multiple-choice questions, students can raise their hands in agreement as each option is considered. Clickers may be used in place of raising hands. The use of clickers in the classroom is especially helpful for faculty to determine students' understanding of the material. The clickers provide more reliable answers than students raising their hands to indicate their choices (Jones, Henderson, & Sealover, 2009). The teacher can clarify any concepts that are misunderstood. Formative quizzes also provide students with the opportunity to practice taking test items written by the teacher. This improves their test-taking abilities and reduces anxiety about what types of questions the teacher asks. A fun variation of this strategy is to turn the questions into a game, such as, *Who Wants to be a Registered Nurse?* It works like this:

- Choosing a student: Use two decks of cards. Each student receives a card upon entering the classroom from the first deck. The teacher pulls a card

from the second deck. Whichever student has the card that matches gets the question.
- The question is asked.
- Students are given a reward, such as a piece of chocolate, if the question is answered without any lifelines.

If students need assistance, three lifelines are available:
- They can ask their neighbor (if the neighbor gets the answer right, they both get candy).
- They can ask the teacher to remove two of the answers.
- They can poll the class.

**Focused listing.** Focused listing is used to determine if students recall the most important points associated with a particular topic. For example, have students create a list of the advantages and disadvantages of an issue, e.g., hemodialysis versus peritoneal dialysis. After lecturing on these two types of dialysis, have students fill in the list. This helps students develop analytical and evaluative skills. *A Pro and Con Grid* is another name for this strategy. This activity helps students develop an awareness of more than one side of an issue.

**Create your own skills checklist.** Prior to demonstrating a new clinical skill, have students develop their own skill checklist based on the principles they have learned. For example, when teaching an advanced nursing skill – such as administering medications through a gastric tube – have students develop their own skill checklist based on the principles related to infection control and medication administration. Students can be divided into two groups. Each group develops a checklist. Then the groups compare their checklists and revise them to make one polished list. The students then read their checklist to the faculty who performs the skills step-by-step as the students have written. Finally, they revise their checklist again after watching the faculty perform the skill. If a checklist is used for their return demonstration, students can then compare their written checklist with that provided for their return demonstrations to compare and contrast. This activity moves students from passive rote memorization of the checklist to actively thinking through the steps and building their own checklist. This is a much higher level thinking activity than rote memorization.

**Role playing physiology and pathophysiology.** Dr. Marie Colucci from Riverside Community College in Riverside, California, shared her activity for teaching diabetes mellitus. The activity is played as follows:

- Volunteers stand at the front of the classroom. These students are assigned the roles of cell, insulin, and sugar. The students are given hats to wear with the words **cell, insulin,** or **sugar.**
- The cell players hook arms and make a circle.
- As the teacher describes the mechanism of normal metabolism, the students playing insulin hook up with sugar, and together they enter the cell to provide energy.
- The group then acts out insulin-dependent diabetes mellitus, non-insulin-dependent diabetes mellitus, and insulin resistance.

**Acting.** In both acting and teaching, the goal is to communicate ideas and feelings to an audience (Burns, 1999). Skillful teachers often dramatize the moments of discovery. A very skillful teacher is Gail Baumlein, formerly a professor of nursing at MedCentral College in Ohio and now a dean at Chamberlain College of Nursing. To teach neurological assessment, this teacher enters the classroom looking disheveled, with make-up smeared, and a shuffled gait. She uses slurred, garbled speech and acts confused. After a few minutes, she hands a note to a student to read to the class. She then leaves the room. The note directs the students to list all the indications of neurological impairment they just witnessed. The students are surprised and engaged. The lesson not only teaches neurological assessment but the importance of observation skills. This type of learning puts the information into a context. Contextual learning provides opportunities for learners to reflect on situations and develop critical thinking skills (Baldwin, 2007; Forneris & Peden-McAlpine, 2006).

**Simple games.** One method for reviewing content at the knowledge/comprehension level is to incorporate simple games. Games such as Thumbs Up (Caputi, 2002b) from College of DuPage are used to present an answer and the students respond with the question. These are projected using a computer. Students enjoy these games while actively using the information they just heard in lecture. Although gaming creates a competitive environment that may seem threatening, it can promote competition that can make learning more interesting, stimulating, and motivating to students (Royse & Newton, 2007).

**Concept mapping.** Mapping is a process that can be used in a variety of ways and can be very simplistic or complex. A concept map can be used to graphically represent a concept or idea in lecture. On a blank area on the chalkboard or overhead transparency, develop a concept map throughout the lecture, with the students giving ideas on what concepts to link where. The students are actively involved in building the concept map. Once this process is role-modeled in class, students can build their own maps as they read their texts as a way to learn, remember, and then review the material.

Concept maps can also be used to develop a concept throughout a course. Serial concept maps are used for this purpose and demonstrate the evolution of the individual student's understanding of a concept as that understanding grows (All & Huycke, 2007). For more on developing concept maps see Caputi (2010) and Caputi and Blach (2008).

**Ad design.** Have students work in groups of two or three and take five to ten minutes to design a magazine or newspaper ad for a product they are learning about. They can be instructed to stress the product's main features and benefits. One group of students produced an ad for "colorectal chips" when studying about the gastrointestinal system. They noted variations of the color of stool then obtained paint chips from the local paint store and named each of the colors. They decided the benefit of this product was to have a common color scheme so all nurses' documentation would be consistent. Very creative!

**Lecture Bingo.** Develop a Bingo card that contains the key terms, concepts, etc., of a lecture. These cards can be developed using the table function of any word processing program. Place one item in each of the boxes on the Bingo card. Create additional Bingo cards with some of the same and some different items. The cards should all be arranged differently. Laminate the cards. Distribute the cards to the students. Provide them with a strip of self-sticking dots. As the lecture proceeds students place a dot on their cards the first time they hear the item. When they get a Bingo they yell "Bingo!" At the end of class, ask students to remove all the dots. The cards are then ready for reuse. This activity engages the students in active listening.

**Flashcards.** Give each student several blank index cards. Throughout the lecture, pause, giving a few minutes for the students to each make a flashcard from a piece of information presented in the lecture. Collect all the cards and, at the end of the lecture, put them in a common place where all students have the greatest access to them, such as the nursing skills laboratory or in the teacher's office. Collecting the cards provides a deck of dozens of flashcards for all students to use. Students then use these cards to study whenever they have some free time while at school. This activity provides time for students to immediately review their notes and decide what information is important to include on a flashcard. The sooner students review their notes, the better retention of the lecture content.

**Quick review.** Throughout the lecture, have students make notes on a piece of paper of key points or interesting information they learned in the lecture. Then, at a select time, have everyone stand in a circle, then toss a soft ball to one of the students. Ask that student to quickly share an item written during lecture. That person then tosses the ball to another person, who then shares information. The process is repeated until everyone has participated. This is a good before-break activity, because the quicker they do this, the sooner they can have break!

**Role play review.** Students are provided with a nursing scenario they are asked to role play. An example is a patient teaching situation where the student "nurse" is teaching a student "patient" about some aspect of nursing care. Students in the class watch the role play and then summarize what they saw. The teacher may develop questions prior to the session that address specific points about the role playing scenario.

## Using Humor as an Enhancement

The value of humor as an instructional strategy is gaining interest. The notion of intentionally incorporating humor as an instructional strategy to promote learning, as opposed to merely attracting attention and entertaining, is believed to be of equal importance to selecting the right audiovisual aid (Vance, 1987).

Not only can humor assist with learning in the classroom, it has also been suggested that a humorous experience during learning can enhance the subsequent learning of nonhumorous information on the same subject. That is, if a teacher uses humor in the classroom while teaching the pathophysiology of the endocrine system, students learn more when they are studying this same subject matter at a later time. In other words, the in-class humor has a facilitating effect on the students' subsequent learning (Vance, 1987). For more ideas on using humor refer to London (2010).

## Using Visuals as an Enhancement

What do you think of when you hear the word cat? Do you think of a small furry animal with whiskers? Most people picture an image of the animal. They do not think of the letters C-A-T. The reason for this is that people tend to think in images (Rayfield, 1996). Hanks and Pulsipher (1991) suggested that a lecture should dominate the students' sense of sight. Even simple visuals are highly effective. This idea of thinking in images or visuals can be integrated into the lecture format.

Unfortunately, visuals are typically a complementary, rather than a dominant, form of communication during a lecture. The dominant form is the spoken word, which is invariably open to miscommunication. Words often fail to precisely communicate the intended message. Several factors, involving both the teacher and students, must be present for information to be verbally communicated correctly. First, the teacher must have a command of the content being taught, an accurate understanding of student characteristics, and an impeccable mastery of the language in order to transmit a complete and accurate representation of the intended information. Second, students must possess a complete understanding of all required prerequisite information and be able to manipulate the audible symbols well enough to internalize them into their cognitive schema. This cognitive schema is based on the students' background knowledge (Dwyer, 1978). Interference with any of these factors results in incomplete and/or inaccurate transmission of information.

One way to resolve the problem of verbal communication is to design the instruction to include visuals. Visuals provide a concrete experience that facilitates student learning of an oral presentation. Visuals assist students in the work of interpreting the spoken word and modifying their existing mental schema to include the new information.

Wileman (1993) offered these advantages for using visual images over verbal communication. Visuals can:
- Present more information in a given amount of time
- Simplify complex concepts
- Clarify pieces of an abstract, language-based concept
- Increase learning retention

Designing lectures to include both verbal and visual communication has the additional advantage of stimulating two senses. This is known as multi-channeling. Multi-channel communication that combines words and relevant visuals results in greater learning than communicating with words alone. The more senses stimulated, the greater the receptivity and retention. Also, the more difficult or complex the verbal message, the greater the need for a visual image to assist the learner in interpreting the information. The real challenge facing the teacher is to produce an interesting, yet educational, combination of verbal and visual communication in the lecture.

## Types of Visuals

There are many types of visuals. One type includes illustrations such as charts, graphs, and tables. These visuals are helpful in arranging verbal information in a logical manner, showing relationships among various items of information.

Pictures are another type of visual. Humans have an extraordinary ability for remembering pictures. Pictures vary in complexity, ranging from abstractions to line drawings to photographs. The more information available in a picture, the more time is needed to examine it. Keep this in mind when selecting pictures for use in lectures. Sometimes it is wiser to use a simple line drawing with labels rather than a complex, highly realistic picture. This is especially true when teaching novices. More complexity can be added as the students become familiar with the concepts being taught.

The use of computers and presentation packages such as PowerPoint® have eliminated the need for the older media of overhead transparencies, 35 mm slides, and cassette tapes. All these forms of media can be wrapped into one presentation and projected with the computer.

The computer has several advantages over the older overhead projector related to using visuals. First, items on a list can be highlighted and faded as the teacher progresses through each item. This can be accomplished with an overhead projector using overlay transparencies, but can be very clumsy. The colorful display of the computer makes the highlighted items more vivid.

Second, animation can be used to introduce topics or add items to a list. This can be stimulating to the eye and provide variety. However, be careful not to overdo. Too much animation that is just for variety and does not support the instruction can be distracting.

Third, animation and video can also be used to support instruction. Overhead projectors are static; computers can be dynamic. Presentation software makes it relatively easy to incorporate all types of animation and video into a lecture.

Access to the Internet opens a whole world of possibilities for classroom teaching that were not available with the old technology. Rather than downloading graphics and video to include in a presentation, the teacher merely accesses the sites during class time. Students can also review those sites prior to or after class. Of course, faculty must review these sites close to the class time to ensure they remain available. This uncertainly in the instability of websites must be considered. It is probably unwise to use a website as the core of your presentation or you may be very disappointed if the site is not available when you need it.

### Factors Affecting the Selection of Visual Support for a Lecture

As you can see from the previous discussion, there are many types of visuals with varying degrees of realism. Some of the factors that influence the choice of visuals include:

- Instructional objectives
- Content analysis
- Audience characteristics
- Time and resources (Wileman, 1993)

**Instructional objectives.** Instructional objectives influence the type of visual chosen. For example, if the objective is to have students identify various types of urinary catheters, actual photos or accurate drawings that depict catheters should be used. A picture or graphic of each catheter labeled with its specific characteristics may be helpful.

**Content analysis.** The type of content taught in the lecture also influences the choice of visuals. If a psychomotor skill is taught, use pictures with varying degrees of realism. Video is well suited for psychomotor skills. If the content is more theoretical in nature, such as the nursing process or stages of a disease, graphic symbols, tables, or charts are more applicable. Models are useful when talking about three-dimensional items. Viewing a model of the heart or the brain while discussing pathology enhances both attention and retention.

**Audience characteristics.** Nursing students are fairly homogenous in many ways. At the very least, they are generally highly motivated adults with a common knowledge base. This makes the task of selecting visuals easier than it would be if teaching a general education course with students of many different ages, backgrounds, and goals.

However, be alert for any characteristics that make the members of the audience vary in their perception of visuals. For example, ethnic background may be a variable that influences how a visual is interpreted. This is important when a graphic is representative of a process or situation, as in the case of icons. Members of one culture may view the meaning of a picture differently from members of another culture. For example, an owl may represent wisdom to one culture but may represent danger and evil to another.

**Time and resources.** Time and resources are practical issues that may limit the choice of visuals. Although a computer-generated presentation can be relatively easy to create, it requires initial learning on the part of the teacher. However, time and resource constraints can be used to stimulate creativity. Once committed to making the lecture a unique blend of verbal and visual communication, creativity can help to overcome any restrictions imposed by time and resources.

## Varying Activities

Varying activities during a lecture session helps to maintain student attention (Gagné, 1988). As discussed earlier, attention begins to wane very early in the lecture period, dropping off sharply within the first half hour. The purpose of varying activities is to extend the attention span of the learner and sustain interest in learning for a longer period of time. When a teacher is known to use many different kinds of media, students are more attentive merely because they are interested in seeing what is coming next. Attention is further sustained by the various activities introduced.

It is helpful to introduce a new stimulus at least every 30 minutes when attention begins to diminish. Examples of new stimuli include slides, video clips, and computer assisted instruction programs. However, it is not always necessary to use such extensive media at each 30-minute interval. A brief change of pace is often all that is needed to provide students a chance to relax their minds and writing hands.

A popular activity during lectures involves a drawing for prizes. As students enter the classroom, they write their names on a piece of paper and then place the paper in a box.

At the start of the lecture and every 30 minutes thereafter, a name is drawn for a prize. The drawings take only half a minute to carry out, yet they provide a brief rest period after which students are once again attentive.

Prizes can consist of items collected from nursing conferences and conventions. Most of these meetings have exhibitors willing to give items that advertise their products. The students love to win these items, mostly because they are nursing or health care related. Examples of some of the items I have collected include mouse pads, paperclip dispensers in the shape of a medicine bottle, a video on handling stress in the nursing profession, issues of various journals, pens, pads of paper, flashlights, a copy of the Nightingale pledge suitable for framing, sunglasses, insulated lunch bags, tote bags, and car license plate holders that say *Learn CPR, Save a Life.*

## Music

One factor that can accelerate learning is music (Rayfield, 1996). Music can be soothing, relaxing, and/or emotionally stimulating. Each of these effects can be used to enhance the lecture session.

It has been noted that students who are comfortable and relaxed during a teaching session are in a better state of mind for learning than students who are stressed. Stress blocks learning (Rayfield, 1996). Research has shown that music that relaxes and soothes has a positive effect on learning (Hutchinson, 1991).

Emotionally charged music produces a physical response that involves shudders, back-of-the-neck tingles, and even chills up the spine. Hutchinson (1991) calls this response the "goose-bump quotient." This goose-bump quotient is directly related to a release of endorphins. That is, when the goose-bump quotient increases, the amount of endorphins released increases. Endorphins result in increased attention, retention, and recall of information. Endorphins solidify information into long-term memory. Playing music enhances learning through the emotion-endorphin connection (Hutchinson, 1991).

Music can be used in a lecture session to meet both objectives. To relax students, music can be played before a class begins or during breaks. Videos that incorporate music and pictures can be very emotionally charged. One example is *Tucked in Tight* (Caputi, 2002c). This video shows a nurse caring for an elderly patient while a gentle voice sings about the life of the patient and the importance of caring for the elderly. After watching the video, the students are asked to write a one-page reflection paper and to discuss what they learned from the video. Reflection provides a means of self-examination which is important for professional growth (Ruth-Sahd, 2003; Van Horn & Freed, 2008).

## Designing Instruction to Incorporate Lecture Enhancements

The major reason for designing instruction is to incorporate strategies that engage students and assist with the learning process. It is not enough merely to stand in the front of the room and talk, hoping students will learn.

Designing instruction to include all the enhancements addressed in this chapter requires additional time and work beyond preparing the lecture content. However, it is well worth the effort for both students and teacher. The students benefit by learning more and by enjoying the learning experience. The teacher also benefits. Lecture time is more enjoyable because of the variety of stimuli and fun activities. The teacher shares in the students' enjoyment.

## Designing the Instruction

Designing instruction involves two tasks: selecting the content and determining the instructional strategies.

### Selecting the Content

The specific information to be included in the lecture is based on the learning objectives. Many nursing faculty struggle with this task. It is often difficult to determine what to include and what to leave out. A well-written set of lesson objectives helps isolate and focus the content.

Preparing the lecture notes comes next. Preparing lecture notes is a critical activity that must be carefully completed. It is imperative to deliver sound instruction covering all the stated objectives. No degree of enhancements can compensate for a lack of good instruction. A few helpful pointers for preparing lecture notes for faculty reference during a lecture include:

- Use 16 point font for lecture notes for easy reading
- Make notes referencing enhancements such as when to show slides or play a video clip if not embedded into the presentation
- Save the notes in multiple places not just on one disc that may get lost or malfunction

### Determining the Instructional Strategies

Instructional strategies are deliberately selected techniques used to ensure certain cognitive processing activities take place in the learner. Faculty must consider the kinds of thinking processes the learner is using to process the material. This is extremely important to promote thinking at a higher level than rote memorization. Instructional strategies transform the delivery of content into a learning experience and encourage the kinds of thinking processes expected of the student nurse.

In this phase, the information to be taught in the lesson is organized. Next, plan the strategies you will use. Finally, plan when and how to use each strategy. Two types of strategies are learning strategies and enhancement strategies.

**Learning strategies.** Strategies in this group are used for the sequencing of the presentation so learning takes place. The sequencing of material can be from general to specific, simple to complex, or concrete to abstract. Determine from the content which type of sequencing would be best for the lecture content.

**Enhancement strategies.** Once the content is sequenced, determine where to incorporate the lecture enhancements. Keep in mind the importance of varying activities. Use many different kinds of enhancements that stimulate both auditory and visual senses. Use models and sample equipment to provide tactile stimulation.

Following are suggestions for incorporating enhancements into a lecture. This list may seem overwhelming, but start small, incorporating one or two suggestions, adding additional enhancements with each subsequent presentation of the same lecture.

- Present information in small chunks based on the learning objectives. After each objective, offer a practice item for students to answer.
- Select graphics and visuals that embellish the verbal information presented. These visuals provide a link between the verbal information and the cognitive processing of the learners.
- Find cartoons specific to the lecture information.
- Decide how to incorporate music. Perhaps play a video with peaceful, serene background music as students are entering the room. Another option is to select a nursing-related humorous song to introduce the topic of the lecture.
- Determine if a top-10 list would be appropriate for this particular content. A humorous top-10 list is a good way to start a lecture.
- Select areas of content that could be enhanced by the use of colored pictures or three-dimensional models.
- Look through your school's software collection for an instructional program that can be used for projecting some of the lecture content.
- Determine if a video, or part of a video, would reinforce the content.

## Developing the Instruction

This step consists of creating a blend of commercially produced materials and unique teacher-made productions. This section starts with a discussion of lecture handouts. After preparing the basic handouts, enhancements are created. Keep in mind all the enhancements discussed in this chapter, and remember the teacher is limited only by time and resources, and that creativity can overcome these limitations.

**Lecture handouts.** The slimmest form of handout is a topical outline. This is helpful to students because it gives an overview of the lecture and a way to determine how the teacher is progressing through the lecture. Think of adding the following to the basic outline.

- **Copies of the lecture presentation.** One PowerPoint® slide per page provides plenty of room for note-taking. If there is a limit to the number of pages that can be duplicated for student handouts, provide three slides to a page with blank lines on the right. With this type of handout, be sure the text is large enough to be read. Be careful not to distribute any copyright material you display in your presentation. The difficulty with using a PowerPoint® presentation as your handout is the problem that arises when trying to include other print materials throughout the presentation.
- **Illustrations, charts, and tables.** Include lots of pictures whenever possible in the handouts. Organize verbal information in charts and tables for easier and quicker processing by the learners.
- **Summary.** Conclude the handout with a summary of the information presented.

**Visuals.** In addition to the visuals contained in the lecture handouts, consider incorporating projected visuals. All formats can be used, including all types of graphics such as photographs, drawings, and illustrations.

Videos have long been used in the classroom. Videos can portray real-life experiences. Many commercially available videos are excellent and reasonably priced. For example, the National Kidney Foundation has excellent patient education videos. One video shows patients performing peritoneal dialysis in their homes. It is extremely helpful for students to watch this procedure being performed because many students do not have prior experience with this procedure.

It is not necessary to show an entire video if time does not permit. Review the video for the section that fits the lecture content, then play only that section of the video.

Another option is for faculty to produce their own video segments. Videos are easy and inexpensive to produce. In-house productions can be very effective. Students enjoy watching their faculty and lab personnel on the screen. Teacher-made videos allow the option of writing a script with the exact content the teacher wishes to present.

With Internet access available in most classrooms, a whole world of video is now available for faculty. Faculty should carefully review any video used from the Internet. Some schools of nursing provide video they have produced to be viewed by other faculty for use with students. For example, Saddleback Community College provides dozens of short video clips demonstrating nursing procedures at www.saddleback.edu/alfa that can be viewed free of charge on the Internet.

**Student participation.** The importance of actively engaging students during a lecture session was addressed earlier in this chapter. This active engagement must be planned. At the very least, periodic questioning should be used. Multiple-choice questions in current NCLEX® style are extremely helpful. Clickers may also be used for this activity as previously explained.

Another form of questioning used to elicit student participation is the open-ended, thinking question. In this form of questioning, a patient situation is posed; the students must construct their own solutions to the situation rather than having options from which to choose. Of course, only brief scenarios can be included unless there is time to incorporate lengthier case studies. This type of questioning fosters critical thinking skills.

A fun experience to encourage student participation is the use of hinky-pinkies. A hinky-pinky is a pair of rhyming words that fits a certain definition. The students are presented with the definition, and they must then give the term defined. Hinky-pinkies should relate to the content of the lecture. Following are a few examples:

Definition: "A man with a low hemoglobin."
Answer: "A pale male."

Definition: "The last test on the spinal column."
Answer: "A spinal final."

### After-Class Help

There is so much to teach and so much to learn that it is often helpful to extend the educational process beyond the initial classroom experience. Following are several suggestions posted on the Nurse Educator's Listserv archives that may assist with the after-class encounter:

- Have available a variety of media that covers the topic. Media such as videos, texts, computer-assisted education programs, and websites provide a variety that can accommodate many different learning styles.
- Review the websites offered throughout the textbooks used in the course. Many publishers have additional activities available free to students who bought their books. Fewer than 30% of students with access to these sites actually use this material, although the material may be very helpful (Missildine, Fountain, & Summers, 2009).
- Create self-paced study modules that students can access on the web.

- Set up a discussion board and post critical thinking scenarios for students to discuss.
- Encourage the formation of study groups. Have students with different learning styles work together so issues might be considered from a variety of points of view.
- Provide a weekly or biweekly review session with the entire class to review the content presented the previous week. This is especially helpful prior to a test. Perhaps a few of the week's allotment of office hours could be used for this purpose.

## Student Evaluation of Lecture Enhancements

It is always important to provide students with a means to evaluate the lecture enhancements. These evaluations are used to guide further planning. Two simple but effective evaluation techniques are the one-minute paper and the critical incident questionnaire (CIQ).

**One-minute paper.** Students are asked to spend one minute writing their responses to one or two questions. Typical questions are:
- What is the most important thing you learned in class today?
- What is the question that is uppermost in your mind?

**Critical incident questionnaire (CIQ).** Brookfield (1995) described a means for discovering how students are experiencing their learning and your teaching. The CIQ provides a look at your teaching through the students' eyes. Critical incidents are vivid happenings that for some reason people remember as being significant. Every class contains such moments, and teachers need to know what these moments are.

The CIQ focuses students on specific, concrete happenings that were significant to them. The students take five to ten minutes to complete the questionnaire at the end of the week. Figure 1 is an example.

Please take five minutes to respond to the questions below about this week's class(es). Do not put your name on the form. When you have finished writing, put the questionnaire on the table by the door. Thanks for taking the time to do this. What you write will help me make the class more responsive to your concerns.

1. When in class this week did you feel most interested with what was happening?
2. At what moment in the class this week did you feel most bored with what was happening?
3. At what moment in class did you feel most confused?
4. What action that anyone (teacher or student) took in class this week did you find most helpful?
5. What about the class this week surprised you the most?

**Figure 1.** Student Critical Incident Questionnaire

Both forms of evaluation give the teacher feedback throughout the course that can be used to make the class better for students currently enrolled. The evaluations also send a message that the teacher cares about what the students think regarding the way the class is conducted.

## Summary

Face-to-face classes remain the primary method used in the educational process. This chapter offered many suggestions that teachers can use to make classroom instruction inviting, exciting, and meaningful. However, to become a great classroom teacher takes time, effort, and patience. And, finally, remember, good teaching is but many small littles.

## Learning Activities

1. For both a lecture you have given and a lecture you have attended, list the advantages and disadvantages of your experience with this method.
2. For a topic you will be teaching, plan four classroom enhancements. Explain why each was chosen.
3. Teach a class using the enhancements developed in #2, and then use the one minute paper to evaluate your teaching.

4. For a topic you recently taught, consider using visuals. What kind would you use? How would you access them?

## Educational Philosophy

My educational philosophy is succinct: Give the best educational experience possible. I believe faculty should continuously challenge themselves to provide creative, interesting, and sound education – students soon learn that education doesn't have to be boring; they become self-motivated, enthusiastic, and interested... learning then follows. — Linda Caputi

## References

All, C. A., & Huycke, L. I. (2007). Serial concept maps: Tools for concept analysis. *Journal of Nursing Education, 46*(5), 217-224.

Anderson, L. W., & Krathwohl, D. R. (2001). *A taxonomy for learning, teaching, and assessing: A revision of Bloom's taxonomy of educational objectives.* New York: Addison Wesley Longman.

Baldwin, K. (2007). Friday night in the pediatric emergency department: A simulated exercise to promote clinical reasoning in the classroom. *Nurse Educator, 32*(1), 24-29.

Bonwell, C. C. (1996). Enhancing the lectures: Revitalizing the traditional format. *New Directions for Teaching and Learning, 67,* 31-44.

Bonwell, C. C., & Eison, J. A. (1991). *Active learning: Creating excitement in the classroom* (ASHE-ERIC Higher Education Report No. 1). Washington, DC: The George Washington University, School of Education and Human Development.

Bonwell, C. C., & Sutherland, T. E. (1996). The active learning continuum: Choosing activities to engage students in the classroom. *New Directions for Teaching and Learning, 67,* 3-16.

Brookfield, S. D. (1995). *Becoming a critically reflective teacher.* San Francisco, CA: Jossey-Bass.

Burns, M. (1999). Thriving in academe: All the world's a stage! *NEA Higher Education Advocate, 17*(1), 508.

Caputi, L. (2002a). *Add pizzazz to your lectures.* St. Charles, IL: L. Caputi, Inc.

Caputi, L. (2002b). *Thumbs Up!* Glen Ellyn, IL: College of DuPage.

Caputi, L. (2002c). *Tucked in tight.* Glen Ellyn, IL: College of DuPage.

Caputi, L. (2010 in press). *Using concept maps to foster critical thinking.* In L. Caputi, Teaching Nursing: The Art and Science, Vol. 2. (2nd ed.). Glen Ellyn, IL: College of DuPage Press.

Caputi, L., & Blach, D. (2008). *Teaching nursing using concept maps.* Glen Ellyn, IL: College of DuPage Press.

Dwyer, F. (1978). *Strategies for improving visual learning.* State College, PA: Learning Services.

Fuszard, B. (1995). *Innovative teaching strategies in nursing* (2nd ed.). Gaithersburg, MD: Aspen Publishers.

Forneris, S. G., & Peden-McAlpine, C. J. (2006). Contextual learning: A reflective learning intervention for nursing education. *International Journal of Nursing Education Scholarship, 3*(1), Online at www.bepress.com/ijnes/vol3/iss1/art17

Hanks, K., & Pulsipher, G. (1991). *Getting your message across.* Los Altos, CA: Crisp Publications.

Hutchinson, M. (1991). Megabrain. New York: Ballatine Books.

Jones, S., Henderson, D., & Sealover, P. (2009). "Clickers" in the classroom. *Teaching and Learning in Nursing, 4*(1), 2-5.

London, F. (2010, in press). Using humor in the classroom. In L. Caputi, *Teaching Nursing: The Art and Science, Vol. 1*. (2nd ed.). Glen Ellyn, IL: College of DuPage Press.

Missildine, K., Fountain, R., & Summers, L. (2009). Textbook companion electronic study materials: Are students using them? *Nurse Educator, 34*(3), 107-108.

Rayfield, S. (1996, November). *Nursing made insanely easy.* Presentation given at the meeting of the National Organization for Associate Degree Nursing, Denver, CO.

Ridley, R. (2007). Interactive teaching: A concept analysis. *Journal of Nursing Education, 46*(5), 203-209.

Royse, M. A., & Newton, S. E. (2007). How gaming is used as an innovative strategy for nursing education. *Nursing Education Perspectives, 28*(5), 263-267.

Ruth-Sahd, L. (2003). Reflective practice: A critical analysis of data-based studies and implications for nursing education. *Journal of Nursing Education, 42*(11), 488-497.

Ryan, D. (2010, in press). Effective presentation skills. In L. Caputi, *Teaching Nursing: The Art and Science, Vol. 1*. (2nd ed.). Glen Ellyn, IL: College of DuPage Press.

Stalheim-Smith, A. (1998). Focusing on active, meaningful learning. Idea Paper No. 34, Kansas State University, Manhattan, KS.

Sutherland, T. E. (1996, Fall). Emerging issues in the discussion of active learning. *New Directions for Teaching and Learning, 67,* 83-95.

Vance, C. (1987). A comparative study on the use of humor in the design of instruction. *Instructional Science, 16,* 79-100.

Van Horn, R., & Freed, S. (2008). Journaling and dialogue pairs to promote reflection in clinical nursing education. *Nursing Education Perspectives, 29*(4), 220-225.

# CHAPTER 36

# REVITALIZING FOR SUCCESS WITH ACTIVE LEARNING APPROACHES

## Kathleen Ohman, MS, EdD, RN, CCRN

---

The content of this chapter relates to the following major content area and subconcepts on the Certified Nurse Educator Examination Detailed Test Blueprint:

**Facilitate Learning**

- Implement a variety of teaching strategies appropriate to content; learner needs; desired learner outcomes
- Use teaching strategies based on evidence-based practices related to education
- Modify teaching strategies and learning experiences based on consideration of learners' past educational and life experiences
- Create opportunities for learners to develop their own critical thinking skills
- Create a positive learning environment that fosters a free exchange of ideas

---

### Introduction

Those teaching nursing are faced with many challenges. The nursing profession requires that students think critically and conceptually, reflect, question, generalize, think beyond the immediate situation, and immerse themselves in abstract and technical language (Beers & Bowden, 2005). Student nurses also must be prepared for the licensed nurse role in a variety of settings. They are expected to be knowledgeable, competent in psychomotor skills, adept at accessing and using information, and capable of clinical reasoning and higher-level thinking (AACN, 2008; Ironside, 2004; Pullen, Murray, & McGee, 2003; Simpson & Courtney, 2002; Smith & Johnson, 2002). To accomplish these expectations in a short amount of time, attention must be paid to how faculty teach and how students learn.

Research suggests the most successful learning methods are those that promote active learning (Beers & Bowden, 2005; Ironside, 2004; McKeachie, 2002; Royce, 2001; Schell, 2006; Weimer, 2002; Youngblood & Beitz, 2001). Additionally, it is more likely that content will be learned when it is attended to, remembered, and reinforced in a "fun setting" (Herrman, 2002). The selection of active, student-centered learning methods, however, should not be haphazard but guided by theories and frameworks of learning and current research findings (Billings &

Halstead, 2009; Ironside, 2006; NLN, 2005). Not every method is appropriate to each situation. There should be a fit between a particular active learning approach and:

- A nursing faculty's philosophical beliefs on teaching and learning
- The evidence base for the approach selected
- Characteristics of the learners
- The outcomes to be achieved during a class period

Because student learning styles and preferences differ, a particular method may have a different effect on learning outcomes for each student. While some students may be engaged, others may resist, especially if the traditional more passive approach of receiving instruction is their preferred method. However, using a variety of active learning approaches helps to engage students and encourage them to diversify their learning preferences.

Learning theories and frameworks applicable to nursing education can be used to guide the selection of active learning approaches (Bastable, 2008; Billings & Halstead, 2009; Caputi, 2010; Jayasekara, Schultz, & McCutcheon, 2006). These include:

- Cognitive learning theory
- Humanistic learning theory
- Adult learning theory

The use of critical, feminist, and phenomenological pedagogies also have been reported to be helpful in creating more egalitarian and cooperative learning environments in nursing education (Baumberger-Henry, 2005; Ironside, 2003). The reader is referred to Vandeveer (2009) and Ironside (2001; 2003; 2006) for a complete discussion of these theories and pedagogies, including the roles of the faculty and student, advantages and disadvantages, and application.

The purpose of this chapter is to provide ideas to re-energize student-centered teaching to promote student learning. A few active methods for classroom instruction within the theoretical frameworks addressed above will be described and a few examples presented.


## Arousal: Creating an Anticipatory Set

An important aspect of engaging learners in the learning process is arousal (Bradshaw & Lowenstein, 2007). Arousal is using positive emotion to capture the learners' attention. Using positive emotions avoids stimulating learners' negative emotions, such as anxiety, anger, or boredom. An arousal activity takes a minimal amount of class time and merely sets the stage for learning. Effective learning, however, extends beyond the role of faculty as entertainer. The effective faculty is a facilitator of student learning and must move the learners beyond the expectation of being entertained as passive participants in the learning process.

Many examples of stimulating arousal to engage learners are reported in the literature (Deck, 2003; Herrman, 2002; London, 2010; Rowles & Russo, 2009). Beginning class with a short reading, demonstration, humorous anecdote, or even a physical activity can engage the learners. For example, prior to initiating a discussion about assessment of a patient with altered cardiac tissue perfusion, the students can be instructed to jog in place. While students are jogging, ask them to plug their nose. Then, ask them to hold their breath. The teacher should be engaged in this activity along with students to know how long to sustain the jogging. Once students are seated following the activity, discuss symptoms the students experienced after jogging. The discussion can be expanded by asking students regarding additional symptoms that might be noted if they were experiencing altered tissue perfusion as a result of coronary artery disease or acute coronary syndrome. Physical activity is highly effective in initiating arousal.

This same type of activity works well for teaching concepts related to impaired oxygenation. In addition to plugging their nose, students are provided with straws through which they are instructed to breathe orally. Students quickly learn what it feels like to try to breathe with a compromised airway, whether it results from a medical condition such as asthma or from medical interventions such as endotracheal intubation with ventilatory support.

Ironside (2003; 2005) uses stories to stimulate thought. Students are asked to write a story about the lived experience related to a specific topic area. Stories are then shared and discussion generated. The sharing and discussion of these stories encourage questioning the meaning and significance of experiences rather than interrogative questioning in which a set answer is expected.


## Think Aloud

Think aloud is a methodology in which students verbalize their thinking while they are thinking. This learning strategy encourages students to assimilate old meanings with new meanings and is an example of cognitive learning theory. This method may be particularly helpful when guiding students in clinical or service learning experiences (Bradshaw, 2007) and group learning situations. It should, however, be discouraged when students are with patients in a clinical setting.

# Photographs, Pictures, and Video Clips

Photographs and pictures can be used to promote critical thinking and evaluate the depth and breadth of students' knowledge (Dearman, 2003; Ulrich & Glendon, 2005). Computerized images on a variety of topics can be easily found using an Internet search engine such as Google (2008). With proper citation, these images can be printed or copied for use as a hard copy, transparency, PowerPoint® slide, or Web enhanced instruction. The addition of visual animations and sound, available in computerized presentation packages like PowerPoint® or free via the Internet, can be helpful in making a point, initiating a discussion, or making comparisons.

Animated computer images, streaming video, and video clips also can be included in presentations to promote class discussion. These enhancements can be procured from a variety of websites with the aid of a search engine by entering the search term images, animation, or video clips and a topic area. Examples of these include those found at HeartPoint Gallery, The Heart: An Online Exploration, 3D Medical Animation Library, and YouTube. The search engine, Google, has an option for YouTube.

One approach to using computerized enhancements is to incorporate streaming video or a video clip to help students teach and prepare patients for diagnostic tests. A video clip of an echocardiogram and a cardiac catheterization can be used (Echocardiogram and Cardiac catheterization from YouTube or from HeartSite.com). After projecting the video in class, ask two or more students to discuss how they would explain these tests to patients. Then other students may be asked to identify the commonalities in patient preparation and note specific differences. This methodology is useful to actively engage students and promote critical thinking. The aphorism "A picture is worth a thousand words" is especially relevant.

# Mnemonics

A mnemonic is a visual or verbal device that enhances efficient memorization and easy access to stored memory because of its novelty or familiarity (Sarvis, 2007; Schumacher, 2005). Though they have been denounced as low-level learning, mnemonics strengthen memory of key concepts and contextual information and facilitate faster "chunking" of material into memory and create a cognitive pattern for making linkages with higher-level concepts (Rummel et al., 2003). Because nursing students need to know certain facts before they can apply and critically reflect on the information, using mnemonics helps students to remember the facts.

The ability to quickly retrieve critical information enhances clinical decision making, problem solving, and test taking (Rummel et al., 2003; Ulrich & Glendon, 2005).

An example of a mnemonic for learning the names and location of cardiac auscultation points is *Auscultation Points To Monitor*. This phrase combines words with a visual image. The first letter of each word represents the valve areas to auscultate: aortic, pulmonic, tricuspid, and mitral (A, P, T, and M) (See Figure 1.) The visual component is to visualize the number two on an adult's chest starting above the right nipple line (auscultate aortic), move horizontally about 2 inches to a point left of the sternum (auscultate pulmonic), move down the left of the sternum about 4 inches (auscultate tricuspid), and extend horizontally below the left nipple about 2 inches (auscultate mitral). This approximates starting auscultation at the second intercostal space to the right then left of the sternum (aortic and pulmonic), auscultating at the fourth intercostal space to the left of the sternum (tricuspid), and finally auscultating at the left fifth intercostal space at the left midclavicular line (mitral). Anecdotal feedback from students indicates they had a hard time remembering the auscultation points until they learned this mnemonic.

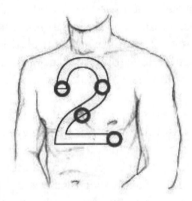

**Figure 1.** Illustration of Mnemonic for Auscultating Heart Sounds

Another helpful mnemonic can be used to learn the side effects of an ace inhibitor. Recall that all ace inhibitors end in the suffix, "-pril." Use the ace inhibitor captopril to remember the adverse effects: **c**ough, **a**naphylaxis, **p**alpitations, **t**aste alterations, orthostatic hypotension, potassium increases, renal impairment, infertility, and leukocytosis (Byrne, 1999).

Meyers and Choka (2008) use a helpful mnemonic for assessment of a change in the patient's mental status, *ODDES*: What are the ODDES? Each letter represents an area to assess as a potential cause for a patient's altered mental status. The letter O represents assessing the patient's oxygenation status. The two letter Ds representing checking two areas pertaining to drugs, assessing for new drugs added to the patient's regime and assessing for drug interactions and determining how long a patient has been taking a medication. The letter E represents assessing the patient's electrolyte status for imbalances that can affect mental status. Finally, the letter S represents sugar, checking the patient's blood sugar level as a cause for mental status change.

## Games

Integrating games into class sessions is another teaching strategy that can infuse fun into the teaching-learning process, enhance students' critical thinking abilities, create community among students, and reinforce content. Games reduce student stress and anxiety and enable students to relax while learning (Henderson, 2005). Board games, card games, computer shell games, Internet games, instructional puzzle games, matrix games, metaphorical simulation games, paper-and-pencil games, simulation games, and television games are just a few of the various types of games possible for inclusion in classroom activities.

**Name that Drug.** This is a one of a variety of games described by Glendon and Ulrich (2005), is formatted similar to a former television game show, **Name that Tune.** The faculty develops 5 to 7 clues about a medication and students on two opposing teams state the number of clues in which they could name that drug. The student team that selects the least number of clues is provided the opportunity to name the drug with the number of clues selected. Points are accumulated based on naming the drug within that number of clues. If incorrect, the opposing team has the opportunity to name the drug using all of the clues provided and earning a point if correct. The team that wins the point starts the next round. This format can be used for a variety of other activities, such as **Name that Nursing Diagnosis or Name that Disease.**

Other games have also been developed based on traditional board games, such as Candyland or Monopoly. Games can also be generated using templates which can be found by using an Internet search engine, such as Google. One such template, using the Jeopardy game format, has been used successfully in incorporating questions and content related to chest and neurological trauma. Student feedback suggests this method has been successful in engaging students in class and helping them to learn information. Questions developed by the teacher or available within textbook resources, such as a study guide accompanying a textbook, can be easily worked into Jeopardy. A template is available at: www.nursing.umich.edu/facultyresources/ bestPractices/games/quiz.html.

For the games previously described, faculty time is needed to write the questions for the games and design the game-board or other elements to be included in the game. Another option is to obtain already developed games. Table 1 identifies resources for obtaining or developing games used in nursing education. Most of those included below are free-access.

| Resources for making your own games: http://nursestoner.com/online_games.html |
| --- |
| Marilyn Smith-Stoner; http://nursestoner.com/online_games.html |
| Nurselearn; http://nurselearn.com/info-word_games.htm?gclid=CJm8tsebp5YCFQNKxw odBm4lxg; http://nurselearn.com/free_game_&_tips.htm |
| Student Nurse Playbook; www.studentnurseplaybook.com/ |
| The Thinking Nurse; www.dupagepress.com<br>ThumbsUp: www.dupagepress.com |
| University of Michigan School of Nursing, Faculty Instructional Technology Resources - Games<br>www.nursing.umich.edu/facultyresources/bestPractices/games.html |
| Welcome to Jeopardy; markedamon@hotmail.com or |
| Nursing Fun: www.nursingfun.com/games.htm |
| Cyber Nurse: www.cybernurse.com/games.html |
| Eclipse Crossword.com; www.eclipsecrossword.com/ |

**Table 1.** Resources for Obtaining Nursing Education Games

Clickers, interactive response devices, have been used in the classroom as an instructional gaming strategy. Students use these devices to select responses to questions. The teacher can then read a display of their responses. The faculty can use student responses to clarify content, engage students in a debate about the correct answer, or to verify student understanding of information. Using these devices engages students in the content, promotes interactivity, and allows the faculty to take advantage of teachable moments during a class period (Skiba & Barton, 2006).

## Simulations

Simulations are representations of actual life events. They may be presented through media, computer software (virtual reality, computer-assisted instruction, CD-ROM), role play, case study analysis, or games that actively involve learners in applying the course content (Gaberson & Oermann, 2007; Rowles & Russo, 2009).

Movie segments, commercials, or clips from television shows can be shown to simulate experiences and reinforce concepts (Herrman, 2002). For example, a segment from the television show *ER* can be used to help students learn medical and nursing management for complications from pregnancy-induced hypertension. Faculty must obtain copyright permission to use a taped episode of a television show. However, YouTube may have usable segments that do not require copyright permission. Wikimedia Commons also has video segments in the public domain that may be useful (http://commons.wikimedia.org/wiki/Category:Video).

When using media be sure to develop a handout that addresses scenes from the episode. For each scene include the following elements:
- Information about the patient being viewed in the episode
- Information about some of the actions the students will be observing
- Questions that relate to medical and nursing management

Before viewing the scenes, have students read through the handout so they are familiar with the questions. After viewing the media segment, discuss the questions and any additional information not covered in the media segment.

Interactive multimedia has been used successfully to teach basic nursing skills. A study by Jeffries, Rew, and Cramer (2002) found no significant difference in cognitive gains between one group of students taught basic nursing skills by the traditional lecture and demonstration approach and another taught through interactive CD-ROMs and interactive classroom laboratory stations. Students in the study group worked in pairs to practice the designated skills, discussed focused study questions and research-based material on the selected skill, and practiced at interactive stations facilitated by the teacher. Findings indicated the groups were similar in their ability to demonstrate the basic skills correctly in the learning laboratory. However, student satisfaction was significantly different by group ($P=0.01$), with the interactive, student-centered group more satisfied than the group experiencing the traditional teaching method.

Simulations with standardized patients (SP) also have been reported in the literature (Merrick et al., 2000; Nehring & Lashley, 2004; Peteani, 2004; Schwind et al., 2001; Yoo, 2003). SPs are individuals recruited and trained to perform in a particular patient role. Yoo and Yoo (2003) studied the effect of two teaching methods on the clinical competence of nursing students enrolled in a nursing fundamentals course. One method used the traditional teaching approach with lecture and laboratory practice with a mannequin. The other method used live SP models. The study found that students in the SP group had significantly higher scores in clinical judgment, clinical skill performance, and communication than the traditional group. The consistency of findings with other studies suggests the SP methodology is more conducive to internalizing psychomotor skills than the traditional method. The SP method allows students to experience more realistic problem solving.

Role playing can also be included to compare and contrast concepts. For example, when comparing concepts related to alterations of arterial perfusion versus peripheral perfusion, patient scenarios can be developed. One student is asked to role play a patient with arterial perfusion problems and another student is asked to role play a patient with peripheral perfusion problems. The faculty presents the scenario for each patient and students "attach to the patient" instructor-prepared drawings of significant history findings and patient signs and symptoms as the scenario unfolds. Because the information is viewable on a "patient," students are able to easily identify the similarities and differences in the patient's history information, and begin to discuss the needed nursing interventions and treatment options.

Nursing faculty at the College of Saint Benedict/Saint John's University (St. Joseph, MN) have also developed scenes for DVD vignettes, recorded at a local hospital, in which faculty portray the role of the nurse and patient. These vignettes are used to augment classes or as part of a clinical examination to evaluate the critical thinking of students in response to actual patient situations. A medical record is developed for the patients portrayed and portions provided to the student. When used in evaluation, the students view a scene and use the medical record to answer questions. For example, in one scene a patient is experiencing chest pain at the change of shift. The day shift nurse asks the night shift nurse to administer morphine sulfate. After viewing the scene the students then determine if the procedure was correct, that the correct dose was administered based on the patient's medication administration record (MAR), and then state additional interventions based on the patient's orders. These vignettes have been exceptionally helpful in evaluating students' application of theory to clinical. For example, although the medical record does not include a beta-blocker or aspirin on the MAR, students often include administering these without a physician's order. Additionally, these vignettes have been useful in determining the students' ability to identify breaches in confidentiality and in providing ethical care because some scenes also incorporate these concepts.

Within the past few years, full-scale simulation (medium to high fidelity) has been introduced into nursing education with the use of a computerized, full-body manikin programmed to provide realistic physiologic responses. The simulations portrayed require careful planning, a realistic environment, and using actual medical equipment and supplies. Advantages to using full-scale simulation include providing a risk-free environment where learners can integrate theory and practice without the fear of patient harm. These also can be used to enhance or evaluate competencies, critical thinking, clinical judgment, knowledge synthesis, technical and communication skills, and interdisciplinary teamwork in the management of a patient with complex problems (Bantz et al., 2007; Decker et al., 2008; Jeffries, 2005; Jeffries, 2006).

Jeffries (2006) identifies a four-step process for constructing a simulation. The first step is developing the blueprint. Important considerations in this step include completing a literature review and determining the design features such as the objectives of the simulation, fidelity (authenticity of the simulation), problem-solving components, learner support, and guided reflection or debriefing after the simulation. The second step is procuring the materials and room. Next, assemble the structure, define the teacher's and student's role, and design the guided reflection. The last step is finishing the project which includes revising the simulation as needed, evaluating learning and process outcomes, and disseminating findings. Instruments such as those presented by Jeffries (2005; 2006), the *Education Practices in Simulation Scale (EPSS)* or *the Simulation Design Scale (SDS)*, can be used to evaluate the educational practices embedded within a simulation or evaluate the major design features needed when developing the simulation.

The challenges of using full-scale, high-fidelity simulation include cost and time commitments, development of evaluation methods, appropriate selection or development of simulated experiences, experiences during simulation not being totally realistic, and the need to validate whether proficiencies demonstrated in the simulated environment are transferable to actual patient care situations (Decker et al., 2008; Dillon et al., 2004). Research is needed to determine if the life of the simulated manikins is sufficient to offset investment costs and eventually result in instructional cost-savings.

An example of a simulated lab experience with multiple stations is available for your review on the CD accompanying this book. The stations are intended for a 4-hour laboratory experience to refresh nursing skills for students who have been out of the hospital clinical setting for an extended time (usually 3 to 9 months). This laboratory experience provides a safe and collaborative environment for students to care for simulated patients. Stations were designed with high-fidelity manikins, stationary manikins, and hospital equipment that students typically encouter. Students are paired for the stations and complete the stations using the handout provided and accompanying questions. At one station students viewed a DVD and practiced suctioning a tracheostomy, inserted an oral airway, and answered questions. At another station, students crushed and administered medications through a feeding tube. A debriefing session followed the laboratory experience. Student comments indicated the experience was very helpful, but they were exhausted and recommended completing this over two, two-hour days rather than over four hours in one day.

## Concept Mapping, Mind Mapping, and Drawings

Concept mapping and drawings are other learning methods supported by cognitive learning theory. Other names for concept mapping include mind mapping, clinical maps, correlation maps, and mapped care plans. Mapping is using a graphic or pictorial tool to illustrate key concepts and their relationships (Caputi & Blach, 2008; Donald, 2002; King & Shell, 2002; Oermann & Gaberson, 2006; Schuster, 2008; Taylor & Wros, 2007). Students can use this tool independently, in small-group work, or in large-classroom situations. This methodology is useful in assisting students to think critically about the interrelatedness of new and previously learned information (Caputi & Blach, 2008). Concept mapping has been used as an approach to teaching and learning about care planning in healthcare settings, organize class notes and guide study time, to organize papers, develop thoughts, or experiment with linking ideas in new ways. Research indicates that concept mapping improves all levels of student performance in nursing and critical thinking (Caputi & Blach, 2008; Irvine, 1995; Schuster, 2008; Taylor & Wros, 2007; Wilgis & McConnell, 2008).

Successful use of drawings as a learning method for courses in pathophysiology and healthy aging was reported by Masters and Christensen (2002). Students were asked to complete a series of drawings to depict their own conceptualization of assigned material. Reproducing textbook illustrations was prohibited. For the pathophysiology course, students completed the reading assignment and then depicted through drawings the effects of specified pathophysiology on normal anatomy and physiology. In the healthy aging course, students were required to draw overlays of changes that occur with aging and how these changes relate to pathophysiology. Christensen (2002) reported positive student and faculty responses to the project and noted that the quality of classroom discussion and student retention had improved.

Concept maps have been integrated into the clinical preparation required by students. Students gather information about a patient and begin developing a concept map that includes the reason for the patient's hospitalization, history, nursing diagnoses, supporting data (which includes diagnostic and laboratory results), outcomes, interventions, and potential complications. Students are expected to aggregate the data around the patient's problem or nursing diagnosis. Once completed, students draw arrows to show the relationships between concepts. After the second day of providing care to the patient, students evaluate the attainment of the outcomes established for the patient and make recommendations for modifications. An example of a concept map is provided on the CD accompanying this book.

## Case-Based Learning

Case-based learning is a student-centered learning method in which students actively solve complex problems that mimic actual clinical practice. Case-based learning enables students to integrate theoretical knowledge and skills of clinical reasoning, critical thinking, problem solving, and interpersonal skills, and apply these to hypothetical or real-case scenarios (Delpier, 2006). Case-based learning is supported by principles derived from cognitive theories and the caring framework.

The first step in development of a case begins with determining clear objectives of what the student is supposed to learn. The next step is to develop the case or story. Delpier (2006) provides examples of cases used in a child and family health nursing course that can be easily incorporated. Ready-made cases can be obtained from current textbooks, journals, and publishers such as College of DuPage Press (www.dupagepress.com); or, the faculty may develop an original case from clinical experience or a review of the literature.

The effectiveness of case-based learning has been studied by DeMarco, Hayward and Lynch (2002). A weekly, one-hour, small-group, case-based learning experience was included in the course "Leading and Managing in Nursing." One case-based scenario presented by the authors was a managerial situation that dealt with interpersonal and/or intraprofessional conflict, delegation decisions in a multiskilled work force, and quality improvement processes in a patient situation. To complete the case, students consulted multiple sources including texts, class notes, the Internet, and professionals in the field. Students submitted formal reports describing their findings, recommendations, and rationales, and presented their papers to the group. Research findings suggest case-based methods stimulate knowledge development from the clinical to the classroom setting and vice versa. Additionally, the study found that working with cases increased students' confidence related to class material and working successfully with others.

## Problem-Based Learning

Problem-based learning (PBL) originated at McMaster University in Canada in the late 1960s for medical education and is now being used in nursing education (Alexander, et al., 2002). Problems reflecting real clinical situations are designed to challenge students to probe deeply and think rigorously to determine possible solutions to the problem. A characteristic of PBL is the content for solving the clinical situation or problem is not presented to the students but must be identified by the group, researched by individual students, and presented to the group for discussion. The faculty role involves developing the problem situations, establishing the climate for learning, encouraging problem solving, and promoting group discussion and debate rather than providing expert content information. Problem-based learning promotes active learning and may be the primary approach used in a nursing program or may be combined with other learning methods (Alexander, et al., 2002; Cannon and Schell, 2001; Solomon, 2005). The evidence, however, regarding knowledge acquisition is mixed (Hwang & Kim, 2006; Rideout et al., 2002).

Hwang and Kim (2006) developed seven case scenario packages based on an analysis of relevant learning to teach cardiorespiratory content for an adult health nursing course using the problem-based learning (PBL) method (see Table 2). The authors also studied the effects of the PBL method as compared to the traditional lecture method on learning the cardiorespiratory content. The authors found the level of knowledge in the PBL group was significantly higher than that of students in the lecture group ($t = 2.007$, $p = .045$). All PBL students with higher and lower grades showed a significant increase in the posttest score. Only students with higher grades in the lecture group showed a notable increase in the posttest score. Learning motivation was also found to be significantly higher in the PBL group ($t = 2.608$, $p = .012$).

| Patient Scenarios Developed by Hwang and Kim (2006) | |
|---|---|
| 1 | A 78-year-old male patient with COPD, asthma, and chronic bronchitis, who complained of dyspnea |
| 2 | A 52-year-old male patient who complained of continued cough and fever and was diagnosed with pneumonia and pleurisy |
| 3 | A 55-year-old male patient who complained of persistent cough and was diagnosed with small cell lung cancer |
| 5 | A 16-year-old male patient with a spontaneous pneumothorax |
| 5 | A 48-year-old male patient who complained of chest pain with a diagnosis of acute myocardial infarction |
| 6 | A 78-year-old female who complained of shortness of breath and general edema and was diagnosed with congestive heart failure |
| 7 | A 45-year-old female patient who had valve replacement surgery with left ventricular constriction |

**Table 2.** Sample Patient Scenario's

## Team-Based Learning

Another variation of small group learning is team-based learning. This is a small group-based instructional strategy that is relatively new to nursing education (Clark et al., 2008). Students are placed into learning teams where they remain for the duration of the course. Units or modules are taught in three-step cycles which require student preparation for assignments, readiness assurance through a quiz with immediate feedback, and an application-focused activity where challenging clinical problems are given to student teams to solve. Several multiple-choice questions are given to the teams and each team arrives at a consensus regarding the answer. Each team holds up a card identifying their answer. Intrateam debates ensue to discuss the rationale for answers provided.

This team-based strategy is theoretically based and empirically grounded, and ensures the effectiveness of small groups working independently in classes where there may be a high student-to-faculty ratio without losing the benefit of faculty led small groups with lower ratios. For some learners, not only is this method more energizing, but it also has been associated with greater assimilation of subject matter (Clark, et al., 2008; Kelly et al., 2005; Michaelsen et al., 2004).

Students in a study by Clark, et al. (2008) using the team-based learning strategy reported more in-class participation than did students in a comparison lecture course. However, although all the students achieved the learning objectives by team-based learning, some students expressed fear that out-of-class learning without complementary lectures put them at risk for missing important content. A disadvantage voiced by some students was not having PowerPoint® presentations to guide studying and some students stated more uncertainty about what they should focus on and learn.

## Reflection

Reflection is a process of purposeful thinking to develop understanding, insight, clinical judgment, and critical thinking (Gray, 2003). Reflection incorporates principles from adult learning theory, humanism, cognitive-development theory, feminism, and phenomenology. Through focusing on past and current learning experiences, students use reflection to enhance and extend their learning. New ideas and ways of thinking are promoted through an internal dialogue with one's self (Scheckel, 2009). Techniques for reflection need to include thoughtful analysis and evaluation. Suggestions include writing assignments, journals, portfolios, reaction papers, classroom discussions, focus groups, and shared readings. As with any learning method, time for reflection needs to be built into the design of selected assignments.

Scanlan, Care, and Udod (2002) completed a qualitative study to understand more fully the meaning and use of personal reflection in teaching and how reflection contributes to the development of classroom teaching expertise. Findings from this study suggest that faculty experiences are integral to the use of reflection in teaching. Reflection is useful for faculty to make connections between the discussion content and students' experiences. The authors found that role modeling and questioning were common techniques used to help students make connections with the content. However, understanding the influence of context on reflection requires further study.

## Narrative Pedagogy

Narrative pedagogy, developed by Diekelmann (2001), is a teaching-learning approach in which faculty and students publicly share and interpret stories of their experiences. Its use requires the teacher to be well-versed in the content area.

However, narrative pedagogy decenters the content and encourages teachers and students to think about the meanings of the content being learned and its significance to the students' emerging practice (Hayden-Miles, Young, & Brown, 2010; Ironside, 2004; 2005).

Ironside (2003) reported implementing and evaluating the use of narrative pedagogy in a one-credit introductory nursing course offered to students during their first undergraduate semester. On the first day of class students completed the College Classroom Environment Scale (CCES) to rate their anticipated perceptions of the learning environment for the course and for later data comparisons. The course began with students and faculty writing and sharing stories of caring for another person or being cared for by someone else. The process of interpreting stories allowed for exploration of the topic. Various questions were posed by the teacher. Reflection led to further exploration of the topic for the next class meeting.

Following completion of the course, students again completed the CCES to determine if there were significant differences between their perception of the learning environment and the actual experience. Qualitative data also was collected via nonstructured interviews. Students were asked to reflect on the course just completed and to describe a particular event that stood out because it reflected what it meant to be a student in the course. Students were asked to share an example of what worked or did not work in the course. The data were analyzed for themes.

Findings of the study indicated there was no statistically significant difference between the pre- and posttest scores on the CCES for 84 percent of the items. This meant there was no difference between what students anticipated and what they actually experienced. Ten of the 62 items showed a significant change, indicating the students found the learning climate worse than expected.

In some situations, however, mean scores on the semester-end CCES were directly opposite the experiences students reported during the interviews. For example, a highly significant decrease was found on the questionnaire item, "Students in this class have gotten to know each other well." Yet, in interviews, students' comments indicated they got to know their peers well. The authors concluded that further research is needed to develop evaluation tools that are congruent with the pedagogy being used.

One possible modification to narrative pedagogy for use in an adult nursing course involves asking students to write a story about a specific topic such as head trauma, from their own or an acquaintance's experience. Because students may be reluctant to read their stories, the teacher also writes a story to help students feel comfortable with sharing their accounts. From the stories, the teacher draws themes of signs and symptoms, diagnostic measures, medical and nursing management, and psychosocial responses. The teacher can ask questions such as, "Besides the signs and symptoms you have mentioned, what else might be important to assess?" This question can be modified to address the other themes of a story. Once the discussion is completed, students compose nursing diagnoses and outcomes for their own story and write them on the board. Students then examine the nursing diagnoses to determine if the major diagnoses for a patient with head trauma have been addressed. For the next class period, students are assigned to read about a research-based nursing intervention and be prepared to present the intervention to the class.

## Experiential Learning

Experiential learning is another effective method to promote learning in nursing students (Ulrich & Glendon, 2005; Welch et al., 2001). In experiential learning, people learn from experience and build upon what they have learned through practice.

Welch, et al. (2001) reported incorporating an experiential learning assignment into an undergraduate nursing course. Students completed a group project that focused on integrating stress theory and research. Research and monograph readings about stress and student stress were assigned and a class seminar on the findings of stress research was presented. Following these activities, individual students interviewed subjects of varying age, gender, and ethnicity. During interviews, the students were to identify stressors, symptoms, coping strategies, emotions, and a subjective sense of wellness or illness. Following the interviews, the students analyzed the data, wrote pertinent nursing diagnoses, identified research-based interventions, and selected applicable community resources.

Once students had completed the assignment, they were assigned to groups of eight or nine to analyze the group data and complete oral and poster presentations. Many students incorporated skits, games, panel discussions, videotapes, and slides into their presentations.

Student and faculty evaluations over four courses indicated this was an exceptional learning experience. Furthermore, the experiential assignment stimulated research among undergraduate nursing students. The authors reported that some nursing students in the sophomore year contacted faculty to inquire about becoming involved in research.

An experiential learning activity found to be highly effective with junior nursing students is a lived experience of an older adult. The activity generates empathy and compassion, and enhances knowledge about a content area. This assignment combines a writing assignment and an experiential assignment. Students write a paper that includes a patient problem, two patient populations who might experience this problem, and recommended assistance or adaptations for the problem. Sample problems are altered mobility, impaired communication, or altered sensation. For 24 hours, students experience what it is like to have this problem. Students are required to have the assistance of an unimpaired individual to prevent injury. Students attend classes and activities, for example, with a walker or in a wheelchair, mimic inability to talk, wear mittens, or include pebbles in their shoes. Upon completion of the activity, students write about their experiences and the responses of others. Students consistently write about how this experience changed their attitudes toward people with a disability.

## Role Play, Discussion, Debate, Use of Questioning, and Use of Materials that Present an Opposing Opinion

Role play, discussion, debate, use of questioning, and use of materials that present an opposing opinion are supported by cognitive-development theories of learning. These learning methods promote faculty-student interactions and student-student interactions where students are exposed to alternative ways of thinking, reasoning, and viewing the world. Content and teaching-learning experiences are chosen to foster the cognitive development of the student, encouraging and even forcing students to think.

A 10 to 15-minute role play can be used to actively involve students in communicating with a simulated patient with a deficit. Student pairs are given a piece of paper which describes a role and actions for that role. Students are not permitted to see their partner's paper. The role play is explained in Table 3.

Following completion of the exercise, the class should discuss the experience, emphasizing essential data for assessment, interventions to promote safety, and communication methods for the different types of aphasia.

Woods and Jordan (2008) present a clever role-play activity for women in labor, developed after the television program *American Idol*. Faculty or staff members role-play seven scenarios which include lip sync to songs for the stages of labor. Other faculty members serve as the judges of *American Idol* and students are the audience who give input to the panel of judges. Following the lip sync, the individual contestants hope to hear the judges say, "You're being admitted to L&D!" The songs provide an indication of readiness for L&D and if not ready the audience answers questions from the judges. These questions may include what the nurse should teach the contestant about the labor process or nursing interventions, rationale, and outcomes.

| A Communication Exercise | |
|---|---|
| **Nurse Role** | **Patient Role** |
| **Scene 1 (five minutes)** | **Scene 1 (five minutes)** |
| You are the nurse assigned to care for a patient who has had a stroke. Following the handout provided, complete a health history and assessment of your assigned "patient." During data gathering, you need to protect the safety of your patient.<br><br>Scene 2 (five minutes) | You are a patient who has experienced a stroke. You have one of the following motor deficits of your choosing: arm paralysis, leg paralysis, or other paralysis. Your "nurse" will be completing a health history and assessment. During data gathering, you begin to slip in your chair and lean to one side.<br><br>Scene 2 (five minutes) |
| Your patient now has aphasia. Continue with the health assessment on your patient. You need to determine the type of aphasia your patient is experiencing and develop strategies to communicate so that you can finish your assessment. | The nurse needs to continue with the assessment; however, you have developed aphasia. The first color listed below that corresponds to a color of your clothing is your aphasia type: **black** is expressive aphasia, **blue** is receptive aphasia, and **other** is mixed. You need to roleplay your communication deficit and respond only when appropriate communication strategies are used by the nurse. |

**Table 3.** Explanation of Neuro-deficit Role Play

## Cooperative Learning Experiences or Collaborative Learning

In cooperative learning experiences or collaborative learning, teams of learners work on assignments and assume responsibility for group learning outcomes (Rowles & Russo, 2009; Stiles, 2006). This learning method encourages teamwork and reflective learning. Large learning assignments can be accomplished efficiently. The Internet and group-conferencing software have been successfully used in cooperative learning experiences. Cooperative learning also has been used in nursing laboratory practice activities, such as physical assessment. Not only does cooperative learning promote the cognitive domain of knowledge development and the psychomotor domain of skill development, it promotes affective learning in which students need to demonstrate a willingness to engage in practice with peers.

Stiles (2006) identifies four steps in facilitating formal cooperative learning. These steps include:

1. Make preinstructional decisions regarding group formation and size, resources, and information processing tasks
2. Explain the tasks and roles to the learning groups
3. Monitor group progress and intervene if needed related to group functioning or group interpretations of the material
4. Evaluate the group work and individual group members in terms of individual performance within the group and learning attained

Research suggests that cooperative approaches result in higher achievement and greater productivity by all students, more positive relationships among students, and greater psychological health (Baumberger-Henry, 2005). However, potential disadvantages of cooperative learning approaches include student resistance to frequent group assignments and unequal student participation.

## Think-Pair-Share

Think-pair-share is a cooperative learning strategy that can be used in seminars or presentations. The professor poses a problem or question and gives students 60 seconds of "think time." Students then share their thoughts and responses with a peer. Pairs of students, or a random selection of students, present their responses to the class (Ulrich & Glendon, 2005). This strategy can be used to enhance rapid thinking in situations requiring immediate action.

## Jigsaw

Jigsaw is also a cooperative learning strategy in which multiple groupings are used to enhance critical thinking (Ulrich & Glendon, 2005). Charania, Kausar, and Cassum (2001) report using jigsaw with a group of nursing students studying concepts related to fractures:

- Pain
- Inflammation
- Immobility
- Stress management

Students are assigned to research one of the four concepts. The students are then grouped with other students who studied the same concept to discuss their findings and develop expertise in the concept. Next, the group members are rearranged so each new group has an expert on each concept. Each group member discusses and clarifies for the group the information about her or his assigned concept. Each group is asked to formulate a nursing approach to caring for a patient with a fracture, integrating all four concepts. Finally, each group makes a brief presentation about their nursing approach.

The students and faculty using jigsaw regarded this approach as an enjoyable, stimulating, meaningful, and effective learning method which enhanced critical thinking and meaningfulness of the information. A few students noted insecurity because jigsaw inhibited their note-taking which raised concerns about preparation for the examination on the topic.

## Learning Communities

Learning communities are "a delivery system and a facilitating structure for the practice of collaborative learning" (Smith & MacGregor, 1998, p. 593). One model of a learning community involves linking a course or courses between different disciplines with faculty members co-planning syllabi and sharing responsibility for teaching the course. This model has been used between the nursing and nutrition departments for a healthy lifestyles course at the College of Saint Benedict and Saint John's University in Minnesota.

Another model of a learning community links a few class periods between different disciplines rather than an entire course. The students are given common assignments and learning activities for a segment of a course.

Other models can be more ambitiously configured with clusters of courses developed around broad interdisciplinary themes. Though the structures may vary for collaborative learning, there is a common intention of building both academic and social communities for students (Smith & MacGregor, 1998).

Daley, et al. (2008) describe learning communities established between two different universities for a collaborative leadership seminar. One learning community, involving two baccalaureate nursing programs at two midwestern universities, used videoconferencing. The other learning community, between a Midwestern university and students in the United Kingdom, was web-based. Both videoconferencing and web-based conferencing allowed for expansion beyond the walls of the local learning community and promoted development of partnerships among peers in other locations. Student facilitators for the conferencing researched the literature about assigned topics, wrote discussion questions, prepared creative learning activities about seminar themes, and e-mailed assigned readings, projected activities, and handouts to the participating group. The faculty advised the students and facilitated the discussion with occasional interjections to stress important points.

The authors note that students, overall, were highly positive about the experience, stating the collaborative leadership seminar "enhanced their learning, exposed them to diverse thinking, increased their ability to collaborate, and made them more likely to work with others in their nursing careers" (Daley, et al., 2008, p. 80). This type of learning community allows students from differing locations to exchange perspectives and gain a more global understanding of nursing.

## Service Learning

Service learning is supported by most learning theories. It has been incorporated into nursing education though it can present a challenge because most nursing curricula are credit-hour heavy. Service learning is directed toward a goal of social responsibility and involves work that meets actual community needs, fosters a sense of caring for others, and includes time for reflective thinking. It is different from other types of experiential learning, such as cooperative learning, internship, field practicum, and clinical experience (Carpenter, 1999). Examples of service learning presented in the literature include volunteering in an introductory nursing course at the local Boys and Girls Clubs of America, participating in the local American Red Cross during a community health course, and helping outreach workers distribute HIV prevention information as a limited component in a nursing course (Bentley & Ellison, 2005; Harrington, 1999).

Nursing students at the College of Saint Benedict and Saint John's University enroll in three, one-credit elective courses during the curriculum. One component of these courses often includes service learning. Students have served meals at homeless shelters, conducted food and clothing drives, participated in screenings, and organized community events.

The positive impact of service learning is illustrated by Bassi, Cray, and Caldrello (2008). The authors engaged nursing students in a collaborative tobacco-free pilot project between a New England school of nursing and a local elementary school in southeastern Connecticut. The school was selected because of the presence of poverty and health disparities and the large number of single-parent homes in the population.

The tobacco-free project included age-appropriate tobacco-use education for the elementary students and their parents. One hundred percent of students in 4th and 5th grade achieved the learning objectives. Four hundred and fifteen students participated in a school-wide poster contest reproducing the content learned. Ten parents enrolled in a smoking cessation program offered on site; two completed the program and one remained tobacco-free.

## Summary

Faculty face many challenges in adopting teaching-learning methods that energize students and focus on learning. Only a few of the many options available to faculty were presented in this chapter. In an era of increased educational accountability, faculty need to decide which learning methods best facilitate student learning. Before any method is implemented, the learning outcomes to be achieved must be carefully and purposefully considered.

## Learning Activities

1. Identify an arousal activity you can use to engage learners in a class on a topic of your choice. Use the activity and discuss with a colleague the students' response to the activity.
2. Teach a class using a PowerPoint® presentation with just text and graphics. Ask students to complete an evaluation of your class addressing the teaching method. Then, teach another class with a PowerPoint® presentation that uses animation, graphics, and video. Have students evaluate this class using the same criteria on the previous evaluation. Compare and contrast the students' evaluations.
3. Ask students to develop a mnemonic to help them learn a topic of their choice. Ask them to explain their mnemonic and how it helps them recall the information.

## Educational Philosophy

A nursing faculty is a designer of creative, lively, and engaging learning experiences where students and faculty are mutually involved in the learning process. Students should be challenged to think critically, integrate concepts, and perform beyond their expectations. Optimism, commitment, and respect are equally important and expected by faculty and students alike. — Kathleen Ohman

# References

Alexander, J., McDaniel, G., Baldwin, M., & Money, B. (2002). Promoting, applying, and evaluating problem-based learning in the undergraduate nursing curriculum. *Nursing Education Perspectives, 33*(5), 248-253.

American Association of Colleges of Nursing (2008). *The essentials of baccalaureate education for professional nursing practice.* Retrieved October 12, 2008 from http://www.aacn.nche.edu/

Bantz, D., Dancer, M., Hodson-Carlton, K., & Van Hove, S. (2007). A daylong clinical laboratory: from gaming to high-fidelity simulators. *Nurse Educator, 32*(6), 274-277.

Bassi, S., Cray, J., & Caldrello, L. (2008). A tobacco-free service-learning pilot project. *Journal of Nursing Education, 47*(4), 174-178.

Bastable, S. (2008). *Nurse as educator: Principles of teaching and learning for nursing practice.* Sundbury, MA: Jones & Bartlett.

Baumberger-Henry, M. (2005). Cooperative learning and case study: Does the combination improve students' perception of problem solving and decision-making skills? *Nursing Education Today, 35*(3), 238-246.

Beers, G., & Bowden, S. (2005). The effect of teaching method on long-term knowledge retention. *Journal of Nursing Education, 44*(11), 511-514.

Bentley, R., & Ellison, K. (2005). Impact of a service-learning project on nursing students. *Nursing Education Perspectives, 26*(5), 287-289.

Billings, D., & Halstead, J. (Eds.). (2009). *Teaching in nursing: A guide for faculty.* Philadelphia: Saunders Elsevier.

Bradshaw, M. (2007). Philosophical approaches to clinical instruction. In M. Bradshaw & A. Lowenstein (Eds.), *Innovative teaching strategies in nursing and related health professions* (4th ed.), pp. 303-310). Sudbury, MA: Jones and Bartlett.

Bradshaw, M., & Lowenstein, A. (2007). *Innovative teaching strategies in nursing and related health professions* (4th ed). Sudbury, MA: Jones and Bartlett Publishers.

Byrne, P. (1999). Mnemonics for medicine and surgery. Retrieved October 4, 2008 from: http://www.scribd.com/doc/19829/Medical-Mnemonics.

Carpenter, D. (1999). The concept of service-learning. In P. Bailey, D. Carpenter & P. Harrington (Eds.), *Integrating community service into nursing education: A guide to service-learning* (pp. 1-18). New York: Springer.

Caputi, L. (2010, in press). An overview of the educational process. In L. Caputi (Ed.), *Teaching nursing: The art and science, Vol. 1.* Glen Ellyn, IL: College of DuPage Press.

Caputi, L., & Blach, D. (2008). *Teaching nursing using concept maps*. Glen Ellyn, IL: College of DuPage Press.

Charania, N., Kausar, F., & Cassum, S. (2001). Playing jigsaw: A cooperative learning experience. *Journal of Nursing Education, 40*(9), 420-421.

Cannon, C., & Schell, K. (2001). Problem-based learning: Preparing nurses for practice. In B. Duch, S. Groh & D. Allen (Eds.). *The power of problem-based learning*. Sterling, VA: Stylus Publishing.

Clark, M., Nguyen, H. Bray, C., & Levine, R. (2008). Team-based learning in an undergraduate nursing course. *Journal of Nursing Education, 47*(3), 111-117.

Daley, L., Spalla, T., Arndt, M., & Warnes, A. (2008). Videoconferencing and Web-based conferencing to enhance learning communities. *Journal of Nursing Education, 47*(2), 78-81.

Dearman, C. N. (2003). Using clinical scenarios in nursing education. In M. Oermann & K. Heinrich (Eds.), *Annual Review of Nursing Education. Vol. 1* (pp. 341-355). New York: Springer.

Deck, M. (2003). Instant teaching tools. *Journal for Nurses in Staff Development, 19*(2), 106-107.

Decker, S., Sportsman, S., Puetz, L., & Billings, L. (2008). The evolution of simulation and its contribution to competency. *Journal of Continuing Education in Nursing, 39*(2), 74-80.

Delpier, T. (2006). CASES 101: Learning to teach with cases. *Nursing Education Perspectives, 27*(4), 204-209.

DeMarco, R., Hayward, L., & Lynch, M. (2002). Nursing students' experiences with and strategic approaches to case-based instruction: A replication and comparison study between two disciplines. *Journal of Nursing Education, 41*(4), 165-176.

Diekelmann, N. (2001). Narrative pedagogy: Heideggerian hermeneutical analyses of lived experiences of students, teachers, and clinicians. *Advances in Nursing Science, 23*, 53-71.

Dillon, G., Boulet, J., Hawkins, R., & Swanson, D. (2004). Simulations in the United States Medical Licensing Examination (USMLE). *Quality & Safety in Health Care, 1*(Suppl. 1), i41-i45.

Donald, J. (2002). *Learning to think: Disciplinary perspectives*. San Francisco: Jossey-Bass.

Echocardiogram. Available at: http://www.youtube.com/watch?v=TwA0LM5_1dE

The Franklin Institute (2008). *The heart: An online exploration*. Retrieved October 4, 2008 from http://www.fi.edu/biosci2/heart.html

Gaberson, K., & Oermann, M. (2007). *Clinical teaching strategies in nursing* (2nd ed.). New York: Springer.

Glendon, K., & Ulrich, D. (2005). Using games as a teaching strategy. *Journal of Nursing Education.* *44*(7), 338-339.

Google (2008). Retrieved October 5, 2008 from http://www.google.com

Gray, M. (2003). Beyond content: Generating critical thinking in the classroom. *Nurse Educator, 28*(3), 136-140.

Harrington, P. (1999). Integrating service-learning into the curriculum. In P. Bailey, D. Carpenter & P. Harrington (Eds.), *Integrating community service into nursing education: A guide to service-learning* (pp. 19-41). New York: Springer.

Hayden-Miles, M., Young, P., & Brown, P. (2010, in press). Narrative pedagory. *Teaching Nursing: The Art and Science, Vol. 2.* Glen Ellyn, IL: College of DuPage Press.

HeartPoint Gallery. (2008). Retrieved October 4, 2008, from HeartPoint www.heartpoint.com/gallery.html

Henderson, D. (2005). Games: Making learning fun. In M. Oermann & K. Heinrich (Eds.). *Annual Review of Nursing Education, 3,* (p. 165-183), New York: Springer.

Herrman, J. (2002). The 60-second nurse educator: Creative strategies to inspire learning. *Nursing Education Perspectives, 23*(5), 222-227.

Hwang S., & Kim, M. (2006). A comparison of problem-based learning and lecture-based learning in an adult health nursing course. *Nurse Education Today, 26*(4), 315-321.

Irvine, L. (1995). Can concept mapping be used to promote meaningful learning in nursing education? *Journal of Advanced Nursing, 21,* 1175-1179.

Ironside, P. (2001). Creating a research base for nursing education: An interpretative review of conventional, critical, feminist, postmodern, and phenomenological pedagogies. *Advances in Nursing Science, 23*(3), 72-87.

Ironside, P. (2003). Trying something new: Implementing and evaluating narrative pedagogy using a multimethod approach. *Nursing Education Perspectives, 24*(3), 122-128.

Ironside, P. (2004). "Covering content" and teaching thinking: Deconstructing the additive curriculum. *Journal of Nursing Education, 43*(1), 5-12.

Ironside, P. (2005). Teaching Thinking and Reaching the Limits of Memorization: Enacting New Pedagogies. *Journal of Nursing Education, 44*(10), 441-449.

Ironside, P. (2006). Using narrative pedagogy: learning and practicing interpretive thinking. *Journal of Advanced Nursing, 55*(4), 478- 478-486.

Jayasekara, R., Schultz, T., & McCutcheon, H. (2006). A comprehensive systematic review of evidence on the effectiveness and appropriateness of undergraduate nursing curricula. *International Journal of Evidence-Based Healthcare, 4*(4), 191-207.

Jeffries, P., Rew, S., & Cramer, J. (2002). A comparison of student-centered versus traditional methods of teaching basic nursing skills in a learning laboratory, *Nursing Education Perspective, 23*(1), 14-19.

Jeffries, P. (2005). A framework for designing, implementing, and evaluating simulations in nursing. *Nursing Education Perspectives, 26*(2), 28-35.

Jeffries, P. (2006). Designing simulations for nursing education. In M. Oermann & K. Heinrich, *Annual Review of Nursing Education, 4,* (pp. 161-177), New York: Springer.

Kelly, P., Haidet, P., Schneider, V., Searle, N., Seidel, C., & Richards, B. (2005). A comparison of in-class learner engagement across lecture, problem-based learning, and team learning using the STROBE classroom observation tool. *Teaching and Learning in Medicine, 17,* 112-118.

King, M., & Shell, R. (2002). Teaching and evaluating critical thinking with concept maps. *Nurse Educator, 27*(5), 214-216.

London, F. (2010, in press). Using humor in the classroom. In L. Caputi (Ed.), *Teaching nursing: The art and science*, Volume 1. Glen Ellyn, IL: College of DuPage Press.

Masters, J., & Christensen, M. (2002). What is a picture really worth? Old teaching techniques and the "new" nursing student. *Nurse Educator, 27*(1), 41, 46.

McKeachie, W. (2002). *Teaching tips: Strategies, research, and theory for college and university teachers* (11th ed.). Boston: Houghton Mifflin.

Merrick, H., Nowacek, G., Boyer, J., & Robertson, J. (2000). Comparison of the objective structured clinical examination with the performance of third-year medical students' surgery. *The American Journal of Surgery, 179,* 286-288.

Meyers, J., & Choka, K. (2008). What are the ODDES? Assessment of Mental Status and Use of the Nursing Process. *Nurse Educator, 33*(5), 192.

Michaelsen, L., Knight, A., & Fink, L., (Eds.). (2004). *Teambased learning: A transformative use of small groups in college teaching.* Sterling, VA: Stylus.

National League for Nursing. (2005). *Position statement: Transforming nursing education.* New York: Author.

Nehring, W., & Lashley, F. (2004). Current use and opinions regarding human patient simulators in nursing education. *Nursing Education Perspectives, 25*(5), 244-248.

Oermann, M., & Gaberson, K. (2006). *Evaluation and testing in nursing education* (2nd ed.), New York: Springer.

Peteani, L. (2004). Enhancing clinical practice and education with high fidelity human patient simulators. *Nurse Educator, 29*(1), 25-30.

Pullen, R., Murray, P., & McGee, K. S. (2003). Using care groups to mentor novice nursing students. In M. Oermann & K. Heinrich (Eds.), *Annual review of nursing education. Vol. 1* (pp. 147-161), New York: Springer.

Rowles, C., & Russo, B. (2009). Strategies to promote critical thinking and active learning. In D. Billings & J. Halstead (Eds.), *Teaching in nursing: A guide for faculty* (pp. 238-261). Philadelphia: Saunders Elsevier.

Royce, D. (2001). *Teaching tips for college and university instructors*. Needham Heights, MA: Allyn & Bacon.

Royse, M., & Newton, S. (2007). How gaming is used as an innovative strategy for nursing education. *Nursing Education Perspective, 28*(5), 263-267.

Rummel N., Levin J., & Woodward, M. (2003). Do pictorial mnemonic text-learning aids give students something worth writing about? *Journal of Educational Psychology, 95*(2), 327-334.

Sarvis, C. (2007). Calling on NERDS for critically colonized wounds. *Nursing 2007, 37*(5), 26-27.

Scanlan, J., Care, W., & Udod, S. (2002). Unravelling the unknowns of reflection in classroom teaching. *Journal of Advanced Nursing, 38*(2), 136-143.

Scheckel, M. (2009). Selecting learning experiences to achieve curriculum outcomes. In D. Billings, & J. Halstead (Eds.), *Teaching in nursing: A guide for faculty* (3rd ed.), (pp. 154-172). Philadelphia: Saunders Elsevier.

Schell, K. (2006). A delphi study of innovative teaching in baccalaureate nursing education. *Journal of Nursing Education, 45*(11), 439-448.

Schumacher, D. (2005). Do your CATS PRRR?: A mnemonic device to teach safety checks for administering intravenous medications. *The Journal of Continuing Education in Nursing, 36*(3), 104-106.

Schuster, P. (2008). *Concept mapping: A critical-thinking approach to care planning* (2nd ed.). Philadelphia: F. A. Davis.

Schwind, C. J., Boehler, M., Folse, R., Dunnington, G., & Markwell, S. J. (2001). Development of physical examination skills in a third-year surgical clerkship. *The American Journal of Surgery, 181*, 338-340.

Simpson, E., & Courtney, M. (2002). Critical thinking in nursing education: Literature review. *International Journal of Nursing Practice, 8*, 89-98.

Skiba, D., & Barton, A. (2006). Adapting your teaching to accommodate the net generation of learners. *OJIN: The Online Journal of Issues in Nursing, 11*(2), Manuscript 4. Available at: www.nursingworld.org/ojin/topic30/tpc30_4.htm

Smith, B., & Johnson, Y. (2002). Using structured clinical preparation to stimulate reflection and foster critical thinking. *Journal of Nursing Education, 41*(4), 182-185.

Smith, B., & MacGregor, J. (1998). What is collaborative learning? In K. Feldman & M. Paulsen (Eds.), *Teaching and learning in the college classroom*. Needham Heights, MA: Simon & Schuster.

Solomon, P. (2007). Problem-based learning. In M. Bradshaw & A. Lowenstein (Eds.), *Innovative teaching strategies in nursing and related health professions* (4th ed.), (pp. 131-140). Sudbury, MA: Jones and Bartlett.

Stiles, A. (2006). Cooperative learning: Enhancing individual learning through positive group process. In M. Oermann & K. Heinrich, *Annual Review of Nursing Education*, (p. 131-159), New York: Springer.

Taylor, J., & Wros, P. (2007). Concept mapping: A nursing model for care planning. *Journal of Nursing Education, 46*(5), 211-216.

Ulrich, D., & Glendon, K. (2005). *Interactive group learning: Strategies for nurse educators* (2nd ed.). New York: Springer.

Vandeveer, M. (2009). From teaching to learning: Theoretical foundations. In D. Billings & J. Halstead (Eds.), *Teaching in nursing: A guide for faculty* (3rd ed.), (pp. 189-226), Philadelphia: Saunders Elsevier.

Vizino, H. (1998). Old shoe stimulation. In M. Deck (Ed.), *More instant teaching tools for health educators*. St. Louis: Mosby.

Welch, J., Jeffries, P., Lyon, B., Boland, D., & Backer, J. (2001). Experiential learning: Integrating theory and research into practice. *Nurse Educator, 26*(5), 240-243.

Weimer, M. (2002). *Learner-centered teaching*. San Francisco, CA: Jossey-Bass.

Wilgis, M., & McConnell, J. (2008). Concept mapping: An educational strategy to improve graduate nurses' critical thinking skills during a hospital orientation program. *The Journal of Continuing Education in Nursing, 39*(3), 119.

Woods, J. (2008). Number 1 in the ratings: A television-based learning activity. *Journal of Nursing Education, 47*(6), 287-288.

Yoo, M., & Yoo, Y. (2003). The effectiveness of standardized patients as a teaching method for nursing fundamentals. *Journal of Nursing Education, 42*(10), 444-448.

Youngblood, N., & Beitz, J. (2001). Developing critical thinking with active learning strategies. *Nurse Educator, 26*(1), 39-42.

# CHAPTER 37

# USING HUMOR IN THE CLASSROOM

## Fran London, BSN, MS, RN

The content of this chapter relates to the following major content area and subconcepts on the Certified Nurse Educator Examination Detailed Test Blueprint:

**Facilitate Learning**

- Implement a variety of teaching strategies appropriate to content; learner needs; desired learner outcomes
- Use teaching strategies based on evidence-based practices related to education
- Show enthusiasm for teaching, learning, and the nursing profession that inspires and motivates students
- Use knowledge of evidence-based practice to instruct learners

## Introduction

Do your students:

- Look forward to attending your class?
- Stay awake while you teach?
- Actively participate in class activities?
- Remember the key points of your presentation?
- Evaluate your teaching positively and recommend you to their peers?

**Scoring:** If you answered **no** four or five times, read on; this chapter may be very helpful. If you answered **no** two or three times, you're on the right track. This chapter may add to your expertise. If you answered **no** once or not at all, you're wonderful! Share your secret!

Using humor in the classroom may help turn **no** responses into **yes** responses. This chapter covers the why and how-to of using humor in teaching.

## Using Humor is Serious Business

Some teachers refrain from using humor because they want to be accepted as serious academic professionals. These teachers believe their deans and other professors will think they are unprofessional **if they are less than serious.** They may even fear they will not be granted tenure.

The best way to be accepted as a serious academic professional is to consistently maintain an evidence-based practice. Oddly, some people confuse the professional seriousness of high academic standards with a serious demeanor.

> *Life does not cease to be funny when people die any more than it ceases to be serious when people laugh.*—*George Bernard Shaw (Moss, 2000, p. 90)*

The use of humor in teaching poses an interesting paradox. A look at the literature reveals no definitions of professionalism, scholarship, or academia that include an absence of humor. Likewise, there is no research that correlates poor academic outcomes with the use of relevant and appropriate humor in teaching. On the other hand, studies that correlate the use of relevant and appropriate humor with effective teaching have been around for decades. Here are just a few:

- Berk, R. A. (2006). Laughterpiece theatre: Humor as a systematic teaching tool, *The Professional & Organizational Development Network in Higher Education,*17(2). Online.
- Bowles, D. J. (2006). Active learning strategies. Not for the birds! *International Journal of Nursing Education Scholarship,* 3(1). Online.
- Hillman, S. M. (1995). Laugh and learn: Humor in nursing education. *Journal of Nursing Jocularity,* 5(1), 32-34.
- Hayden-Miles, M. (2002). Humor in clinical nursing education. *Journal of Nursing Education,* 41(9), 420-424.
- McLaughlin, D. E., Freed, P. E., et al. (2006). Action methods in the classroom: Creative strategies for nursing education. *International Journal of Nursing Education Scholarship,* 3(1), Online.
- Parkin, C. J. (1989). Humor, health, and higher education: Laughing matters. *Journal of Nursing Education,* 28(5), 229-230.
- Pease, R. A. (1991). Cartoon humor in nursing education. *Nursing Outlook,* 39(6), 262-267.
- Rosenberg, L. (1989). A delicate dose of humor . . . in the practice of teaching of nursing. *Nursing Forum,* 24(2), 3-7.
- Ulloth, J. K. (2002). The benefits of humor in nursing education. *Journal of Nursing Education,* 41(11), 6-81.
- Warner, S. L. (1991). Humor: A coping response for student nurses. *Archives of Psychiatric Nursing,* 5(1), 10-16.
- Warnock, P. (1989). Humor: A didactic tool in adult education. *Lifelong Learning,* 12(6), 22-24.

- Watson, M. J., & Emerson, S. (1988). Facilitate learning with humor. *Journal of Nursing Education, 27*(2), 89-90.
- Ziv, A.(1988). Teaching and learning with humor: Experiment and replication. *Journal of Experimental Education, 57*(1), 5-15.

Consequently, those who do not apply humor when teaching demonstrate a personal bias toward seriousness that is unsubstantiated by the literature.

> *Seriousness is the only refuge of the shallow.*
> —Oscar Wilde (Nisker, 2001, p. 35)

Therefore, one attribute of a serious academic professional is the application of humor to one's teaching.


## Relevant and Appropriate Humor

When incorporating humor into nursing education, it is important the humor is both relevant and appropriate. Relevant humor relates to the topic of the classroom presentation. This humor keeps the learner's attention and contributes to, or enhances, the lesson.

Humor in the classroom is like a song in a musical stage production. In a good musical, each song tells you a bit more about the characters or advances the plot. The music is not an interruption of the play to provide some musical entertainment. It changes the pace of the program and entertains as it moves the story along. Similarly, relevant humor within teaching moves the lesson forward but on a lighter note.

Appropriate humor is slightly more subjective in definition but definable, nonetheless. It applies not to political correctness but to therapeutic usefulness. Bill Cosby, a comedian with a Doctor of Education degree, generally demonstrates appropriate humor. Don Rickles, who specializes in the comedy of insult, demonstrates humor that is inappropriate for the classroom.

Appropriate humor laughs with people. It can be aimed at the teacher, the teacher's foibles, or things in the environment. Appropriate humor also:
- Shares frustrations
- Decreases stress and anxiety
- Promotes hope
- Establishes emotional bonds between people and brings them together, and/or puts a problem into perspective

Inappropriate humor laughs at people, increases stress and anxiety, and decreases hope. It hurts others, distances people from one another, and creates problems.

Choosing appropriate humor is a learned skill. Because this quality is more subjective, the inappropriateness of humor may not be apparent until evidenced by the students' reactions. If it becomes apparent that humor is inappropriate, the teacher should apologize immediately, briefly, and sincerely. The teacher then self-reflects on why the humor was inappropriate and applies this knowledge to using humor in the future.

Teaching with relevant humor keeps the learner engaged and helps the learner follow the line of thought used in the presentation. Inappropriate humor disengages that connection between teacher and learner by creating discomfort. Humor is an effective teaching tool because it feels good while it keeps the learner awake, aware, and open to new information.

## Education is Serious Business

Education is serious business; it is not entertainment. Students should learn because they want to learn and not because the teacher sneaks information in with a laugh. Don't get stuck in the muck of shoulds. Yes, education is serious business, but capturing and holding the attention of the learners is a characteristic of good teachers. Sometimes this is best accomplished with humor.

Intelligence and motivation enhance learning, but so does readiness to learn, which relates to the emotional state of the learner. To some, the phrases **calculus** or **organic chemistry** or, in the case of nursing, **deadly disease** create enough fear to shut down the learner's ability to accept new information. The screaming thought of "I can't do that" blocks out all other information, no matter how well it is presented.

> *Humor can be planned and executed to rivet your students' attention in a nanosecond and sustain a level of engagement that can facilitate learning.*
> *(Berk, 2002, p.6)*

Educating while entertaining overcomes this fear. This is not dumbing down, which means the message has been oversimplified and diluted. Edutainment – a blend of education and entertainment – relaxes learners so they are open to new information.

Television chef Alton Brown, who uses props and analogies to illustrate cooking science, edutains with great expertise. For example, in a show on grilling, he presented the various ways to light the charcoal. He said his neighbor prefers to use lighter fluid. "There he is now!" In the background, the audience can see a cloud of smoke coming up from behind a fence, see a fire flare up, and hear a man scream. Alton Brown showed the dangers of using lighter fluid to start an outdoor grill rather then lecture about those dangers. He went on to describe safer methods.

Abraham Maslow said, "Education is in a palatable form" when teaching is done with humor. Connecting teaching objectives to a light-hearted activity creates an environment that facilitates learning. In addition, it will be fun.

> *Choose to have fun.*
> *Fun creates enjoyment.*
> *Enjoyment invites participation.*
> *Participation focuses attention.*
> *Attention expands awareness.*
> *Awareness promotes insight.*
> *Insight generates knowledge.*
> *Knowledge facilitates action.*
> *Action yields results.*
> *– Oswald B. Shallow (Wooten, 1994, p. 31)*

## Humor and Quality Teaching

Some readers may be thinking, "Sure, humor feels good. I can't argue with that. But show me the evidence that humor is a factor in quality teaching." Or put another way, "If you're asking me to seriously consider humor, which could radically alter my proven time-tested approach to teaching, known technically as the Non-Critical-Thinking-Passive-Comatose-Boring Method, show me the hard evidence that it works" (Berk, 1998, p. 5).

This chapter opened with the proposal that using humor in the classroom helps students:

- Look forward to attending class
- Stay awake while teachers teach
- Actively participate in class activities
- Remember the key points of the presentation
- Evaluate the teaching positively and recommend teachers to their peers

A brief look at some of the literature supports the positive effects of using humor in the classroom. Laughter has physiologic effects that arouse then relax (Fry, 1992). The first phase of laughter stimulates (increases the pulse and respiratory rates), and the second phase of laughter relaxes the muscles, reduces blood pressure, and eases tension. Laughter enhances blood oxygen levels. This arousal and relaxation physiologically prepares learners to pay attention and relax, preparing the internal environment to accept new information. Using humor in teaching helps students stay awake and remember the key points of the presentation.

Psychologically, humor creates an environment that promotes learning. Ziv (1983) found that when humor was used throughout the school day, learning increased by 15%. Other researchers (Droz & Ellis, 1997) discovered that when humor is used to introduce a new topic and capture the learner's complete attention, an increase in learning results. In a sense, humor opens the mind to see things in new ways.

> *Humor in education sets the tone for a caring environment*
> *that promotes openness and facilitates communication . . .*
> *[The learner is more willing to] shift patterns of thinking,*
> *generate creative solutions to problems,*
> *perceive double meanings,*
> *understand analogies,*
> *and examine paradoxes.*
> *Flexible and creative ways of thinking emerge;*
> *the corollary benefits are*
> *critical thinking and independent problem-solving.*
> *– Cannella, Missroon, and Optiz, (1995, p. 61)*

Ulloth (2002) summarized a review of the literature by saying, "Using humor to stimulate mental processes and control fear and anxiety helps students retain the content they have learned. In addition, when anxiety is reduced, students are more likely to open their minds to learning and enjoy the experience." (p. 477)

## Adding Humor to a Presentation

Although adding humor to a presentation does require additional work, it is a fun part of course-building. It is an opportunity to be creative and express individuality. However, this is not a career in stand-up comedy. Students should not leave class feeling they have just walked out of a show at a comedy club. A major goal is to ensure students are not bored with the presentation or, even better, that the students leave feeling energized about what they have just learned.

Teachers can think of humor as a teaching condiment. The content of what is taught is like the nutrition in food. Humor is the condiment of education. As much as you enjoy any one condiment, you would not want to eat a meal of it. Imagine a soup of salad dressing, a bowl of mustard, or a meal of sliced garlic. Too much! And not very satisfying.

One difference between the food at a fine restaurant and a fast-food chain is the use of condiments. Fast-food chains use salt. Fine restaurants carefully adjust the herbs and spices to bring out the best in food. Similarly, adding a pinch of select humor to each class brings out the best of the content.

## How to Add Humor When Teaching

Applying one rule and following two steps can help guide the incorporation of humor into teaching. The rule is: Don't do anything that makes you uncomfortable. Be yourself and relax.

The two steps are:

1. Choose the comfortable level of risk.
2. Choose the specific humor to use.

Fortunately, there is a wide range of ways to add humor to a presentation. These ways also come in a full range of risk. Low-risk humor is very safe to try; if no one laughs, the moment is quickly forgotten. On the other hand, high-risk humor is humor that is potentially embarrassing when it flops. The teacher tries to be funny, and no one laughs!

Teachers who feel uncomfortable about adding humor should start with low-risk humor. Fortunately, low-risk humor provides the same benefits as risky methods. After experiencing success using low-risk humor, teachers can consider new ways to add humor. Embarrassment is really all in one's head!

Students recognize when teachers choose humor beyond their comfort level. The humor seems forced. Teachers may overreact to the embarrassment and never teach with humor again. This would be a great loss. Instead, teachers should keep within their own comfort level.

Following are some ways to add humor to teaching. Teachers should note the methods that seem the most comfortable for them.

### Step 1: Choosing the Level of Risk

Following is a list of types of humor. The list is arranged from low-risk to high-risk humor. Teachers should choose the level at which they feel most comfortable.

**Low-risk Humor:**
- Quotations
- Analogies
- Metaphors
- Questions
- Cartoons
- Photographs, drawings, or other art
- Multiple-choice items used during class
- Top-10 lists
- Anecdotes
- Humorous material in the syllabus including items such as:
  - Prerequisites
  - Professor's credentials
  - Office hours
  - Teaching strategies
  - Reading list
  - Sidebars
  - Footnotes
- Humorous problems or assignments
- Add humor to the environment:
  - Descriptors, cautions, warnings, or quotations on handouts
  - Picture frame around a funny quote
  - Bulletin board with humorous theme

**Medium-risk Humor:**
- Spontaneous humor:
  - In response to student questions
  - In response to your mistakes
  - In response to interruptions

**Higher-risk Humor:**
- Costumes
- Skits, dramatizations
- Games
- Opening jokes
- Funny song lyrics or poem

## Step 2: Choosing the Specific Humor to Use

Once the risk level is determined, choose the specific humor to use. Just as the audiovisuals are planned, so is the humor. Ziv (1988) proposed that when identifying the main concepts of a lecture, humor should be used to make those main concepts clearer and to increase students' recall of the material.

Educators must know their students and choose humor that is appropriate. Caputi (2002) stated that the closer the teacher and students are in age, the more congruent is their taste in humor. She described a lecture that included a cartoon based on the characters from the Bonanza television series. Only the students who were old enough to have seen the series got the joke; the younger students did not. When the teacher hummed the theme song, the older students hummed along. The younger students then joined in on the laughter, but they were laughing at the humming, not the cartoon.

Educators need to remember to use humor as a condiment. Less is more. Humor is used to wake up brains. Teachers should start out small in the first session of the course. This will engage the students but keep their expectations for future humor reasonable. Thus, each use of humor throughout the term will be a surprise and have more impact. Teachers need to remember that there is work involved in adding humor well, and so they should minimize the humor-adding workload.

The above types of humor can be introduced into a classroom for inspiration. Humor is all around; all teachers need to do is collect it. They can read cartoons in newspapers, magazines, and books and keep copies of those relevant to classroom topics.

## Listening for Relevant Humor

Humor is all around us. Relevant humor can be found in jokes, funny conversations, anecdotes, and newspaper stories. Also, the Internet is a great source for humor. Following is a list of some websites for both general and nursing-related humor:

- www.ucomics.com
- www.unitedmedia.com/comics
- www.comics.com
- www.learnwell.org/laugh.htm
- www.wakeuplaughing.com
- www.nurstoon.com/
- www.ncpamd.com/mcjokes.htm
- www.angelfire.com/wa/nursejokes/index.html

- www.nursinghumor.com

The CD-ROM that accompanies this book includes these websites for easy access.

Teachers can keep a file folder with humor resources. As their collections grow, they can start databases, creating humor files in programs such as Access®, FileMaker Pro®, or Excel®, entering the items, documenting the sources, and categorizing each item by theme. This makes searching for humor an easier task when preparing for class.

## Humor in Action: Concrete Examples

### Quotations

Quotations can be added to projected images as students enter the classroom. When teaching patient advocacy with a scientific bend, the following may be used: "If you're not part of the solution, you're part of the precipitate" (Steven Wright, live performance, 5/8/2002). On the topic of nutrition: "How much Healthy Choice ice cream can I eat before it's no longer a healthy choice?" (Anonymous). On the topic of patient-centered care: "I'm getting an MRI tomorrow to find out if I have claustrophobia" (Steven Wright, live performance, 5/8/2002).

### Visual Humor

Teachers can use photographs, drawings, or other pieces of art to visually inject humor. A picture can be used to relieve a tense moment. After presenting a lot of detailed information, such as the Kreb's cycle, teachers can try projecting a picture of the Edvard Munch's painting *The Scream*, also know as *The Cry*. The familiar image exaggerates the tension in the classroom and, by acknowledging this, releases it.

### Humor Incorporated into Handouts

A bit of humor on the syllabus can help set a relaxed tone and test to see if anyone reads it! Following is an adaptation of a warning written by Berk (1998) that might work at the top of a reading list:

*Warning: Reading the following articles, which contain a drillion killion research findings and citations, could cause drowsiness, nausea, bloating, numbness, various mutations, and a substantial penalty for early withdrawal. Cruel? Sick? Inhumane? Perhaps. But I couldn't help it. My name is Ron and I'm a professorholic. (p. 7)*

## Cartoons

Cartoons are easy to incorporate into your presentation. Because they are copyrighted, permission must be obtained from the author first. Authors' names can be found on the Internet for contact information – either e-mail addresses or addresses of the syndicates. State specifically which cartoon you want to use, in what context, and the size of your audience. Most do not charge a fee, as long as they are given credit.

If there is no cartoon that precisely meets classroom needs, you can change the caption on an existing cartoon. For example, Caputi (2002) reported that during a lecture on sexually transmitted diseases and safe sex, she used a picture of the manager of a baseball team and an umpire arguing. She rewrote the caption so that under the umpire it read, "Latex condoms, better protection!" and under the manager it read, "Natural membrane, feels best!" She put this cartoon on the handout that reviewed the types of condoms available.

## Riddles, Jokes, and Funny Definitions

Educators can use jokes or riddles that relate to the class content to open the class or wait until a dull moment to inject it to wake up their students. For example, here are some from Caputi (2002) that may work when covering the urinary system:

Question: What does a urologist spend the day doing?
Answer: Curin' urine.

Or, when talking about care of patients with GI problems:

Question: What do you call a gastric tube inserted through the nose?
Answer: A nose hose

Or, on the topic of blood disorders:

Question: What do you call a man with anemia?
Answer: A pale male.

Or, toward the end of the term:

Question: What results from studying too hard?
Answer: Brain strain.

## Anecdotes

Anecdotes can be funny stories that teach and can be collected from life experiences of teachers and their colleagues. Following is a funny story from Caputi (2002) that illustrates how important it is to assess a patient's learning needs before teaching.

A nurse was teaching an 80-year-old widower how to take care of his indwelling urinary catheter after returning home. He lived by himself in a small apartment and had no family caring for him, making him totally responsible for his own care. The nurse taught him how to use a leg bag during the day and a drainage bag at night. She taught him how to empty the bag. She also taught him signs and symptoms of a urinary tract infection and when to call the physician. The patient was able to return-demonstrate all the necessary skills and verbalize knowledge of all the information she had taught. She felt very satisfied with her teaching.

The next day he called her with a question. The nurse was surprised to hear from him because he seemed to understand it all so well.

Could your students guess what question this gentleman had when he called the nurse?

His question: "My girlfriend is here and wants to know what I do with this catheter when we are having sex."

The nurse was embarrassed. Because this man was 80 years old, a widower, and living alone, it never occurred to her that he might be sexually active.

## Top-10 Lists

You can create a funny Top-10 list for nearly any topic. Be creative! Here is one from Caputi (2002) that is used at the end of the term:

**Top 10 Things You Can No Longer Say After Finishing Nursing School**
10. I'll do that when the term is over!
9. Wait, let me get you the real nurse.
8. But I gained those 5 pounds because I sit around studying all day!
7. I'm only a nursing student, doctor. It does no good to yell at me!
6. No, you can't listen to your punk rock music on the car tape player. I have to listen to my nursing lectures. . . . I have a test tomorrow!

5. Maybe that green halo the patient is seeing isn't really digitalis toxicity but a reflection off my green student uniform.
4. Turn the television down; I'm trying to study!
3. But I **deserve** that hot fudge sundae; I've been studying all day!
2. How many days left until graduation?
1. Sorry, I can't administer that enema to the patient; I haven't passed my return on that skill yet!

## Games

Adapt television game show formats (such as Jeopardy, Family Feud, or Name That Tune) or board games (such as Trivial Pursuit or Cranium) to add fun to the classroom experience. Games teach content, create community among students and faculty, and encourage students to interact to solve problems collectively (Glendon & Urlrich, 2005). They offer a good relief when reviewing information before an exam. For some example game shows adapted for education go to http://www.murray.k12.ga.us/teacher/kara%20leonard/Mini%20T's/Games/Games.htm.

## Funny Raps and Songs

Higher on the risk continuum are humor delivery systems that involve audience participation. Rap songs require only rhyme and rhythm, songs involve, well, singing. Figure 1 is an example from Caputi (2002) of a rap used for a test review. An audio file of this rap is located on the CD-ROM accompanying this book.

Now that it's test time, Let's look at pathophys.
Let's review. Sick it's got to be
Gallbladder, liver, When liver has hepatitis,
And pancreas, too. A, B, C or D?????
Look at the liver Don't forget steatorrhea.
It's very complex. What's this you say?
Over 400 functions Floating, frothy, foul-smelling?
At its best. Why not just flush it away!
The gallbladder's simpler, Straight up or on the rocks?
Only a few. Inflammation on the way.
Storage makes one, Just say "No, I've gotta go,"
And concentration makes two. Or cirrhosis, one day!
Exocrine pancreas? Liver flap, restlessness,
So what's this all about? Irritability, lethargy.
Exocrine … "through the duct" Wonder what this could be?
Is how it all gets out. En-cepha-lop-athy!
Now that it's test time, Now that it's test time,
Let's review. Let's review.
Gallbladder, liver, Gallbladder, liver,
And pancreas, too. And pancreas, too.
Portal circulation Pain in the upper right,
From the GI tract. Going around to the back?
Takes it to the liver, Could be gallstones,
All the nutrients extract. Better check it out, Jack!
Hepatocytes and Kupffer cells Elevated amylase
And bile canaliculi. And lipase, too?
All found in the liver Pancreatitis might be
With a microscopic eye. The diagnosis for you.
Bile flow from the liver ducts, Murphy's, Cullen's, Turner's,
To the gallbladder to be stored. Oh, no, what should I do?
Ready for that meal of fat, Vis-u-ali-zation
But don't forget there's more. Can help get you through.

**Figure 1.** Gallbladder, Liver, and Pancreas, Too!

Bile carries along the bilirubin Put Cullen's C around the umbilicus,
For excretion from that fellow. Turn them over for Turner's flanks,
If something gets in the way, A positive Murphy's tells you
That fellow turns all yellow! It's in the gallbladder's ranks.
Now that it's test time, Now it's REALLY test time,
Let's review. That's it for the review.
Gallbladder, liver, Just let me take the time
And pancreas, too. To wish good luck to you!

**Figure 1 continued.** Gallbladder, Liver, and Pancreas, Too!

Teachers can compose their own funny song lyrics, or find appropriate humor by a nursing humor singing group, such as Too Live Nurse or The NurSing Notes (1993).

Search the Internet for other humorous healthcare-related musical performers, including Chordiac Arrest! at http://www.singers.com/barbershop/chordiacarr.html and Deb Gauldin at www.debgauldin.com.

### Learning More about Using Humor to Teach

The best way to learn about using humor to teach is to jump in and do it. Feedback from students teaches more than any peer-reviewed, fully referenced book can.

However, more concrete information about incorporating humor, *Professors Are from Mars, Students Are from Snickers: How to Write and Deliver Humor in the Classroom and in Presentations* (Berk, 1998) is recommended. Following is a summary of Berk's suggestions to optimize the delivery of humor:

- Edit humorous material to assure it is not offensive to anyone
- Memorize the material
- Practice the timing
- Involve the audience
- Vary voice modulation, intonation, and speed
- Enunciate every word
- Use facial expressions
- Gesture with your hands and arms
- Move your body around

- Use audiovisual aids
- Make eye contact
- Practice
- Recover from a bomb gracefully
- Critique your delivery

Ulloth (2003, p. 36) offers these rules for developing and implementing humor in nursing classrooms:
- Be yourself
- Use humor regularly
- Avoid offensive humor
- Be sensitive to emotional students
- Be spontaneous
- Remember that humor is a tool to convey information, not the primary purpose of the class
- Use relevant humor to emphasize the educational point
- Add humorous material to course syllabi, tests, and handouts
- Remember to enjoy yourself
- Remember, humor is a condiment

*If you're finding it is hard work to add humor to your teaching,*
*you are working too hard at it.*
*– Fran London*

Ziv (1998) advised not to distract students with humor. If they are too aroused, they may be distracted by too many cues and will not spend enough time processing the content presented. Never use more than three or four instances of humor in an hour.

Lomax and Moosavi (2002) reported they opened each class with a piece of humor that related to a concept previously taught or to be taught in the class. Occasionally they presented students with a humorous piece and asked them to describe the related concept, either verbally or in a written assignment.

Teachers should not encourage students to focus on the teacher's wit rather than the subject matter. Even one injection of humor in a class is enough to enhance effective teaching.

Try it! During the next presentation or lecture in class, add some relevant and appropriate humor. Teachers enjoy laughter, too!

*A classroom without humor is like a cake without sugar.*
*– Lori Ellis and Marilyn Droz (1997)*

As you role model the appropriate use of humor in the classroom, take the opportunity to explain what you are doing and why. Tell your students about the evidence relating to the therapeutic benefits of humor.

## Summary

Adamle and Chiang-Hanisko, et al. (2007) surveyed faculty members from four nursing programs about the inclusion of humor in the nursing curriculum, and found students were taught substantially more about humor in clinical settings than in the classroom. They believe "The nurse's ability to recognize humor, interpret its usage, and respond to it may be one of the most critical points in the assessment and care of a patient" (page 13), and by introducing the topic in class, students will be more likely to recognize humor and apply it in practice.

## Learning Activities

1. Think about instructors you have had who used humor well in the classroom. Write a description of how humor was used and the reaction of the students.
2. Prepare a classroom presentation for students and incorporate humor into the beginning, middle, and end. Survey students at each point and ask about the effectiveness of this instructional strategy
3. Locate a teacher who uses humor. Ask that teacher to discuss what effect using humor has had on his/her teaching.

## Educational Philosophy

Adult learning principles are at the core of everything I teach. Formal lectures are as boring to listen to as they are boring to prepare. — Fran London

## References

Adamle, K. N., Chiang-Hanisko, L. et al. (2007). Comparing teaching practices about humor among nursing faculty: An international collaborative study. *International Journal of Nursing Education Scholarship, 4*(1), online.

Berk, R. A. (1998). *Professors are from Mars, students are from Snickers: How to write and deliver humor in the classroom and in presentations.* Madison, WI: Mendota Press.

Berk, R. A. (2002). *Humor as an instructional defibrillator: Evidenced-based techniques in teaching and assessment.* Sterling, VA: Stylus Pub, LLC.

Cannella, K. S., Missroon, S., & Optiz, M. P. (1995). Humor—An educational strategy. In K. Buxman (Ed.), *Nursing perspectives on humor* (pp. 51-86). Staten Island, NY: Power Publications.

Caputi, L. (2002). *Add pizzazz to your lectures: Using humor and other nontraditional strategies to enhance your lecture sessions.* St. Charles, IL: L. Caputi, Inc.

Droz, M. & Ellis, L. (1997). Humor and its implications in the classroom. *Therapeutic Humor, 11*(4), 3, 5.

Fry, W. F. (1992). The physiologic effects of humor, mirth, and laughter. *JAMA, 267*(13), 1857-1858.

Glendon, K., & Urlrich, D. (2005). Using games as a teaching strategy, *Journal of Nursing Education, 44*(7), 338-339.

Heinz, C. (2002). Use of the "plugged up ketchup bottle" metaphor in educational research. *Journal of Condiment Behaviors, 12,* 66-91.

Hillman, S. M. (1995). Laugh and learn: Humor in nursing education, *Journal of Nursing Jocularity, 5*(1), 32-34.

Lomax, R. G., & Moosavi, S. A. (2002). *Using humor to teach statistics: Must they be orthogonal?* [online]. Available: http://www.leaonline.com/doi/abs/10.1207/S15328031US0102_04?journalCode=us

Moss, A. (2000). *Zen paths to laughter.* North Clarendon, VT: Turtle Publishing.

Nisker, W. S. (2001). *The essential crazy wisdom.* Berkeley, CA: Ten Speed Press.

Parkin, C. J. (1989). Humor, health, and higher education: Laughing matters. *Journal of Nursing Education, 28*(5), 229-230.

Pease, R. A. (1991). Cartoon humor in nursing education. *Nursing Outlook, 39*(6), 262-267.

Rosenberg, L. (1989). A delicate dose of humor . . . in the practice of teaching of nursing. *Nursing Forum, 24*(2), 3-7.

The NurSing Notes. (1993). *Health and humor through harmony.* Syracuse, NY: NurSing Notes. For information, contact: Larry Brennan RN, (315) 463-8971, LBrennan@twcny.rr.com, www.thenursingnotes.com

Too Live Nurse. (2001). *Ineffective individual coping.* New Lebanon, NY: Too Live Nurse Productions, www.toolivenurse.com.

Ulloth, J. K. (2002). The benefits of humor in nursing education, *Journal of Nursing Education, 41*(11), 476-81.

Ulloth, J. K. (2003). Guidelines for developing and implementing humor in nursing classrooms. *Journal of Nursing Education, 42*(1), 35-37.

Warner, S. L. (1991). Humor: A coping response for student nurses. Archives of *Psychiatric Nursing, 5*(1), 10-16.

Warnock, P. (1989). Humor: A didactic tool in adult education. *Lifelong Learning, 12*(6), 22-24.

Watson, M. J., & Emerson, S. (1988). Facilitate learning with humor. *Journal of Nursing Education, 27*(2), 89-90.

Wooten, P. (1994). *Heart, humor, and healing.* Mount Shasta, CA: Commune-A-Key.

Wright, S., Quotes. Accessed February 11, 2008. http://thinkexist.com/quotes/stephen_wright/

Ziv, A. (1983). The influence of humorous atmosphere on divergent thinking. *Contemporary Educational Psychology, 8*, 68-75.

Ziv, A. (1988). Teaching and learning with humor: Experiment and replication. *Journal of Experimental Education, 57*(1), 5-15.

# CHAPTER 38

# EFFECTIVE PRESENTATION SKILLS

## Dianne Ryan, MA, RN, BC

---

The content of this chapter relates to the following major content area and subconcepts on the Certified Nurse Educator Examination Detailed Test Blueprint:

**Facilitate Learning**

- Practice skilled oral communication that reflects an awareness of self and relationships with learners
- Communicate effectively orally and in writing with an ability to convey ideas in a variety of contexts
- Create a positive learning environment that fosters a free exchange of ideas

---

## Introduction

*"As long as there are human rights to be defended; as long as there are great interests to be guarded; as long as the welfare of nations is a matter for discussion, so long will public speaking have its place."*
—William Jennings Byran

In the early 1980s Wallace and Wallechinsky conducted a survey among the American public regarding their worst fears in life, then published their responses in the *Book of Lists* (Wallace, Wallechinsky, & Wallace 1983; 1993; 2005). The list consisted of fears that included flying, insects, heights, deep water, and dogs, but what surprised them was the number one fear – speaking before a group! Death was seventh. So basically what this says is that the average American would rather die than stand before a group and speak! Since then, the survey has been conducted several more times, and although death has climbed upwards to the number two fear, public speaking still reigns as the king of the fears. This prompts the question, "Why are so many people afraid to speak before a group?"

At some point in our lives, most of us will be faced with having to give a presentation, whether it be at work, church, school, a meeting, a social club, for a campaign, or for some other cause. Hopefully, by virtue of your chosen career as a nurse educator, public speaking is not one of your fears, although it can be nerve racking. Making an effective presentation is more than just standing in front of an audience and speaking; it takes skill and practice. Whether you are a novice or an experienced presenter, there is always room for improvement.

This chapter addresses the skills, strategies, and techniques used to develop and deliver effective presentations including preparation and practice, overcoming stage fright, visual and vocal dimensions, room set-up, and entertaining questions. Teaching in a classroom setting necessitates the same skill set as a presenter in front of an audience. Therefore, these same techniques can be used by faculty. This chapter presents many tips and guidelines I have learned through my years of public speaking. A bibliography is included at the end for additional reading.

## Preparing for the Presentation

*"It takes three weeks to prepare a good ad-lib speech."*
—*Mark Twain*

Preparing a well-designed presentation is crucial to the overall effectiveness of the message the presenter wants to deliver to the audience. Preparation can also improve the speaker's physical presence. Time and energy must be invested into the presentation's design, impacting how the presentation is delivered and what the audience learns. Fifty percent of your focus should be on the preparation of the presentation and the other fifty percent on practicing the delivery. Following are some important aspects to consider when preparing for your presentation.

### Know Your Audience

*"The simplest way to customize is to phone members of the audience in advance and ask them what they expect from your session and why they expect it. Then use their quotes throughout your presentation."*
—*Alan Pease*

So often, a presenter is not fully aware of the demographics of the audience or class who will be attending the presentation, or their level of experience with the topic being discussed. To make your presentation more interesting and more effective, it is helpful to know as much as you can about your audience prior to the delivery of your presentation so you can tailor the content to their needs and interests. Remember, you are presenting for their benefit! Some questions to consider include:

- What is their knowledge level of and/or experience with your topic?
- What is their interest in your topic?

- What is their profession; their gender; their age?
- What is their educational background?
- Are they friendly or hostile?
- Are they attending the presentation freely or because they must attend?
- What do they 'want' to learn from the presentation?
- What do they 'need' to learn from the presentation?

So how can these questions be answered? Some of this information may be known via the presentation's registration process or the location of the presentation, such as an anatomy and physiology class for first year nursing students in a school of nursing.

To obtain more detailed information, a written questionnaire or survey can be developed and distributed ahead of time to elicit some feedback from the learners regarding what they want to learn from you. Or, you can phone the future participants and conduct a small verbal survey to ascertain the information you desire. The more you know about your audience, the more effective your presentation will be. If the above options are not feasible, then you can greet and talk with participants as they arrive to the presentation. Just be prepared to make changes right then and there if you discover the learners want to go in a different direction than the one you had planned. If attendees believe there is nothing in your presentation for them, they very quickly will lose interest in what you have to say. A good presenter makes every attempt to provide the audience what they want, in addition to what they need.

## Time Allotment

Be aware and respectful about how much time you have to present your topic and then stay within the timeframe. If you exceed the time allotted, you may end up delaying presenters who follow you resulting in their being denied the amount of time they were given to speak. Include your **Question and Answer (Q and A)** session in the allotted timeframe when calculating how much time you will have for each objective and related content. For a one-hour presentation there should be fifty minutes of content and ten minutes of Q and A. Once your presentation is developed, practice its delivery and how it fits into your timeframe; if you exceed your timeframe, edit your content. To assist you with staying within the timeframe when presenting, check for a clock in the room that will be within your view. If not, keep a watch on the podium so you can check your timing throughout the presentation. Or, have a timekeeper who will keep you apprised of how much time has either passed in your presentation versus how much time you have left in the presentation. This way, someone else is responsible for tracking your pace, leaving you to focus on the delivery of the content.

You should plan to have more than half your presentation delivered before reaching the midway point of your allotted time. For example, for a sixty minute presentation, 65 % should be delivered within the first thirty minutes. This allows for some 'catch-up' if needed, plus a Q *and* A session if one is planned for the end. Also keep in mind that any presentation that exceeds ninety minutes should have a five to ten minute break planned into the timeframe.

## Organize Your Ideas/Formulate Your Notes

When preparing your presentation it is important to organize your ideas about what you want to say in a logical sequence. This is best done by creating an outline using key words and phrases that will assist in guiding you through the major points of your presentation. The content should flow from the simple to the complex. Know what you are going to say and how you are going to say it. Develop a strong opening and a reiterated ending, both of which will be discussed in this chapter.

If you decide to use notes during the presentation they should be easy to handle and easy to read. Keep your notes brief; having too much written material makes extracting out what you want to say more difficult. In addition, writing your presentation word for word makes you tempted to read it which in turn discourages eye contact, limits your freedom of movement, and tends to foster a monotone delivery. Again, use key words and phrases, leaving space between them so they are easier to read and locate should you lose your place. You will speak more spontaneously when your notes are constructed in an outline format. It is acceptable to use either sheets of paper or index cards for your notes, whichever is more comfortable for you to manipulate while presenting. Notes should be either computer generated or hand printed, neatly and large enough to read when glanced upon. Number the pages so if they should separate, they can be easily reordered.

## Practice Makes Perfect

*"There are always three speeches, for every one you actually gave.*
*The one you practiced, the one you gave, and the one you wish you gave."*
—Dale Carnegie

After investing so much time and energy into planning, designing, and developing your presentation, you should not be overly confident that you can now stand before your audience and "wing it". You worked too hard not to give the delivery of the presentation the attention that it deserves. As previously mentioned, rehearsing is important; in fact, 55% of your allotted preparation time should be spent rehearsing your presentation. Rehearsing will decrease your nervousness, increase your confidence, and assist you to become comfortable with your presentation so you will be prepared. Practice the presentation exactly as it is to be given. This means delivering the presentation out loud, in a conversational tone at an average rate of 150 to 200 words per minute. Reading your notes does not equate to practicing the presentation. Keep in mind that it takes longer to deliver the presentation than it does to read it.

The most preferred way to practice is to videotape your presentation. Practicing in front of a mirror is distracting as you start to focus on your facial expressions or imperfections, which can alter your delivery pace. While a friend or family member can make for a good audience, they may be reluctant to be honest with their critique of your performance. To improve your delivery, you need honest feedback. Of these three, the video is the most likely to provide the most accurate feedback. The videotape will reveal your non-verbal communication, such as degree of eye contact with the audience, use of gestures, overall appearance, voice quality and use of fillers such as "um"; use of notes, degree of movement, etc. Rehearsal of your presentation also assists with editing. As you practice, time the presentation, including the question and answer session to determine its length. If necessary, edit by either trimming or adding content. Practice in the room in which you will be presenting to become comfortable with the environment.

## Overcoming Stage Fright

*"According to most studies, people's number one fear is public speaking.*
*Number two is death. Death is number two. Does that sound right?*
*This means to the average person, if you go to a funeral,*
*you're better off in the casket than doing the eulogy."*
—*Jerry Seinfeld*

So the average American would rather die than speak before a group. Why is that? What are we afraid of? That the audience won't like us? They won't listen to what we have to say? Anxiety, nervousness, jitters, stage fright, apprehension, whatever you want to call it, comes from within ourselves, no where else. It is a self-conscious emotion that is conjured up in the mind of the presenter, often as a result of the 'fear of failing.' Giving a talk can be an exhilarating experience once you overcome your preliminary nervousness. A mild degree of anxiety is essential because it is what puts you "on stage"; it gives you the zest and vitality that makes your presentation interesting. When you are anxious, your adrenalin flows, which heightens your perception and increases your concentration levels. It gives you energy that is waiting to be used. However, too much anxiety can impede your concentration and natural flow of speech. Symptoms of anxiety include increased heart rate, sweaty palms, shaking hands and/or knees, butterflies in the stomach, dry mouth, nausea, shortness of breath, stammering, and facial twitches, which you may experience at various levels before a presentation. Never, ever, announce your nervousness to the audience or in any way call attention to it. Most people won't even notice, but once you tell them, they will look for your symptoms. Following are techniques to assist you with overcoming stage fright.

## Be Prepared!

*"If you fail to prepare, you are prepared to fail."*
—*Author Unknown*

Know the content that you are presenting inside and out; in other words, prepare, prepare, prepare. Being prepared helps you to feel confident. Over rehearse the introduction so if you feel anxious in the beginning, you will be able to get through it without difficulty. It is important to remember that you know more than the audience does about your topic; they came to hear what you have to say, not to criticize you. With excessive preparation, you will be the most qualified and informed person there.

## Think Positively

Since anxiety originates within the mind, positive self-talk can help to reduce it. Negative thoughts are destructive and demoralizing. Don't tell yourself how nervous you are about presenting. The subconscious remembers and will feed into the negativism, increasing your anxiety level. Instead, tell yourself how prepared and confident you are about your topic; that what you have to say is important and useful to the audience.

## Relaxation Techniques (Mild Anxiety is Good!!)

The use of relaxation techniques prior to presenting can relieve anxiety. The most common and easiest technique to employ is deep breathing exercises. Deep breathing a few minutes before you begin speaking will control nervousness while slower breathing will assist with relaxation. A deep breath immediately before you start talking will give a boost to your voice quality and projection. To perform controlled breathing, inhale deeply through your nose with pursed lips and then slowly blow the air out of your mouth as if blowing out candles.

Other techniques to employ include visual imagery and physical exercise. Before presenting, find a quiet location, close your eyes, and imagine yourself in a 'special place' that you enjoy or where you feel comfortable. Spending a few minutes at that place will help to relax you. While you don't want to break out in repetitions of select calisthenics in front of your audience or jog outside the room, physical exercise, such as bending, stretching, or going for a walk, will release pent up energy and reduce your anxiety level.

## Stimulate Audience Participation

To help you feel more at ease, focus on the audience instead of yourself by asking them a question or using an ice breaker that will encourage social interaction. This will engage the group and stimulate a conversation between the speaker and audience members. Make sure that you talk 'with the group' and not 'at the group'. Remember, the learners are nice people responding to you and what you are saying, not monsters trying to sabotage you.

## Keep Moving!

An antidote for nervousness is action! Don't hide behind a podium; this may add to your anxiety level. Walking around coupled with the use of hand gestures provides an outlet for your anxiety and can create an illusion of confidence and calm. Be energetic, be natural, be unpredictable in your movements. Within a few minutes you will feel the symptoms of your anxiety begin to subside. At the same time, your movement also relieves the visual boredom of the audience.

## The Opening

*"The best way to make a speech is to have a good beginning and a good ending -- and have them as close together as possible."*
—*George Burns*

It has been said that learners remember the first thing and the last thing they are told. The opening to your presentation is vital because it sets the tone with the audience. Once the tone is set, it is difficult to change. To ensure that you will be off to a good start, you want an opening that will attract the attention of your audience immediately. Plan your opening as much as you plan the entire presentation. Following are techniques to employ that can assist you with a great opening.

## Warm Up the Audience

Work the room before the presentation begins by greeting the learners as they arrive and introducing yourself. This will establish friendly faces that you can focus on when presenting. This also provides the opportunity to inquire what they hope to learn from the presentation. Use ice breakers to help loosen them up and get excited for what you are about to present.

## Open with a Bang!

This is your opportunity to grab the audience's attention and establish a rapport. Avoid sleepy openers such as, *"Today I would like to talk to you about . . ."*, or *"I've been asked to speak to you on . . ."*. These openers often result in a loss of interest in what you have to say and set a tone that will be difficult to change. You want to break down that psychological barrier between presenter and audience and create a friendly and relaxed environment. Employ your special talents and use anecdotes, quotes, video clips, pictures, humor, ice breakers, or pose questions. Just remember to be yourself, not something that you're not. And don't overdo it. Once you have gotten their attention, move ahead with your presentation.

## Tell Them What They Will Learn

Believe it or not, sometimes learners arrive to a presentation not knowing why they are there or what the presentation is about. Therefore, it is your job as the presenter to tell them what they will learn and why. And then do so, step by step, keeping it simple and to the point so you generate interest among the learners.

## Delivery

*"Three things matter in a speech: Who says it, how he says it, and what he says . . . And, of the three, the last matters the least."*
—John Morley

Now that you have prepared and practiced your presentation, it is time to focus on the visual dimensions, of your delivery. Your delivery is the most visible component of your presentation. Fifty-five percent of your message is communicated to the audience through your appearance and your body language. Fifty-five percent! There are specific visual dimensions on which you need to focus your attention that will impact your delivery and how successful you will be with communicating your message to the audience.

## Visual Dimensions

### Attire/Grooming

*"They expect a professional presentation, so they expect to see a "professional." Dress appropriately for the occasion, but don't be one of the crowd."*
*—Wess Roberts*

As the speaker, it is a given that you will be scrutinized by some members of your audience. From a visual perspective, that includes how you are dressed. This is ultimately what will establish your credibility and identify you as the speaker, giving you an executive presence, even before your first word is spoken. Dress neatly, comfortably, appropriately, and professionally, always dressing one level **above** your audience. Don't worry how dressed up you may look; you can never be faulted for looking too **professional,** but you will be faulted for looking too **non-professional.** Your clothes should not call attention to themselves. Bright, flashy outfits and jewelry can distract the audience, making it difficult for them to focus their attention on what you are saying rather than what you are wearing. In most instances, business suits are an appropriate form of dress. Keep coat jackets unbuttoned because it denotes a friendly receptiveness. For men, facial hair should be neatly trimmed. For woman, hair below shoulder length should be tied back. You want to look neat and put together. When you look your best, you will feel good. If you feel good, you will be confident. If you feel confident, you will deliver a great presentation!

### Gestures

Have you ever watched other individuals on the street or throughout your work environment when they are engaged in conversation with each other? What are they doing with their hands? They are using their hands to express their message in addition to their verbal communication. Gesturing is a natural process that both enhances and reinforces what we are trying to say when we communicate verbally.

When presenting, the audience needs to see your hands, so it is important to keep them in view. Don't hide them behind your back or under a podium or in your pockets. We are a visual society that responds favorably to movement to maintain our interest. Gesturing provides this visibility, as long as you gesture in moderation. Excessive use of your hands can be annoying and distracting to the audience; they'll quickly lose interest in what you have to say. It is better to not use any gestures at all than to have your hands flailing all over the place. To gain a comfort level with gesturing, practice in front of a mirror, a video camera, or a friend. Just do what comes naturally, don't force it, but be as animated as possible.

It is permissible to keep one hand in your pocket, so long as you take it out and gesture with it on a periodic basis. If necessary, you can hold small items in your hand for comfort reasons, but be careful not to hold items that can be distracting, such as a pen that 'clicks' or a paper clip that ends up being bent 'straight' by the time your presentation is over!  Another thing to remember, never point at anyone in the audience. It is demeaning and turns your audience off.

### Facial Expressions

In addition to the importance of gesturing with your hands, your facial expressions contribute to the message you are trying to deliver to your audience. Those who are listening will focus on the face of a presenter more often than any other part of the body because it is from facial expressions that congruency in verbal and non-verbal messages occur. The best facial expressions are those that come from normal conversation and are natural, not exaggerated. When possible, match your facial expressions to the tone of the presentation. For example, you don't want to appear angry when speaking about the birth of a baby, or appear euphoric when lecturing on how to care for a patient who has experienced physical trauma. When appropriate, smile at your audience – a lot!

### Eye Contact

When presenting, it is important for the speaker to connect with the learner. This is accomplished by establishing a relationship with your learners through the use of eye contact. This means looking directly into the eyes of your audience and not above their heads, to the floor, or worse yet, reading from your notes.

Whether you are presenting before a large group or a few people, you want to have eye contact with as many people as you can; it makes those in the audience feel as if you are speaking directly to them. As you are speaking, intermittently scan left to right and then right to left; working different parts of the room as you are doing so. You want to look as natural as possible, not as if watching a ping-pong match with your head and gaze darting back and forth. When you lock eyes with someone, maintain the contact for one full sentence or complete thought. Then move on to another person and do the same. Continue this process with as many audience members as possible. In a small group, you should be able to establish eye contact with all members. However, if the audience is very large, it will be impossible to make eye contact with everyone in the room, so it is best to do so in sections, following the same pattern as described above. If you have difficulty looking at your audience while talking, try to make a game of it. Look for people with blonde hair, blue shirts, or eye glasses and make eye contact with them. This way you work the room as you begin to develop a comfort level with looking at your audience as you are presenting.

Eye contact provides you with feedback because you can visualize the faces in your audience to see if they are in agreement with what you are saying or if they appear lost or confused. It also lets your audience know that you are paying attention to them and that you care about their response to your presentation.

## Use of Notes

As mentioned previously, the use of notes as a presenter is permissible and is acceptable by your audience as long as you don't read them verbatim. When referring to your notes look up at your audience 95% of the time and maintain eye contact. Do not fumble with the pages; it is distracting to the audience and makes you appear to be unorganized.

If using a podium, keep your notes on top and use the thumb of your dominant hand to move down the notes in order to maintain your place. Use your non-dominant hand to slide the top page to the side when finished, exposing the next page. If you are not using a podium, you can hold the notes in one hand and then discreetly move the page to the back with the other when finished. It is important to keep one hand free for gesturing. Be careful not to get ahead of your notes, because if you get stuck in the presentation and need to refer to them, you may not be able to find your place on the note pages. Then you will have to stop and sort through your notes to find your place, which can result in a decrease in audience interest and an increase in your anxiety level.

# Posture/Positioning

*"What you do speaks so loudly, I can not hear what you say."*
*—Old Proverb*

While presenting, you want your physical posture and positioning to denote that you are the speaker, and a confident one at that. How you stand and hold yourself before the group will determine how effective you are with communicating your message to the learners. (Remember: It was mentioned earlier that 55% of your message is delivered via your non-verbal communication, i.e. physical presence). The positions described below can make a lasting impression on the audience about you as the speaker, such as, being too serious, unapproachable, not serious enough, nervous or anxious, unfriendly, or even unsure of self or the topic being presented. You may have seen them portrayed by other presenters in the past which should prompt you to ask yourself, *"How many have I used when I was giving a presentation?"* Following are positions to avoid.

## Good Soldier

In this position, the presenter stands one of two ways. The first stance is when the presenter stands "at attention" with legs together and both arms straight down at his/her side while speaking. There is no use of gestures or movement. The presenter appears stiff, even afraid. The second stance is the "at ease" position, in which the presenter is standing with hands and arms behind the back and legs slightly apart. Again, no gestures are used and since the hands are not visible, the audience perceives this speaker has something to hide.

## Fig Leaf

This position is one of the more popular among presenters, both novice and experienced. The presenter stands with legs straight, either together or slightly apart, with hands either folded or clasped together and positioned in front of the groin area for an extended period of time, possibly for the entire presentation. Once again, no gestures are used. The speaker is perceived as either not open, defensive, or uncomfortable before the group. Other hand positions that take-off from the fig leaf position that should also be avoided include one or both hands lying on or clasped over the lower abdomen, diaphragm, or chest areas.

## Stern Parent

There are two versions of this stance to be leery of practicing. The first is presenting with your arms folded in front of your chest. This portrays a speaker who is closed and unreceptive to anyone or anything. It is often used by those who do not know what to do with their hands or are uncomfortable gesturing. The second version takes the first version one step further. Periodically, one of the folded arms comes loose so that the presenter can point at someone in the audience, often shaking his/her finger up and down as if scolding someone. This is not viewed favorably by the audience. In fact, this position can anger those on the receiving end.

## Rocking Horse

This position requires balance and coordination to execute accurately. The presenter rocks from side to side, shifting from one foot to the other, while speaking. This can be a result of pent up energy that needs to be released or even a certain degree of nervousness. It would be best for this type of presenter to move around as described earlier, which will release energy and reduce anxiety. I once had an employee who, while presenting, rocked front to back, from heel to toe and was totally unaware of what she was doing. I was so intrigued by her agility and the fact that she didn't fall over, that I did not hear anything she was saying!

## Caged Lion

Often a subconscious practice, those who pace back and forth while presenting resemble a caged lion at the zoo. As mentioned earlier in this chapter, moving around in front of the audience while you are presenting is a good thing. However, pacing back and forth is not only distracting, but exhausting to watch! And while it may relieve excess energy in the presenter, it can irritate the audience members. When moving, come to a position and stop for a complete thought or sentence. Then move again, stop, and so on.

## Helicopter Hands

Presenters who excessively gesture with their hands sometimes take on the appearance of a helicopter about to take off. Imagine their hands whirling around in circles masquerading as effective gesturing, while instead it is distracting to the audience. Gesturing is important, but don't overdo. To reiterate, gesturing must arise naturally as it does when you are speaking with someone one-to-one.

## Jangler

This type of presenter keeps one or both hands in his/her pockets that contain coins or keys and, in most cases, unknowingly jangles them inside the pocket while presenting. This is a result of mild anxiety and gives the presenter something to do with the hands. This is not only distracting, even annoying, to the audience, but it also prohibits the natural gesturing that arises from normal communication. So, before presenting, empty your pockets of any loose change, keys, or any other items that can cause noise. If you like to have one hand in your pocket and have something inside to hold onto, consider having either one coin or one key inside so you can grasp it without making any extraneous noises.

So what is the correct way to stand in front of a group when presenting? The answer is simple. Correct posture and positioning while standing before a group, that will identify you as the speaker, is as follows:

Stand up straight, shoulders squared and pushed back, with your head held high. Do not tilt your head to the side as if you have a kink in your neck; this gives the impression that you are not fully convinced of what you are saying. Imagine an invisible wire suspended from the ceiling that pulls your head up, almost stretching your neck a little, so that you look at the audience straight-on. Keep both your feet firmly planted on the ground with them pointing forward and spread about twelve to fifteen inches apart, distributing your weight evenly. Knees are to be slightly bent for stability and comfort. Avoid standing at an angle or crossing your ankles as if striking a pose. You are presenting not modeling. Arms are to be kept at your side with elbows bent at waist level and hands open and visible to the audience. When you move, do as naturally as possible, allowing your movements to coincide with your words. You must display a certain degree of physical vitality. It will energize your audience and help to maintain their interest in you and the message that you are trying to relay. Expose yourself to the audience as much as possible, let them see you; all of you. Don't hide behind a podium or other object. This fosters a relationship of openness and trust between the presenter and the learners. It is as if you are saying *"Look at me, I have nothing to hide. What you see is what you get!"*

Avoid the temptation to lean on, sit on, or droop over items such as tables, the backs of chairs, the podium, or audiovisual equipment. Doing so gives the impression that you do not have the necessary energy or desire to communicate your message to those in attendance. If you send a message that you don't have the energy, or the enthusiasm, to be presenting then why should the audience show any interest in what you have to say?

A presenter's movement, posturing, and positioning will also help to establish the formality or informality, and the level of intimacy with the group. In a formal setting, the presenter stands in front of the group, either in the front of the room or up on a platform stage. There is no intimacy with the group; clearly you are the speaker and they are the learners. As a presenter starts to move toward the group and enters the group's personal space on their level, walking amongst them, the setting becomes less formal and a level of intimacy begins to develop. Pulling up a chair and sitting at eye level within the group is a very intimate and informal way of presenting; you are now one of them. Match your delivery style to your purpose, audience, and content.

## Vocal Dimensions

*"The trouble with some speakers is that you can't hear what they're saying; the trouble with others is that you can."*
—*Author Unknown*

The most powerful asset that you possess as a presenter is your voice. Thirty-eight percent of your message is communicated to your audience through your vocal cords, which means it is how you say what you are saying. Add that to the 55% of your visual dimensions that we previously discussed and you discover that 93% of your message actually comes from your appearance, body language, and voice. Ninety-three percent! This means that only 7 percent of your message is communicated to your audience by what you say. Amazing! A quality presentation is dependent on the presenter's ability to control and vary the pitch, tone, pace, and volume of his/her voice while speaking passionately and persuasively. Therefore, points specific to your vocal dimensions need to be considered before presenting to a group so your message may be communicated in the most effective way.

### Tone/Pitch

As a speaker, the tone of your voice plus its pitch is important and requires attention when delivering a presentation. A monotone voice is very hard to listen to, much like that of hearing the same key played over and over again on a piano. It is difficult for the learner to concentrate on what is being said when there is no variation to the sounds coming from a presenter's mouth. There are exercises that can be employed to help change the tone of your voice and make it more interesting. Count from one to ten, then from one to twenty, and then from one to thirty in variable ways: louder, softer, higher, lower. With practice, you will see a difference in your tone during various points throughout your presentation. The pitch (high or low) of your voice needs to change according to the level of enthusiasm you are exerting while speaking. A patterned pitch, which goes up and down in regular intervals in a sing-song type of pattern is often indicative of a memorized presentation. You can vary your pitch by increasing the volume of your voice, your rate of delivery, and your level of enthusiasm. An exercise to lower the pitch of your voice and make it deeper and stronger involves humming the scale to the lowest note and then holding it for as long as possible. Do the exercise three times a day. Practice using a tape recorder to get a true indication of how you sound. Over time you will notice the improvement in both your tone and your pitch. Increasing your lung capacity will deepen the pitch, enrich the tone, and strengthen the volume, making your voice more powerful. To do this, take a deep breath in and then as you hold it, count as high as you can. Repeat and with each attempt you should be able to count higher.

### Volume

When presenting, it is imperative to ensure that everyone in the audience can hear you. If you are not using a microphone, then you need to speak louder than a normal conversational tone. However, if you are soft spoken or presenting in a large room to a large audience, a microphone should be used. When using a microphone, speak in a normal conversational tone. Be careful not to shout. As you make specific points during your presentation, alternate the volume of your voice, which will keep the audience interested in what you have to say. If you are excited, the volume of your voice will get higher. When you are trying to make an important point, lower your voice to a whisper.

### Pace

The pace of your presentation should be at the same rate of speed as when talking on the telephone. Vary the pace to match the content or mood of the presentation's message. When excited, speak faster; when serious, slow it down. Don't speak too slowly or you will bore the audience to the point of sleep. If you speak too quickly, your audience will not catch everything you are saying. The average delivery is 150 to 200 words per minute. Keep in mind that people listen faster than you can speak, so don't be a speed demon. Speak clearly, don't slur, and be aware of the time during your presentation so you don't race at the end to cover all your content.

## Pauses

It is necessary during the delivery of a presentation to give yourself and the audience some breathing space. This can be done by using pauses. Pausing after certain statements throughout the presentation accentuates the points you are making, helps you to gather your thoughts, and provides for the digestion of what was just said. Pauses need to come from natural conversation and cannot be planned. When pausing, look at the members of the audience, not away from them. You need to develop a comfort level with using pauses which takes practice. Avoid filling the pauses with "um, you know, like, okay", etc.

## Articulation

I just addressed the importance of pacing the delivery of your presentation, ensuring that everyone can hear you, speaking in a varying pitch and tone, and interjecting pauses to allow for reflection. It is extremely important the learners can understand what you are saying. Speak slowly, clearly, and distinctly. Pronounce words correctly, use proper grammar, and know the meaning of the words you use. Avoid the use of slang, jargon, and sexist or ethnic language, and clichés. Be careful when using acronyms; explain what they mean to avoid any confusion. Heavy accents and regional dialects need to be toned down so your audience can understand what you are saying. To improve the clarity of your voice, practice by using assonance, the repetition of vowels, **"The rain in Spain . . ."**, and alliteration, the repetition of consonants, *"Susie sells seashells . . ."*. In time, you will hear a noticeable difference.

## Techniques

*"The lecturer should give the audience full reason to believe that all his powers have been exerted for their pleasure and instruction."*
—*Michael Faraday*

There are various techniques to consider when preparing and delivering a presentation in order to make it interesting and more effective: simplicity, enthusiasm, humor, anecdotal stories, and inviting the audience to participate. Use of some or all of these techniques can enhance your presentation and assist you with relating to your audience in a positive manner.

## Simplicity

*"Be sincere, be brief, be seated."*
*—Franklin D. Roosevelt*

When trying to get a point across, do it in as few words or sentences as possible. Sometimes we feel we need to elaborate on points that we are making to get our message through to the recipients, when in actuality we may lose their interest, even confuse them. When possible, the less said the better. As you plan your presentation always remember KISS: Keep It Simple Speaker!

Avoid using complex, showy words. This is not the way to impress your audience; in fact, it could be a turn-off, especially if they do not know the meaning of the words you use. Your goal is to teach your audience so they will benefit from what you have to say, rather than have them distracted by trying to decipher the meaning of the words you are using.

## Enthusiasm

*"I always think a great orator convinces us not by force of reasoning,*
*but because he is visibly enjoying the beliefs which he wants us to accept."*
*—William Butler Yeats*

The presenter must have passion for the topic being presented in order to be dynamic and well received by the audience. If you are genuinely enthusiastic about the presentation topic and demonstrate that enthusiasm in your delivery, than you will generate enthusiasm amongst your audience members as well; it is contagious.

Keep in mind that the audience should never be more enthusiastic about the topic than the presenter. If you have been repeatedly delivering the same presentation and feel you can not be genuinely excited about the topic, than you must feign your enthusiasm. Presenters who are not into the topic will lose credibility as well as the audience's interest.

Employing the **visual** and **vocal dimensions** that were discussed previously will help stimulate enthusiasm in your learners. They need to see and hear how much you enjoy the topic that you are sharing with them. Be a cheerleader!

## Humor

An effective technique that can enhance a presentation, even make it unique and interesting, is humor. Humor can be in the form of personal anecdotes, jokes, cartoons, pictures, props, quotes, and stories interjected at either the beginning, throughout, or at the end of a presentation. When used appropriately it can warm up your audience and grab their attention, even relax them. It helps to link the presenter to the audience. Keep in mind the use of humor is not for everyone and should only be used if the presenter feels comfortable with it. For example, when writing the presentation, the speaker can not add jokes afterwards, plugging them in wherever she/he wants to get a laugh; that will just not work. In fact, the jokes or humorous anecdotes need to arise from the presentation in order to be effective.

Humor should never be insulting, offensive, or at the expense of one of the audience members. To be effective, it must be constructive, not destructive. So be careful! If anyone is to be the brunt of the speaker's humorous anecdote, it needs to be the speaker. This way there is no opportunity for an audience member to be hurt or ridiculed in any way.

Use humor sparingly. Too much humor interjected into your presentation will overpower the underlying message that you are trying to get across to the audience. If you feel that you can not use humor in a way that will enhance your presentation or assist with getting your message across to the audience, then don't use it.

## Anecdotes

*"Speakers who talk about what life has taught them never fail to keep the attention of their listeners."*
—*Dale Carnegie*

Audience members are human, just like the presenter, and they relate to real life experiences the presenter shares with them. These experiences, or anecdotes, can connect the audience members to the speaker and assist them to understand the information presented. Space the anecdotes out during the presentation, but don't overdo it. Your primary intention is to delivery content, not tell stories.

## Invite Participation

When possible, engage the audience by getting them involved in your presentation. This will not only stimulate their interest but will contribute to their learning experience by making it active, not passive. Engage participation with questions, icebreakers, group activities, case studies, games, personal anecdotes, or written exercises. Encourage them to ask questions or to share their experiences. It is important to remember you can learn from your audience as well.

# Environment

*"Lecturers should remember that the capacity of the mind
to absorb is limited to what the seat can endure."*
—*Author Unknown*

There is nothing more disturbing to an audience or more frustrating to a presenter than an environment that distracts from the presentation. Therefore, to facilitate the delivery of an effective presentation it is important to be familiar with the room set-up. All the conditions below, if not to your satisfaction, can have a significant impact on your presentation and your audience's ability to maintain interest in your topic and connect with you as the presenter.

## Room Size/Seating/Tables

When possible, it is important to scan the room you will be presenting in prior to the delivery of the actual presentation. You can become familiar with its location, size, layout, seating options, noise level, lighting, etc. This prevents any surprises the day of the presentation and allows you the opportunity to have things changed or rearranged if necessary. The number of participants will determine the type of seating most conducive for learning. The size of the room will determine how many participants can attend the presentation comfortably and how much space is available for you to move around. Things to note include:

- What is the layout of the room? Is it auditorium style, amphitheater style, or basic classroom style (Figure 1)?
- Is the seating fixed or are the chairs mobile? There isn't anything that you can do to alter fixed seating, but mobile tables and chairs can be arranged in various formats to facilitate the learning experience so the learners have both a view of the presenter and of each other (see Figures 2 and 3). These arrangements make for a more interactive and collaborative learning environment.

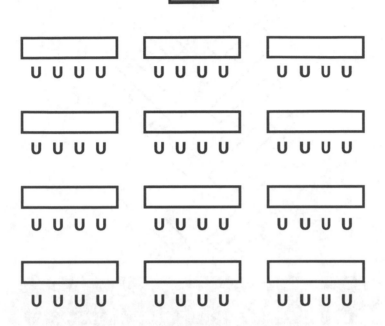

**Figure 1.** Classroom-style Seating

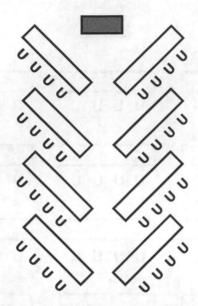

**Figure 2.** Chevron-style Seating

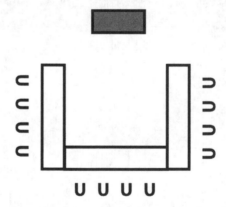

**Figure 3.** U-shaped Style Seating

- Are there writing surfaces such as tablet arms or tables? When possible, it is important for the participants to have a writing surface to lean on to aid with the note-taking process. If you have a small number of participants for your presentation but find yourself in a large auditorium or amphitheater style room, you can tape off the back rows as a way to encourage the learners to sit closer to you. Participants tend to sit in the back of the room rather than in the front when in this type of setting. If you are in a room that has mobile seating, remove excess seats in the back to encourage the learners to sit closer to the front. However, make sure excess seating is available if needed, in the event you have more participants than anticipated.

## Lighting/Acoustics

There should be ample lighting, especially if the participants will be taking notes. Check that all lighting is working properly and familiarize yourself with the location and operation of all light switches and dimmers. When surveying the room size and seating arrangement, sit in various locations to determine if any of the participants will have an obstructed view. Obstructed views may occur in rooms with support columns or poles. If so, discourage participants from sitting in those locations by either removing the chair if possible, or taping off the area. Can you be heard by those in the back of the room? Are there any distracting noises in the room, such as air conditioners or fan vents? Is the room located next to a high traffic area? Can you hear doors opening and closing or people talking outside the room? Plan how to deal with the distractions before the day of the presentation. If the room is equipped with an acoustical system, turn it on and test your voice projection.

## Podium/Microphone

Most formal presentation rooms are equipped with a podium and microphone. Other rooms may have a podium but no microphone. It is the personal preference of the presenter whether or not to use either one. However, standing behind a podium hides up to two thirds or more of the presenter from view. We discussed earlier how we live in a visual society; participants want to see the individual presenting to them. By showing your whole body you are sending a message that you are confident, open, and receptive. Standing behind a podium also prevents the speaker from moving around, which maintains learner interest. A podium sometimes serves as a security for those who are mildly nervous before the presentation; it hides shaking knees and trembling hands. This is acceptable as long as the presenter does not lean on the top or grab on to the sides of the upper portion of the podium. Being able to present without the use of a podium takes time and practice. Try with each presentation to gradually move away from the podium. Start by standing to the side of the podium. This way, the participants will be able to see you and you will still have the security of the podium next to you.

Microphones are necessary if the presenter has a soft spoken voice that will not project within the room. There are two styles of microphones that may be available. A hand-held microphone is held by the presenter, but can also be mounted in a holder on a podium. A lavaliere is clipped onto the presenters' lapel or shirt.

When using a microphone, speak in your normal tone of voice, do not shout. When using a hand-held microphone, either mounted to a podium or actually in your hand, keep it at a level slightly below your chin. This will not only provide better projection of your voice, but will prevent you from obstructing the view of your mouth or altering the quality of your voice if the microphone is held to close to your lips. Lavaliere microphones are meant to be clipped to a presenter's clothes at a level slightly below the clavicle. It should not be held in the hand when presenting, which is distracting to the audience.

## Audiovisuals/Equipment

When using audiovisual equipment, you need to ensure it is working properly. Turn the equipment on and off. Are the lights working? If the bulb in a projector burns out do you know how to change it? If not, is there someone available on site who can? Do you need extension cords or power strips? Are the plugs safe? It is important to familiarize yourself with the location of outlets, how the projection screens work (portable versus wall mounted versus motorized), the use of remote controls, and any other troubleshooting techniques that may be necessary in the event of equipment failure.

Besides working properly, ensuring laptops can accommodate the unique features of a presentation, e.g., videos and audio, is essential particularly since some planning committees require submission of the presentation ahead of time.

## Temperature

The number of participants in the room determines how warm or cool the room temperature should be. If the room is too warm, the participants may begin to doze and/or lose their ability to concentrate. If the room is too cold, the participants will focus on ways to keep warm, including getting up and leaving. The room should be at a comfortable temperature of between 68 and 70 degrees. It is important to note if the room is equipped with a thermostat that can be manually controlled by anyone in the room, or if it is part of a bigger system that requires maintenance personnel to adjust the temperature when necessary.

## Drinking Water

Excessive talking can result in a dry mouth which will ultimately have an effect on your vocal dimensions. It is recommended to have drinking water available to keep hydrated and maintain voice quality during long presentations.

## Entertaining Questions

*"No question is so difficult to answer as that to which the answer is obvious."*
*—Bernard Shaw*

As part of preparation for the presentation, it is important to decide if you plan a question and answer session. Questions from the audience are a good indication of the level of their awareness, attention, and interest in your subject. They also indicate if the participant learned from the presentation and gives the speaker the opportunity to clarify misunderstanding or confusion on the learner's part. Determine if you will entertain questions during the presentation or if you will have a question and answer session only at the end of the presentation. This decision is often based on the content you are presenting and the amount of time allotted for the presentation. A general guideline is approximately ten minutes of questions and answers for every 50 minutes of didactic content.

Many presenters dread the question and answer session. Why? They are fearful they will not be able to answer a question that is posed to them. While this is usually not the norm, there will be times when a presenter is faced with a question that he/she can not answer. However, in most instances, if the presenter knows the content and is well prepared, that will not be the case. To avoid this possibility, the presenter needs to anticipate questions that may be asked by the learners and then plan how to answer them. Some points to remember that will help you when answering questions are:

- Do not stray from your objectives. Questions outside the realm of the topic being taught will occasionally be raised. If responded to, these questions can be very distracting and can greatly disturb the learning at hand, even cause confusion amongst other learners. It is advised that you tactfully inform the participant that you will discuss the matter after the presentation and continue toward achieving the objectives of your presentation.

- Rephrase the question when necessary. When the question presented appears unclear to the rest of the group, or if the questioning participant speaks too softly so others can not hear, it is important for the presenter to repeat or rephrase the question so the whole group is aware of what is being asked and can appreciate the answer. Chances are there are other participants who have a similar, or the same, question. This also gives the speaker the opportunity to clarify what the participant is asking, while gaining extra time to formulate an answer.

- Direct your answer to the audience. Although one participant may ask a question, direct your answer to all those in attendance so everyone benefits from your response. Several may have wanted to ask the same or a similar question. Never guess at the answer. Even the well-prepared presenters will be asked questions they will be unable to answer. It is essential that you never guess at the answer, hypothesize an answer, or, even worse, make up an answer, just to be able to have an answer to the question. There are two strategies you can employ if you find yourself faced with a question you can not answer. You can respond, "That is a very good question. Does anybody know the answer"? This turns the question back to the participants to determine if anyone knows the answer. Chances are someone will. Or, you can simply state you do not know the answer but you will attempt to find it, explaining that you will get back to the participant at a later time. This shows that you care and will gain respect from the participants. But make sure that you do follow-up with the answer. If you do not follow-up, you will lose credibility as a speaker.

- Avoid debating or arguing. It is not unusual for an occasional participant to disagree with points being covered, particularly when they have had exposure to conflicting material. A simple solution in this case is to quote your source, e.g., Grey's Anatomy, American Journal of Nursing, etc. and then continue with the material. If the participant is persistent, you can suggest discussing the issue off line rather then spending the question and answer session justifying your answer. It is appropriate to agree to disagree with the participant. No matter what, just remember, you are the presenter, so keep your cool.

- Use appropriate language. A good presenter is a good communicator. When answering questions or presenting a topic, it is critical for the presenter to use language appropriate to the group. Sophisticated medical terminology is acceptable when addressing a group of nurses but can have detrimental effects on the learning process of a lay person.

- Avoid over-answering questions. When a question has been answered, stop talking about the question. Say as little as possible to get the point across. If the answer is a simple yes or no, then leave it at that. Over-explaining may quickly lead to boredom and disinterest.
- Give everyone equal time. Make sure you cover the entire room when calling on participants who have questions, especially if time is limited. Avoid those that monopolize the question and answer session. Should this occur, it is appropriate to say, "I know you have a lot of questions but let's give someone else a try". Questions specific to one individual can be addressed after the session to save time.
- Do not overlook questions. A good presenter keeps a watchful eye on the audience, being careful not to allow the intensity of presenting to cause you to miss a waving arm or a puzzled expression. An unanswered question is a major block to learning and can result in even more questions being asked as the level of uncertainty amongst participants increases.
- Be respectful and considerate. Everyone wants to feel their contribution to the class, whether it is a question or an answer, is meaningful. Therefore, it is important that a presenter never ridicules or demeans a participant, but rather exercises sensitivity and care. Remember: there is no such thing as a stupid question!
- Pose your own questions. Asking the audience questions enlists their participation and lets the presenter test what they have learned from the presentation. It also provides the presenter with information about any areas that need clarification or further review.

## The Finish

*"Let it never be said of you, 'I thought he would never finish.'*
*Get off while you're still ahead; always leave them wanting more."*
—Dorothy Sarnoff

The information presented in a lecture can be overwhelming; therefore, a brief summary at the finish can assist the learners to organize their thoughts and their notes; it helps to pull everything together. It has been said that learners remember the first thing that they hear and the last thing, so to maximize the impact at the end of your presentation, take the opportunity to restate your message and summarize the key points you want them to take away. Don't overdo it; only a few sentences are necessary. Remind the participants what was accomplished during the presentation.

This allows the participants to focus on the most salient points you presented, and being the last thing they hear, will most likely be what is remembered.

Make your ending attention getting by ending on a strong note. If applicable to communicating your message, use anecdotes, quotes, or phrases. It is appropriate to memorize your ending so you can concentrate on the delivery. It is acceptable to use phrases such as, *"So, in conclusion . . ."*, or *"In closing I'd like to . . ."* which will get your audience's attention and alert them that you are about to finish the presentation.

## Summary

*"All the great speakers were bad speakers at first."*
—*Ralph Waldo Emerson*

As with any skill, being able to present improves with practice; it is a learning process. Practice, along with solid preparation, an organized approach, and attention to the skills and techniques that were discussed in this chapter, will help you become an effective speaker and deliver winning presentations every time!

## Learning Activities

1. Attend a professional presentation. Using the attributes of a presenter discussed in this chapter, rate the presenter.
2. Prepare a presentation or lecture you will be providing to a group. Ask a friend to watch your rehearsal and provide feedback. Videotape a rehearsal of your presentation. Compare and contrast the feedback from your friend and what you view on the videotape. How is the feedback the same? Different?
3. Watch a television program of a politician giving a speech. Describe the speaker's style. How does it conform to the guidelines presented in this chapter?

## Educational Philosophy

Healthcare is continuously changing. Therefore, nurses need to be responsible and accountable for enhancing their professional development in order to maintain a current level of proficiency when practicing nursing. To assist with the process, nurse educators need to provide viable, cost-effective, outcome-oriented, and creative

educational programs that provide nurses with the knowledge and skills required to effectively function in a variety of complex and specialized clinical nursing services.
— Dianne Ryan

## References

Atkinson, C. (2005). *Want to persuade? Tell a story*. Presentations, September, 27-30.

Bienvenu, S. (2000). *The presentation skills workshop: Helping people create and deliver great presentations*. New York City: AMACOM.

Bobo, J. (2004). How to repair and resuscitate an audience abused by boredom. *Presentations*, January, 58.

Booher, D. (2003). *Speak with confidence*. New York: McGraw-Hill.

Boyd, S. (2003). For a more powerful performance, say it short and say it well. *Presentations*, January, 62

Bristol-Smith, D. (2001). Nervous? Learn how to manage preshow jitters. *Presentations*, April, 78.

Cunningham, R. (2000). Good presenters are never content with their content. *Presentations*, April, 102.

Desana, J. (2005). Inspiring an audience begins with speaker's vision. *Presentations*, January, 50.

Egan, M. (1998). *Would you really rather die than give a talk?* New York: AMACOM.

Esar, E. (1996) *20,000 Quips and quotes*. New York: Barnes & Noble.

Helms, M. (2003). The key to a strong presentation is in the details. *Presentations*, May, 58.

Hill, J. (2004). The writing on the wall. *Presentations*, February, 37-40

Kalies, B. (2004). Take the fear out of giving presentations. *Presentations*, February, 58.

Kerr, M. (2002). Adding humor to high-tech presentations has some serious advantages. *Presentations*, November, 82.

McInnes, K. (2001). "Adding pizzazz." A presentation skills workshop for health-care professionals. *Journal for Nurses in Staff Development*, May/June, 151-158.

McKenzie, S. (2002). Break nervous habits before they become distractions. *Presentations*, February, 62.

Richardson, P. (2000). Use these tricks to speak all day without getting hoarse. *Presentations*, May, 90.

Ryan, D. (2001). Effective creation and use of visual aids. Chapter 8. In, *Basics and beyond: An educator's reference*. (2nd ed.). Emergency Nurses' Association.

Sherman, R. (2001). *Sherman's 21 laws of speaking*. Blacklick, OH: Cedar Creek Press.

Stack, L. (2004). 10 time-management tips to aid presenters. *Presentations*, November, 50.

Varga, M. P. (1996). *Great openings and closings*. Mission, KS: Skillpath.

Waldrop, D. E. (2000). What you wear is almost as important as what you say. *Presentations*, July, 74.

Walinska, K. (2000). Technical subjects need that human touch and feel. *Presentations*, September, 84.

Wall, T. (2004). PowerPoint pitfalls that can kill an audience's will to stay awake. *Presentations*, October, 46.

Wallace, I., Wallechinsky, D., & Wallace, A. (1983, 1993, 2005). *The book of lists*. New York: Bantam Books.

Wofford, M. (2004). You don't have to be perfect to be effective as a speaker. *Presentations*, December, 90.

Zielinski, D. (2005). Cracking the dress code. *Presentations*, February, 26-30.

Zielinski, D. (2003). Perfect practice (How the pros rehearse). *Presentations*, May, 30-36.

Zielinski, D. (2002). Clock work (How to make the most of your presentation preparation time). *Presentations*, February, 32-40.

Zielinski, D. (2000). Stop joking . . . and start using humor to communicate better. *Presentations*, January, 34-42.

378, 379, 384, 393, 394, 395, 397, 402, 417, 423, 471, 497, 502, 508, 511, 518, 544, 546, 553, 562, 563, 568, 570, 571, 573, 575, 579, 581, 582, 583, 584, 585, 586, 587, 588, 589, 590, 591, 592, 593, 594, 595, 596, 597, 598, 599, 600, 601, 607, 614, 615, 633, 648, 658, 668, 679, 701, 722, 726, 731, 732, 745, 751

caring activities 568

caring behaviors 417, 573, 583, 589, 590, 595, 598, 599

caring factors 588, 589, 590, 591, 593

caring knowledge 590, 591, 593, 595, 596

caring pedagogies 591, 596

case-based learning 722

certified nurse educator 3, 4, 6, 9, 27, 48, 68, 88, 100, 113, 123, 127, 146, 167, 183, 198, 230, 239, 256, 267, 285, 306, 334, 367, 403, 424, 441, 459, 483, 502, 525, 559, 582, 600, 620, 631, 642, 659, 686, 711, 740, 759

core competencies 16

detailed test blueprint 9, 27, 48, 68, 88, 100, 113, 127, 146, 167, 183, 198, 230, 239, 256, 267, 285, 306, 334, 367, 403, 424, 441, 459, 483, 502, 525, 559, 582, 600, 620, 642, 659, 686, 711, 740, 759

change agent 4, 5, 49, 183, 198

CINAHL 119, 310, 327, 663, 675, 680, 681, 682

clickers 261, 278, 279, 692, 705, 709, 717

climate for affective learning 565

clinical component 57

clinical evaluation 43, 56, 158, 390, 404, 405, 407, 416, 432, 436, 438, 475, 480, 490, 660

clinical evaluation tool (CET) 416, 436

clinical log data 490

Clinical Nurse Specialist (CNS) 484, 499

clinical practice guidelines (CPG) 672

Cochrane Collection 669, 675

cognitive-development theories 728

cognitive learning theory 34, 35, 712, 713, 721

cognitive retention 564

cognitive schemata 28

cognitive skills 432, 436, 564, 650, 652, 691

collaboration 117, 122, 201, 202, 203, 206, 214, 215, 234, 274, 279, 288, 299, 376, 378, 404, 412, 470, 473, 499, 539, 553, 577, 584, 585, 588, 589, 590, 660

collaborative learning 203, 259, 261, 262, 465, 729, 731, 739, 778

collaborative relationships 418, 470, 477, 586

college philosophy 370

collegiality 9, 50, 234, 368, 404, 406, 502, 582

competency testing 403, 404, 405, 407, 416

complex health systems 584, 596

computer literacy 289, 301

concept-based curriculum 365, 441, 443, 444, 445, 448, 449, 452, 453, 456, 458

concept mapping 21, 35, 595, 635, 694, 721, 736, 738, 739

conceptual teaching approaches 452

conflict resolution 404, 406

content analysis 32, 429, 431, 433, 699

content saturation 388, 389, 442, 456, 458

continuous quality improvement 5, 9, 48, 100, 113, 124, 127, 146, 167, 183, 198, 544

cooperative learning experiences 729

core competencies 4, 5, 6, 7, 16, 123, 201, 231, 371, 373, 408, 661

course planning 55, 58

Critical Incident Questionnaire (CIQ) 43, 706

critical thinking 15, 18, 33, 35, 37, 59, 135, 149, 253, 281, 285, 288, 300,

**D**

**E**

style editors 180

educational environment 5, 6, 16, 41, 127, 241, 242, 253, 269, 313, 373, 583

educational process 1, 27, 28, 29, 41, 43, 45, 94, 96, 114, 220, 689, 705, 707, 734

educational research 13, 83, 85, 111, 112, 120, 122, 123, 124, 145, 439, 596, 757

educational settings 48, 483

Education Resources Information Center (ERIC) 150

edutainment 743

effective presentation skills 685, 688, 689, 709

end of life issues 574

enhancement strategies 702, 703

ESL/EFL 308

ESL student 311

essential educational competencies 365, 424, 425, 426, 427, 428, 429, 432, 433, 434, 435, 436, 475

ethics 105, 106, 107, 108, 110, 111, 119, 165, 244, 246, 247, 249, 250, 253, 292, 303, 304, 377, 379, 449, 476, 480, 488, 489, 519, 563, 581, 618, 620, 621, 622, 623, 624, 625, 626, 627, 628, 629, 630, 634, 636, 637, 638, 639, 640, 641, 659, 681

ethnically diverse faculty 312, 318

ethnically diverse student profile 311

ethnicity in nursing 308

Eurocentric 308, 310, 312, 315, 316, 512

Eurocentric curriculum 312, 315

evaluation 4, 5, 16, 19, 28, 43, 44, 48, 53, 54, 55, 56, 58, 59, 60, 66, 83, 84, 104, 105, 113, 114, 115, 117, 121, 122, 124, 145, 147, 149, 158, 159, 160, 164, 193, 199, 211, 217, 230, 234, 235, 245, 261, 263, 288, 297, 305, 318, 328, 333, 359, 360, 362, 367, 369, 370, 384, 386, 389, 390, 393, 397, 401, 403, 404, 405, 407, 416, 417, 418, 419, 420, 421, 424, 425, 426, 427, 428, 430, 432, 433, 434, 435, 436, 438, 439, 441, 447, 451, 452, 455, 456, 458, 463, 466, 468, 469, 472, 473, 474, 475, 476, 477, 478, 479, 480, 483, 487, 490, 500, 502, 525, 528, 531, 532, 536, 540, 542, 543, 544, 546, 547, 548, 549, 558, 559, 561, 564, 567, 570, 572, 576, 577, 578, 582, 590, 594, 595, 596, 598, 600, 614, 620, 639, 642, 644, 659, 660, 666, 668, 706, 707, 719, 720, 725, 726, 733, 737

formative evaluation 43

summative evaluation 43

evaluation strategies 4, 5, 16, 113, 386, 424, 441, 525, 559, 567

evidence-based care 378, 384, 665, 681

Evidence-based Care Sheets 672

evidence-based findings 114, 118

evidence-based nursing education 1, 13, 125, 371, 373, 539

evidence-based nursing practice 560, 652

evidence based practice (EBP) 113, 116, 118, 328, 642, 643, 644, 659, 660, 661, 662, 663, 664, 665, 666, 667, 668, 669, 670, 671, 672, 673, 674, 675, 676, 677, 678, 679, 682

evidence-based research 114, 650

evidence-based teaching 1, 114, 115, 116, 118, 124, 125, 126, 328, 435, 436

expectancy value theory 72, 80

experiential learning 37, 584, 727, 732, 739

experiential learning environments 37

extrinsic motivation 69, 73

**F**

faculty development 5, 6, 21, 28, 33, 56, 65, 66, 115, 118, 144, 204, 390, 435, 453, 454, 610

faculty engagement 453

faculty evaluation 54, 456

Institute of Medicine  113, 114, 125, 199,
200, 202, 205, 226, 376, 394, 410,
425, 438, 442, 458, 460, 480, 661,
681
Institute of Medicine (IOM)  113, 114, 124,
125, 200, 201, 376, 378, 394, 410,
412, 425, 438, 480, 661, 681
Institute of Medicine Studies (IOM)  376
instructional design process  28, 29
instructional objectives  39, 394, 438, 559,
699
instructional strategies  31, 32, 34, 35, 36,
38, 75, 131, 138, 257, 260, 416, 689,
702
integrative learning  200, 205, 206, 225,
584, 588, 592, 598, 599
interactive learning  135, 143, 262, 274,
275, 276, 326
inter-rater reliability  528, 530, 531, 534,
538, 539
intrinsic motivation  73, 80, 83, 86

**J**

Jeopardy  276, 278
jigsaw  452, 730, 731, 735

**K**

knowledge brokers  218
knowledge workers  216, 218, 387, 394

**L**

learner analysis  29
learner development  4, 5, 27, 306, 334,
459, 559, 686
learning communities  143, 203, 213, 215,
479, 592, 731, 735
learning expectations  274
learning strategies  73, 76, 78, 115, 134,
262, 274, 306, 323, 324, 329, 346,
369, 386, 388, 442, 559, 568, 639,
689, 690, 691, 692, 702, 739, 741
learning styles  15, 25, 27, 31, 36, 46, 260,
273, 285, 306, 411, 423, 459, 597,

705, 706, 712
learning theories  33, 36, 38, 712, 732
legacy journals  177
Leininger's Sunrise Model  508
liberatory pedagogy  269
licensure/certification pass rates  368, 390,
391
limited-cohort distance-education programs
495
Living Book  278
low confidence learners  74

**M**

mainstreaming  317
marginalized student  312
medical ethics  519, 626
Medline  150, 152, 327, 675
mentorship program  293, 299
meta-analysis  115, 663
Millennials  30, 47, 257, 258, 259, 260,
261, 262, 263, 265, 268, 270, 272,
273, 274, 275, 277, 278, 281, 283,
658
mnemonics  714, 734
moral principles  627, 628, 629, 632, 636,
637
motivation  31, 68, 69, 72, 73, 75, 76, 80,
81, 82, 83, 84, 85, 86, 87, 92, 96,
148, 205, 217, 237, 246, 264, 286,
465, 510, 512, 563, 564, 567, 575,
598, 608, 723, 743
multimedia technology  274
multisite approaches  494
music  40, 91, 171, 219, 278, 573, 574,
592, 689, 701, 703, 742, 751

**N**

narrative pedagogy  620, 633, 635, 640,
641, 725, 726, 735, 736
national certification  123, 486, 491, 492,
496, 499
National Council of State Boards of Nursing (NCSBN)  376, 410

394

screening process 460, 461, 462

second degree nursing students 459

self-efficacy 69, 70, 71, 74, 80, 81, 85, 86, 143, 567

self-regulated learning 73, 75, 83

service learning 115, 262, 464, 588, 592, 713, 732

share pairs 324

Silent Generation 256

simulations 35, 66, 81, 210, 219, 263, 265, 275, 276, 280, 350, 508, 593, 718, 719, 720, 735, 737

skills laboratory component 58

Skinner's learning theory 34

social cognitive motivation theory 69

socialization 4, 5, 9, 16, 27, 48, 68, 88, 100, 230, 239, 256, 267, 272, 285, 289, 290, 302, 306, 312, 334, 459, 512, 559, 560, 573, 579, 621, 624, 639, 641, 686

social learning theory 35

Spellings' Report 526

spiritual assessment 610, 611, 612

spiritual care 600, 601, 602, 603, 604, 605, 606, 607, 608, 609, 610, 612, 613, 614, 615, 616, 617, 618, 619

spiritual distress 604, 605, 613, 616

spiritual formation 604, 605, 608

spirituality 369, 505, 514, 581, 600, 601, 602, 603, 604, 605, 606, 607, 608, 609, 610, 611, 612, 613, 614, 615, 616, 617, 618, 619

spiritual needs 604, 607, 612, 615, 618

spiritual self-assessment 610, 612, 616

spiritual well-being 604, 608, 611, 613

staff development 49, 66, 172, 621, 624, 686, 735, 787

stage fright 760, 763, 764

standardized patients 719, 739

Star Model of Knowledge Transformation 665, 666

StartRight in Nursing School 30, 31

student-faculty relationships 230, 236

student learning outcomes 368, 369, 370, 371, 372, 373, 374, 376, 377, 378, 382, 383, 385, 387, 388, 389, 392, 446, 447, 544, 548, 560

Student Portfolio Rubric 533, 534, 536, 538, 539, 550, 555

students with disabilities 334, 335, 336, 337, 338, 339, 340, 342, 343, 346, 347, 348, 349, 350, 352, 353, 355, 356, 357, 358, 359, 360

student-teacher relationship 101, 102, 586, 598

study buddy 347

systematic review 480, 662, 663, 664, 673, 674, 675, 676, 677, 736

**T**

teaching assignments 12, 50, 51, 237, 264

teaching caring 582, 584, 585, 591, 598

teaching evidence based practice (EBP) 581, 659

teaching evidence-based practice (EBP) 115, 682

teaching-learning process 27, 28, 29, 32, 114, 318, 323, 373, 462, 716

team-based learning 724, 725

team building 404, 406, 422, 645

team teaching 49, 63, 235

Technology Informatics Guiding Education Reform (TIGER) 203, 227

tenure track 54, 485

tenure-track positions 14

test blueprint 6, 7, 9, 27, 48, 57, 68, 88, 100, 113, 123, 127, 146, 167, 183, 198, 230, 235, 239, 256, 267, 285, 306, 334, 367, 403, 424, 441, 459, 483, 502, 525, 559, 582, 600, 620, 642, 659, 686, 711, 740, 759

test item writing 17, 18

   analysis levels 18

test review 235, 321, 752

The Boomers 256